International and Cultural Psychology

Series Editor: Anthony J. Marsella

For further volumes:
http://www.springer.com/series/6089

Laurence J. Kirmayer
Jaswant Guzder · Cécile Rousseau
Editors

Cultural Consultation

Encountering the Other
in Mental Health Care

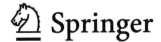 Springer

Editors
Laurence J. Kirmayer, M.D.
Institute of Community & Family
  Psychiatry
Jewish General Hospital
Montreal, QC, Canada

Jaswant Guzder, M.D.
Institute of Community & Family
  Psychiatry
Jewish General Hospital
Montreal, QC, Canada

Cécile Rousseau, M.D., M.Sc.
CSSS de la Montagne
Montreal, QC, Canada

ISSN 1574-0455
ISBN 978-1-4614-7614-6 (Hardcover)   ISBN 978-1-4614-7615-3 (eBook)
ISBN 978-1-4939-2692-3 (Softcover)
DOI 10.1007/978-1-4614-7615-3
Springer New York Heidelberg Dordrecht London

Library of Congress Control Number: 2013944571

Springer is part of Springer Science+Business Media (www.springer.com)

Preface

Cultural diversity poses many challenges to mental health care. These stem from the ways that culture configures illness experience, contributing to the causes and mechanisms of psychopathology, the modes of expressing suffering, and the strategies of coping, help seeking, healing, and recovery. There is increasing recognition of the importance of culture for mental health services, exemplified by the notions of cultural competence in the training of professionals and the organization of health care institutions. DSM-5 introduced a cultural formulation interview to encourage clinicians to contextualize diagnosis. This book puts flesh on the bones of DSM-5 by showing how knowledge of culture can be applied in everyday practice to produce more refined and effective diagnostic assessments and clinical interventions. The model we propose uses outpatient consultation as a vehicle to deliver cultural expertise throughout the health care system, with an emphasis on supporting primary care through collaboration.

The Cultural Consultation Service described in this volume began as a response to the growing diversity of the catchment area of our hospital. Cultural consultation is a way to bring some of the richness and complexity of the histories and social contexts of mental health problems into clinical work, through reformulating the nature of problems and devising solutions that fit the context. Our approach has been framed within the language of Canadian multiculturalism, inflected by the "intercultural" perspective of Quebec and the cosmopolitan world of Montreal. Every year, Canada receives about 250,000 immigrants and 25,000 refugees so that, at any given time, almost 20 % of Canadians were born outside the country, with a high proportion of newcomers in most metropolitan areas. About 4 % of the population identify as Indigenous peoples, and awareness of historical injustices toward their communities has driven renewed attention to issues of culture to achieve equity in health services.

Our subtitle, "Encountering the Other," points toward the basic existential fact of alterity—meeting with people with different lifeworlds and geographies of belonging. In a sense, this is always the case; the fact of cultural difference only magnifies or makes it more obvious. We hope our work shows the relevance of a Levinasian ethic of recognition, hospitality, care, and concern for the other in their humanness and difference.

As the subtitle indicates, the focus of this book is on practice: on practical issues in clinical work, both technical and scientific, pragmatic as well as political. We have aimed to describe the process of cultural consultation in sufficient detail to allow others to develop similar services. In addition to framing guidelines and strategies for consultation, we have tried to bring the work alive through brief clinical vignettes. These are based on cases seen at the CCS and other similar programs, but all have been disguised in ways that preserve their gist and protect patient confidentiality.

Chapter 1 provides an overview of different approaches to addressing diversity in mental health services. There are many clinical strategies and models of service for addressing culture. We show how the particular ways of construing culture and identifying the cultural "Other" as well as the ways of constructing dimensions of social identity like race and ethnicity reflect local demography, histories of migration, ideologies of citizenship, and the dominant paradigms in culture and mental health. One country's strength is another's weakness, so we can learn much from looking beyond our borders. We outline the distinctive features of the cultural consultation approach and its fit with multiculturalism. Finally, we discuss some of the ways in which cultural knowledge can enhance empathy, providing a basis for building a clinical alliance in order to deliver effective care.

Chapter 2 describes the history of the Cultural Consultation Service against the backdrop of other intercultural programs in Montreal. This is followed by a description of the key steps in the implementation of the service from identifying the need and choosing the model through assembling resources and training key people. We then present the main findings from formative and outcome evaluations of the service. The initial evaluation of the CCS demonstrated the acceptability of its procedures to clinicians and patients. The service uncovered high rates of misdiagnosis and inadequate treatment among the cases referred to the CCS, which undoubtedly represent only a small proportion of these problems in the general health care system. The majority of referring clinicians found the service helpful and recommended the service to their colleagues.

In Chapter 3, we describe the actual process of conducting a cultural consultation in detail, from initial intake and triage, through assembling the consultation team and the process of interviewing and assessment and working with interpreters and culture brokers, to cultural formulation, case discussion, and the communication of recommendations to referring clinicians. We present the key dimensions of the cultural formulation used by the CCS consultants and culture brokers, which is an expansion of the outline originally developed for DSM-IV as well as templates for recording intake information and presenting consultation reports.

The CCS based at the Jewish General Hospital was developed in partnership with the Transcultural Child Psychiatry Team of the Montreal Children's Hospital led by Cécile Rousseau. Chapter 4 describes the experience of that service along with a similar program developed by Marie Rose Moro at the Avicenne Hospital in France. The chapter draws out some ways in which approaches to culture reflect local sociocultural contexts while emphasizing the central role of cultural systems of meaning in psychiatric care for immigrant children and their families.

Cultural consultation relies on close collaboration with mental health interpreters and culture brokers. Chapters 5 and 6 discuss ways of working with these essential resources. Chapter 5 lays out the different models of interpreting and advocates for the use of community interpreters who are trained professionals but able to take on an advocacy role for patients within the health care system. Cultural consultation requires more than linguistic interpretation, however, and Chapter 6 describes the role of culture brokers or mediators who can act as go-betweens in the process of assessment and treatment delivery. Models of cultural mediation developed in various settings are discussed along with the ethical and pragmatic challenges associated with this essential group of health care workers.

Cultural formulations generally involve understanding problems in social contexts, which require systemic thinking. Chapter 7 discusses the relevance of family systems theory to cultural consultation. Cultural variations in family configurations, age and gender roles, developmental trajectories, and expectations can be integrated into a structural and systemic formulation that can guide strategic interventions. Attention to family structure and process is relevant and revealing for most cases but absolutely essential in understanding and intervening with children and adolescents.

Although cultural consultation does not rely exclusively on ethnic matching, bilingual/bicultural clinicians play an important role as consultants and culture brokers as well as in training. However, the presence of a clinician with an identifiable ethnic minority or racialized identity raises complex issues of transference and countertransference. Chapter 8 explores some of the ways that gender and ethnicity interact with hierarchies of power using the example of South Asian consultants working with individuals and families from India, Pakistan, Bangladesh, and Sri Lanka. The ambivalent responses of patients and professionals to female clinicians who are members of minority groups but who embody institutional power and authority can include both resistance and positive expectations. Recognition of these patterns can provide important diagnostic information and therapeutic leverage. However, effective assessment and treatment demand that the clinician be aware of the range of possible responses to their identities and work through their own reactions of internalized racism and gendered hierarchies. Peer supervision through a case conference or reflecting team is essential for the clinician to maintain a therapeutic stance and address gaps in understanding cultural agendas.

Although much of the work described in this volume is based at hospital outpatient clinics, cultural consultation can be delivered in nonclinical settings. Chapter 9 describes consultation for racialized or marginalized groups in contexts that include community organizations, legal and social service institutions, and work-related programs. The identity of the consultant figures prominently in negotiating issues of trust that stem from experiences of systemic racism and discrimination. Models drawn from community development and empowerment, including the work of Paulo Freire, are useful in orienting the consultant toward addressing larger issues of structural violence that are reflected in the struggles of individuals.

Primary care is a major target for cultural consultation which fits well with current models of collaborative or shared care. Chapter 10 describes the principles of collaborative care and the ways that attention to cultural diversity can be integrated into this approach. The authors present their experiences providing child psychiatric consultation in collaborative care for communities with high levels of immigrant and refugee and families. The chapter discusses the Ethnocultural Toolkit developed by the Canadian Collaborative Mental Health Initiative and the guidelines for prevention of common mental health problems among newcomers developed by the Canadian Collaboration for Immigrant and Refugee Health. Finally, training methods to support collaborative care are summarized.

The CCS is based in an urban center but aims to provide support to a wide region. This can be extended to include rural and remote communities through telepsychiatry. Chapter 11 discusses the particular challenges of cultural consultation work in rural and remote communities. In Canada, the population in remote communities is predominantly indigenous, so the practical issues of providing care to small, distant communities are interwoven with more specifically cultural issues surrounding the history of colonization, sedentarization, and forced assimilation for Indigenous peoples. Examples from work with Inuit in the arctic of Quebec illustrate some of the key principles of culturally safe and competent practice with Indigenous populations.

About one-third of the patients seen by the CCS are refugees and Chapter 12 discusses some of the issues specific to their predicament. People applying for asylum often go through a prolonged period of uncertainty that is enormously stressful. Although the clinicians providing basic medical care at the regional refugee clinic are expert in issues of migration health, some cases pose very complex diagnostic or treatment issues which cultural consultation can help clarify. In some cases, a letter from a psychiatrist or other mental health professional can be helpful in the adjudication of refugee status, and the complexities of preparing such documentation are reviewed. Many refugees have been exposed to high levels of traumatic violence including torture, and this may also make special demands on the clinicians' skill and require additional support.

Migration can have different effects across generations and certain patterns of migration, with family separation and reunification, may put youth at risk for social and mental health problems. Chapter 13 considers cultural consultation for courts and youth protection. These consultations aim to inform the legal and social service system about the impact of culture on adaptation and social integration so that more appropriate sentencing and interventions can be devised. This work requires understanding the specific mandate, skills, and limitations of workers in legal, forensic, and child protection settings. Approaches to training judges, police, and others in these settings are also discussed.

Chapter 14 considers cultural consultation in general hospital psychiatry, including the emergency department and inpatient wards. These settings pose special challenges for cultural consultation due to the acuteness and severity of illness and the time constraints and other pressures. Nevertheless, attention to culture and context can make a major contribution to resolving seemingly intractable problems. Often this involves understanding the systemic issues of the treating team, the ward, or the hospital itself.

These same issues affect general medical care and Chapter 15 broadens the discussion to cultural consultation in general internal medicine and specialty medical or surgical settings. Examples drawn mainly from the Transcultural Consultation Service of Geneva University Hospitals in Switzerland serve to illustrate how attention to culture can inform the care of patients with complex medical problems and uncover institutional weaknesses in the delivery of care to cultural minority patients.

The final chapter discusses the implications of our experiences with the CCS and similar services for mental health policy, research, training, and practice. The resources needed to set up a service like the CCS are quite modest so that, with a few key people, a similar program can be developed in many settings. The approach is scalable to address any level of clinical need. The service can readily provide a research and training setting, equipping the next generation of clinicians with the tools to improve cultural safety and competence in diverse settings.

Addressing culture in mental health care is not only a matter of accurate and effective person-centered care but also a question of human rights and of the vision of the kind of society and communities we want to create. We believe that cultural consultation provides an important arena for building pluralistic societies and hope that this volume will encourage others to explore this approach.

Montreal, QC, Canada   Laurence J. Kirmayer
                                                                             Jaswant Guzder
                                                                             Cécile Rousseau

Acknowledgements

We have many people to thank for their creative contributions to the evolution of the CCS and for the quality of care we have been able to deliver. The CCS is based at the Institute of Community and Family Psychiatry of the Jewish General Hospital, one of several teaching hospitals, affiliated with McGill University in Montreal. The Jewish General Hospital has a long tradition of care and research responsive to the needs of the community. Our network of colleagues, students, and community partners enriched this work immeasurably. We are privileged to work within a highly diverse group of professionals characterized by deep respect for and interest in difference as well as sameness. The ways that we engage and address our own differences deeply inform our approach to greeting those who come (or are sent) to us for help.

The Department of Psychiatry of the Jewish General Hospital has been a supportive environment for developing the CCS from its inception. We thank the department heads who made this project possible, Philip Beck who was the head during the first years of the service, and Michael Bond who has provided continued support for the service up to the present. The original CCS project involved partners from many organizations including the Division of Social and Transcultural Psychiatry of McGill University, affiliated teaching hospitals, and community clinics as well as the regional board of health and social services. In addition to the editors, the main partners were: from the Jewish General Hospital, G. Eric Jarvis, Ruta Westreich, Judy Gradinger, Liliane Spector, and Judy Malik; from the Montreal Children's Hospital, Klaus Minde, Louise Auger, Heather Clarke, Toby Measham, Lucie Nadeau, Deogratias Bagilishya, Nicole Heusch, Louise Lacroix, and Fiona Key; from Hôpital Jean-Talon, Carlo Sterlin, Louise Corbeil, and Celia Rojas-Viger; from Hôpital Ste. Justine, Sylvaine de Plaen and Jean-François Saucier; from the Psychosocial Research Unit, Douglas Hospital Eric Latimer; from the CLSC Côte-des-Neiges, Pierre Dongier, Ellen Rosenberg, and Vania Jimenez; and from the Régie régionale de la santé et des services sociaux de Montreal-Centre, Isabelle Hemlin.

The work of the CCS reflects the contributions of many people. We would like to acknowledge the current CCS staff, Antonella Clerici, Kay Berckmans, and Chrissi Galanakis. The original staff included Caminee Blake, Margaret O'Byrne, Sadeq Rahimi, Radhika Santhanam-Martin, and Suzanne Taillefer. Other research assistants associated with the project have included Sudeep Chaklanabis, Virginia Fauras, and Tomas Jurcik.

The work of the CCS depends crucially on the knowledge and skill of the many culture brokers who build bridges between different worlds: Sohail Abbas, Abdel Hamid Afana, Lida Aghasi, Rana Ahmed, Elena Alvarado, Pascale Annoual, Shafiqa Awj, Deogratias Bagilishya, Saliha Bahig, B.J. Barua, Evgueni Borokhovski, Roya Daneshmand, Nathalie Dinh, Marcel Durham, Gertrude Edem, Habib El-Hage, Therese Eustache, Hirut Eyob, Virginia Fauras, Marie-Rose Kalanga, Theodora Katerelos, Myrna Lashley, Marie Nathalie Leblanc, Judy Malik, Humera Manzoor, Alessandra Miklavcic, Luisa Molino, Yogini Nath, Kristin Norget, Mealea Ong Chan, My-Huong Pham, Andrena Pierre, Sadeq Rahimi, Mahbobeh Sadria, Gity Shirzad, Krishnaswamy Srinivasan, Maziar Taleshi, Jose Francisco Cuayas Tapia, Brett Thombs, Param Vairamuthu, Marta Valenzuela, Shirlette Wint, Siu Yuk (Louisa) Leung, Yue Zhao, and Xiaolu Zhou.

Many visiting scholars, residents, and students have contributed vitally to the work of the CCS over the years, including Sohail Abbas, Ademola Adeponle, Abdel Hamid Afana, Rana Ahmed, Faisal Al-Nowais, Cedric Andres, Luladay Asseku, Lauren Ban, Michaela Beder, Gaëlle Bélanger, Imen Ben Cheikh, Paul Benassi, Venkataramana Bhat, Caecilie Buhmann, Jessica Carlsson, Nick Carson, Yuexi Chen, Mathieu Chicoisne, Carl Chiniara, David Cohen, Rob Comey, Zoe Cost-Von Aesch, Helen Costin, Ghenwah Dakhallah, Vittorio De Luca, Melissa Dominice Dao, Irene Falgás Bagué, Reza Fallah, Marion Foissac, Rebecca Ganem, Cristiana Giordano, Kate Hibbard, Xiaojue Hu, Tomas Jurcik, Yasir Khan, Shu Kondo, Lonzozou Kpanake, Vincent Laliberté, Yvan Leanza, Anne-Marie Leblanc, Karim Lekhal, Annie Levesque, Annie Li, Eric Lis, Yogini Nath, Denise Noël, Jerryne Mahele Nyota, Federica Micucci, Alessandra Miklavcic, Peter Muthenge Munene, Ana Neto, Katerina Nikolitch, Masa Noguchi, Michel Okitapoy, Rimma Orenmann, Auralyd Padilla, Anton Parker, Judith Peranson, Rasitha Perera, Sadeq Rahimi, Anna Lanken Rasmussen, Priya Raju, Malika Robichaud, Carla Romano, Sarah Roosen, Coline Royant, Radhika Santhanam-Martin, Kelly Saran, Kemal Sayar, Daisy Singla, Vincenzo Spigonardo, Radhika Sundar, Hamida Tairi, Bouny Te, Irene Toniolo, Don Tran, Constantin Tranulis, Anda Vintiloiu, Fatima Unwala, Rob Whitley, Christina Wipperman, Meredith Woermke, Rahel Wolde-Giorghis, Esther Yakobov, Naofumi Yoshida, Lorin Young, Waël Youssef, Meng Yu, Mehdi Hassan Zadeh, and Xiaolu Zhou.

Anthony Marsella invited this volume for the series he edits and we thank him for his patience and encouragement during its long gestation. We also thank our international colleagues who have explored cultural consultation in other contexts and helped to show the relevance of this approach to diverse health care systems: Sofie Bäärnhielm, Rachid Bennegadi, Kamaldeep Bhui, and Sushrut Jadhav. Finally, we thank our families for their love, patience, and support as we have labored long and hard to bring this project to fruition.

Contents

Contributors

Isabelle Boivin, D.Ps. is a clinical psychologist. Since 2007, she has been a research assistant for Dr. Yvan Leanza in the field of community interpreting in intercultural clinical encounters. Her research interests are intercultural psychology, adult developmental psychology, and qualitative research.

Janet Cleveland, Ph.D. is a psychologist, anthropologist, and legal scholar. Since 2003, she has conducted research on the impact of Canada's policies toward refugee claimants on their health and human rights. In particular, she has studied the role of psychological reports in the context of refugee status determination procedures, the impact of administrative detention on refugee claimants' psychological health, and most recently, the impact of changes to the Interim Federal Health Program on refugee claimants' access to health care.

Marie-Eve Cotton, M.D. is Professeure Adjointe de Clinique at Université de Montréal. She works as a psychiatric consultant for the Inuit population at the Inuulitsivik Health Center, Povurnituq, and the Tulattavik Health Center of Ungava, Nunavik, Northern Quebec. She also works as a psychiatrist in the program of assertive community treatment (PACT) team at Hôpital Louis-H. Lafontaine, Montreal. Her clinical and academic interests include Inuit explanatory models of mental illness, racism toward Indigenous peoples, and the representation of mental illness in movies and novels.

Melissa Dominicé Dao, M.D., M.Sc. is an assistant professor, Division of Primary Care Medicine, Department of Community Medicine and Primary Care, Geneva University Hospitals. After specializing in general internal medicine in Geneva, Switzerland, she trained at McGill University in transcultural psychiatry. She now practices as a primary care physician and teaches primary care and cultural competence issues at the Geneva University Hospitals, where she founded and directs the Transcultural Consultation Service since 2007.

Danielle Groleau, Ph.D. is an associate professor in the Division of Social and Transcultural Psychiatry at McGill University, FRSQ senior research fellow, and senior investigator at the Lady Davis Institute, Jewish General Hospital. She is a medical anthropologist with a doctorate in Public Health and postdoctoral training in Cultural Psychiatry. Her research focuses on the social and cultural determinants of health behaviors in reproductive health. She teaches qualitative methods and public health in the Faculty of Medicine.

Danielle was responsible for the process evaluation of the Cultural Consultation Service. She does consultation and training for national and international agencies, including the Government of Québec, PAHO, and WHO.

Jaswant Guzder, M.D. is an associate professor of psychiatry and of social work, McGill University, and head of Child Psychiatry and director of the Childhood Disorders Day Hospital at the Jewish General Hospital. She was co-director of the Cultural Consultation Service from its inception. From 1980 to 1984, she worked in Mumbai, India, as a psychiatric consultant and psychoanalyst and continues to consult in India for Ummeed, Angaan, and Tata Institute of Social Services. Her current academic activities include cross-cultural training, family therapy training, and child trauma projects in Canada, India, Nepal, Sri Lanka, Turkey, Israel, and Jamaica.

Ghayda Hassan, Ph.D. is a clinical psychologist and professor of Cultural Clinical Psychology at the University of Quebec at Montreal (UQAM). Dr. Hassan believes that we cannot develop expertise in any specific cultural group, but rather that clinical cultural psychology is more about a clinical stance, a "way of being," "a way of being with the other," and an approach to "meaning making within the context of an encounter with the other." Her clinical and research activities focus on the interplay of culture, identity, mental health, and violence in a variety of clinical and community settings. She has worked with Arab-Canadian Muslim and non-Muslim groups, Filipino-Canadian youth, Caribbean-Canadian youth mostly of Haitian origin, and Latin American families.

Felicia Heidenreich-Dutray, M.D. is a psychiatrist at the Équipe mobile psychiatrie et précarité, Centre Hospitalier de Rouffach, Alsace, France. She worked as a medical anthropologist in Senegal before doing clinical work and research in transcultural psychiatry with Marie Rose Moro in Paris (2000–2007) and with Cécile Rousseau in Montreal (2007–2009). Her research interests include refugee children and families, psychiatric diagnosis in immigrant families, and development of mental health services for immigrant populations.

G. Eric Jarvis, M.D., M.Sc. is an assistant professor and director of the Cultural Consultation Service at the Jewish General Hospital. His clinical work involves the psychiatric evaluation and treatment of immigrants and refugees. His current research interests include the relation between psychosis and culture and the process of cultural consultation. Dr. Jarvis also writes about the history of psychiatry.

Laurence J. Kirmayer, M.D. is James McGill Professor and Director, Division of Social and Transcultural Psychiatry, McGill University, and editor-in-chief of *Transcultural Psychiatry*. He directs the Culture & Mental Health Research Unit at the Jewish General Hospital where he conducts research on the mental health of Aboriginal peoples, mental health services for immigrants and refugees, and the cultural basis of psychiatric theory and practice. He was founding director of the Cultural Consultation Service.

Myrna Lashley, Ph.D. is an assistant professor in the Division of Social and Transcultural Psychiatry at McGill University and project director at the Lady Davis Institute for Medical Research at the Jewish General Hospital in Montreal. She is a counseling psychologist with 15 years of experience as a psychological consultant for the courts in youth corrections and has been involved in training in multiculturalism for police and other professional groups. She is the vice-chair of the board of the École nationale de police du Québec and chair of the Canadian Cross-Cultural Roundtable on Security. Her current research is focused on cultural competence as a strategy to prevent radicalization leading to violent extremism.

Yvan Leanza, M.Ps., Ph.D. is a former postdoctoral fellow in the Division of Social and Transcultural Psychiatry and the Department of Family Medicine, McGill University (2004–2005). After many migratory moves between Switzerland and Canada, he is now an associate professor in the School of Psychology, Laval University (Québec City), where he teaches cross-cultural psychology and intervention and leads the Psychology and Cultures lab (www.labo-psychologie-cultures.ca). His research focuses on working with interpreters and intercultural relations in health care settings and on sleep in cross-cultural perspective. He is a founding member and the current director of *Alterstice—International Journal of Intercultural Research* (www.alterstice.org).

Marie Nathalie LeBlanc, Ph.D. is an anthropologist and professor in the Department of Sociology of Université du Québec à Montréal. Her main ethnographic fieldwork has been conducted in West Africa and in Québec. Her research interests focus on religious dynamics in postcolonial contexts (mainly in relation to Islam and Christianity), the roles of youth and women in the moralization of contemporary public spheres, new forms of cultural citizenship in relation to popular culture, and the construction of social identities in intercultural contexts. She is the head of the research unit on democratization, civil society, and social movements at the Centre interdisciplinaire de recherché sur le développement international et société (CIRDIS, UQAM). Her involvement with the Cultural Consultation Service has been as a culture broker in cases involving patients of African origin.

Begum Maitra, M.D., M.R.C.Psych. is a child and adolescent psychiatrist and adult psychotherapist in private practice. As a consultant child psychiatrist in the British National Health Service, she worked in inner city London for 16 years, developing her long-standing interests in cultural meanings and devising consultation, supervision, and training for mental health professionals. She continues to work as an independent expert for children at risk, and their families, in court proceedings and has done so for 23 years. She writes and teaches in the UK and India.

Toby Measham, M.D., M.Sc. is an assistant professor at McGill University and a member of its Division of Social and Transcultural Psychiatry and Child Psychiatry. Her clinical and research interests include transcultural child psychiatry and the development of collaborative community-based mental health care services for children and their families.

Alessandra Miklavcic, Ph.D. is a medical anthropologist and sociolinguist. She is currently a senior qualitative researcher at St. Mary's Hospital Research Centre, Montreal. She received her doctorate from the University of Toronto, and completed a postdoctoral fellowship at the Division of Social and Transcultural Psychiatry, McGill University in 2010. She has worked on mental health research with immigrants and refugees as well as first-episode of psychosis both in academia and in volunteer sectors in Europe, India, and North America. Her research interests include qualitative methods discourse analysis, media representation of mental illness, social inequalities, and global health.

Lucie Nadeau, M.D., M.Sc. is an assistant professor in the Divisions of Social and Transcultural Psychiatry and Child Psychiatry of the Department of Psychiatry, McGill University. She works as a child psychiatrist at the Montreal Children's Hospital, Jewish General Hospital, CSSS de la Montagne, and the CSSS Cavendish. She is also a child psychiatry consultant for the Inuulitsivik Health Center in Inuit communities of the Hudson Coast of Nunavik, Quebec. Her current research focuses on collaborative care in youth mental health in multi-ethnic neighbourhoods, and community-based and school-based projects in Aboriginal communities.

Ellen Rosenberg, M.D. is an associate professor, Department of Family Medicine, McGill University and staff physician, Family Medicine Centre, St. Mary's Hospital where she conducts research on doctor-patient communication with trained and lay interpreters.

Cécile Rousseau, M.D., M.Sc. is an associate professor, Department of Psychiatry, and director, Transcultural Psychiatry Service, CSSS de la Montagne, where she has built a team addressing refugee and immigrant children's mental health, with particular interest in children of war. She has conducted epidemiological and ethnographic research on the personal, family, and cultural determinants of refugee children's mental health. She has developed innovative school prevention programs for refugee and immigrant children and adolescents using creative expression workshops. In partnership with researchers in international law and community organizations, she has analyzed the cultural and psychological construction of immigration policies and their consequences for the mental health of refugees.

Radhika Santhanam-Martin, Ph.D. is a clinical psychologist who works in the field of trauma. She has more than two decades of experience in clinical practice in institutions in India, Canada and Australia. In Australia, she has worked in tertiary hospitals, universities and health services as a clinical consultant and senior lecturer. Currently, she works in collaboration with organizations in Melbourne that provide services for refugees, asylum seekers, culturally and linguistically diverse groups, and Indigenous families.

Shirlette Wint, M.S.W. is a social worker and a cultural consultant to the Caribbean community. She has worked with diverse black community groups, among them the Côte-des-Neiges Black Community Association, Women on

the Rise, and Little Burgundy Urban Mediation and Prevention and has been
involved in several Youth and Parent Support Groups and has spearheaded
efforts to liaison with schools and community social and health centers. She has
coordinated and written on research in the Caribbean community both at the
community organization and school liaison levels. She is a consultant with the
Cultural Consultation Service of the Jewish General Hospital.

Introduction: The Place of Culture in Mental Health Services

Laurence J. Kirmayer, Cécile Rousseau, and Jaswant Guzder

Cultural diversity presents an important challenge for health care services in every society around the world. Although contemporary anthropology has rejected the view of cultures as tightly integrated systems that produce individuals who are all alike in their values and perspectives, it remains clear that cultures—as systems of knowledge and practice that give our lives identity, meaning, and purpose—shape every aspect of experience including health and illness. Indeed, through the psychobiological processes of development, culture is inscribed on our brains, bodies, families, and communities. Even when migration or other events lead to profound changes in the ways we live, our cultural backgrounds leave traces in our behavior like accents, styles of gesture, and communication, as well as habitual or automatic responses to specific symbols, words, or expressions of emotion. In addition to these traces of our collective histories, the confluence and intermixing of cultures in our globalizing world create new possibilities for self-fashioning. Culture is the constantly evolving medium through which we articulate our deepest values and greatest aspirations. Human biology, behavior, and experience are culturally shaped and mental health practice must respond to the resulting diversity.

There is now a large body of evidence on the impact of culture on illness behavior and experience. Social and cultural processes shape the mechanisms of disease, the symptoms of distress, and subsequent ways of coping or help seeking (Kirmayer, 2005). Systems of healing reflect cultural models of body, self, and person that are grounded in distinctive ontologies or notions of what constitutes the individual and the world (Kirmayer, 2006). Although one might think that universal aspects of biology trump cultural influences in serious illness, the crisis of illness itself challenges our everyday assumptions. Experiences of physical or emotional distress and other types of conflict mobilize cultural systems of knowledge and meaning in an effort to make sense of the problem or affliction. These systems of knowledge then shape the experience, course, and outcome of illness. Studying this cultural shaping of illness experience is at the core of research in medical anthropology and cross-cultural psychiatry and psychology, which in

L.J. Kirmayer, M.D. (✉)
Culture and Mental Health Research Unit,
Institute of Community and Family Psychiatry,
Jewish General Hospital, 4333 Cote Ste Catherine
Road, Montreal, QC, Canada H3T 1E4
e-mail: laurence.kirmayer@mcgill.ca

C. Rousseau, M.D., M.Sc.
Centre de recherche et de formation,
CSSS de la Montagne, 7085 Hutchison Street,
Local 204.2, Montréal, QC, Canada H3N 1Y9
e-mail: cecile.rousseau@mcgill.ca

J. Guzder, M.D.
Center for Child Development and Mental Health,
Institute of Community and Family Psychiatry,
4335 Cote St. Catherine Road, Montreal, QC,
Canada H3T 1E4
e-mail: jaswant@videotron.ca

turn, have supported the development of strategies for addressing cultural diversity in health care (Kirmayer & Minas, 2000). In this chapter, we will summarize some of these strategies to provide a backdrop for the model of cultural consultation described in detail in this book.

What Is Culture?

We have begun by using the word culture quite loosely—and we will continue to take much license—but "culture" deserves a closer look. The word culture has a variety of meanings covering a broad territory and its use has changed over time, reflecting changes in scientific knowledge as well as politics. At the outset it is useful to distinguish three broad meanings of culture (Eagleton, 2000): (1) as the social matrix of every aspect of human biology and experience, (2) as the ways in which human groups or communities with a shared history or identity are distinguished from each other, and (3) as the cultivation of our collective creative capacities, expressed in large part by language but also through music, the arts, and other media.

Culture is a basic dimension of human biology and experience—reflecting the fact that we are social beings and that the ways we live shape our brains and bodies. This definition of culture encompasses all of the humanly constructed and transmitted features of the environment, including both material aspects, systems of knowledge, and institutions—like marriage, professional roles, and the legal system—that rest on shared agreements or social conventions. Recent work in cultural neuroscience is beginning to show the ways in which culture is inscribed on the nervous system, but the greater part of culture remains outside any individual in the social world, ready to hand to be taken up and used in appropriate social contexts (Choudhury & Kirmayer, 2009). Culture therefore involves not only cognitive models or representations but also situated knowledge, discourse, and practice, which may reside in patterns of interaction and social institutions.

The second meaning of culture involves "otherness"—the marking off of a group or community as distinct from others, defined in terms of some shared lineage, geographic origin, or other characteristics, including language, religion, and way of life. This meaning of culture includes the notion of ethnicity, from the Latin *ethnos* or nation (Banks, 1996). Ethnicity is shaped by the ways that groups are defined within a culture and by the sense of distinctiveness that comes from encountering others different from one's own familiar group or community. While culture is an inevitable consequence of our biology as social animals with immense capacities for learning and memory, ethnicity reflects the dynamics of territorial boundary marking and belonging. In the contemporary world, ethnicity raises important political problems of voice and recognition within societies that contain diversity as a result of their histories of formation and subsequent migration. Ethnocultural diversity is thus both a political fact and a biosocial reality demanding attention in health care on both grounds.

Race is another way that groups are marked off from each other by attributing superficial differences in appearance or geographic origin to intrinsic differences in biology or some other "essence." Racial distinctions reflect the history of violent encounters between groups and support racist ideologies associated with systems of discrimination, marginalization, and oppression that continue to result in significant health disparities in many societies (Fredrickson, 2002; Gee, Spencer, Chen, Yip, & Takeuchi, 2007; Gravlee, 2009; Surgeon General, 2002). Contemporary molecular biology has deconstructed the notion of race, showing how visible differences between individuals or groups usually are inconsistently associated with small differences in the genome (Koenig, Lee, & Richardson, 2008). As a result, race is an unreliable marker of biological difference. However, because of the social and psychological consequences of racial labels and their impact on health, racialized identities remain an important issue in understanding health disparities of populations and the social predicaments faced by individuals subject to structural violence and discrimination. In the last decade, religion has been propelled to the forefront of international and intercommunity conflicts and has become a renewed source of tension and discrimination and a marker of social exclusion for some minority communities (Rousseau, Hassan, Moreau, & Thombs, 2011).

The third meaning of culture as cultivation stems from the notion of societies achieving some higher value through civilizing processes associated with the elaboration and refinement of language, religion, ritual etiquette, science, and the arts. In European history, this civilizing process supported hierarchical systems of status distinguishing those with greater refinement from the uncultured or uncultivated masses (Elias, 1982). Through colonization, this European value system was applied to other peoples and nations as well as slaves and other categories of subalterns or subordinate groups (Lindqvist, 1996; Spivak, 2006). Colonial blinders led psychiatrists and other mental health practitioners to see the world along a single hierarchy with the Western way of life at the top and others at the bottom representing more or less primitive, barbaric, or childlike versions of humanity (Bhugra & Littlewood, 2001).

Postcolonial thinkers, notably Frantz Fanon and Edward Said, have thoroughly critiqued and challenged this Eurocentric hierarchy, which has been used to justify oppression, exploitation, and even genocide. Along with the challenges to this hierarchy has come an effort to consider diverse traditions on an equal footing, as alternative ways of being human, to be understood on their own terms. This respect for diversity does not entail moral or conceptual relativism. However, it does demand that we systematically challenge assumptions of a single developmental hierarchy or monolithic definitions of health and well-being and asks that we examine the roots of our ideas about human nature and our moral values in a particular cultural history and way of life. This reflective approach allows us to understand how our values and way of life justify each other and opens the door to consider alternatives.

This critique extends to the basic models and practices that organize mental health services and interventions. Although contemporary mental health professionals aim to ground their practice in scientific evidence, clinical psychology and psychiatry are rooted in Western cultural traditions (Rose, 1996). Values drawn from Northern European and Euro-American notions of individualism and autonomy pervade psychiatry's diagnostic nosology, theory, and therapeutic interventions (Gaines, 1992; Kirmayer, 2007). Although the focus on individual autonomy, competence, and well-being may have a liberating effect by creating new options for people trapped in untenable social situations, it has also created new dilemmas with serious tensions and contradictions. To act in the best interests of the vulnerable individual, clinicians must see beyond the individual to consider the wider social context from which their lives draw meaning and on which they may depend to realize their aspirations. The concept of social suffering, introduced by medical anthropologists Kleinman, Das and Lock (1997), highlights the ways that mental illness reflects larger processes of adversity and inequity rooted in problems of power, violence, and oppression that beset families and communities. This points to a central theme throughout this book: the need to understand mental health problems and their solutions in social, cultural, historical, and political contexts. As practitioners, this includes reflection on the cultural embedding of health services, systems, and institutions.

Approaches to Diversity in Mental Health Services

In every society, culture influences the major social determinants of health giving rise to significant differences and disparities across groups. The social categories and identities constructed through culture, like race, ethnicity, and religion, are associated with differences in social position and health status. Some groups are advantaged, while others are marginalized. There is good evidence that ignoring cultural difference and diversity in health care contributes to health disparities (Alegria, Atkins, Farmer, Slaton, & Stelk, 2010; Kirmayer, Weinfeld, et al., 2007; Smedley, Stith, Nelson, & Institute of Medicine U.S. Committee on Understanding and Eliminating Racial and Ethnic Disparities in Health Care, 2003).

Broadly speaking, health services respond to the fact of cultural diversity in one of two ways: either working to assimilate patients into standard practice by normalizing and ignoring difference or acknowledging and responding to difference by developing more varied models and practices. Within mental health services, these alternatives are played out in corresponding clinical strategies: assuming that newcomers can quickly adapt to conventional services or developing specialized clinics and programs for those who have particular needs because of differences in culture, language, religion, or other aspects of their background and identity. Adaptations in services may represent technical changes in procedures (e.g., the use of interpreters), alternative forms of assessment and treatment, or changes in our models of psychopathology and corresponding interventions.

One common approach to diversity attempts to match the service to the patient, on the assumption that ethnic or cultural matching will allow optimal delivery of effective services. Efforts to match services to the ethnocultural background of the patient can occur at the level of technical interventions, the person of the clinician, or the whole institution (Weinfeld, 1999). The effectiveness of these different types of matching depends on their meaning for the specific group, which in turn depends on their political position within the larger society. For those who are politically marginalized, insuring they have some measure of institutional control may be a far more effective response than providing a traditional form of healing or a clinician from a similar background.

When culture is recognized in mental health care, most often it is invoked to explain failures of communication, treatment adherence, and mutual understanding between clinician and patient. Culture in this sense is something that the clinician attributes to the patient and is a sort of baggage or barrier to communication and cooperation. Attaching culture to the patient ignores the ways in which institutional practices may reflect cultural values of the dominant social groups and devalue, marginalize, or exclude other groups. Ignoring the cultural identity of others does not insure equity but simply hides the culturally rooted biases and assumptions inherent in standard clinical practices, bureaucratic routines, or "common sense." As Suman Fernando has argued, this can result in forms of institutional racism or discrimination, characterized by:

> the collective failure of an organization to provide an appropriate and professional service to people because of their colour, culture or ethnic origin. It can be seen or detected in processes, attitudes and behaviors which amounts to discrimination through the unwitting prejudice, ignorance, thoughtlessness and racist stereotyping which disadvantages minority ethnic people. (Fernando, 2009, p. 14)

More positively, notions of culture may be used to acknowledge the characteristics of ethnic groups and their shared needs, values, and predicaments. Information about culture has been introduced into the training of health care professionals in the form of handbooks summarizing patterns of illness behavior in specific ethnic groups (e.g., Harwood, 1981; Waxler-Morrison, 1989). This fits with a general tendency in person perception to form stereotypes. Unfortunately, it often fails to capture either the range of variation within any given ethnocultural group or the fact that cultural practices are tied to personal and family histories in complex and idiosyncratic ways.

Of course, cultural difference also involves the personal and professional background of the clinician and the cultural assumptions of medical practice. An analysis of cultural difference in terms of the relative power, social position, and interaction of the local worlds of clinician and patient is likely to be more useful than stereotypic portraits of patients' ethnocultural background. This sort of analysis requires attention to the ideologies and institutions of the dominant society as much as any consideration of the background and trajectory of minority groups or individuals. Medicine too is a cultural institution and understanding its cultural assumptions opens up a space to begin to engage others on a more equal footing. Several decades of work in medical history and anthropology have begun to lay bare the cultural roots and assumptions of biomedicine and psychiatry (Kleinman, 1980; Lock & Gordon, 1988; Lock & Nguyen, 2010). The perspectives of the humanities and social sciences can help clinicians move beyond the frameworks of conventional mental health practice to appreciate the unique predicaments of individuals as well as the alternative visions of health and healing that are part of the riches and resources of a diverse society.

Differences in lay and professional perspectives about health and illness occur in larger social and political contexts in which certain groups are singled out as culturally different and targeted for special consideration. This process of "othering" depends on local histories of migration, definitions of citizenship, and social constructions of identity. Understanding something of these histories is essential for appreciating why specific models have been developed or become dominant in particular national contexts.

Although some nations have defined themselves in terms of specific ethnic identities, cultural diversity has been a characteristic of many societies. History records several different types of political regimes that have tolerated cultural and religious diversity. The political philosopher Michael Walzer (1997, p. 14) identified multinational empires, consociations, certain nation states, and immigrant societies as examples of regimes of toleration, along with international society as a whole.[1] Although small communities have been homogenous throughout history, the creation of ethnic nation states has sometimes

involved reimagining identity and rewriting history to elide the true diversity of geographic regions and peoples (Anderson, 1991; McNeill, 1986). The ways that a country defines itself can have profound implications for the social position, security, and integration of newcomers. A society that sees itself as united by some common blood or lineage may leave migrants in a prolonged or perpetual state of marginalization.

Multiculturalism and other ideologies of citizenship that support ethnocultural communities actively acknowledge and support cultural diversity as a value in itself. This provides pathways of integration for ethnocultural communities into a society that is defined as inherently diverse (Kymlicka, 1995). Political values like multiculturalism can inform the range of social institutions including the health care system (Kivisto, 2002). Health services reflect local ideologies of citizenship and modes of communal life. In the area of culture and mental health, theory and practice have evolved in somewhat different directions in different countries owing to many factors including the composition of the population, notions of citizenship, and the political status of ethnocultural minorities as well as local schools and traditions within psychiatry and psychology.

Castles and Miller (1998) distinguish four broad models of citizenship: (1) the *imperial* model (e.g., the British Empire) brings together diverse peoples under one ruler; (2) the *folk* or *ethnic* model (e.g., Germany) defines citizenship in terms of common descent, language, and culture; (3) the *republican* model (e.g., France) defines the state as a political community based on a constitution and laws so that newcomers who adopt the rules and the common culture are accepted as full citizens; and (4) the *multicultural* model (e.g., Canada, Australia) shares the political definition of community with the republican model but accepts the formation of ethnic communities within the polity. The health systems created on the basis of these conceptions of citizenship and unique histories of migration have influenced both the direction of cultural psychiatry and the development of mental health services in each country.

---

[1] Here is how Walzer (1997, p. 44) describes Canadian society:

> Canada is an immigrant society with several national minorities—the Aboriginal peoples and the French—that are also conquered nations. These minorities are not dispersed the way the immigrants are, and they have a very different history. Individual arrival doesn't figure in their collective memory; they tell a story, instead, of long-standing communal life. They aspire to sustain that life, and they fear that it is unsustainable in the loosely organized, highly mobile, individualistic society of the immigrants. Even strong multiculturalist policies are not likely to help minorities of this sort, for all such policies encourage only "hyphenated" identities—that is, fragmented identities, with each individual negotiating the hyphen, constructing some sort of unity for him or herself. What these minorities want, by contrast, is an identity that is collectively negotiated. And for that they need a collective agent with substantial political authority.

Countries like Britain and France, which were major colonial powers, have had substantial immigration from former colonies. Based on their experiences within colonial systems of education and power that bear the legacy of colonial times, such immigrants often come with positive expectations of "returning to the center," but they have met with systemic racism and discrimination which has had significant impact on their mental health (Littlewood & Lipsedge, 1982). The distinctions between the imperial and republican models, as well as the different national histories of psychiatry and psychoanalysis, have led to somewhat different responses in cultural psychiatry and models of service.

In the UK, the prototypical cultural "Other" was termed "Black" and this term covered a much broader range of backgrounds than in Canada (Fernando, 1995). In recent years, the term "BME," "Black and Ethnic Minority," has become popular (Fernando, 2005). Being Black is not a neutral social category but is associated with significant social adversity and ill health. For example, there is evidence that Afro-Caribbean migrants to the UK and some other European countries experience elevated rates of schizophrenia compared to the rates in the population in their countries of origin (Cantor-Graae & Selten, 2005). This is not due to selective migration and the rate is even higher in the second generation. The effects of discrimination and social exclusion are likely contributing factors (Cantor-Graae, 2007) and these may be viewed as forms of structural violence (Kelly, 2005). In recognition of this problem, cultural psychiatry in the UK has focused on inequalities in care for immigrants and in providing services that are explicitly antiracist (Fernando, 2005). Following a national inquiry into a racially motivated attack in 1993 on Steven Lawrence, a Black youth, the government mandated a program of professional training and quality assurance to address issues of discrimination in the workplace, including mental health centers. While the inquiry focused on needs within the police and justice systems, Fernando (2005) has underlined how this unmasking of cultural agendas with the formulation of institutional racism remains crucial to pro-

vide equitable mental health practice. However, the translation of these principles into actual clinical practice is uneven (Bhui, Ascoli, & Nuamh, 2012), and debate continues on the merits of specialized services vs. improving the response of primary care and general psychiatry.

France faced similar migration from former colonies, notably from North Africa (the Maghreb). In France, the republican ideal downplays the significance of culture to assert the common values of political participation in the state. Ethnocultural identity is something individuals are supposed to be free to express in their homes but is not actively supported by the state, which is conceived of as a neutral space that accommodates all citizens. Despite the ideal of inclusion, however, many people from former colonies in North Africa have experienced continued discrimination and marginalization (Ben Jelloun & Bray, 1999). Mental health services in France have been strongly influenced by a psychoanalytic tradition that tends to situate problems in the individual psyche with unconscious dynamics shaped by cultural representations minimally acknowledging the major dimensions of the social realities. In the clinical approach of Tobie Nathan, consultations with specialized ethnopsychiatric teams composed of practitioners from diverse backgrounds aim to create a transitional space where the clinician's interventions can mediate the collective symbolic worlds of the immigrants' country of origin and France (Corin, 1997; Nathan, 1986, 1991; Sargent & Larchanche, 2009; Sturm, Nadig, & Moro, 2011). Through the theory of complementarity, this approach recognizes the contribution of different ontologies, conceptual universes, and systems values to the healing process. At the same time, however, by locating the problem of intercultural interaction in a symbolic intrapsychic space, this approach risks sidestepping the problem of social change needed to create public spaces that accommodate newcomers and promote effective exchange among groups (Fassin & Rechtman, 2005).

In recent years, the prototypical Other in England and France has shifted from individuals defined in racialized terms as "Black," "African," or "Asian" to those categorized as Muslim or

Islamic. This shift reflects the post-9/11 environment in which the threat of terrorism has been attached to a whole religion and the religion in turn conflated with language (Arabic), ethnicity, and geographic origins. This is an extremely important issue for migrants, even those not from an Islamic background, who now face an increasingly suspicious reception and are viewed as holding values that are fundamentally incompatible with the liberal, democratic, or republican values of European countries (Rousseau et al., 2011; Rousseau, Jamil, Hassan, & Moreau, 2010).

Canada and Australia are immigrant or settler societies with explicit policies of multiculturalism. In both cases, this is reflected in efforts to respond to cultural diversity in mainstream settings. In Australia, multiculturalism promoted the development of services responsive to the diverse needs of Aboriginal and immigrant communities (Ziguras, Stankovska, & Minas, 1999). With respect to immigrants, the cultural "Other" has been framed as someone who is linguistically different, and the general term used in many research studies and policy documents was non-English-speaking background or "NESB"; in recent years, this has been supplanted by the acronym "culturally and linguistically diverse". In relation to immigrant communities, the development of services initially emphasized the importance of surmounting communication barriers and an extensive system of interpreting services was developed, with public health information available in many languages. Both the national- and state-level governments have mental health policies and programs designed to respond to the fact of cultural diversity. Refugees and those seeking asylum have constituted a more contentious category of cultural "Other" and have met with harsh policies aimed at deterring migration (Silove, Steel, & Watters, 2000). There has also been a very active network of centers involved in the treatment of survivors of torture and strong advocacy for the plight of asylum seekers held in detention (Cleveland & Rousseau, 2012; Kronick, Rousseau, & Cleveland, 2011; Silove, Austin, & Steel, 2007).

In Canada, multiculturalism was made an official policy in 1971 with the explicit aim of main-

taining ethnic languages and cultures and combating racism (Kamboureli, 1998). Subsequent legislation has attempted to promote pluralism and diversity in the workplace and insure equal access to health care services. In a sense, everyone in Canada—with the crucial exception of Indigenous peoples—is an immigrant, so the sharp distinction between newcomers and those of older stock is hard to sustain. There is a tendency to view culture and ethnicity in positive terms, and it is common for people to identify themselves as "hyphenated" Canadians, including mention of their country of origin or heritage (Mackey, 1999). This rosy picture is challenged, however, by the history of selective migration policy influenced by racist efforts to maintain a "White Canada" (Ward, 2005) and, more explicitly, by the ongoing struggle of French Canadians to assert their distinct identity as a founding people rather than a linguistic minority (Bibeau, 1998). Perhaps as a result, compared to Australia, there has been less development of interpreting in health services in much of Canada. This has begun to change with the influx of large numbers of Chinese and other Asians to Vancouver and Toronto. In response to the size of these communities, ethnospecific services have been developed in Toronto and Vancouver, often with funding from ethnocultural minority communities (Ganesan & Janze, 2005; Lo & Chung, 2005). Nevertheless, the dominant approach to cultural diversity in mental health care has been to apply standard models, with limited efforts to consider the impact of ethnicity on illness experience. Although the goal of multicultural health care remains treating everyone in mainstream settings with due recognition of their cultural background, this is honored more often in the breach. Recently, the Mental Health Commission of Canada (2009) produced a framework for transformation of the mental health care system in Canada that includes responding to diversity as one of seven key principles. The resultant mental health strategy for Canada identifies six strategic directions which include (1) attention to diversity and disparities in the mental health of immigrants, refugees, ethnocultural communities, and racialized groups and (2) the mental health of Indigenous peoples (First Nations, Inuit, and Métis) (Mental Health Commission of Canada, 2012). Although the strategy lays out a set of priorities in each of these areas, it remains unclear whether and how this will be translated into actual policy and practice.

Within Canada, the design and delivery of health care services is under provincial jurisdictions, and there are some important regional differences in how services are addressing cultural diversity. In Quebec, concern about maintaining French language and culture in the context of the dominance of English in North America has led to a rejection of the tenets of multiculturalism, in favor of the construct of "interculturalism." On one interpretation, interculturalism stands for the recognition that when cultures encounter each other, they influence each other and are both transformed. The outcome is not a society composed of multiple islands or ghettos of ethnocultural groups but a vibrant exchange in which new cultural forms are created. In reality, because French Quebecois are a local majority but a small minority in the sea of Canadian and American-Anglo culture, interculturalism has been translated into policies of selective immigration, obligatory French-language education for newcomers' children, and tests of professionals' language competency that strive to maintain French as a working language and priority in health care institutions. Concerns about the extent to which Quebec society should adapt to the needs and values of newcomers have been framed as a problem of "reasonable accommodation" (Bouchard & Taylor, 2008), and discussed in relation to the need to protect and promote French language as central to Quebecois identity and culture.

The United States shares elements of republican and multicultural models. It is an immigrant society but has been profoundly marked by its history of slavery and racism. Despite a policy of assimilation, successive waves of migration have resulted in the presence of large distinct groups defined by race, ethnicity, and language. This has been framed in terms of ethnoracial blocs grouping together African-Americans, Asian and Pacific Islanders, Hispanics or Latinos, American Indians and Alaska Natives, and Caucasians or Whites (Hollinger, 1995). This way of demarcating major groups has led to recognition of marked disparities in health and access to services (Smedley et al., 2003; Surgeon General, 2002). The response has been the development of ethno-specific clinics where patients can be treated by clinicians with requisite language skills and cultural knowledge and more general implementation of training and practice models to achieve "cultural competence" (Betancourt, Green, Carrillo, & Ananeh-Firempong, 2003; Yang & Kagawa-Singer, 2007). Both the American Psychiatric Association and the American Psychological Association have developed standards for cultural competence in professional training and quality assurance in service delivery. Initiatives at the level of federal and state governments are addressing mental health service delivery issues for diverse populations. For example, California has established regulations requiring community health clinics to have staff capable of working in any language present in the community above a specified threshold. Managed care companies are increasingly concerned to demonstrate their responsiveness to cultural issues in order to meet the needs of a diverse population. Cultural competence in the USA has been framed largely in terms of the composition of the professional work force, and this speaks directly to issues of political representation.

Commitments to multiculturalism may develop even in formerly nonimmigrant societies. For example, Swedish society, which was relatively homogeneous until the 1940s (aside from the indigenous Sami population and such ethnocultural minorities as Finn-Swedes and Romani), received many immigrants after WWII, so that approximately 15 % of Swedes are first- or second-generation immigrants and one-third of these are non-European. Since the mid-1970s, newcomers to Sweden have been almost exclusively refugees, and Swedish efforts in cultural psychiatry have focused on research and services that address the sequelae of trauma. Swedish immigrant policy since 1975 has been based on three major principles: (1) equality (providing immigrants the same standard of living as Swedes), (2) freedom of choice (giving members of ethnic minorities the opportunity to retain their cultural identity or adopt Swedish cultural identity), and (3) partnership (promoting working together) (Bäärnhielm, Ekblad, Ekberg, & Ginsburg, 2005). The protection of Swedish as a minority language in the European and global context is coupled with the protection of minority languages. Current language policy in Sweden recognizes five official minority languages: Finnish, Meänkieli, Sami, Romani, and Yiddish. Everyone has the right to language—specifically, to learn Swedish and to use one's mother tongue or minority language.[2] Despite the policy of freedom of choice and partnership, immigrants are underrepresented among health care and social work professionals. In 1999, the County Council of Stockholm sponsored the development of a Centre for Transcultural Psychiatry, which provides specialized clinical consultations and training programs to improve the quality and accessibility of mental health services for the immigrant and refugee population. The center has worked to raise awareness of issues of diversity and recently published guidelines on the treatment of asylum seekers that argue for the provision of psychiatric services as an issue of human rights.

Each of these models of mental health service is a reflection of local political and social factors that have mandated particular forms of recognition and response. Each society defines certain groups as "Other" and certain forms of otherness as worthy of formal recognition and investment of resources; more marginal groups are excluded, ignored, or expected to find their own way through the maze of available services. Common across all of these settings is the tendency to view the norms, values, and standards of the dominant social group not as "culture" but simply as "the proper way to do things" or common sense. This use of the rhetoric of common sense to obscure the cultural basis of the practices of the dominant group is compounded in medicine by appeals to evidence-based practice. In the larger society, appeals to common sense and technocratic ratio-

nality are often part of claims that public space is somehow culturally (and religiously) neutral. Unfortunately, most of the available evidence in mental health has been developed and evaluated on samples of patients that are not representative of the diversity of the population in terms of gender, ethnicity, and the social contexts of their problems (Whitley, Rousseau, Carpenter Song, & Kirmayer, 2011). Despite this limitation, there is a strong tendency to assume that the available evidence is sufficient and that standard clinical methods and interventions can be applied across cultures and settings without questioning their appropriateness, efficacy, and effectiveness. Moreover, even when methods of assessment or intervention have been culturally adapted, most have not been subjected to systematic evaluation. Absence of evidence is not evidence of no benefit. There are many reasons to believe that systematic attention to culture can improve the accessibility, acceptability, quality, and outcomes of mental health services. Some of the clearest demonstrations come from the work of the Cultural Consultation Service (CCS) on individual cases where cultural knowledge becomes pivotal to effective care.

Cultural Consultation as a Response to Diversity

In this book we present cultural consultation as one approach to addressing cultural diversity in mental health services. The CCS that we will describe was developed in the specific context of Montreal, within the bilingual province of Quebec, which has its own distinct history, demography, patterns of migration, configurations of community, and politics of identity. However, we believe that the CCS model is widely applicable because it was developed in a culturally diverse metropole, is highly adaptable, and makes few assumptions about the patient population, the nature of the health care system, or larger political contexts. Indeed, all of these dimensions of patients' experience and the context of care can become the explicit focus of the consultation process.

---

[2] See www.sprakradet.se/about_us.

Table 1.1 Key features of the cultural consultation approach

- Focus on the social context of the patient's predicament and the clinical encounter
- Recognize the ubiquity of culture in the lives of patients, clinicians, and institutions
- Explore culture as explicit knowledge, values, and practices but also as implicit, embodied, and enacted
- Use a systemic and self-reflexive view of mental health problems
- Emphasize issues of power, position, and communication
- Consider culture and community as resources for helping and healing
- Work within the system while attempting to challenge and change it through advocacy, education, and critique

The CCS sees cases referred from primary care and other health or mental health practitioners (Kirmayer, Groleau et al., 2003). In the CCS approach, patients are referred by clinicians who believe that issues of cultural difference are complicating their care, either in terms of diagnostic assessment, treatment planning, and adherence or, most basically, in the unfolding of the clinician–patient relationship itself. The aim is to provide a more comprehensive assessment to identify relevant social and cultural dimensions of the case and so to assist the referring clinician and, ultimately, the patient. The CCS assessments use interpreters and culture brokers to collect background information necessary to understand the patient's narrative and experience in cultural context. Information is collected and organized with the aid of the cultural formulation. The case is discussed at a multidisciplinary conference, and the resulting assessment, recommendations, and potential resources are conveyed to the referring clinician.

Several key orientations distinguish the orientation of cultural consultation from that of conventional psychiatric practice (Table 1.1). Most of these are consistent with the principles of person-centered, systemically oriented mental health care, but they differ substantially from the focus on diseases and disorders that currently dominates psychiatric care in North America. While cultural consultation often produces information about symptoms, signs, and behaviors that result in a revision of conventional psychiatric diagnoses (see Chapter 2), it also addresses the broader dimensions of life predicaments that are among the real reasons that patients consult clinicians and the social, structural, and contextual problems that are some of the most important causes of illness severity, disability, and chronicity.

Focus on social and cultural contexts. People come for help not only to diagnose symptoms or treat disorders but also to understand and deal with predicaments. Cultural consultation aims to understand these predicaments by adding attention to social and cultural dimensions that are often missing in conventional mental health practice. Mental health emerged as a psychological and psychiatric discipline with a focus on individual psychopathology. Whether this is attributed to biological or psychological characteristics of the individual, this tends to ignore the local and global social contexts of family, community, and wider networks in which individuals live. Understanding these social contexts is essential to appreciate the developmental trajectories and interactional processes that contribute to mental health problems as well as the potential sources of help and pathways to healing and recovery.

The ubiquity of culture. Culture is the backdrop, matrix, and medium of all experience. In clinical work, therefore, culture is an essential dimension of patients' illnesses and clinicians' responses, both at the level of their own identities and in the social roles and practices they draw from. Recognizing the ubiquity of culture works against the tendency to view culture as a defining feature of the other—while our own ways of doing things are taken for granted, viewed as commonsense, or seen as grounded in science and rationality. Cultural consultation looks at culture in the everyday thinking of clinicians and the functioning of institutions. Misunderstandings and conflicts can occur because of different values and perspectives between patients and clinicians, and this requires a two-sided analysis of the divergent assumptions and expectations.

Culture as embodied and enacted. Culture involves explicit knowledge, values, attitudes, beliefs, and behaviors that individuals can describe. But culture also involves embodied practices or ways of doing things that individuals may find difficult to describe because they have become part of habits and routines that occur outside of awareness or automatically. Culture includes procedural knowledge that may be difficult to put into words, like knowing how to ride a bike, dance, or cook a meal. Much of culture depends on the knowledge of others in the social world and on familiar contexts that put specific tools and resources ready to hand. Cultural knowledge and practices are built into institutions and social environments in ways that call forth particular responses from individuals. Recognizing these tacit, embodied, enacted, and interactional dimensions of culture requires observation of actual behavior in family, community, and other social contexts.

Systemic, interactional, and self-reflexive view. Cultural consultation emphasizes a systemic-interactional view. The social contexts in which people live consist of webs of interaction with others within families, communities, and social institutions. Many mental health problems may be caused, exacerbated, or maintained by vicious circles of interpersonal interaction. These systemic patterns can cause a potentially transient problem to become chronic and refractory to treatment. Identifying the family, community, or wider social dynamics that contribute to problems is essential to devising an effective intervention. Clinicians, health care institutions, and the cultural consultation team itself are all part of the system that includes the identified patient. Systemic thinking therefore requires self-reflexivity in which clinicians and consultants consider their own roles in the ongoing interactional dynamics of illness and healing.

Emphasis on power, position, and communication. Historically, cultural differences have been used to create and justify systems of power and domination in which some groups experience privilege while others suffer disadvantage, disempowerment, and silencing. Cultural consultation aims to recognize the current positions of power, domination, and subordination relevant to patients' predicaments. This may involve tracing the historical roots of constructions of identity and difference that shape current relationships between ethnocultural groups. This leads to another level of self-reflexivity in which we recognize the ways in which our position in the health care system, and as individuals with particular ethnocultural backgrounds, is part of a larger history that may maintain structural inequalities, evoking explicit as well as implicit and unconscious attitudes that influence the clinical interaction.

Culture and community as resources. Culture is not simply a source of idiosyncratic ideas about illness that constitute a challenge or barrier to the delivery of routine mental health care. Culture and community provide crucial sources of meaning, identity, and resilience for individuals and families. Such resources may include religious congregations, spiritual traditions, and many other forms of collective belonging and meaning making. Cultural consultation approaches culture as an essential resource, exploring with the patient strategies for accessing social support, as well as specific forms of self-help, coping, and both lay and professional interventions that can foster healing and recovery.

Working with and within the system. Cultural consultation works with the existing health care system while challenging it through advocacy, education, and critique. The goal is to improve the quality of clinician–patient interaction. As engaged practitioners, we are interested in trying to make an immediate difference for our clients, who include both patients and their families, as well as other clinicians who are struggling to provide humane and effective care. At the same time, cultural consultation often identifies structural and systemic problems of inequality, discrimination, and violence that demand a more political response to impel social change. We contribute to this by using individual cases as opportunities for broader education and advocacy and through research, documentation, and knowledge translation activities that attempt to influence health and social policy.

Throughout this volume we will use clinical vignettes to illustrate the basic issues in cultural consultation. The following brief examples illustrate some of the great variety of cases referred and the diverse interpretive strategies and interventions developed through the process of cultural consultation:

- A woman is referred from a psychiatric clinic because her depression is not improving despite treatment with many antidepressant medications. A family interview in her mother tongue reveals that she is caught in a feud over family honor that has cut her off from all contact with her daughter and granddaughter. Simply bringing this predicament to light in a family session opens up communication and improves her condition.
- A man is brought to the emergency room by police after loudly declaiming his religious concerns in a public place. He is initially treated for psychosis. Evaluation reveals that his behavior was not psychotic but rather a dissociative episode and that he is actually depressed. His treatment is changed to antidepressant medication and he recovers.
- An adolescent is referred by a family physician concerned that her parents are preventing her from having a normal social life, dating boys, and developing greater autonomy. Through the consultation, the referring physician is helped to enlarge his one-sided view of the intergenerational issues and to understand what is at stake for this young woman, who risks estrangement from her family and community. He is thus better able to help her think through her predicament.
- The parents of a young man with a psychotic illness want to take him to see a traditional healer. The psychiatrist is adamantly opposed, convinced that this will cause a relapse in his condition. A culture broker from their own background is able to explore the family's concerns and convince the psychiatrist that the treatment options do not have to be framed as either/or. The family takes the young man to the healer and he improves.
- A woman facing eviction from her home because of her "paranoid" behavior is assessed and the consultant finds she is suffering from the effects of racism in her community. He writes a letter to the court to raise this issue as a mitigating circumstance.
- A social service organization requests advice on how to help families concerned about their youth deal with racism in Canadian society. They are linked with the organizations of other ethnocultural communities to discuss strategies for helping youth adjust to the North American context.
- A person seeking asylum is referred for assessment because of episodes in which he became disoriented and incoherent. The consultant writes a letter to the immigration review board indicating that his difficulty in narrating his personal history reflects the effects of psychological trauma and does not imply he is lying.

The patients in these stories had migrated from Ethiopia, Haiti, India, Pakistan, Rwanda, Sri Lanka, and Trinidad. Even from these brief vignettes, it is clear, however, that the cultural dimensions of their difficulties stem as much from features of Québec society and its health care system as they do from any distinctive aspects of their cultures of origin.

These examples show that the intercultural clinical encounter requires enlarging the role of psychiatric expertise to include technical interventions (reassessing complex cases, revealing biases in diagnosis), psychoeducation (articulating multiple perspectives drawing from social sciences and the expertise of culture brokers from the community), mediation (negotiating interventions with other health care institutions, schools, employers, and community agencies), and advocacy (representing the patients' interests in juridical and other institutional settings like the immigration review board). The resources brought to bear to improve the care of these diverse patients include bilingual/bicultural clinicians, interpreters, culture brokers or mediators, religious and community leaders, anthropologists, and reviews of relevant social science and ethnographic literature.

One of the significant effects of the CCS has been the recognition of the language skills and cultural knowledge of clinicians and culture brokers who are themselves from diverse backgrounds. By addressing cultural and linguistic differences as both technical issues of understanding the impact of social processes on mental health and illness and also as political issues of voice and representation, the CCS creates a professional context in which clinicians can use their cultural knowledge for advocacy without risking being stereotyped or marginalized themselves. The CCS thus works to increase the representation of diverse voices within the health care system.

Many of the cases seen by the CCS involve difficulties that the referring clinicians are having in understanding the logic or imagining the rationale for patients' behavior. Meaningful communication requires a common language and shared background knowledge. To the extent this is missing, it must be developed, either from within the clinical conversation over time, building on areas of mutual understanding, or by an outside mediator or culture broker who supplies the missing contextual information needed to help patient and physician understand each other. This mutual understanding may not always resolve differences, but it allows them to be clearly articulated, setting the stage for meaningful negotiation.

Many problems that are initially attributed to characteristics of patients or their family are better understood in terms of the biases or assumptions of biomedicine; these biases include the tendency to view help seeking and treatment as either/or (traditional or biomedical), rather than as using many sources in a complex hierarchy of resort, depending on the perceived nature and severity of the problem; a view of religion and spirituality as irrelevant or pathological rather than sources of comfort, strength, and resilience; and the tendency to stereotype others rather than understanding their stories as unique or, on the contrary, to treat each individual's story as wholly personal rather than understanding it as culturally embedded.

Elaborating the cultural meanings of individual identity, illness experience, coping, and adaptation goes beyond linguistic translation to include an appreciation of the impact of collective history and current social context. The additional information and perspectives generated

through cultural consultation serve to enlarge the clinical imagination, enabling the professional to understand the patient's predicament in new ways. This, in turn, opens up new lines of action, expanding the clinician's repertoire and introducing an element of pluralism into a monolithic medical system.

What Culture Adds to Clinical Assessment

The clinical encounter is a situation of unequal power and authority. The patient is usually in a state of vulnerability and uncertainty, dependent on the clinician for information, clarification, legitimation, comfort, and care. The clinician is operating in a context defined by institutional and professional authority and technical expertise. Research on doctor–patient interaction makes it clear that physicians tend to dominate the clinical encounter, directing the conversation, limiting patients' ability to present aspects of their illness experience and lifeworld that the clinician deems irrelevant to the task of diagnosis (Mishler, 1984). The refinement of psychiatric nosology that began with DSM-III has exacerbated this problem, because symptom reports are now viewed not as ways to get a picture of the person's illness experience but simply as criteria for diagnosis. At its worst, the exploration of patients' illness experience is replaced by the routinized collection of symptoms and signs.

While psychiatric diagnosis provides a way to explain symptoms and suffering, it differs in important ways from the biographical and social accounts that are common in everyday explanations of misfortune. Psychiatric diagnostic systems contain information about diseases and disorders. The act of diagnosis maps the patient's individual story and clinical presentation onto a generic set of categories. The clinician making a diagnosis does this by identifying the relevant details in the patient's history of the illness and clinical presentation, ignoring irrelevant details, as well as most idiosyncrasies of illness behavior or narration. The result is a diagnostic label that names a pathological process that is associated with a specific treatment and prognosis. Of course, specifying the precise treatment and prognosis usually requires considering additional information about the patient's life context.

To convey a meaningful diagnosis to a patient and plan an appropriate clinical response, the clinician must link the diagnosis to explanations that make sense in terms of language, culture, and context. Often, however, clinicians simply present a generic story to patients and hope this is intelligible. Insofar as the patient's experience does not fit the generic textbook account, the discrepancies may be viewed as irrelevant or the patient may be viewed as an unreliable historian, unable to give a clear account of their condition or understand its true nature (Kirmayer, 1988). Unfortunately, this reduction of illness experience to diagnostic categories does not fulfill the basic mandate of medicine. There is little place in this scheme for identifying problems (or solutions) that reside primarily or exclusively in the interpersonal or social world. By ignoring social context, crucial elements of the clinical presentation and underlying problems may be missed.

The Contextual Framing of Psychiatric Disorders

A basic assumption of current psychiatric nosology is that there is a straightforward link between pathophysiological mechanisms and clinical symptomatology. Hence, one can work backward from the clinical interview to identify core syndromes or disorders and, ultimately, underlying mechanisms. However, there is much evidence that the translation of physiopathology and psychopathology into specific symptoms and behaviors is mediated by cognitive and social interactional processes that reflect specific culture models and practices (Kirmayer & Sartorius, 2007). Patients focus on specific aspects of illness experience because cultural models or narratives make them salient or because they fit with expectations in the health care system. As a result, cultural context affects both the pragmatics of diagnosis and the basic architecture of the system. Some brief examples of types of problems

commonly seen among patients referred to the CCS will serve to illustrate how social and cultural context makes a difference to illness experience, diagnosis, and treatment.

Many patients in primary care present with bodily symptoms for which there is no clear medical explanation (Kirmayer, Groleau, Looper, & Dao, 2004). In DSM-IV-TR or ICD-10, these are classified as somatoform disorders, implying a specific form of psychopathology. In fact, somatic symptoms accompany most forms of emotional distress (Simon, VonKorff, Piccinelli, Fullerton, & Ormel, 1999). Many common symptoms reflect cultural idioms of distress used to express a wide range of personal concerns (Kirmayer & Young, 1998). People in many parts of the world employ sociosomatic theories that link adverse life circumstances to physical and emotional illness (Groleau & Kirmayer, 2004). However, patients' disclosure of the emotional and social dimensions of their predicament depends on cultural concepts of the person and views on what is appropriate to express to others within the family, in the community, and in health care settings. Social and emotional dimensions of distress may be suppressed or hidden because of the potential for social stigmatization. The category of somatoform disorders, which is applied to any somatic condition for which there is no clear physiological explanation on the assumption that psychological factors must therefore account for the condition, reflects both the mind-body dualism of biomedicine and the clinician's difficulty in accessing the social meanings of the patient's suffering (Kirmayer, 2000; Mayou, Kirmayer, Simon, Kroenke, & Sharpe, 2005). Instead of simply identifying a somatoform disorder, we can go further in assessing and treating persistent somatic symptoms—medically explained or not—by understanding the meanings and consequences they have in couple, family, community, and health care systems that shape illness behavior and experience (Kirmayer & Sartorius, 2007).

The CCS sees a number of patients with dissociative symptoms that may resemble psychotic disorders but that follow cultural scripts that invoke distinctive notions of possession by spirits or other agents. Contemporary psychiatry understands these symptoms as indications of dissociative disorders, which include recurrent experiences of derealization and depersonalization, psychogenic amnesia, and dissociative identity disorder. Across cultures, however, dissociative experiences are extremely common and, when they occur in culturally prescribed times and places, usually do not indicate individual pathology (Kirmayer, 1994a). Trance and possession commonly occur as part of religious cults and healing practices, where such behavior is expected and follows cultural scripts (Seligman & Kirmayer, 2008). In spiritual or religious contexts, dissociation demonstrates that the person is being controlled by or speaking for a god, spirit, or ancestor. Dissociative behavior therefore can serve to communicate feelings of distress, powerlessness, or lack of control that arise from rigid and oppressive social circumstances (Kirmayer & Santhanam, 2001). Dissociation may be pathological when it persists outside the bounds of locally accepted behavior and disrupts adaptation. The diagnosis of pathological dissociation therefore requires careful consideration of social contexts, including when and where the behavior first emerged, how others responded to it, and what social consequences followed. Dissociative symptoms may be readily misdiagnosed as psychotic in cross-cultural settings, complicating the recognition of other co-occurring conditions.

Many of the patients referred to the CCS have been exposed to civil war, genocide, torture, or other forms of violence. Posttraumatic stress disorder (PTSD) has become a common way to identify some of the lasting effects of psychological trauma. However, traumatic situations evoke a wide range of responses not captured under the rubric of PTSD (Kirmayer, Lemelson, & Barad, 2007). Silove (1999) identified several distinct biobehavioral and biosocial systems that may be affected by exposure to torture and massive human rights violations including systems regulating safety, attachment, sense of justice, existential meaning, and identity. The same events that cause intense fear, however, may also be associated with the loss of loved ones, home, and community. These ruptures of attachment can lead to grief, nostalgia, homesickness, and depression. Capricious violence, torture, and genocide can also radically disrupt the sense that one lives in a just world, leading to mistrust, survivor guilt, and persistent anger. Torture and chaotic violence directly attack the individual's sense of coherence, trust, and connection to others, creating feelings of alienation and emotional isolation. These effects of violence reflect the impact on adaptation of social and psychological predicaments that are not explicitly included in current psychiatric nosology. Yet for many refugees or survivors of torture, they may be among the most important clinical concerns and determinants of long-term adaptation.

Major depression and anxiety disorders are among the most common mental health problems around the world, but there are significant variations in the symptoms, clinical presentation, and ways of coping (Kirmayer, 2001). Clinical depression and anxiety may occur due to psychological and interpersonal processes and be effectively resolved with cognitive or interpersonal therapy that focuses on interactions with others (Bass et al., 2006). Grief after bereavement is presumably a normal response to an inevitable aspect of the human condition, but it has been increasingly pathologized in psychiatry (Horwitz & Wakefield, 2007). In many cultural contexts, depressed mood and anxiety may be viewed not as forms of illness that warrant help seeking or treatment with medication but as moral or character development that requires self-mastery and endurance (Kirmayer, 2002a). Our understanding of the nature of depression and anxiety and their appropriate treatment has been influenced by the economic contexts of psychiatric practice (Healy, 2004; Tone, 2009). The promotion of medication treatments of depression has been heavily subsidized by the pharmaceutical industry, and this has lead to broadening of the category of depression and exaggerations of the evidence for medication efficacy (Horwitz & Wakefield, 2007; Kirsch et al., 2008). Across cultures there are a wide range of strategies for mood and anxiety regulation that are incorporated in local forms of healing or religious practice and that may provide therapeutic options for patients from diverse backgrounds.

There is evidence that the prevalence, course, and outcome of schizophrenia and other psychotic disorders are strongly influenced by social and cultural factors (Cantor-Graae, 2007; Morgan, McKenzie, & Fearon, 2008). The unusual or bizarre experiences of initial psychosis often prompt an intensive search for meaning. Biomedical explanations of psychosis in terms of brain pathology may result in loss of self-esteem, conflict with others, and social stigmatization and so may contribute to chronicity. In contrast, some religious or cultural systems of meaning may give positive meaning to psychotic experiences, allowing the person to maintain self-esteem and social integration, and therefore contribute to better outcome (Kirmayer, Corin, & Jarvis, 2004). The clinician's ability to negotiate shared meaning with the patient depends not only on the quality of the clinical alliance but also on the cultural fit of the illness explanation for the patient and for others in the patient's family or entourage (Tranulis, Corin, & Kirmayer, 2008).

Empathy and the Politics of Alterity

Attention to culture and context is not only essential for accurate diagnostic assessment and effective treatment; it is at the root of clinical practice based on an ethics of recognition (Kirmayer, 2012a). Recognition of cultural identity may be essential for well-being and allowing individuals to realize their cultural identities is a basic human right (Kirmayer, 2012b). At the political level, this recognition requires tolerance of diversity and pluralism. At the interpersonal level, it requires a particular ethical stance that is most evident when we face someone whom we experience as radically other.

As the philosopher Emmanuel Levinas (1998; Lévinas & Poller, 2003) argued, the vulnerability of the other calls forth from us moral consciousness, conscience, and responsibility. This insight can be applied to the pragmatics of intercultural encounter through the recognition that each life draws its texture from the minute particulars of cultural and personal history. Translating our awareness of the other's vulnerability into compassionate action demands detailed knowledge of

their predicament and the ability to shift perspective. Empathy is both a motive and a vehicle for acquiring this knowledge. But, even in the absence of empathy, Levinas insists we must acknowledge our responsibility for the other. Indeed, it is precisely where empathy fails that this injunction has its greatest ethical implication.

Empathy has both affective and cognitive prerequisites: affectively, it depends on creating safety to allow us to feel the other and to enter the difficult places where they dwell; cognitively, empathy demands that we acquire detailed information about the other's lifeworld in order to imaginatively reconstruct their experience. Thus, empathy is not an automatic consequence of our capacity for vicarious emotion in the presence of another person; it depends on detailed knowledge and understanding as well as a nondefensive, open stance and effort to engage. As such, empathy contributes to a way of being together that changes the quality of relatedness in everyday life. When others' life experience is radically different, it may be difficult for us to empathize; when their experience is painful or threatening to us, we may suppress our own capacity for empathic understanding and turn away. In clinical work with refugees and asylum seekers, we have noted how difficult it is for some clinicians to credit their patients' stories of violence chaos and betrayal (Kirmayer, 2001). The process of cultural consultation provides some of the background knowledge or "mental furniture" needed to construct a picture of the others' world and a professional framework that calls the clinician to empathize with others having radically different or uncanny experiences (Kirmayer, 2008).

No amount of empathy or recognition can take the place of respect for the others' agency, so pluralism also demands a political process of creating social institutions that anchor, support, and valorize the other, recognizing the others' voice and vision as an independent fact and imperative. This recognition has multiple effects on the patient, on the clinician, on their respective communities, and on society as a whole. Taking the other seriously, listening to and working with them, allows us to explore new ways of being, both individually and collectively, exchanging knowledge, putting into play new ideas, values, and concepts, that then circulate in the larger society. As they circulate, these new ideas begin to splice and recombine with other ideas creating hybrid forms of identity, new frameworks for moral reasoning, and new forms of healing. To give one prominent example, in recent years the spread of Buddhism to the West has encouraged the development of new strategies for the control of pain and anxiety and the prevention of depression. Dialectical behavior therapy and mindfulness-based therapies have borrowed from Buddhism without wholesale adoption of Buddhist values or a monastic way of life. As this example illustrates, cultural hybridization, with the incorporation of specific ideas and techniques, is reshaping clinical practice as social systems interact ever more rapidly and intensively in our globalizing world.

Recently, there has been much critique in European countries of the idea of multiculturalism and concern that the efforts to accommodate newcomers from diverse backgrounds are eroding civil society. Political leaders have declared that multiculturalism has failed. This is deeply ironic, since as an explicit political policy multiculturalism is very new, and in most of the countries where it has been said to fail, it has scarcely been tried. Multiculturalism is blamed for problems of social integration that might be more fairly attributed to a lack of recognition and dialogue, to postcolonial or historical legacies, and to ongoing structural inequalities both locally and in global society. Indeed, the critique of multiculturalism seems to be fueled by a broader attitude of xenophobia aimed at justifying policies of exclusion (Ryan, 2010). This critique can also be seen as an indication that majorities are feeling threatened by globalization and by the shifts in power and privilege in the world, including in high-income countries. Collective fears have been shown to influence clinicians' capacity to be empathic (Rousseau & Foxen, 2010; Brunner, 2000) and this may fuel a reluctance to adapt services to respond to cultural diversity.

When it takes culture and context seriously, the clinical encounter can work against these forces of xenophobia and social exclusion, enacting and enabling pluralism in several ways: acknowledging the vulnerability and needs of the other as a moral imperative; creating bonds of empathy that allow one to feel with and understand the other's experience; reshaping institutions to recognize the agency and voice of the other, but also acknowledging the fears associated with otherness and the hidden feelings of vulnerability of the majority; and so allowing multiple ways of knowing and being to coexist, implementing forms of tolerance, hospitality, peaceful coexistence, and practical conflict resolution.

Conclusion

In this introductory chapter, we have reviewed some ways in which different societies have responded to cultural diversity in mental health services, outlined some key principles of the cultural consultation approach, illustrated the importance of cultural context for diagnostic assessment and treatment, and considered the ethical foundation of attention to culture as a basic human right and need for recognition. Multicultural mental health care allows us to work toward dialogue, pluralism, and inclusion in society at large in several ways: recognizing the other in our practice and our institutions, bearing witness to their suffering, intervening in a differentiated way, carrying the implications of their experience with us into the world, advocating for them in the larger sphere, ceding power and control of institutions to them or supporting their own efforts at building social institutions, and allowing ourselves to be changed and transformed. The last is the most profound outcome because it means we must give something up but also that we transmute the meaning of our own experience by hybridizing it with that of the other. This can only occur in a way that is not exploitative or mere appropriation if there has been some leveling of power. This requires active engagement with communities so that open discussion and negotiation of ways to meet the needs of the community occurs and health care institutions are driven not solely by technical or bureaucratic goals of efficiency and effectiveness but by values that reflect communal aspirations. This dialogue can begin in the clinical encounter, where it is naturally framed by attention to the individual's most basic needs and concerns.

References

Alegria, M., Atkins, M., Farmer, E., Slaton, E., & Stelk, W. (2010). One size does not fit all: Taking diversity, culture and context seriously. *Administration and Policy in Mental Health, 37*(1–2), 48–60.

Anderson, B. R. (1991). *Imagined communities: Reflections on the origin and spread of nationalism* (Revisedth ed.). New York, NY: Verso.

Bäärnhielm, S., Ekblad, S., Ekberg, J., & Ginsburg, B. E. (2005). Historical reflections on mental health care in Sweden: The welfare state and cultural diversity. *Transcultural Psychiatry, 42*(3), 394–419.

Banks, M. (1996). *Ethnicity: Anthropological constructions*. London, England: Routledge.

Bass, J., Neugebauer, R., Clougherty, K. F., Verdeli, H., Wickramaratne, P., Ndogoni, L., et al. (2006). Group interpersonal psychotherapy for depression in rural Uganda: 6-month outcomes: Randomised controlled trial. *The British Journal of Psychiatry, 188*, 567–573.

Ben Jelloun, T., & Bray, B. (1999). *French hospitality: Racism and North African immigrants*. New York, NY: Columbia University Press.

Betancourt, J. R., Green, A. R., Carrillo, J. E., & Ananeh-Firempong, O., II. (2003). Defining cultural competence: A practical framework for addressing racial/ethnic disparities in health and health care. *Public Health Reports, 118*(4), 293–302.

Bhugra, D., & Littlewood, R. (Eds.). (2001). *Colonialism and psychiatry*. New Delhi, India: Oxford University Press.

Bhui, K., Ascoli, M., & Nuamh, O. (2012). The place of race and racism in cultural competence: What can we learn from the English experience about the narratives of evidence and argument? *Transcultural Psychiatry, 49*(2), 185–205.

Bibeau, G. (1998). Tropismes Québecois. Je me souviens dans l'oubli. *Anthropologie et Sociétés, 19*(3), 151–198.

Bouchard, G., & Taylor, C. (2008). *Building the future: A time for reconciliation (abridged report)*. Quebec, Canada: Commission de consultation sur les pratiques d'accommodement relies aux differences cultural, Gouvernment du Quebec.

Brunner, J. (2000). Will, desire and experience: Etiology and ideology in the German and Austrian medical discourse on war neuroses, 1914–1922. *Transcultural Psychiatry, 37*(3), 295–320.

Cantor-Graae, E. (2007). The contribution of social factors to the development of schizophrenia: A review of recent findings. *Canadian Journal of Psychiatry, 52*(5), 277–286.

Cantor-Graae, E., & Selten, J.-P. (2005). Schizophrenia and migration: A meta-analysis and review. *The American Journal of Psychiatry, 162*(1), 12–24.

Castles, S., & Miller, M. J. (1998). *The age of migration: International population movements in the modern world* (2nd ed.). New York, NY: Guilford.

Choudhury, S., & Kirmayer, L. J. (2009). Cultural neuroscience and psychopathology: Prospects for cultural psychiatry. *Progress in Brain Research, 178*, 261–281.

Cleveland, J., & Rousseau, C. (2012). Mental health impact of detention and temporary status for refugee claimants under Bill C-31. *Canadian Medical Association Journal, 184*(15), 1663–1664.

Corin, E. (1997). Playing with limits: Tobie Nathan's evolving paradigm in ethnopsychiatry. *Transcultural Psychiatry, 34*(3), 345–358.

Eagleton, T. (2000). *The idea of culture*. Oxford, England: Blackwell.

Elias, N. (1982). *The civilizing process*. New York, NY: Pantheon Books.

Fassin, D., & Rechtman, R. (2005). An anthropological hybrid: The pragmatic arrangement of universalism and culturalism in French mental health. *Transcultural Psychiatry, 42*(3), 347–366.

Fernando, S. (Ed.). (1995). *Mental health in a multi-ethnic society: A multidisciplinary handbook*. New York, NY: Routledge.

Fernando, S. (2005). Multicultural mental health services: Projects for minority ethnic communities in England. *Transcultural Psychiatry, 42*(3), 420–436.

Fernando, S. (2009). Meanings and realities. In S. Fernando & F. Keating (Eds.), *Mental health in a multi-ethnic society: A multidisciplinary handbook* (2nd ed., pp. 13–26). London, England: Routledge.

Fredrickson, G. M. (2002). *Racism: A short history*. Princeton, NJ: Princeton University Press.

Gaines, A. D. (1992). From DSM-I to III-R: Voices of self, mastery and the other: A cultural constructivist reading of U.S. psychiatric classification. *Social Science & Medicine, 35*(1), 3–24.

Ganesan, S., & Janze, T. (2005). Overview of culturally-based mental health care in Vancouver. *Transcultural Psychiatry, 42*(3), 478–490.

Gee, G. C., Spencer, M., Chen, J., Yip, T., & Takeuchi, D. T. (2007). The association between self-reported racial discrimination and 12-month DSM-IV mental disorders among Asian Americans nationwide. *Social Science & Medicine, 64*(10), 1984–1996.

Gravlee, C. C. (2009). How race becomes biology: Embodiment of social inequality. *American Journal of Physical Anthropology, 139*(1), 47–57.

Groleau, D., & Kirmayer, L. J. (2004). Sociosomatic theory in Vietnamese immigrants' narratives of distress. *Anthropology & Medicine, 11*(2), 117–133.

Harwood, A. (Ed.). (1981). *Ethnicity and medical care*. Cambridge, MA: Harvard University Press.

Healy, D. (2004). *Let them eat prozac: The unhealthy relationship between the pharmaceutical industry and depression*. New York, NY: New York University Press.

Hollinger, D. A. (1995). *Postethnic America: Beyond multiculturalism*. New York, NY: Basic Books.

Horwitz, A. V., & Wakefield, J. C. (2007). *The loss of sadness: How psychiatry transformed normal sorrow into depressive disorder*. New York, NY: Oxford University Press.

Kamboureli, S. (1998). The technology of ethnicity: Canadian multiculturalism and the language of law. In D. Bennett (Ed.), *Multicultural states: Rethinking difference and identity* (pp. 208–222). London, England: Routledge.

Kelly, B. D. (2005). Structural violence and schizophrenia. *Social Science & Medicine, 61*(3), 721–730.

Kirmayer, L. J. (1988). Mind and body as metaphors: Hidden values in biomedicine. In M. Lock & D. Gordon (Eds.), *Biomedicine examined* (pp. 57–92). Dordrecht, Netherlands: Kluwer.

Kirmayer, L. J. (1994a). Is the concept of mental disorder culturally relative? In S. A. Kirk & S. Einbinder (Eds.), *Controversial issues in mental health* (pp. 1–20). Boston, MA: Allyn & Bacon.

Kirmayer, L. J. (2000). Broken narratives: Clinical encounters and the poetics of illness experience. In C. Mattingly & L. Garro (Eds.), *Narrative and the cultural construction of illness and healing* (pp. 153–180). Berkeley, CA: University of California Press.

Kirmayer, L. J. (2001). Failures of imagination: The refugee's narrative in psychiatry. *Anthropology & Medicine, 10*(2), 167–185.

Kirmayer, L. J. (2002a). Psychopharmacology in a globalizing world: The use of antidepressants in Japan. *Transcultural Psychiatry, 39*(3), 295–312.

Kirmayer, L. J. (2005). Culture, context and experience in psychiatric diagnosis. *Psychopathology, 38*(4), 192–196.

Kirmayer, L. J. (2006). Beyond the 'new cross-cultural psychiatry': Cultural biology, discursive psychology and the ironies of globalization. *Transcultural Psychiatry, 43*(1), 126–144.

Kirmayer, L. J. (2007). Psychotherapy and the cultural concept of the person. *Transcultural Psychiatry, 44*(2), 232–257.

Kirmayer, L. J. (2008). Empathy and alterity in cultural psychiatry. *Ethos, 38*(4), 457–474.

Kirmayer, L. J. (2012a). Rethinking cultural competence. *Transcultural Psychiatry, 49*(2), 149–164.

Kirmayer, L. J. (2012b). Culture and context in human rights. In M. Dudley, D. Silove, & F. Gale (Eds.), *Mental health and human rights* (pp. 95–112). Oxford, England: Oxford University Press.

Kirmayer, L. J., Corin, E., & Jarvis, G. E. (2004). Inside knowledge: Cultural constructions of insight in psychosis. In X. F. Amador & A. S. David (Eds.), *Insight in psychosis* (2nd ed., pp. 197–229). New York, NY: Oxford University Press.

Kirmayer, L. J., Groleau, D., Guzder, J., Blake, C., & Jarvis, E. (2003). Cultural consultation: A model of mental health service for multicultural societies. *Canadian Journal of Psychiatry, 48*(2), 145–153.

Kirmayer, L. J., Groleau, D., Looper, K. J., & Dao, M. D. (2004). Explaining medically unexplained symptoms. *Canadian Journal of Psychiatry, 49*(10), 663–672.

Kirmayer, L. J., Lemelson, R., & Barad, M. (Eds.). (2007). *Understanding trauma: Integrating biological, clinical, and cultural perspectives.* New York, NY: Cambridge University Press.

Kirmayer, L. J., & Minas, H. (2000). The future of cultural psychiatry: An international perspective. *Cannadian Journal of Psychiatry, 45*(5), 438–446.

Kirmayer, L. J., & Santhanam, R. (2001). The anthropology of hysteria. In P. W. Halligan, C. Bass, & J. C. Marshall (Eds.), *Contemporary approaches to the study of hysteria: Clinical and theoretical perspectives* (pp. 251–270). Oxford, England: Oxford University Press.

Kirmayer, L. J., & Sartorius, N. (2007). Cultural models and somatic syndromes. *Psychosomatic Medicine, 69*(9), 832–840.

Kirmayer, L. J., Weinfeld, M., Burgos, G., Galbaud du Fort, G., Lasry, J.-C., & Young, A. (2007). Use of health care services for psychological distress by immigrants in an urban multicultural milieu. *Canadian Journal of Psychiatry, 52*(4), 61–70.

Kirmayer, L. J., & Young, A. (1998). Culture and somatization: Clinical, epidemiological and ethnographic perspectives. *Psychosomatic Medicine, 60,* 420–430.

Kirsch, I., Deacon, B. J., Huedo-Medina, T. B., Scoboria, A., Moore, T. J., & Johnson, B. T. (2008). Initial severity and antidepressant benefits: A meta-analysis of data submitted to the Food and Drug Administration. *PLoS Medicine, 5*(2), e45.

Kivisto, P. (2002). *Multiculturalism in a global society.* Oxford, England: Blackwell.

Kleinman, A. M. (1980). *Patients and healers in the context of culture.* Berkeley, CA: University of California Press.

Kleinman, A., Das, V., & Lock, M. (Eds.). (1997). *Social suffering.* Berkeley, CA: University of California Press.

Koenig, B. A., Lee, S. S.-J., & Richardson, S. S. (2008). *Revisiting race in a genomic age.* New Brunswick, NJ: Rutgers University Press.

Kronick, R., Rousseau, C., & Cleveland, J. (2011). Mandatory detention of refugee children in Canada: A public health issue? *Paediatrics & Child Health, 16*(8), e65–e67.

Kymlicka, W. (1995). *Multicultural citizenship.* Oxford, England: Oxford University Press.

Levinas, E. (1998). *Entre nous: Thinking of the other.* New York, NY: Columbia University Press.

Lévinas, E., & Poller, N. (2003). *Humanism of the other.* Chicago, IL: University of Illinois Press.

Lindqvist, S. (1996). *Exterminate all the brutes.* New York, NY: New Press.

Littlewood, R., & Lipsedge, M. (1982). *Aliens and alienists.* Harmondsworth, England: Penguin.

Lo, H. T., & Chung, R. C. (2005). The Hong Fook experience: Working with ethnocultural communities in Toronto 1982–2002. *Transcultural Psychiatry, 42*(3), 457–477.

Lock, M., & Gordon, D. (Eds.). (1988). *Biomedicine examined.* Dordrecht, Netherlands: Kluwer.

Lock, M., & Nguyen, V.-K. (2010). *An anthropology of biomedicine.* Malden, MA: Wiley-Blackwell.

Mackey, E. (1999). *The house of difference: Cultural politics and national identity in Canada.* London, England: Routledge.

Mayou, R., Kirmayer, L. J., Simon, G., Kroenke, K., & Sharpe, M. (2005). Somatoform disorders: Time for a new approach in DSM-V. *The American Journal of Psychiatry, 162*(5), 847–855.

McNeill, W. H. (1986). *Polyethnicity and national unity in world history*. Toronto, Ontario, Canada: University of Toronto Press.

Mental Health Commission of Canada. (2009). *Toward recovery and well-being: A framework for mental health strategy for Canada*. Ottawa, Ontario, Canada: Mental Health Commission of Canada.

Mental Health Commission of Canada. (2012). *Changing directions, changing lives: The mental health strategy for Canada*. Ottawa, Ontario, Canada: Mental Health Commission of Canada.

Mishler, E. G. (1984). *The discourse of medicine*. Norwood, NJ: Ablex Publishing Corporation.

Morgan, C., McKenzie, K., & Fearon, P. (2008). *Society and psychosis*. New York, NY: Cambridge University Press.

Nathan, T. (1986). *La folie des autres. Traité d'ethnopsychiatrie clinique*. Paris, France: Dunod.

Nathan, T. (1991). Modifications techniques et conceptuelles récemment apportées à la psychopathologie par la clinique ethnopsychoanalytique. *Psychologie Française, 36*(4), 296–306.

Rose, N. S. (1996). *Inventing our selves: Psychology, power, and personhood*. New York, NY: Cambridge University Press.

Rousseau, C., & Foxen, P. (2010). Look me in the eye: Empathy and the transmission of trauma in the refugee determination process. *Transcultural Psychiatry, 47*(1), 70–92.

Rousseau, C., Hassan, G., Moreau, N., & Thombs, B. D. (2011). Perceived discrimination and its association with psychological distress among newly arrived immigrants before and after September 11, 2001. *American Journal of Public Health, 101*(5), 909–915.

Rousseau, C., Jamil, U., Hassan, G., & Moreau, N. (2010). Grandir et vivre ensemble dans un contexte de mondialisation conflictuelle. *Enfances et Psy, 48*(3), 56–63.

Ryan, P. (2010). *Multicultiphobia*. Toronto, Ontario, Canada: University of Toronto Press.

Sargent, C., & Larchanche, S. (2009). The construction of "cultural difference" and its therapeutic significance in immigrant mental health services in France. *Culture, Medicine and Psychiatry, 33*(1), 2–20.

Seligman, R., & Kirmayer, L. J. (2008). Dissociative experience and cultural neuroscience: Narrative, metaphor and mechanism. *Culture, Medicine and Psychiatry, 32*(1), 31–64.

Silove, D. (1999). The psychosocial effects of torture, mass human rights violations, and refugee trauma: Toward an integrated conceptual framework. *The Journal of Nervous and Mental Disease, 187*(4), 200–207.

Silove, D., Austin, P., & Steel, Z. (2007). No refuge from terror: The impact of detention on the mental health of trauma-affected refugees seeking asylum in Australia. *Transcultural Psychiatry, 44*(3), 359–393.

Silove, D., Steel, Z., & Watters, C. (2000). Policies of deterrence and the mental health of asylum seekers. *Journal of the American Medical Association, 284*(5), 604–611.

Simon, G. E., VonKorff, M., Piccinelli, M., Fullerton, C., & Ormel, J. (1999). An international study of the relation between somatic symptoms and depression. *The New England Journal of Medicine, 341*(18), 1329–1335.

Smedley, B. D., Stith, A. Y., Nelson, A. R., & Institute of Medicine (U.S.) Committee on Understanding and Eliminating Racial and Ethnic Disparities in Health Care. (2003). *Unequal treatment: Confronting racial and ethnic disparities in health care*. Washington, DC: National Academy Press.

Spivak, G. C. (2006). *In other worlds: Essays on cultural politics*. New York, NY: Routledge.

Sturm, G., Nadig, M., & Moro, M. R. (2011). Current developments in French ethnopsychoanalysis. *Transcultural Psychiatry, 48*(3), 205–227.

Surgeon General. (2002). *Mental health: Culture, race, and ethnicity*. Rockville, MD: U.S. Department of Health and Human Services.

Tone, A. (2009). *The age of anxiety: A history of America's turbulent affair with tranquilizers*. New York, NY: Basic Books.

Tranulis, C., Corin, E., & Kirmayer, L. J. (2008). Insight and psychosis: Comparing the perspectives of patient, entourage and clinician. *The International Journal of Social Psychiatry, 54*(3), 225–241.

Walzer, M. (1997). *On toleration*. New Haven, CT: Yale University Press.

Ward, W. P. (2005). *White Canada forever: Popular attitudes and public policy toward orientals in British Columbia* (3rd ed.). Montreal, Quebec, Canada: McGill Queen's University Press.

Waxler-Morrison, N. E. (1989). *Cross-cultural caring: A handbook for practitioners*. Vancouver, British Columbia, Canada: University of British Columbia.

Weinfeld, M. (1999). The challenges of ethnic match: Minority origin professionals in health and social services. In H. Troper & M. Weinfeld (Eds.), *Ethnicity, politics, and public policy: Case studies in canadian diversity* (pp. 117–141). Toronto, Ontario, Canada: University of Toronto Press.

Whitley, R., Rousseau, C., Carpenter Song, E., & Kirmayer, L. J. (2011). Evidence-based medicine: Opportunities and challenges in a diverse society. *Canadian Journal of Psychiatry, 56*.

Yang, J. S., & Kagawa-Singer, M. (2007). Increasing access to care for cultural and linguistic minorities: Ethnicity-specific health care organizations and infrastructure. *Journal of Health Care for the Poor and Underserved, 18*(3), 532–549.

Ziguras, S. J., Stankovska, M., & Minas, I. H. (1999). Initiatives for improving mental health services to ethnic minorities in Australia. *Psychiatric Services, 50*(9), 1229–1231.

Development and Evaluation of the Cultural Consultation Service

Laurence J. Kirmayer, Danielle Groleau, and Cécile Rousseau

In this chapter, we describe the development, implementation, and evaluation of the Cultural Consultation Service (CCS). We begin with some background on the development of intercultural services in Montreal. The next section describes the rationale for the CCS approach and the steps involved in setting up the service. The third section provides an overview of the cases seen by the service in the first decade of its operation, including sources and reasons for referral, as well as sociodemographic and clinical characteristics. This provides a sense of the portfolio of cases from which vignettes are drawn throughout this book to illustrate key issues in cultural consultation. The remaining sections summarize findings from qualitative process and outcome evaluations of the service.

L.J. Kirmayer, M.D. (✉) • D. Groleau, Ph.D.
Culture & Mental Health Research Unit,
Institute of Community & Family Psychiatry,
Jewish General Hospital, Montreal,
QC, Canada H3T 1E4
e-mail: laurence.kirmayer@mcgill.ca; danielle.groleau@mcgill.ca

C. Rousseau, M.D., M.Sc.
Centre de recherche et de formation,
CSSS de la Montagne, 7085 Hutchison, Local 204.2,
Montréal, QC, Canada H3N 1Y9
e-mail: cecile.rousseau@mcgill.ca

Background

McGill University has a long history of involvement in cultural psychiatry, dating back to the 1950s when the Division of Social and Transcultural Psychiatry was established (Prince, 2000). In the early 1970s, under the leadership of H.B.M. Murphy at McGill and Guy Dubreuil at the Université de Montréal, an interuniversity research group on medical anthropology and ethnopsychiatry (GIRAME) fostered collaboration and exchange among social scientist (anthropologists and sociologists) and health professionals (psychologists, psychiatrists, doctors, and nurses) from universities in Quebec and other Canadian provinces. This group focused mostly on international research in psychological and medical anthropology, to promote, coordinate, and disseminate research and teaching concerning sociocultural factors in health (Bibeau, 2002). GIRAME published a bilingual (French/English) journal, *Santé/Culture/Health*, which included much work in culture and mental health. Toward the end of its life as a network, the scholars associated with GIRAME began to focus on the issues of providing effective mental health care for the population of Québec (Bibeau, Chan-Yip, Lock, & Rousseau, 1992; Corin, Bibeau, Martin, & Laplante, 1991). GIRAME reflected the geopolitical and ethnocultural specificities of Montreal, a place of encounter of the Latin and the Anglo-Saxon world, and highlighted the richness associated with the intermingling of European and North American academic and clinical traditions. The use of diverse languages and bilingual communication was at the center of GIRAME activities, in its conferences, seminars, and publications. This inclusion of diverse perspectives within an active interdisciplinary exchange is one of the important legacies of GIRAME for the Division of Social and Transcultural Psychiatry and the establishment of our clinical-academic programs including the CCS.

Montreal is a city of almost two million situated in the Province of Quebec in eastern Canada.[1] The city is located on an island in the St. Lawrence River. The greater metropolitan area, including many surrounding municipalities both on and off the island of Montreal, totals almost four million residents—almost half the population of the whole province. The population of greater Montreal includes a very diverse mix of people with about 21% of the population born outside Canada. A high proportion of those born outside the country (22%) are recent newcomers who arrived in the last 5 years, including both immigrants and refugees. The languages spoken at home include French for 70% and English for 19%, but about 22% are allophones, a local term used to designate those with languages other than French or English. The most frequent mother tongues are French (66%), English (14%), Arabic

(3.5%), Spanish (3%), Italian (3%), Chinese (2%), and Haitian Creole (1%). About 16% of the city are "visible minorities," including 5% Black, 2% Latin American, 2% South Asian, and 2% Chinese. In terms of ethnicity, the majority of Montrealers describe their origins as Canadian or French with the remaining top ten identities including Italian, Irish, English, Scottish, Haitian, Chinese, German, First Nations, Québécois, and Jewish.[2]

Prior to the establishment of the CCS, Montreal was home to several specialized services directed to immigrants and refugees. These included the transcultural program of the Hôpital Jean-Talon (HJT), the Montreal Children's Hospital (MCH) program for immigrant and refugee children, a network of professionals involved in the treatment of individuals who have suffered organized violence (RIVO), and a provincial social service department for refugees, refugee claimants, and unaccompanied minors called SARIMM. This service was integrated into a community health center servicing immigrant neighborhoods, the CSSS de la Montagne, and changed its name to become PRAIDA. Because of the important mental health needs of its clientele, PRAIDA, which offers services to refugee families and has a supra-regional role, was an early partner of all of the transcultural programs including the CCS. In parallel, Montreal saw the emergence of programs and consultants offering training in intercultural work to professionals.

All of the services developed in response to demographic changes over the past 20 years in Montreal, which has seen a large increase in the cultural diversity of both the general and patient

---

[1] The data in this paragraph reflect the census metropolitan area of Montreal. Data on language (mother tongue and language spoken at home) is from the 2011 census (Statistics Canada, 2012. Montréal, Quebec (Code 462), and Quebec (Code 24) (table). Census Profile. 2011 Census. Statistics Canada Catalogue no. 98-316-XWE. Ottawa. Released October 24, 2012. http://www12.statcan.gc.ca/census-recensement/2011/dp-pd/prof/index.cfm?Lang=E). Data on ethnicity and immigration was not available from the 2011 census, and the 2006 census was used (Statistics Canada, n.d.). *Population by immigrant status and period of immigration, 2006 counts, for Canada and census metropolitan areas and census agglomerations -20% sample data* (table). "Immigration and Citizenship." "Highlight tables." "2006 Census: Data products." *Census.* Last updated March 27, 2009. http://www.statcan.gc.ca/pub/12-591-x/2009001/02-step-etape/ex/ex-census-recensement-eng.htm#a2 (accessed February 21, 2013).

[2] Statistics Canada. No date. *Visible minority groups, 2006 counts, for Canada and census metropolitan areas and census agglomerations -20% sample data* (table). "Ethnocultural Portrait of Canada." "Highlight tables." "2006 Census: Data products." *Census.* Last updated October 6, 2010. http://www12.statcan.gc.ca/census-recensement/2006/dp-pd/hlt/97-562/pages/page.cfm?Lang=E&Geo=CMA&Code=01&Table=1&Data=Count&StartRec=1&Sort=2&Display=Page (accessed February 21, 2013).

populations in the city. The MCH and HJT responded to increased diversity among the specific populations served (e.g., 50% of children seen at the MCH are allophone and 33% of the Jean-Talon catchment area is allophone, i.e., non-English or French mother tongue). The Côte-des-Neiges area, where the CCS is located, is one of the most ethnically diverse neighborhoods in Montreal, with more than half the population born outside Canada. As such, the services are rooted in the recognition of diversity as an important issue for health care because of concern about inequities in access and in the delivery of culturally appropriate care. Indeed, there was evidence from our own work in this neighborhood for underutilization of mental health services due both to lower rates of referral from primary care and direct resort (Kirmayer et al., 2007). The CCS project was, in part, a response to this observation.

Each of the services was initiated by professionals with experience in cultural psychiatry, whose particular perspective shaped the orientation of services, along with input from other professionals and social scientists working with each group. Reflecting the different backgrounds of the clinicians and their institutional settings, the services have followed different models of care. Despite the different orientations of the services, their common goal has been to work within the broader frameworks of psychiatry and collaborate with existing services. While the conceptual models of the services were initially tentative and open, all services have changed significantly over time as they learned from and adapted to their milieu, patient populations, and institutional constraints.

RIVO

In 1984, a group of Quebec health professionals who were involved in different Latin-American countries founded "L'association Médicale pour l'Amérique Latine et les Caraibes" which was a group of professionals committed to fighting health inequalities in Quebec and in Latin America. The mental health committee of this association began to work on appropriate services for refugees, which, at the time, were largely coming from Central and South America. Reaching out to community organizations that were providing first-line support to refugees, like the House of friendship founded by the Mennonite Church of Eastern Canada (http://www.maisondelamitie.ca), this group organized a network to provide care for the persons who had experienced organized violence in their countries of origin.

This network was formalized as "Le réseau d'intervention pour les personnes ayant vécu la violence organisée" (RIVO) with the following premises: (1) it explicitly avoided the notions of "victims" or "survivors" as a way of acknowledging that the experience of organized violence was not necessarily framed in those terms for those who suffer from it. In seeking alternate language, RIVO wanted to emphasize the agency and strength of refugees as persons, families, and communities and take a critical stance toward the dominance of trauma-centered approaches; (2) a politically committed clinical stance was central to its philosophy; (3) it was conceived as a broad network, bringing together professionals from different disciplines, in private practice or in institutions, with diverse clinical orientations, including practitioners of ethnopsychiatric, humanistic, cognitive-behavioral, and psychodynamic psychotherapies.

RIVO has provided a referral network for patients seen in the community or various institutional settings who required care that took into account their histories of exposure to violence, torture, and forced migration. The network has also served as professional support groups with peer supervision through case conferences and educational activities. Although the cultural dimensions of care were not at the forefront for all the clinicians affiliated with RIVO, the case discussion seminars always emphasized the interaction between traumatic context and the cultural background of patient and clinician. After a period of rapid growth during which RIVO was delivering therapy to more than 400 persons each year, cuts in funds for refugee health care by the federal government in 2012 have severely constrained and jeopardized its mission, illustrating the fragility of services which are not considered essential by the policy makers or mainstream health care institutions.

The Hôpital Jean-Talon Transcultural Clinic

The Jean-Talon Hospital Transcultural Clinic (HJTC) was created in 1993 to respond to the needs of the large immigrant population in the hospital's catchment area. The clinic was established by Dr. Carlo Sterlin, a psychiatrist originally from Haiti, who had worked in the area of transcultural psychiatry since the 1960s, starting at McGill (Sterlin, 2006). The origins of this clinic stemmed from the observation that many patients of Haitian origin who attended the outpatient clinics of HJT spoke only Creole and had clinical manifestations that did not fit conventional psychiatric diagnostic frameworks. Despite the initial perception by others that the clinic focused solely on the Haitian population, the clinic grew into a well-established transcultural psychiatry service working with a broad diversity of immigrant and refugee patients. Six clinicians attached to the hospital formed the core staff. However, throughout its existence, the clinic has relied on volunteers, and three of the four active clinicians involved donated their services in return for the academic and professional stimulation of peer supervision and collegial support. The HJTC intervention model includes both consultation and clinical services. The service applied two models, one using a small group composed of a principal therapist and two or three co-therapists and the second involving a large group comprised of clinicians from different cultural backgrounds, culture brokers, and an interpreter, as well as members of the patient's entourage. The clinic also provides training and community prevention and mental health promotion programs.

The clinic's therapeutic approach was strongly influenced by the French ethnopsychoanalytic approach originated by Devereux (1970) and further developed by Nathan (1991) and Rose-Marie Moro (Moro & Rousseau, 1998; Sturm, Nadig, & Moro, 2011). According to Nathan, the rationale

for the large group method includes at least four distinctive features (Nathan, 1991, 1994a, 1994b; Streit, 1997; Zajde, 2011):

1. It reassures families in crisis who come from collectivist or communalistic societies who may find the group less threatening than a face-to-face dyadic clinical encounter.
2. It is an effective method to limit the problems of personal and cultural countertransference.
3. Through the intervention of the interpreter, it reduces the risk of misunderstanding the family.
4. The different perspectives, questions, and interpretations of the multiple therapists provide a sort of "semantic bombardment" that unsettles the client, disengages them from their dominant systems of interpretation, and mobilizes their capacity to explore new modes of interpretation and action.

Despite this rationale, this group intervention strikes many as posing the threat of a power imbalance that could be unsettling to patients. Evaluations of this model to date have mainly involved detailed analyses of cases (Sturm et al., 2011; Zajde, 2011). In an effort to better understand the perspective of patients who received treatment at the Jean-Talon clinic with this extended group psychoanalytic model, the initial CCS project supported an initial assessment of the service (Sterlin, Rojas-Viger, & Corbeil, 2001). The goal was to identify the acceptability and impact of the intervention from the patient's point of view. This evaluation reviewed the experience of the HJTC with the 20 patients who had completed therapy at the clinic between November 1995 and September 2000. Most of the respondents appreciated the interventions and found the following aspects helpful: (1) it allowed them to express their suffering in their own language, (2) it was useful to hear proverbs that recalled their countries of origin (cf. Bagilishya, 2000), and (3) it was helpful to speak about their countries and personal history in an atmosphere of attentive listening and respect, which encouraged them to reflect on their past and consider how to refashion their future.

Although the clinical approach of the HJTC borrowed heavily from French ethnopsychiatric models—thus trying to bridge traditional/cultural interpretations with a Western psychoanalytic dimension—the approach has remained flexible. The emphasis is on presenting concepts that make sense to the patient, using only those definitions of "mental health" that fit the client's perspective. The HJTC team thus tries to incorporate psychodynamic intervention models with an anthropological approach that draws on the client's cultural interpretation of the problem by creating a space for the interaction of multiple discourses. The clinic continues to welcome families and is an interesting setting to train professionals interested in cultural intervention.

The Transcultural Child Psychiatry Team of the Montreal Children's Hospital

The transcultural child psychiatry team of the Montreal Children's Hospital (MCH) was established by Dr. Cécile Rousseau, who was also instrumental in setting up RIVO, and whose long involvement and contacts with community organizations working with refugees at multiple levels linked this service to a broad grassroots network and partnership. Rousseau had worked as a general practitioner in Central America and participated in several large community research projects in Montreal, examining issues including racism, access to institutional support, and the social exclusion of immigrants and cultural minorities. As a child psychiatrist, Rousseau saw the need for specialized services designed to meet the mental health needs of refugee and immigrant children and their families, in particular (but not limited to) those having lived through organized violence. The most salient aspects of this service were its commitment to responding to refugee mental health needs in social and political context, integrating concern with socioeconomic issues and broader power dynamics with close attention to the experience of children and their families.

The MCH team began with a very open mandate and initially received referrals for a wide range of problems. Interventions included clinical assessments and ongoing therapy for refugee and immigrant children and their families. The model utilized a team approach toward clinical intervention. The team was confronted with numerous complex cases that they were not equipped to manage but which included cultural issues, for example, developmental disorders among immigrant children. Because the team soon became overloaded, the MCH revised and limited its mandate to cover a circumscribed patient population, in order to reduce patient load and increase efficiency. Referrals to the MCH came primarily from schools, lawyers, a CLSC, or another clinician. A priority was placed on refugee families, particularly those who have lived through organized or other forms of violence, though a large number of children with potential developmental and behavior problems (e.g., ADD) were also seen. In addition, the team worked closely with the psychiatric emergency ward and saw a number of patients with acute psychoses. Although the relevance of cultural issues in cases of psychosis was initially more difficult for clinicians to appreciate (see Chapter 14), the team was able to work as consultants to the inpatient ward at the MCH to develop interventions with these families.

The evolution of the MCH service from broader grassroots accessibility to integration within the hospital also meant changing its practices to adapt to the norms and constraints of the institution. For example, given the hospital's referral and triaging policies, the team had to shift from an informal word-of-mouth referral system from the community to the more formal process required by the psychiatry unit's triage system. Because of reluctance among patients to speak initially with someone from outside the team, an administrative coordinator was hired on the team to take referrals and triage cases. In addition to clinical services, the MCH Transcultural Team was involved in a number of other institutional activities, including providing training for outside institutions (e.g., Department of Youth Protection) as well as working on prevention programs in Montreal-area schools.

The MCH model utilized an eclectic and flexible clinical model that incorporated various theoretical streams in a hybrid "bricolage" of approaches including French ethnopsychiatry of Nathan (1994a, 1994b) and Moro (2000), North American medical anthropology, as in the work of Arthur Kleinman and Byron Good (e.g., Good, 1994; Kleinman & Good, 1985; Kleinman & Kleinman, 1996), and the political dimensions of collective and individual suffering recognized in some versions of Latin-American psychoanalytic thinking and social psychiatry, for example, Marcelo and Maren Vinar (1989) and Elisabeth Lira (Lira & Weinstein, 1984).

As in the case of RIVO and the Jean-Talon Clinic, the nonpsychiatric clinical staff of MCH transcultural clinic were supported through community fund raising efforts. This provided the program with some freedom from institutional constraints but also made it precarious. The community-oriented foundations of the MCH developed into important partnerships and team members eventually moved from the MCH to a comprehensive community clinic where they continue work in close partnership with community organizations, schools, health care institutions, and social service organizations like Youth Protection. The work of the MCH team is described in more detail in Chapter 4.

Origins of the Cultural Consultation Service

The CCS was developed in response to gaps in services identified in earlier epidemiological work, a review of models of care, and a fortuitous research funding opportunity.

Earlier research in Canada identified important inequities in access to mental health services (Beiser, Gill, & Edwards, 1993; Federal Task Force on Mental Health Issues affecting Immigrants and Refugees, 1988). Studies in Quebec also documented the importance of culture as a determinant of mental health needs and service use (Bibeau et al., 1992; Rousseau & Drapeau, 2002, 2003, 2004; Rousseau, ter Kuile, et al., 2008). In Montreal, a community epidemiological study in 1995 examined help-seeking

patterns and health care utilization among immigrant populations in the Côte-des-Neiges district (the catchment area of the Jewish General Hospital and the local comprehensive community clinic, the CLSC Côte-des-Neiges) (Kirmayer, Young et al., 1996). The study compared newcomers from the Caribbean, Philippines, and Vietnam with Canadian-born English- and French-speaking residents in the same neighborhood and found a high degree of unmet need for mental health services. In particular, the study documented underutilization of existing resources by new immigrants (Kirmayer et al., 2007). In many cases, this was attributed to the perception that they would be stigmatized by their community or would face barriers due to language, culture, religion, or racism and discrimination in conventional mental care settings. Other epidemiological surveys have confirmed the specificities of the needs of migrant and refugee communities in Quebec (Rousseau & Drapeau, 2002). Qualitative interviews revealed some of the complex issues of social stress and cultural meanings of symptoms that influenced help-seeking and referrals to mental health (Groleau & Kirmayer, 2004; Whitley, Kirmayer, & Groleau, 2006a, 2006b).

A site review of the Australian Transcultural Mental Health Network afforded the first author the chance to see a variety of models in action in eastern Australia, including programs in Sydney, Melbourne, and Victoria, and web-based resources (Kirmayer & Rahimi, 1998). This led to an overview of approaches to culturally responsive services that linked models of care to local demography, patterns of migration, and political ideologies of citizenship that singled out specific groups as "others" worthy of attention in designing health care services (Kirmayer & Minas, 2000; see Chapter 1). This comparison made it clear that the ethnic matching or ethnospecific clinic approach common in the USA did not fit the Canadian context well. In Canada, the high level of diversity and constant immigration undercut any sharp distinction between newcomers and established ethnocultural communities. The link between long-standing cultural and linguistic communities and newer waves of migration was solidified in the policy of multiculturalism, which suggested that cultural diversity could be acknowledged and respected in mainstream social institutions. The goal then was to find ways to improve the response to diversity across the mental health care system.

An opportunity to pursue this arose with a federal government program funding research aimed at improving continuity of care. The Health Transition Fund (HTF) was a $150-million fund administered by Health Canada (the federal Ministry of Health) from 1997 to 2001, which supported 140 projects across Canada to evaluate innovative ways to deliver health care services. These projects were expected to generate evidence that policy makers in government, health care providers, researchers, and others could use to make informed decisions that would lead to a more integrated health care system. The project "Development and Evaluation of a Cultural Consultation Service in Mental Health" (QC424) was funded from 1999 to 2001. This research grant provided the resources to develop the CCS and conduct a formative evaluation on its implementation and a review of the outcomes of the first 100 cases referred to the service. Further grants insured the maintenance of the CCS, but, as was the case for other cultural programs, funding cultural consultation within mainstream institutions has remained a challenge.

Implementing the CCS

Implementing the CCS involved a bootstrapping process that built on existing clinical programs, research projects, and training activities in cultural psychiatry. The design and implementation of the project followed several steps as listed in Table 2.1.

Assessment of Need for the Service

In the process of preparing the grant proposal for the CCS project, meetings were held with key stakeholders in health and social services institu-

Table 2.1 Steps in implementation of the CCS

1. Assessment of need for the service
2. Selection of appropriate models for service delivery
3. Recruitment and training mental health professionals for intercultural work
4. Development of clinical procedures for consultation
5. Development of information resources for cultural consultations
6. Advertising and recruitment of patients
7. Evaluation of service

tions and the community, including colleagues within the Department of Psychiatry of the Jewish General Hospital (the host institution), the Montreal Children's Hospital Transcultural Team and Multiculturalism Program, the Jean-Talon Hospital Transcultural Clinic, several CLSC's (comprehensive community clinics) located in ethnically diverse neighborhoods that had links with the JGH, the regional refugee clinic (based at the local CLSC), the office of the regional health authority responsible for the bank of interpreters and for issues of access to care for linguistic and cultural minorities, members of the RIVO, and community groups working with Caribbean and South Asian communities. These meetings identified specific needs for services, and the organizations provided letters of support for the grant proposal. This also served to strengthen existing partnerships and collaborations and to identify a steering committee for the project.

In the process of this initial assessment of local needs, a major issue identified was the underutilization of interpreter services. Despite the availability of a bank of interpreters trained and made available by the Montreal regional health authority, hospitals were observed to make little use of this service. Hospitals had to pay for these services out of their general budget, so cost may have been one important barrier. However, efforts to reduce the cost, offering a discount for a period, had limited effect. Another issue identified was general lack of familiarity with cultural issues and a desire for more in-service training at community clinics and organizations. McGill faculty affiliated with Division of Social and Transcultural Psychiatry had done presentations to community clinics and hospitals, but there was a need for more in-depth training to provide practical help with case management and skills to work with specific types of issues or cultural groups. These needs were identified as priorities and considered in the design, staff recruitment, and work plan of the CCS.

Choosing the Appropriate Models for Service Delivery

As discussed in Chapter 1, a variety of models have been developed to meet the challenge of culturally appropriate care:

1. The simplest approach is to insure access to standard care for all patients. At a minimum, this requires readily available interpreter services. However, since many individuals from culturally diverse backgrounds are unaware of mental health services or experience significant barriers, access must include elements of community outreach education. Moreover, health care providers must be trained, and quality assurance standards must be in place, to insure they make appropriate use of interpreters (see Chapter 5).

2. A second approach relies on existing resources within cultural communities. In most communities of any size, there are professionals, religious leaders, traditional healers, elders, and other helpers who often deal with mental health problems. These people have intimate knowledge of the social norms and cultural history of their community. Their modes of intervention are culturally consonant and integrated in the community. They may enjoy greater legitimacy and authority than biomedicine or formal mental health services which may be associated with stigma or fears of coercive treatment. Conventional health care services may refer people to such practitioners or work in close collaboration with them, each providing complementary aspects of patient's care. However, for complex cases and major psychiatric disorders, community helpers may not have the requisite expertise and institutional resources to provide all aspects of care.

3. A third approach involves the development of specialized services to improve access and provide culturally appropriate care. This includes a wide range of models including ethnospecific clinics for specific populations (e.g., Hispanic clinics with Spanish-speaking staff). This model is practical in settings where there is a large population with shared cultural or linguistic background that can be addressed through matching. It has the advantage of making expertise readily available by concentrating it at one site and creating an organizational structure that can institute some form of community control. The disadvantages include a potential lack of influence on the wider health care system and increased stigmatization as patients from specific backgrounds are segregated at one location.

In the case of the CCS, the choice of an outpatient consultation model was based on several considerations related to the composition of the hospital catchment area, health care policy in Quebec, and the larger values of multiculturalism and interculturalism (see Chapter 1):

• The existing emphasis on primary care delivery of mental health services with psychiatry providing outpatient backup consultation or collaboration to strengthen the capacity of frontline services.

• The very high degree of cultural and linguistic diversity in the population making ethnospecific services impractical.

• The relatively small size of communities with a high proportion of newcomers so that for many groups, only limited services were available within the community.

• The cultural values of multiculturalism and interculturalism, which encourage interaction among ethnic groups in a shared social space rather than hiving off groups in specialized settings.

• The recognition that, despite the goal of inclusiveness through mainstreaming, the lack of specialized services means that minorities' issues are often ignored or misunderstood in clinical intervention planning. Hence, there remains a need for bringing together a critical mass of expertise in culturally responsive services both for adequate care and training of professionals to improve their cultural competence and promote cultural safety throughout the health care system.

The CCS adopted an approach to clinical assessment and intervention that focused on knowledge transfer to primary care physicians or other referring clinicians. The aim was to use the consultation not only to address the needs for that specific case but also to transfer knowledge, attitudes, and skills that could be used by the referring clinician to approach similar cases in the future. At the same time, the CCS could serve as a training center for mental health practitioners (psychiatry residents, psychology interns, social work, and nursing students) and a research site for work on refining methods of cultural formulation and assessment.

Recruiting and Training Mental Health Professionals and Staff for Intercultural Work

The CCS built on available expertise in the McGill Division of Social and Transcultural Psychiatry and the wider network of colleagues at other institutions in Montreal. The founders of the CCS were psychiatrists (LJK and JG) with much experience in intercultural clinical work, training, and research. LJK brought research experience in medical and psychological anthropology as well as clinical involvement in consultation-liaison psychiatry, behavioral medicine, and indigenous communities. He trained in psychiatry at University California, Davis, in Sacramento in the late 1970s, where psychiatrist Henry Herrera, anthropologist Byron Good, and sociologist Mary-Jo Good had developed an innovative consultation program working collaboratively with local healers (Good, Herrera, Good, & Cooper, 1982). JG brought extensive experience in family systems-oriented child psychiatry as well as psychoanalysis. Both took part regularly in the case conferences that provided models of systemic and cultural thinking for later work by colleagues and students.

The service recruited a clinical psychologist who functioned initially as the coordinator of the service. In addition to administrative support staff, other people recruited during the initial phase of the CCS included clinicians with consultation experience from the target disciplines (psychiatry, psychology, family medicine, nursing, and social work) to act as consultants and trainers, a webmaster, and an IT person to maintain computer databases and Internet website resources, an evaluation researcher to work with the team to conduct a process evaluation (DG), and research assistants to collect outcome data from patients.

Because the staff involved were unfamiliar with the cultural consultation model—which was, in fact, a work in progress—we used weekly meetings of the service to forge a team, address organizational issues, and create a shared understanding and approach to the work of the service. Although these meetings centered on cultural formulations of referred cases or consultation to organizations, they also devoted time to logistics, discussed problems and dilemmas in the functioning of the service, and identified potential solutions for implementation. This process helped to clarify the role of the CCS and the type of knowledge translation and clinical tasks within its purview.

Building on the existing network developed by the MCH, the CCS established a bank of 73 consultants, predominately psychologists, psychiatrists, and social workers. In fact, a small number of consultants were used repeatedly, both because of the specific background of referred cases and because of the high level of skill they evinced. Consultants integrated directly into the team (as staff at the JGH, postdoctoral fellows, or trainees) were used most frequently.

Culture brokers were recruited as needed for a specific case. Preference was given to bilingual, bicultural clinicians with expertise in cultural psychiatry or psychology. However, in most instances, brokers with all of these attributes were not available. As a result, the culture broker might be someone with limited mental health knowledge who was closely supervised by the CCS consultant throughout the process of data collection and formulation. In effect, training occurred through this experience of on-the-job supervision. The culture broker was required to prepare a cultural formulation report following the Outline for Cultural Formulation in DSM-IV-TR (American Psychiatric Association, 2000). This was augmented with additional topics to address other aspects of identity, migration history, developmental experiences, illness models, and social structural problems (see Chapter 3). The culture broker's work could then be assessed both by observation during the assessment interview process, by their presentation of cultural information during the CCS case conference, and through the quality of their written report. This allowed the CCS consultants to identify culture brokers who were skilled, who would be invited to continue to work with the service, and those who were less skilled or biased, who would not be employed again.

With the end of grant funding, the service scaled back to a more streamlined model with a clinical director working closely with an administrative coordinator who is also highly skilled in interpersonal relations performing intake, triage, and assigning consultants to cases. In addition to the CCS consultants, culture brokers, and referring clinicians, the service allows selected students and trainees from health and social science disciplines to take part in the weekly case conferences contributing diverse perspectives to the discussion and insuring a lively exchange.

Development of Clinical Procedures for Consultation

The clinical procedures of the CCS were modeled on outpatient consultation, with patients referred by primary care or other frontline clinicians seen by the CCS team at the Institute of Community and Family Psychiatry (the location of the outpatient psychiatry clinics of the Jewish General Hospital). The referring clinician or organization was invited to take part in the consultation and subsequent cultural formulation case conference, though most clinicians were unable to attend because of their own schedules. On some occasions, consultants travelled to the referral site to see patients there or to present the results of the consultation to the referring team.

The key participants in the consultation included a CCS clinician (usually a cultural psychiatrist or psychologist), an interpreter (when initial triage suggested one would be needed), and, usually, a culture broker with specific cultural knowledge pertinent to the case. The CCS clinician played a supervisory role and usually took the lead in meeting the patient and organizing the assessment process. The culture broker played varying roles, sometimes taking part in the interview and on other occasions providing contextual information and comments on the case during the subsequent CCS case conference. In many instances, the culture broker prepared a written cultural formulation following an expanded version of the DSM-IV-TR Outline for Cultural Formulation (American Psychiatric Association, 2000; Kirmayer, Thombs, et al., 2008). A handbook was prepared for consultants and culture brokers working with the CCS team, which outlined basic procedures and provided guidelines for the cultural formulation and other resource materials (see Chapter 3).

Development of Resources for Cultural Consultations

Cultural consultation requires mobilizing relevant resources for specific cases. These resources may include interpreters, culture brokers, community organizations, and clinicians or others with specific skills or expertise. To identify these resources, we canvased existing programs, services, and organizations to collect information on individuals and programs relevant to the work of the service. We created databases of community organizations, professionals, and resource persons with expertise in culture and mental health and a website for access to this data and related information in cultural psychiatry. These databases were maintained by the CCS coordinator and updated regularly.

To facilitate cultural consultations, referrals, and identification of appropriate clinical and community resources, we developed three database resources: (1) a community organization resource database; (2) a clinician, interpreter, and culture broker database; and (3) a bibliographic database and library of literature in culture and mental health (with about 1,500 books and 3,000 articles). These databases were made available to CCS consultants and clients in multiple formats: over the Internet, in printed form, and by telephone, fax, or e-mail from the CCS. The CCS website served as a portal with links to online resources for clinicians and consultants, including (1) information on professional training activities and conferences in intercultural mental health; (2) bibliographies and references to online texts and technical documents; (3) patient information handouts, pamphlets, and other documents for users in multiple languages; and (4) information on community resources. This site evolved into the Multicultural Mental Health Resource Centre (http://www.mmhrc.ca) with the support of the Mental Health Commission of Canada.

The community organization resource database was based on earlier work by Heather Clarke and collaborators at the Montreal Children's Hospital Multiculturalism Program who had produced a spiral-bound document of about 80 pages listing organizations that were run by and provided services for specific ethnocultural communities. We transformed this document into a searchable database on a desktop computer. We developed a questionnaire to update the existing database requesting information about community services being offered including the cultural populations served, availability of interpreters, social services (e.g., home visitors, support groups), and mental health-related services. The questionnaire was mailed to 87 organizations in the greater Montreal area and followed up with telephone contact to collect up-to-date information.

We also created a database of clinicians, interpreters, and culture brokers who were available to participate in cultural consultations. The database included contact information, areas of expertise (language, culture, specific patient populations, or types of clinical issues), and our own notes on previous experiences working with that individual.

Advertising and Recruitment of Patients

To make use of the CCS, clinicians must be aware of the service, identify appropriate patients in their practice, and have a simple referral process. The CCS was devised as a regional service, with consultations available for patients from the greater Montreal area. The information resources and referral activities were available more widely, across the province of Quebec, by telephone, fax, or e-mail.

To make clinicians aware of the CCS when it was first launched, a brochure announcing the service was prepared and distributed to the mailing lists of the Quebec Corporation of Psychologists and the Quebec Psychiatric Association (see Fig. 2.1). The brochure described the service and stated: "a cultural consultation is best reserved for cases where there are difficulties in understanding, diagnosing and treating patients that may be due to cultural differences between clinician and patient. Such differences can occur even when patient and clinician are from similar background because of wide variation within social and cultural groups."

Initial referrals to the service were asked how they heard about the service. It appeared that few referrals came about as a result of this mailing. Instead, referrals tended to come from clinicians familiar with the core group of CCS consultants because of either previous work, in-service training, or presentations at hospitals and institutions in the region. As the usefulness of the service became apparent, further referrals came from the same sources and gradually spread by word of mouth to colleagues both locally and at other clinical, social service, and community centers. Hence, the referral sources grew in concentric circles geographically and by collegial links.

Evaluation of the CCS

Evaluation is essential for any new service to determine its effectiveness and limitations and to provide a basis for refinement and justify its place in a health care system that faces ongoing

HOW DO I REQUEST A CONSULTATION?

A consultation request can be made by contacting the CCS Monday to Friday between 8:30 to 4:30. At the time of the request, the consultee should be prepared to provide the reasons for the consultation as well as basic identifying information about the patient (e.g. date of birth, occupation, languages spoken, address, immigration or refugee status, medicare number).

OTHER ACTIVITIES OF THE CULTURAL CONSULTATION SERVICE?

- In-service training and workshops for health professionals.
- Internships and rotations for trainees in psychiatry and other mental health disciplines.
- Development of an internet database of resources on culture and mental health.
- International Consortium for Cultural Consultation

DIRECTOR

G. Eric Jarvis, M.D., M.Sc.

SERVICE COORDINATOR

Antonella Clerici, B.A.

RESEARCH COORDINATOR

Chrissi Galanakis, M.Sc.

Institute of Community & Family Psychiatry
Jewish General Hospital
4333 Côte-Ste-Catherine Road
Montreal, Quebec H3T 1E4
Tel. (514) 340-8222 x5655
Fax: (514) 340-7503
E-mail: antonella.clerici@mail.mcgill.ca
Website: http://www.mcgill.ca/culturalconsultation

WHAT IS CULTURAL CONSULTATION?

A cultural consultation is a comprehensive assessment of the social and cultural factors influencing diagnostic, prognostic and treatment issues of patients with mental health problems.

WHAT IS THE FUNCTION OF THE CCS?

The CCS may provide specific cultural information, links to community resources or formal cultural psychiatric or psychological assessment and recommendations for treatment.

WHAT CONSTITUTES AN APPROPRIATE CASE FOR CULTURAL CONSULTATION?

Cultural consultation is best reserved for cases where there are difficulties in understanding, diagnosing and treating patients due to cultural differences between clinician and patient. Such differences can occur even when patient and clinician are from a similar background because of wide variation within social and cultural groups.

WHO CAN MAKE A REFERRAL TO OUR SERVICE?

Requests for consultation can be made by any physician or licensed mental health practitioner and will be screened to determine if they are appropriate.

CULTURAL CONSULTATION SERVICE

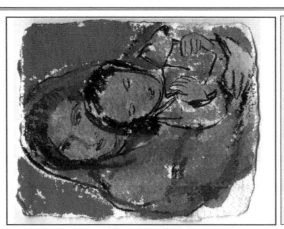

THE CULTURAL CONSULTATION SERVICE (CCS) OF THE JEWISH GENERAL HOSPITAL DEPARTMENT OF PSYCHIATRY OFFERS CLINICAL CONSULTATIONS TO PSYCHIATRIC, MEDICAL AND MENTAL HEALTH PRACTITIONERS, AS WELL AS INSERVICE TRAINING IN CULTURE AND MENTAL HEALTH.

Fig. 2.1 Brochure describing the Cultural Consultation Service

financial constraints. From its inception, the CCS has been a research setting and a variety of studies have been conducted that shed light on the implementation, impact, and effectiveness of the service. The following sections present the results from the initial evaluation of the CCS, which included a formative process evaluation of the implementation of the service and a basic outcome assessment. The goal of the process evaluation was to document the development of the service to identify facilitating factors and barriers to implementation. The process evaluation used a model of participatory action research with a research anthropologist (DG) working as a participant observer in close collaboration with the clinical teams.

The outcome evaluation of the services involved assessing the consultations in terms of (1) patterns of referral from specific institutions and professionals, (2) reasons for consultation, (3) sociodemographic and clinical characteristics of cases referred, (4) use of specific professional and community resources including interpreters and culture brokers, (5) consultation diagnosis and treatment recommendations, (6) themes in cultural formulations, (7) referring clinician satisfaction with the consultation, and (8) concordance with the recommendations. Efforts to assess patient outcomes in terms of symptoms and functioning and cost-effectiveness analysis were stymied by the great heterogeneity of the cases seen and the need to minimize intrusiveness in the consultation context, which sometimes did not involve seeing the patient but only meeting with the referring clinician. This is a common problem in evaluations of consultation services.

Quantitative Evaluation

Over the 13-year period from 1999 to 2012, the CCS service received 636 requests for consultation and completed 491 consultations. Of these, 455 cases were directly assessed by a CCS consultant, and 36 cases were only discussed at a CCS case conference. The majority of consultation requests concerned individuals (86%), but some involved couples or families (12%). A few

Table 2.2 Sources of referral of CCS individual cases ($N=406$)[a]

	n	%
Referral source		
Community health clinic (CLSC)	135	33
Hospital outpatient psychiatry clinic	84	21
Hospital outpatient clinics (nonpsychiatric)	37	9
Hospital inpatient (medical and psychiatric)	35	9
Private practitioner	48	12
Government agency	19	5
Community organizations	16	4
Rehabilitation center	13	3
School	7	2
Hospital emergency room (including ER psychiatry)	6	1
Medical clinic (nonhospital)	5	1
Law firm	1	0
Referring professional		
Physician (primary care, specialty medicine)	126	31
Social workers	97	24
Psychiatrist	78	19
Psychologist/psychotherapist	67	17
Nurse/mental health care nurse	22	5
Other health care professional (nutritionists, OTs, etc.)	7	2
Organization	1	0
Other (legal and lay persons, teachers, interpreters)	8	2

[a]Only individual cases directly assessed by a CCS consultant are represented in Tables 2.2, 2.3, 2.4, 2.5, 2.6, 2.7, 2.8, and 2.9

cases (2%) involved requests from organizations to discuss issues related to their work with a whole ethnocultural group or community. The CCS also received frequent requests for information and links to resources.

Table 2.2 summarizes the referring institutions and professionals.[3] Referrals came from the whole range of health and social service professionals based at hospitals (40%) and comprehensive community clinics (CLSC, 33%). Smaller numbers came from private practitioners (12%), government agencies (5%), and community

---

[3] Tables 2.2, 2.3, 2.4, 2.5, 2.6, 2.7, 2.8, and 2.9 present data on individual cases seen by CCS consultants; couples and families and cases not seen directly by a consultant are not included.

Table 2.3 Reasons for referral and expectations for consultation (N=406)

	n	%
Reasons for referral		
Clarify diagnosis or meaning of symptoms and behaviors	320	79
Help with treatment plan	277	68
Problems with clinician–patient communication	90	22
Help with refugee claim/immigration status	75	18
Problems with treatment adherence	54	13
Other cultural problems	79	19
Expectations for consultation		
One-time consultation	341	84
Follow-up by CCS	70	17
Provide ongoing treatment	27	7
Help locating resources for patient	138	34
Other	33	8

Table 2.4 Sociodemographic characteristics of CCS individual cases (N=406)

	n	%
Age		
0–13	4	1
14–21	37	9
22–40	203	50
41–64	152	37
≥65	10	3
Gender (female)	210	52
Marital status		
Never married	148	37
Married	145	36
Living as though married	18	4
Separated	39	10
Divorced	36	9
Widowed	18	4
N/A[a]	2	0
Education level		
No formal education	13	3
Primary	33	8
Secondary	139	34
Post-secondary	147	36
N/A[a]	74	18
Employment status		
Unemployed	224	55
Employed/full time	58	14
Employed/part time	11	3
Student	37	9
Homemaker	39	10
Disability/sick leave	13	3
Maternity leave	2	0
Retired	6	2
Welfare	6	1
Other	3	1
N/A[a]	7	2
Immigration status		
Refugee or asylum seeker	167	41
Landed immigrant/permanent resident	85	21
Citizen	123	30
Other (student visa, status Indian)	15	4
N/A[a]	16	4
Year of arrival in Canada (of N=377 not born in Canada)		
1950–1959	4	1
1960–1969	3	1
1970–1979	10	3
1980–1989	39	10
1990–1999	104	28
2000–2009	205	54
2010–2013	10	3
N/A[a]	2	0

[a]N/A: Data that were not recorded at intake were categorized as "Not available"

organizations (4%). The majority of cases were referred by physicians, mental health practitioners, or other health professionals. Almost one in four cases was referred by social workers (24%). Most (n=223, 55%) of the referring clinicians indicated at the time of referral that an interpreter would be required for the consultation. Of these, only 60 had used an interpreter with the index patient in the past.

As seen in Table 2.3, the most common reasons for consultation were requests for help with clarifying a diagnosis or the meaning of specific symptoms or behaviors (79%), treatment planning (68%), problems with clinician–patient communication (22%), requests for help with issues related to immigration status (18%), treatment adherence (13%), or other cultural problems (e.g., better understanding of culture of psychosocial factors, assess ability to return to work) (19%). Three quarters of all cases had multiple reasons for requesting consultation reflecting the complexity and interrelatedness of issues. Based on intake assessment, the majority of referrals were classified as either ASAP (n=167) or Urgent (n=136), comprising over 75% of the cases.

Sociodemographic characteristics of the cases are summarized in Table 2.4. The mean age of patients referred was 36.7 years. The overall educational level of patients was high with 36% having completed at least some post-secondary education. However, over half of the patients were unemployed at the time of referral. Of the patients who were born outside of Canada, 104 arrived between 1990 and 1999 and 215 arrived between 2000 and 2012. The earliest year of arrival was 1951. Non-Canadian-born patients had spent a mean of 7.5 years (range 0–58 years, median 4 years, mode 1 year) in Canada, between arrival and referral. A large proportion of the cases seen (41%) were asylum seekers or refugee claimants. This reflects the fact that the CCS is located near the regional refugee clinic, which is a federally funded service that provides basic medical care while claimants are awaiting determination of their status. Although they are very experienced in providing medical and psychosocial care for this population, staff at the clinic call on the CCS for help with complex diagnostic and management issues as well as help with assessments related to claimants' appearance before the Immigration Review Board (see Chapter 12).

The cases represented enormous diversity in terms of countries of origin, languages, ethnocultural groups, and religions as summarized in Table 2.5. Patients came from 70 different countries, with the largest numbers coming from India ($n=51$), Pakistan ($n=34$), and Sri Lanka ($n=25$). When grouped by region of origin, 147 patients (36%) originated from South-Central Asia, followed by 61 patients from sub-Saharan Africa. The rest were distributed between North Africa, the Middle East, East Asia, Latin America, Europe, Southeast Asia, the Caribbean, and North America. Paralleling this geographic origin, the largest set of ethnicity groups was South Asian ($n=128$, 31%), followed by Middle Eastern/North African (16%), sub-Saharan African (13%), and South or Central American (10%). Most patients self-identified as belonging to two major religions, Christianity ($n=144$, 35%) and Islam ($n=120$, 30%), with smaller proportions belonging to Judaism, Sikhism, Hinduism, Buddhism, traditional indigenous religions, or no religion. Separate branches or sects of each religion are not identified (e.g., both Sunni and Shia Muslims are included under the umbrella of Islam). Patients spoke a great variety

Table 2.5 Ethnocultural characteristics of CCS individual cases ($N=406$)

	n	%
Region of origin		
South-Central Asia	147	36
Southeast Asia	12	3
East Asia	19	5
Middle East/North Africa	51	12
Sub-Saharan Africa	61	15
South or Central America	39	10
Caribbean	32	8
Europe	15	4
North America	30	7
Ethnicity (geographic grouping)		
South Asian	128	31
Southeast Asian	11	3
East Asian	25	6
Middle Eastern/North African	63	16
Sub-Saharan African	53	13
European	17	4
Latin American	35	9
Caribbean	28	7
Aboriginal	23	6
North American	1	0
N/A[a]	22	5
Religion		
Buddhism	10	2
Christianity	144	35
Hinduism	27	7
Islam	120	30
Judaism	2	0
Sikhism	37	9
Traditional indigenous	7	2
Other	3	1
None	12	3
N/A[a]	44	11
Mother tongue		
African languages	38	9
Arabic	27	7
Chinese (Mandarin, Cantonese)	19	5
English	38	9
French	13	3
European languages (other than French or English)	15	4
Middle Eastern languages (other than Arabic)	35	9
Spanish	46	11
South Asian languages (e.g., Hindi, Tamil, Urdu)	135	33
Southeast Asian languages (e.g., Khmer, Vietnamese)	8	2
Indigenous languages	3	1
Other	23	6
N/A[a]	6	2

[a] Data that were not recorded at intake upon referral were categorized as "Do not know"

Table 2.6 Resources needed for cultural consultation (N=406)

	n	%
Matching of consultant		
Ethnicity	51	13
Language	18	4
Religion	4	1
Specific clinical skills		
Psychiatric (mental status examination, medication)	251	62
Social work expertise	8	2
Child and family therapy	6	1
Experience with refugees, trauma, and migration issues	5	1
Somatization	2	1
Other (e.g., drug abuse, medical complications)	7	2
Interpreters	153	38
Culture brokers	198	49

of languages and dialects (76 recorded at intake), with the largest single number speaking Punjabi. When grouped by region, most patients spoke South Asian languages (33%), followed by Middle Eastern (e.g., Arabic, Farsi; 16%), Spanish (11%), African (9%), European (7%, including French), and East Asian languages (5%, mainly Chinese). Small numbers of patients spoke indigenous languages (e.g., Mi'kmaq, Lakota, Quechua) and other languages (e.g., Kreyol, Pidgin, and American Sign Language). Less than half (n=167) of all patients spoke at least a little French, and 40% (67/167) of these were fluent in French. Of importance for understanding potential difficulties in navigating the health care system, fully 47% (n=192) of patients had no French language skills at the time of referral. However, almost 75% overall had at least some English language skills and 26% (n=106) were fluent in English; 23% (n=92) patients could speak no English at all.

This culture and linguistic diversity demanded a wide range of resources in terms of consultants, interpreters, and culture brokers (Table 2.6). Some form of matching of the consultants' background (language, ethnicity, or religion) with that of the patient was needed in 18% of cases, and some specific clinical skills (psychiatric expertise,

family therapy training, experience working with trauma, refugees, somatization) was needed in 69% cases. Because it was often not possible to find a skilled clinician with the requisite language skills and cultural background knowledge, it was necessary to use both interpreters and culture brokers to address the specific cultural and mental health issues raised by a case. Interpreters were employed in 38% (n=153) of cases, and culture brokers in 49% (198); 15% of cases (59) had both interpreters and culture brokers. For smaller ethnocultural communities or more recent immigrants, it was sometimes difficult to find a well-trained interpreter or appropriate culture broker to work with a patient or family. Patients were sometimes reluctant to meet with a culture broker or consultant from their own background because the small size of the local community made confidentiality difficult to maintain.

Table 2.7 summarizes the intake and final diagnoses of patients assessed by the CCS. The first column presents the initial diagnosis as reported by the referring clinician at the time of intake to the CCS. Patients had an average of 1.67 diagnoses at referral. The most frequent diagnoses at the time of intake were major depressive disorder, PTSD, psychotic disorders (including schizophrenia and psychotic symptoms NOS), and other anxiety disorders. The level of certainty of these diagnoses varied with the expertise of the referring clinician and the extent of previous evaluation. Of these intake diagnoses, on average 55% were confirmed by the consultation. For most diagnostic categories, the level of confirmation of intake diagnosis ranged from 40 to 76%, but low rates of confirmation were found for some psychotic disorders as well as anxiety, adjustment, and dissociative disorders. The CCS evaluation made new diagnoses in 73% of cases (n=295), with an average of 2.00 diagnoses per case (1.46 new diagnoses per case overall). The final column in Table 2.7 presents the proportion of final diagnoses in each case that were new. Fully 61% of the final diagnoses were produced by the CCS; put another way, 2/3 of the final diagnoses differed from the referral diagnoses. In particular, most diagnoses of psychotic, anxiety, adjustment, and personality

Table 2.7 Intake and final diagnoses of CCS cases ($N=406$)

	Intake	Confirmed		New	Total	New/total
				Diagnosis[a]		
Diagnostic category	n	n	%	n	n	%
Affective disorder	198	143	72	100	243	41
Depression	173	132	76	87	219	40
Bipolar	25	11	44	13	24	54
Psychotic disorder	154	70	45	101	171	59
Schizophrenia/schizophreniform	43	25	58	22	47	47
Schizoaffective	13	5	38	15	20	75
Other psychotic	37	12	32	39	51	76
Psychotic symptoms	61	28	46	25	53	47
PTSD	109	81	74	59	140	42
Anxiety disorder	48	17	35	30	47	64
Adjustment disorder	12	4	33	46	50	92
Somatoform disorder	24	14	58	14	28	50
Personality disorder	20	8	40	43	51	84
Personality traits	16	5	31	44	49	90
Childhood disorder	3	0	0	15	15	100
Learning disorder	7	3	43	13	16	81
Eating disorder	5	0	0	2	2	100
Substance abuse	16	10	63	26	36	72
V-code	20	5	25	43	48	90
Other conditions	6	0	0	8	8	100
Cognitive disorders	13	7	54	15	22	68
Dissociative disorders	7	1	14	2	3	67
Factitious disorders	2	0	0	0	0	0
Impulse control disorders	1	0	0	7	7	100
Sexual and gender identity disorders	2	0	0	1	1	100
Sleep disorders	1	0	0	2	2	100
General medical condition	15	5	33	20	25	80
Total Diagnoses	679	373	55	591	964	61
Average Diagnoses per case	1.67	0.92		1.46	2.37	

[a]*Intake* = Diagnosis by referring clinician provided at intake, *Confirmed* = intake diagnoses confirmed by CCS evaluation, *New* = new diagnoses made by CCS evaluation, *Total* = Confirmed + New CCS final diagnoses in each category, *New/Total* = proportion of diagnoses in each category made by CCS evaluation

disorders as well as V-codes were made by the CCS. The increase in diagnoses of psychoses probably reflects the specific expertise of cultural psychiatry in differentiating psychosis, dissociative disorders, and cultural variations in illness experience (Adeponle, Thombs et al., 2012; see Chapter 14). The fact that the CCS was able to make diagnoses of personality disorders more frequently likely reflects the ability to collect more information about past patterns of behavior and cultural norms. The increased diagnosis of adjustment disorder and the use of V-codes stem from the careful attention to situational or contextual issues including migration, acculturation, family systems, and other social stressors and predicaments. Overall, this table indicates that the CCS plays an important role in basic diagnostic reassessment.

Of course, psychiatric diagnosis is only one aspect of clinical assessment, and the cultural formulations produced by the CCS identified many other issues or problems that required clinical attention. Table 2.8 lists the predominate themes in the cultural formulations many

Table 2.8 Common themes in cultural formulations (*N*=283)

	n	*%*
Family systems issues	77	27
Family and couple conflict		
Changes in configuration of extended family		
Intergenerational issues		
Family honor and obligations		
Exposure to trauma and violence	66	23
Impact of war, torture, and organized violence		
Domestic violence		
Effects of violence on development		
PTSD, depression, and other sequelae		
Migration issues	71	25
Stresses and losses on migration trajectory		
Uncertainty of refugee or immigration status		
Family separation and reunification		
Homesickness and mourning for culture		
Cultural identity, acculturation, and adjustment	123	43
Adjusting to life in host country		
Shifting/hybrid cultural identity		
Changing gender roles and relations		
Changing social roles and community		
Cultural models of illness and healing	47	17
Modes of symptom expression and idioms of distress		
Illness explanatory models and causal attributions		
Cultural influences on social determinants of health		
Treatment choice and expectations for care		
Other social, economic, and structural issues	129	46
Stereotyping, prejudice, and discrimination		
Social isolation, marginalization		
Poverty, socioeconomic uncertainty		
Unemployment or underemployment		

of which influenced diagnosis, treatment recommendations, treatment adherence, or constituted clinical problems in their own right. These issues fall into several broad groups that are often closely related. The most frequent issues included:

- Variations in family systems and structures (e.g., patriarchal families), including changes in age and gender roles (e.g., significance of marriage, divorce, adolescence, or elder status for identity and social status of men and women) and notions of honor and shame as regulatory principles in family dynamics (see Chapter 7).
- The impact of exposure to violence and massive human rights violations (including civil war, genocide, torture and childhood and domestic violence), which may be experienced prior to migration, on the journey to safety or after resettlement.
- The impact of migration itself (e.g., issues of identity, fracturing extended families, changing gender roles, eliminating communal supports and mediators, and creating tensions between generations); the stressful impact of the uncertainty and complexity inherent to the application process, waiting period, and review board hearing for asylum seekers (see Chapter 12); and the impact of prolonged family separation and reunification (see Chapter 13).
- Issues related to changes in social roles, gender relations, hybrid identities, and new configurations of family and community.
- The impact of other social, economic, and structural issues including poverty, unemployment (or underemployment for migrants whose credentials are not recognized), as well as ethnic, religious, or racial stereotyping, prejudice, and discrimination, including everyday micro-aggression, institutional racism, and biases in provision of health and social services as well as interactions with mainstream institutions like the police, youth protection, and the justice system (see Chapters 11 and 13).
- The effects of cultural modes of expressing symptoms, models of illness, and expectations for treatment, including the prevalence of dissociative symptoms leading to misdiagnosis of psychosis, experiences with health care and healing practices in country of origin, and the value of religious practices in coping and healing.

Table 2.9 Referring clinician evaluation of consultation outcomes (N=134)

	n	%
Recommendations		
Recommendations were clear	124	93
Recommendations were feasible	102	76
Impact of cultural consultation		
Influenced the patient keeping appointments more regularly[a]	9	12
Influenced the patient's treatment adherence[a]	16	21
Improved the clinician–patient relationship[a]	28	36
Influenced the use of other services	36	29
Referring clinician satisfaction (N=91)		
Satisfied with the consultation	73	80
Helped to deal with patient's problems	58	64
Recommend service to a colleague	86	95
Use service again	85	93

[a]Data only available for 78 cases because of a change in questionnaire

Table 2.10 Reasons for non-implementation of CCS recommendations (N=287)

	n	%
Patient lost to follow-up	75	26
Patient refused or disagreed with recommendation	64	22
Clinician found recommendation inappropriate or irrelevant	29	10
New circumstances made recommendation irrelevant or inappropriate	37	13
Recommendation implemented but results unsatisfactory	2	1
Recommendation already implemented	6	2
Lack of systemic resources	6	2
Recommendation will be implemented in future	10	3
Patient unable to implement the recommendation	4	1
Clinician did not have opportunity	7	2
Third-party disagreed with recommendation	4	1
Recommendation too costly or difficult to implement	4	1
Recommendation arrived too late	5	2
Lack of communication with third-party needed to implement	2	1
Clinician forgot to implement or does not remember if implemented	36	13

The cultural formulation was presented as a narrative that identified the salient issues and their interactions in an individual case. This was distilled into a brief clinical problem list that could be addressed with specific interventions, which was conveyed to the referring clinician.

To assess the usefulness of the CCS consultations, referring clinicians were contacted about 6 months after the consultation and asked to respond to a brief questionnaire. Each of the recommendations in the consultation report was read to the clinicians, and they were asked whether the recommendation had been implemented and, if not, why. The questionnaire also asked questions about the clarity and feasibility of recommendations in this case and the effect of the consultation on client adherence to treatment and health care utilization as well as on the clinician–patient relationship. Finally, they were asked about their overall satisfaction with the service.

Outcome data are available on 134 referrals from 91 clinicians (Table 2.9). For the great majority of cases, the referring clinicians found the consultation recommendations clear (n=124, 93%) and feasible (n=102, 76%). There was some evidence for impact on clinical care and service use, with 12% reporting the patient was better at keeping appointments and 21% finding that the patient was more adherent to treatment. Out of the total 701 recommendations made to these clinicians, 59% (n=414) were implemented, with a mean of 3.1 recommendations/case. Table 2.10 summarizes the main reasons for not implementing specific recommendations. The most common reason for lack recommendation concordance was patient lost to follow-up, which occurred for 26% (n=75) of recommendations. This was followed by recommendations that were not implemented due to patient refusal (22%). The clinician disagreed with the recommendation in 10% of cases (n=29), and the recommendation became irrelevant in 13% of the cases (n=37). The clinician forgot to implement the recommendation or did not remember if the recommendation was implemented in 13% of cases (n=36). Patient-related reasons for not implementing a recommendation were reported in a total of 49% of the recommendations. In most cases, referring clinicians reported that they were satisfied with the consultation (80%) and indicated that it had helped in the management of their patients (64%). Nearly all who used the service said they would use it again (93%) and would recommend that their colleagues use it (95%).

Formative Process Evaluation of CCS Implementation

Given the innovative nature of the CCS, the principal objective of the qualitative evaluation was to document the process of its implementation. To promote the active participation of the service's members in the evaluation process, the evaluator met with CCS clinical team on several occasions to determine the specific objectives of the evaluation, which included (1) developing a typology of intercultural clinical problems seen by the CCS, (2) identifying themes in the cultural formulations produced by the culture broker and the team, (3) identifying barriers and facilitating factors for the implementation of the service, and (4) describing components of the service which changed as a result of the process evaluation.

The evaluation used a multiple case study method with overlapping levels of analysis (Yin, 2008). In case study designs, the explanatory power derives from the depth of case analysis, not from the number of units analyzed. The formative evaluation was conducted during the initial grant-funded phase of the project and included the initial 52 cases seen by the CCS. The different levels of analysis used in the study were based on the perspectives and explanations of three members of the research team who included an anthropologist, two clinical psychologists, and psychiatrist. Two sources of data were used:

1. The CCS case files were reviewed to compile the following data: (a) the referring clinician's stated (explicit) reasons for the referral, (b) the case notes of the clinical coordinator and CCS consultants from triage through completion of the consultation, (c) the complete text of the cultural formulation and clinical recommendations for the case, and (d) the summary of clinical recommendations produced at the end of the consultation with the CCS team.

2. Participant observation during the clinical case conference provided information on the case and on the process of interaction among consultants, culture brokers, and referring clinicians. The evaluator and the clinical coordinator participated in these meetings and took process notes. The meetings were also audio-recorded and transcribed so that they could be reviewed if needed.

Post-case conference research meetings were held immediately following each weekly CCS case conference meeting. The meetings were chaired by the lead evaluator (DG), an anthropologist with graduate training in public health who was responsible for the evaluation. The other participants were usually the CCS clinical coordinator (a clinical psychologist) and a participating mental health practitioner with experience in qualitative research. We used the technique of triangulation of perspectives in order to maximize the internal validity of the qualitative results (Denzin, 1989; Green & Thorogood, 2004). This group reviewed the participant-observation notes and reflected on the assessment process and clinical conference interactions. During these meetings, these three participants aimed to address the specific research objectives by answering the following key questions:

1. What were the principal themes in the cultural formulation for the case?
2. Did the consultation process identify additional problems related to the case that were not initially recognized at triage?
3. Did the consultation process reveal implicit problems?
4. Based on participant observation during the clinical consultation, are there ways to improve the CCS process?
5. Did the consultation identify training needs?

Discussion among the researchers continued until consensus was reached on each question.

Cultural Issues Motivating Clinician's Request for a Cultural Consultation

Referring clinicians' explicit reasons for requesting a cultural consultation recorded at the time of triage are summarized in Table 2.11. These reasons for referral were stated directly by the clinician or elicited with the help of the CCS coordinator during the triage process. Additional cultural issues that were uncovered later on during the consultation are labeled "emergent." Finally, some clinicians omitted to mention key reasons for referral that were clearly present at the time of referral and motivated the request but only became apparent during the course of the assessment. These unstated reasons for referral are labeled "implicit." Most cases had multiple reasons for referral, and thus the categories are not mutually exclusive.

The most common reasons for referral explicitly indicated by clinicians at the time of triage related to clinical issues they were experiencing with their patient such as cultural difference creating an uncertainty in the choice of treatment including medication choice (92%), uncertainty of diagnosis (50%), and experiencing problems with patient's treatment adherence (40%). The second most important category of explicit reasons presented at triage by referring clinicians involved problems related to clinical and interpersonal communication (communication 71%

and interpreter 12%). Intercultural communication issues occurred between clinicians and patient or between clinicians and the patient's family. Interpreter issues usually involved issues of access or availability, but in some cases, there were communication difficulties between clinician and interpreter with misunderstandings or misalliances (see Chapter 5). Difficulties experienced by the referring clinicians themselves (e.g., feeling lack of skill or competence to deal with problem or emotionally overwhelmed by patient's trauma history) were the explicit reasons for consultation in about 1/3 of cases.

The third most frequent category of problem we termed *systemic*. This involved issues related to bureaucratic procedures, practices, and demands of the health, social, educational, legal, or immigration systems. Systemic problems led in turn to other problems including the need for additional diagnosis, interpreters, and better intercultural communication. For example, a child who was having difficulty adjusting to the French school system (a provincial legal requirement for immigrant children in Québec) needed an educational assessment to determine if he was suffering from a learning disorder that would give clinical grounds to make an administrative appeal to allow him to attend school in English.

The consultation process itself sometimes revealed additional issues that had not been identified at triage that could account for the referral in about 1/3 of cases. These included issues the referring clinician was not aware of (termed *emergent* in Table 2.11) and those that the clinician likely knew but did not explicitly declare (termed *implicit*). These results suggest that in many cases, the specific reasons for referral were too complex to identify at triage and required more assessment. For example, a consultation request was identified at the moment of triage as a demand for clarification of whether the diagnosis of depression was accurate. The patient was the father of a family that had escaped an ongoing war in their country of origin. During the consultation process, the CCS team understood that the interpreter's lack of training in mental health had contributed to the diagnostic confusion because he had concealed information due to his concern

Table 2.11 Reasons for referral to the CCS of initial 52 cases

	Explicit		Emergent		Implicit	
	n	%	n	%	n	%
Treatment choice	48	92	0	0	0	0
Diagnosis unclear	26	50	5	10	0	0
Treatment adherence	21	40	0	0	0	0
Communication	37	71	4	8	2	4
Interpreter problem	6	12	4	8	0	0
Systemic problems	12	23	10	19	7	13
Inherent to patient	0	0	2	4	0	0
Referring professional	18	35	0	0	1	2
Total	168		25		10	

that the patient's family would be harshly judged or stigmatized. Once the CCS consultant addressed the concerns of the interpreter, the information required to make a diagnosis was readily obtained.

While their reasons for consulting the CCS were genuine, some clinicians did not reveal some of the key reasons motivating their referral. These reasons became apparent as information was collected on the case or, in some instances, because of general knowledge about changes in the health care system or obvious gaps in available services. We estimated that close to one-third of the requests for consultation at the CCS were also motivated by implicit reasons involving a hidden agenda. In most cases, it is likely that referring professionals did not disclose these reasons because they knew the CCS only accepted cases that clearly suggested a cultural component and that it did not provide post-consultation treatment for patients. Among the cases presenting implicit reasons, the most frequent issues were associated with the referring professional or to the health care system. Problems associated with the referring professional involved situations where clinicians either lacked confidence in their own ability to treat the patient or questioned the competence of another professional involved in the case. These issues were difficult for the clinician to disclose at the time of referral because doing so would threaten their clinical authority or undermine professional solidarity. Other implicit problems associated with the referring clinician involved cases where clinicians were confronted with challenges to some of their own assumptions, stereotypes, or prejudices regarding the cultural group of their patient. Clinicians may have been reluctant to reveal such biases because they are contrary to ethics or the professional ideal of affective neutrality (Williams, 2005). A second distinct category of implicit problem involved systemic issues. In all of these cases where they arose, implicit systemic problems were related to problems of accessibility to mental health services, particularly for asylum seekers or for those needing services in a specific language.

For 63% of cases, no new reasons were identified during the consultation, suggesting that the triage process often was sufficient to help the referring clinician accurately identify and articulate the basic needs for consultation. New reasons for consultation—of which neither the referring clinician nor the triaging psychologist had been aware—were identified through the consultation process in the remaining 37% of cases. The most common type of new problem was systemic (10/19 cases), involving availability of services, continuity of care, or dilemmas created by specific institutional practices. The systems involved included health and social services, education, legal, and immigration.

The relative lack of recognition of systemic problems may have to do with the tendency to attribute difficulties to characteristics of the patient rather than the system and to become habituated to or normalize everyday difficulties with the system. In five cases, new diagnostic issues were raised, including the need for specialized medical or neuropsychological evaluation to rule out organicity or intellectual impairment. Multiple new reasons (2–4) were identified for 12 cases (23%), indicating the complexity of issues that might have gone unrecognized without cultural consultation.

Implicit reasons for consultation were identified in 15/52 (29%) of cases. The most common implicit reasons involved problems that concerned referring clinicians themselves (10/15) or systemic issues (8/15). Implicit reasons for consultation related to the referring clinician and usually involved their own lack of confidence, comfort, or competence in dealing with the patient. In some cases, the referring clinician's implicit concern was with the competence of another professional, and the cultural consultation was seen as a way to document inadequate care and mobilize an alternative. Subtler cases involved challenges to clinicians' implicit assumptions about including cultural differences in gender roles, religious values, and issues of racism. Implicit problems related to systemic factors (found in 8/52 or % of cases) differed from those we identified as new problems in that there was some reason for the clinician to downplay or hide them. Generally, this was because the referring clinician was hoping to transfer the patient or obtain services for the patient that the CCS was not set up to provide, i.e., psychotherapy, long-term treatment, or case management. These cases are clear indicators both of problems in accessibility to services, lack of use of interpreters, insufficient training in cultural competence for primary care or mental health practitioners, or other gaps in the health care system.

Cultural consultation often facilitated the therapeutic alliance between the referring clinician or team and the patient. The referring clinicians' effort to seek a consultation may have demonstrated to the patient an interest in understanding the patient in his or her own cultural framework. The cultural formulation produced by the consultation made sense of the patient's puzzling or disturbing symptoms and behaviors by placing them in social and cultural context. This clarified the patient's predicament and thus increased the clinician's empathy for the patient. These issues sometimes encouraged agencies or clinics to take an interest in knowledge transfer and training on cultural competence as an underdeveloped agenda and broadened the use of existing community organizations working with minorities or providing additional skills to refugees or immigrants.

Cultural consultation also revealed the complexity of the case, transforming clinician's frustration into an appreciation of the intellectual and professional challenges presented by the case and so increasing clinician's interest and motivation to remain actively involved. Even where patients were not seen, the advice and reinterpretation of events provided by the CCS team worked to improve and maintain the referring clinician's treatment alliance and refine their diagnostic and treatment approach.

Conclusion

The CCS model uses outpatient consultation to support primary care clinicians and frontline mental health workers with the aim of improving the response to diversity in mainstream services. The CCS consultations to individual practitioners as well as case conferences and in-service training to clinics and organizations promote knowledge exchange. The CCS brought together local resources and, through a working group, developed an approach to cultural consultation built around the use of cultural consultants, culture brokers, and interpreters and organized in terms of a cultural formulation with specific recommendations to the referring clinician. The CCS assessment often results in changes in diagnoses and identifies important social and cultural issues that influence treatment and that may constitute important clinical problems in their own right. In general, referring clinicians find the service helpful for understanding complex cases, and there is some evidence the consultations can improve treatment engagement and adherence. Although it has not proved possible to conduct a rigorous outcome assessment at the level of patients health status owing to the great heterogeneity of patients referred and the time-limited intervention the CCS provides, as illustrated throughout this book, cultural consultation can have a dramatic impact on individual cases.

The analysis of cases seen in the Cultural Consultation Service and other transcultural clinics indicates that access to mental health care varies widely by linguistic and cultural background. In a significant number of cases, language barriers and the cultural complexity of the cases had prevented adequate assessment in conventional mental health care settings. The CCS was able to provide clinical reassessment and redirection of treatment in a substantial proportion of cases, and these interventions have been well received by referring clinicians. Although cultural consultations require substantial resources, in terms of specific expertise in cultural psychiatry as well as interpreters and culture brokers, the result of this intensive process is often a change in diagnosis and treatment plan with significant immediate and long-term consequences for patients' functioning, use of services, as well as clinician satisfaction.

References

Adeponle, A., Thombs, B., Groleau, D., Jarvis, G.E. & Kirmayer, L. J. (2012). Using the cultural formulation to resolve uncertainty in diagnosis of psychosis among ethnoculturally diverse patients. *Psychiatric Services, 63*(2), 147–153.

American Psychiatric Association. (2000). *Diagnostic and statistical manual (4th ed.), text revision (DSM-IV-TR)*. Washington, DC: American Psychiatric Press.

Bagilishya, D. (2000). Mourning and recovery from trauma: In Rwanda, tears flow within. *Transcultural Psychiatry, 37*(3), 337–354.

Beiser, M., Gill, K., & Edwards, R. G. (1993). Mental health care in Canada: Is it accessible and equal? *Canada's Mental Health, 41*(2), 2–7.

Bibeau, G. (2002). Fascination with the margin: Some aspects of the intellectual itinerary of Guy Dubreuil. *Transcultural Psychiatry, 39*(3), 376–393.

Bibeau, G., Chan-Yip, A., Lock, M., & Rousseau, C. (1992). *La santé mentale et ses visage: Vers un québec plus rythmique au quotidien*. Montréal, Quebec, Canada: Gaeten Morin.

Corin, E., Bibeau, G., Martin, J.-C., & Laplante, R. (1991). *Comprendre pour soigner autrement*. Montréal, Quebec, Canada: Presses de l'Université de Montréal.

Denzin, N. K. (1989). Strategies of multiple triangulation. In N. K. Denzin (Ed.), *The research act: A theoretical introduction* (3rd ed., pp. 234–247). Englewood Cliffs, NJ: Prentice-Hall.

Devereux, G. (1970). *Essais d'ethnopsychiatrie générale*. Paris, France: Gallimard.

Federal Task Force on Mental Health Issues Affecting Immigrants and Refugees. (1988). *After the door has been opened: Mental health issues affecting immigrants and refugees in Canada*. Ottawa, Ontario, Canada: Health and Welfare Canada.

Good, B. J. (1994). *Medicine, rationality, and experience: An anthropological perspective*. Cambridge, England: Cambridge University Press.

Good, B. J., Herrera, H., Good, M. J., & Cooper, J. (1982). Reflexivity and countertransference in a psychiatric cultural consultation clinic. *Culture, Medicine and Psychiatry, 6*(3), 281–303.

Green, J., & Thorogood, N. (2004). *Qualitative methods for health research*. Thousand Oaks, CA: Sage.

Groleau, D., & Kirmayer, L. J. (2004). Sociosomatic theory in Vietnamese immigrants' narratives of distress. *Anthropology & Medicine, 11*(2), 117–133.

Kirmayer, L. J., & Minas, H. (2000). The future of cultural psychiatry: An international perspective. *Cannadian Journal of Psychiatry, 45*(5), 438–446.

Kirmayer, L. J., & Rahimi, S. (1998). *Evaluation of the Australian transcultural mental health network Internet web site*. Montreal, Quebec, Canada: Division of Social & Transcultural Psychiatry, Department of Psychiatry, McGill University.

Kirmayer, L. J., Thombs, B. D., Jurcik, T., Jarvis, G. E., & Guzder, J. (2008). Use of an expanded version of the DSM-IV outline for cultural formulation on a cultural consultation service. *Psychiatric Services, 59*(6), 683–686.

Kirmayer, L. J., Weinfeld, M., Burgos, G., Galbaud du Fort, G., Lasry, J.-C., & Young, A. (2007). Use of health care services for psychological distress by immigrants in an urban multicultural milieu. *Canadian Journal of Psychiatry, 52*(4), 61–70.

Kirmayer, L. J., Young, A., Galbaud du Fort, G., Weinfeld, M., & Lasry, J.-C. (1996). *Pathways and barriers to mental health care: A community survey and ethnographic study* (Working Paper 6). Montreal, Quebec, Canada: Culture & Mental Health Research Unit, Institute of Community & Family Psychiatry, Sir Mortimer B. Davis—Jewish General Hospital.

Kleinman, A., & Good, B. (1985). *Culture and depression: Studies in the anthropology and cross-cultural study of depression*. Berkeley, CA: University of California Press.

Kleinman, A., & Kleinman, J. (1996, Winter). Social suffering. *Daedalus—Journal of the American Academy of Arts and Sciences, 125*, 1–24.

Lira, E., & Weinstein, E. (1984). *Psicoterapía y represión politica*. Mexico City, Mexico: Siglo Veintiuno.

Moro, M. R. (2000). *Psychothérapie transculturelle des enfants et des adolescents* (2eth ed.). Paris, France: Dunod.

Moro, M. R., & Rousseau, C. (1998). De la nécessité du métissage en clinique. *PRISME, 8*(3), 8–18.

Nathan, T. (1991). Modifications techniques et conceptuelles récemment apportées à la psychopathologie par la clinique ethnopsychoanalytique. *Psychologie Française, 36*(4), 296–306.

Nathan, T. (1994a). *L'influence qui guérit*. Paris, France: Éditions Odile Jacob.

Nathan, T. (1994b). Les bienfaits des thérapies sauvages. Thérapie scientifique et thérapie sauvage. *Nouvelle Revue d'Ethnopsychiatrie, 27*, 37–54.

Prince, R. H. (2000). Transcultural psychiatry: Personal experiences and Canadian perspectives. *Canadian Journal of Psychiatry, 45*(5), 431–437.

Rousseau, C., & Drapeau, A. (2002). Santé mentale. In Institut de la statistique Québec (Ed.), *Santé et bien-etre, immigrants récents au Québec: une adaptation reciproque? Étude auprès des communautés culturelles 1998–1999* (pp. 211–245). Montréal, Quebec, Canada: Les Publications du Québec.

Rousseau, C., & Drapeau, A. (2003). Are refugee children an at-risk group?: A longitudinal study of Cambodian adolescents. *Journal of Refugee Studies, 16*(1), 67–81.

Rousseau, C., & Drapeau, A. (2004). Premigration exposure to political violence among independent immigrants and its association with emotional distress. *The Journal of Nervous and Mental Disease, 192*(12), 852–856.

Rousseau, C., ter Kuile, S., Munoz, M., Nadeau, L., Ouimet, M. J., Kirmayer, L., et al. (2008). Health care access for refugees and immigrants with precarious status: Public health and human right challenges. *Canadian Journal of Public Health, 99*(4), 290–292.

Statistics Canada. No date. *Visible minority groups, 2006 counts, for Canada and census metropolitan areas and census agglomerations -20% sample data* (table). "Ethnocultural Portrait of Canada." "Highlight tables." "2006 Census: Data products." *Census.* Last updated October 6, 2010. http://www12.statcan.gc.ca/census-recensement/2006/dp-pd/hlt/97-562/pages/page.cfm?Lang=E&Geo=CMA&Code=01&Table=1&Data=Count&StartRec=1&Sort=2&Display=Page (accessed February 21, 2013).

Statistics Canada. (2012). *Montréal, Quebec (Code 462) and Quebec (Code 24) (table). Census Profile. 2011 Census.* Statistics Canada Catalogue no. 98-316-XWE. Ottawa. Retrieved October 24, 2012, from http://www12.statcan.gc.ca/census-recensement/2011/dp-pd/prof/index.cfm?Lang=E

Statistics Canada. (n.d.). *Population by immigrant status and period od immigration, 2006 counts, for Canada and census metropolitan areas and census agglomerations −20% sample data* (table). "Immigration and Citenzenship." "Highlight tables." "2006 Census: Data products." *Census.* Last updated March 27, 2009. Retrieved February 21, 2013, from http://www.statcan.gc.ca/pub/12-591-x/2009001/02-step-etape/ex/ex-census-recensement-eng.htm#a2

Sterlin, C. (2006). L'ethnopsychiatrie au Québec: Bilan et perspectives d'un temoin acteur clé [Ethnopsychiatry in Quebec: Assessment and perspective of a key actor and witness]. *Santé Mentale au Québec, 31*(2), 179–192.

Sterlin, C., Rojas-Viger, C., & Corbeil, L. (2001). *Rapport d'Évaluation de L'intervention Clinique du Module Transculturel Hôpital Jean-Talon* [Evaluation report of the clinical intervention of the transcultural module of Jean-Talon hospital]. Montreal, Quebec, Canada: Culture and Mental Health Research Unit.

Streit, U. (1997). Nathan's ethnopsychoanalytic therapy: Characteristics, discoveries and challenges to western psychotherapy. *Transcultural Psychiatry, 34*(3), 321–343.

Sturm, G., Nadig, M., & Moro, M. R. (2011). Current developments in French ethnopsychoanalysis. *Transcultural Psychiatry, 48*(3), 205–227.

Vinar, M., & Vinar, M. (1989). *Exil et torture.* Paris, France: Éditions Denoël.

Whitley, R., Kirmayer, L. J., & Groleau, D. (2006a). Understanding immigrants' reluctance to use mental health services: A qualitative study from Montreal. *Canadian Journal of Psychiatry, 51*(4), 205–209.

Whitley, R., Kirmayer, L. J., & Groleau, D. (2006b). Public pressure, private protest: Illness narratives of West Indian immigrants in Montreal with medically unexplained symptoms. *Anthropology & Medicine, 13*(3), 193–205.

Williams, S. J. (2005). Parsons revisited: From the sick role to…? *Health, 9*(2), 123–144.

Yin, R. K. (2008). *Case study research: Design and methods (applied social research methods)* (Vol. 5). Thousand Oaks, CA: Sage.

Zajde, N. (2011). Psychotherapy with immigrant patients in France: An ethnopsychiatric perspective. *Transcultural Psychiatry, 48*(3), 187–204.

The Process of Cultural Consultation

3

Laurence J. Kirmayer, G. Eric Jarvis,
and Jaswant Guzder

Introduction

In this chapter, we describe the process of
cultural consultations in terms of the specific
steps from intake and triage, through interviewing and clinical data collection, to case formulation, communication of recommendations, and
follow-up. Our aim is to provide sufficient detail
about the nuts and bolts of cultural consultation
and the actual process to help others wishing to
set up similar services.

The CCS team works within the framework of
the cultural formulation introduced with DSM-IV,
to identify ways that cultural background and
current contexts interact to shape the manifestations of illness, its course, and potential interventions. The aim is to complement standard
psychiatric evaluation by focusing on social and
cultural dimensions that may be less familiar and

that tend to get less attention in routine care.
The CCS consultants use models drawn from
cultural psychiatry and psychology, cognitive
behavioral therapy, family systems theory, and
ecosocial systemic approaches that emphasize
the social embedding of illness experience as
well as gender, racialized identity, and ethnicity
(see Chapters 7 and 8). Cases are formulated in
terms of the interplay of personal and social
meanings and dynamics that include interactions
with families, communities, health care, and systems. While the consultations use psychiatric
diagnostic categories (as presented in DSM-5
and ICD-10), they also explore the personal and
social meanings of symptoms and include a
broader problem list of social predicaments as
well as sources of resilience and potential strategies for healing and recovery. The cultural formulation brings together psychiatric and cultural
expertise in an integrated assessment and recommendations for more effective patient care.

The flow of patients through the CCS is
depicted in Fig. 3.1. The process begins with an
initial contact with the service by a referring
clinician. The CCS coordinator does an intake
and initial triage. The resource people needed to
assess the case are assembled, and meetings are
held with the patient and members of their entourage. An initial report and cultural formulation is
prepared, and preliminary recommendations are
conveyed to the referring clinician. The case is
presented at a weekly CCS meeting, where the
cultural formulation and recommendations are

L.J. Kirmayer, M.D. (✉) • G.E. Jarvis, M.D., M.Sc.
Culture and Mental Health Research Unit,
Institute of Community and Family Psychiatry,
Jewish General Hospital, 4333 Cote Ste Catherine Road,
Montreal, QC, Canada H3T 1E4
e-mail: laurence.kirmayer@mcgill.ca;
eric.jarvis@mcgill.ca

J. Guzder, M.D.
Center for Child Development and Mental Health,
Institute of Community and Family Psychiatry,
4335 Cote Ste Catherine Road, Montreal, QC,
Canada H3T 1E4
e-mail: jaswant@videotron.ca

L.J. Kirmayer et al. (eds.), *Cultural Consultation: Encountering the Other in Mental Health Care*,
International and Cultural Psychology, DOI 10.1007/978-1-4614-7615-3_3,
© Springer Science+Business Media New York 2014

Fig. 3.1 Flow diagram of
CCS procedure

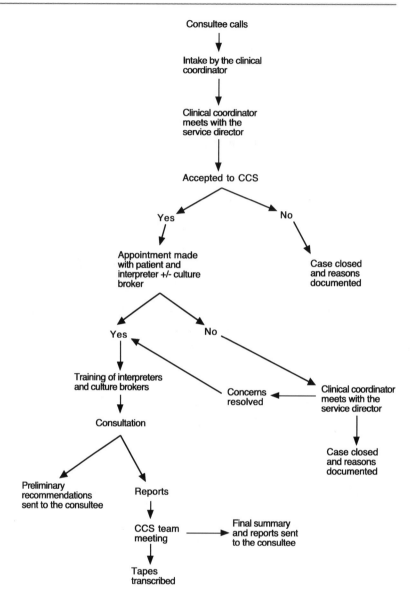

discussed and refined. The full consultation report is prepared and sent to the referring clinician, and appropriate follow-up is arranged. In the sections that follow, we discuss each of these steps in detail.

Before the Consultation Request

As discussed in Chapter 2, when the CCS was established, the availability of the service was announced by sending a mailing to all psychiatrists and psychologists in the province and contacting regional comprehensive community clinics. Since that time, referrals to the CCS have come mainly from institutions located in highly diverse neighborhoods of the city that maintain ongoing links with the CCS. The good experiences of other practitioners in the institution are the most effective "advertising" for the service. Invited talks and presentations at health care and social service institutions and ongoing training activities also serve to make the service visible and stimulate referrals.

The CCS sees many patients referred by clinicians in the community who request clarification of diagnosis and refinement of treatment planning. The need for cultural consultation arises from perceived problems in clinical work with patients and their families. For example, a clinician may encounter a patient with linguistic, religious, or culture differences sufficient to pose a dilemma for routine care or undermine the clinician's usual confidence in making an accurate diagnosis or implementing appropriate treatment. Obtaining an outpatient consultation involves time and effort, and there is no financial incentive for referring clinicians. In general, therefore, cases must be puzzling, severe, or worrisome enough to overcome the time pressures and constraints of routine clinical practice, which encourages efficiency rather than engaging in lengthy consultations. Hence, when a clinician decides to enlist the help of the CCS, the clinical dilemma usually has advanced to a critical point or impasse, and the clinician is casting about for new directions. As a result, referrals to the CCS often occur at a time of crisis and are conveyed with some urgency. Yet the problems are often long-standing and complicated, requiring careful inquiry to understand and address.

Intake and Triage

Initial inquiries about the CCS, as well as intake and triage of all cases, are handled by the CCS clinical coordinator. At the time of the establishment of the CCS, the coordinator was a clinical psychologist who was able to provide information and perform basic triage at the time of first contact. In recent years, the initial contact has been with a nonclinical coordinator who has a clerical/administrative position, and the coordinator has worked closely with the clinical director (a cultural psychiatrist) who performs triage. The administrative coordinator uses a structured intake form to collect information necessary to open a case file and guide initial triage. Separate forms are used to collect information on referrals of individuals, couples and families, and groups (see Appendix A).

The goal of the initial intake is to document the nature of the request and to assess whether it qualifies as an appropriate referral to the service. A standard procedure is followed to collect information and triage all cases:

1. The referring clinician, individual, or organization requesting the consultation is identified along with their contact information, institutional affiliation, and profession.
2. The identity (name, date of birth, migration status, country of origin, languages, ethnicity) and contact information for the patient and, if appropriate, their immediate family are recorded.
3. The primary case manager or practitioner following the patient in treatment is determined as a way of knowing to whom the recommendations should be directed and to ensure that the CCS can maintain its consultative role.
4. Other key people involved in the case are noted, e.g., social worker, lawyer, youth protection worker, and school contacts.
5. The reasons for the consultation request are recorded in an open-ended way, with additional questions to clarify and complete information regarding the circumstances of the patient and referral.
6. The referring clinician is then asked to specify the *cultural* reasons for which they were seeking consultation. If they are unclear, they may be read a list of options from which they can choose. They are encouraged to choose as many categories as apply to their request.
7. Referring clinicians are asked what their expectations are with respect to how the service might assist them. Again, referring clinicians are read a list of options from which they can choose. If they indicate they are requesting that the service takes over treatment of the patient, it is immediately clarified that our role is consultative.
8. In cases where the request for a consultation is not appropriate, the reasons why the request falls outside the role of the CCS is clarified, and the referring clinician is redirected to other resources. In some cases, the request can be addressed by providing information.

For example, common requests involve locating an interpreter or community resources to provide some social support or help navigating bureaucratic systems. Such interventions are recorded on the Limited Intervention Form (Appendix A). The CCS maintains a database of information on these resources and can direct the caller to the appropriate service.

9. If the consultation request falls within the scope of the CCS, the clinical coordinator clarifies whether the patient is aware that this request is being made and whether the referring clinician feels that the patient understands what the cultural consultation will involve. The clinical coordinator tells the referring clinician to advise the patient of the consultation and provides a brief description of the consultation process, as well as an indication of the length of time needed to arrange the consultation. A typical notification includes the following:

> Thank you for having referred your patient to the Cultural Consultation Service. Before Mr./Ms. [name of patient] arrives, we need you to tell him/her a little about our service. Please explain that he/she will be meeting with an evaluation team that may include a psychiatrist, an interpreter, and someone knowledgeable about your patient's culture to help us understand him/her better. There may be a student in attendance. The Cultural Consultation Service is a research clinic and periodically evaluates its effectiveness. In a few months, a research assistant will contact you to ask a few questions.

This procedure is essential to allow the coordinator to contact the patient to schedule an appointment as trouble free as possible.

10. Once the intake information has been gathered, the CCS coordinator contacts the patient by telephone to set up an appointment for the assessment. At this time, the coordinator outlines the steps in the consultation, indicates who will be present, and reassures the patient about confidentiality. The coordinator also greets patients when they arrive for their appointment and introduces patients and their families to the consulting team. At the end of the evaluation session, the research assistant is introduced to the patient to obtain informed consent and collect preliminary information for the ongoing evaluation of the CCS. The coordinator sets up follow-up appointments as needed. If at any stage, either the referring clinician or the patient no longer wishes to proceed with the consultation, the reasons for the refusal are recorded.

Based on the referral request, the clinical director determines the type of cultural consultation needed. Cultural consultations generally take one of three forms:

1. A direct assessment of a patient by a cultural consultant, interpreter, and/or culture broker preferably with the participation of the referring clinician. A complete assessment usually involves 1–3 meetings with the patient, a brief written report transmitting initial preliminary recommendations, followed by a clinical presentation to the team for discussion, and a longer cultural formulation report with a summary of final assessment and recommendations.

2. The second major form of consultation occurs strictly between the referring clinician and the cultural consultant, without the patient being seen directly. Typically, the referring clinician presents the case and the specific questions or concerns to be addressed during a clinical meeting in which the CCS team members and the invited consultant discuss the case to clarify social context, identify cultural issues, and develop recommendations for culturally appropriate clinical management and treatment interventions.

3. Some consultations involve recurrent problems affecting a series of cases, systemic or institutional issues, or the relationship of an organization to a cultural community. In this type of consultation, the focus may be on broader systemic issues rather than an individual case. The formulation, in these cases, aims to identify institutional strategies that can be used to improve cultural competence and safety.

Assembling the Consultation Team

Depending on the type of cultural consultation and details of the case obtained at the time of triage, the coordinator and director determine the specific resources needed for the case. These may include clinical consultants, interpreters, culture brokers, and other professionals or resource people from the community. Guidelines for working with interpreters and culture brokers are present in Table 3.1 and discussed in more detail in Chapters 6 and 7.

Table 3.1 Guidelines for working with interpreters and culture brokers

Before the interview

- Explain the goals of the interview to the interpreter or culture broker
- Clarify the roles of interpreter, culture broker, and clinician (to free the culture broker from language translation, an interpreter participates as well)
- Explain that the culture broker may ask questions during the evaluation depending on need but may also simply observe and provide background information and interpretation afterward during the debriefing or case conference outline the conduct of the interview (sequence of topics, tasks, etc.)
- Discuss the social position of the interpreter or culture broker in their country of origin and in local community in so far as it may influence the relationship with the patient
- Explain the need for literal translation in the mental status examination (e.g., to assess thought disorder, emotional range and appropriateness, suicidal intent)
- Ask for feedback when something is hard to translate
- Discuss etiquette and cultural expectations relevant to the interview process

During the interview

- Arrange seating (usually in a triangle)
- Introduce yourself and the interpreter or culture broker to the patient
- Discuss confidentiality and ask for patient consent to have the interpreter, culture broker, or others present
- Look at and speak to the patient; use direct speech ("you" instead of "she/he")
- Use clear statements in everyday language
- Slow down your pace; speak in short units
- Clarify ambiguous responses (verbal or nonverbal)
- Ask the patient for feedback to insure that crucial information has been accurately communicated
- Give the culture broker ample opportunity to seek clarification for issues that have not been addressed
- Give the patient ample opportunity to ask questions or express concerns that have not been addressed
- Some culture brokers may take over the interview in an inappropriate manner. In such cases, the lead clinician should call for a break in the interview to clarify the roles of the clinician and culture broker

After the interview

- Debrief the interpreter or culture broker to address any emotional reactions and concerns
- Discuss the process of the interview, any significant communication that was not translated, including paralanguage
- Assess the patient's degree of openness or disclosure
- Consider translation difficulties, misunderstandings
- Respond to questions the culture broker may have about the cultural formulation
- Review and itemize salient cultural themes with the culture broker for future reference
- Ask the culture broker if another meeting with the patient and family would be helpful
- Determine if future meetings would be best with the culture broker alone to foster open, uninterrupted communication with the patient and family
- Encourage the culture broker and address any doubts or discomfort about the intercultural work that must be done
- Explain to the culture broker that an honest evaluation of the patient's problems is crucial even if it portrays the culture of origin in a negative light
- Plan future interviews
- Work with the same interpreter/culture broker for the same case whenever possible

Adapted in part from Kirmayer, Rousseau et al. (2008)

When possible, the CCS team identifies a bilingual, bicultural mental health professional from a background similar to the patient to participate in the consultation process. Having a mental health expert who can communicate directly with the patient and provide the cultural context for illness, symptoms, and behaviors streamlines the process of clinical communication and cultural formulation. However, this only works when the clinician has a good understanding of the theory and conceptual models of cultural psychiatry and psychology so that they can link the clinical data with relevant aspects of the social and cultural context. Tacit knowledge of culture is not sufficient to work as a cultural mediator because cultural issues may be taken for granted, distorted, or ignored due to unexamined biases of the clinician. Hence, not every bilingual, bicultural clinician is equipped to contribute to cultural consultations. Moreover, given the high level of diversity among patients referred and the fact that many patients are from newer, smaller communities, patients often cannot be ethnically matched to a clinician. As a result, the CCS depends on a lead consultant who has broad knowledge of cultural psychiatry and who can work closely with an interpreter and culture broker throughout the consultation process.

As discussed in Chapter 5, language interpreting is essential for effective intercultural work and is an ethical imperative in health services. Information on language fluency is gathered for each patient at intake and reassessed during the consultation. As a matter of course, the CCS uses professional interpreters whenever it appears that the patient has less than perfect fluency in English or French. In fact, interpreters are offered even if patients prefer to conduct the interview in limited English or French unless they refuse outright. The availability of interpreters signals to the patient that they have options for communication. They may find it easier to express complex issues in their mother tongue, and in families with varying levels of language proficiency, the presence of the interpreter increases the likelihood that previously silent members of the family system will speak up. Throughout the health care system, interpreters are underutilized, and

for many patients seen by the CCS, this is the first opportunity to speak to professionals in their first language. Some patients have been moved to tears when finally offered services in a language of their choice.

There are many reasons for using professional interpreters rather than family members or other volunteers. Family members or other ad hoc or informal interpreters may not know how to translate language affected by severe symptoms, such as psychosis, and this can impede the diagnostic assessment. Nonprofessional interpreters may be embarrassed by material brought forward in the interview and may elect not to translate items that they feel should remain private. Even professional interpreters may be deeply affected by reports of trauma, suicide, marital infidelity, or aggression. Finally, it is possible that family members may be the direct cause of the patient's symptoms and have a stake in hiding their involvement, as in cases of domestic violence. Despite these issues, volunteer interpreters of convenience are frequently used in hospital settings. A key contribution of the CCS is the systematic use of professional interpreters who, over time, are well known to the service and can collaborate closely in the assessment process.

Cultural consultation often requires information about culture and social context that goes beyond what the patient and their family can provide even with the help of an interpreter. To provide this more detailed contextual information, the CCS employs culture brokers for most cases (see Chapter 6). Culture brokers or mediators are people with inside knowledge of the patient's culture of origin as well as some understanding of the concerns of mental health professionals and the local health care system. Often, culture brokers are professionals with a similar background to the patient. Sometimes they are academics (e.g., anthropologists, other social scientists) with extensive knowledge of the culture of specific geographic regions, ethnic groups, or communities. It is essential that they know about the current local context of the relevant migrant community rather than rely on idealized portraits drawn from the ethnographic literature. Culture brokers are important contributors to the consultation process, providing crucial background information and insights that help to situate the case in social and cultural context. Depending on their level of expertise, they may be asked to prepare the cultural formulation, which then becomes part of the overall assessment by the clinical consultant.

In some cases, the CCS contacts other community resource people including members of community organizations, religious or spiritual leaders, or others to provide additional background information or identify potential solutions for clinical problems. To protect confidentiality, this may involve a general inquiry or discussion without mentioning any details of a specific case. If clinical details need to be discussed, this contact is done with the express permission of the patient. Some patients may want to invite community or religious leaders to the consultation so that their interests and views may be better represented.

Meeting the Patients and Their Entourage

The CCS coordinator contacts the patient to set up a meeting time convenient to them and to the consulting team. Usually these meetings are held at the Institute for Community and Family Psychiatry, a separate building which houses the outpatient psychiatry department of the Jewish General Hospital, including the CCS. The CCS coordinator greets the patients and brings them to the office or meeting room of the consultant. After the first interview, the coordinator, or a research assistant, obtains consent for inclusion of the patient's information in the ongoing research program of the CCS.

The consultant comes to the meeting with a general notion of the consultation request (which may have been clarified by contact with the referring clinician), the sociodemographic background of the patient as conveyed through the triage process, the presenting problems, and a variable amount of history depending on the detail of the referral notes. This information has already been used to identify the appropriate interpreter and

culture broker or other resource people to participate in the assessment interview. However, much of this information may be imprecise and requires clarification with the patient.

Whenever possible, the consultant meets with the referring clinician, interpreter, and culture broker before seeing the patient to clarify their roles and modes of collaboration in the interview process. This is particularly important when the interpreter or culture broker has not worked with the CCS in the past. In some cases, the interpreter, culture broker, or a member of the referring clinical team has accompanied the patient to the interview, and the clinician usually will see them at the start to determine if there are specific issues to clarify or, less commonly, proceed immediately to introduce the patient to the evaluating team to insure they are comfortable with everyone present. Table 3.1 provides an overview of how to work with interpreters and culture brokers.

The initial discussion with the patient explains the nature of the CCS and the consultation process and explores their own understanding of the reasons for referral. This leads naturally to a discussion of patients' major concerns. Establishing the patients' own concerns and desire for help (which may differ substantially from the issues identified in the referral) is a crucial step in building a working alliance and the level of trust needed to collect information and, eventually, to convey recommendations to the patient and the referring clinical team. At the same time, patients are reminded that the consultation is confidential and nothing will be sent to other professionals without their consent.

Families play a central role in help-seeking for patients from many backgrounds. Although health care in North America tends to be focused on patients as individuals, engaging the family is essential both for proper assessment and to insure that interventions are acceptable and effective. Entering, engaging, and joining with the family are clinical skills derived from family therapy that are essential for the assessment process in cultural consultation (see Chapter 7).

Members of the referring treatment team are encouraged to accompany the patient to the consultation. These clinicians have essential information needed to understand the reasons for consultation and to develop solutions. They often have long-standing and complex relationships with the patient and, at times, have their own agendas that may conflict with or eclipse the patient's primary concerns. It is important to strike a balance between collaborating with the referring clinician—seeing the case from their point of view, since they are, in a sense, the client in the consultation and one of the principal aims of consultation is to increase their cultural competence—and recognizing that the referring clinician and team are part of an interactional system with its own dynamics (see, e.g., Chapters 13 and 15). Sometimes the problems identified in cultural consultation are located in interactions of the referring team or institution with the patient or even in the referring team's internal dynamics. These systemic issues must not be misattributed to the patient, but they must be explored in a way that is respectful and nonthreatening for the clinicians who may be implicated and whose involvement will be important for any subsequent intervention.

Culturally Oriented Interviewing

DSM-IV introduced an outline for cultural formulation listing key areas of information useful in clinical assessment (American Psychiatric Association, 2000). This outline is organized in terms of four broad areas: (1) cultural identity of the individual, (2) cultural concepts of illness and help-seeking, (3) cultural dimensions of functioning and psychosocial stressors and supports, and (4) the clinician–patient relationship. Information about these areas is integrated into a case formulation with implications for diagnosis, prognosis, and treatment. The CCS has employed a modified version of this outline with additional issues addressing developmental history, migration trajectory, the role of religion and spirituality, and social structural adversities. Table 3.2 presents the current version of this outline. The outline serves as a useful reminder of key areas to explore in clinical assessment and a standard way to present the findings. However, the sequence in which specific topics are addressed and the way they are phrased will vary depending on the characteristics and concerns of the patient and consultant as well as the unfolding process of the interview.

Cultural Identity of the Individual

This first section of the cultural formulation describes the individual's main ethnic, linguistic, religious, or cultural reference groups. This includes the patient's self-identification and affiliation as well as personal and family background (which they may no longer identify with or, indeed, may be at odds with) and also categories that others may use to label or characterize the patient. Identity may be rooted in place of birth of self or family, religion, caste, spirituality, sexual orientation, occupation, or other affiliations. For migrants and racialized or ethnic minorities, the level of identification and involvement with the culture of origin and with the host culture or majority culture are both important. Answers to questions about identity are relative to the context and the patient's perception of the interlocutor. Thus, someone may identify as "Caribbean" or "West Indian" to a Euro-Canadian interviewer, but give more detail in terms of country, region, or parish to others from the same background. Identity is relevant to clinical care because it may influence patients' relationships with others in local social worlds, links to communities, access to resources, as well as developmental pathways and current predicaments. Language abilities, preferences, and patterns of use are especially important for identifying potential barriers to care, social integration, and the clinical need for an interpreter.

Cultural Conceptualizations of Distress

This section of the cultural formulation describes personal and cultural modes of expressing distress and symptoms, models of illness, and patterns and expectations for help-seeking.

Table 3.2 Outline for cultural formulation

I. Cultural identity of the individual

- Racial, ethnic, or cultural reference groups that may influence the patient's relationships with others, access to resources, and developmental and current challenges, conflicts, or predicaments
- For migrants, the degree and kinds of involvement with both the culture of origin and the host culture or majority culture should be noted separately
- Language abilities, preferences, and patterns of use are relevant for identifying issues access to care, social integration, and the need for an interpreter
- Other clinically relevant aspects of identity including religious affiliation, socioeconomic background, personal and family places of birth, and growing up, migrant status, and sexual orientation

II. Cultural conceptualizations of distress

- Cultural constructs that influence how the patient experiences, understands, and communicates their symptoms or problems to others
- Cultural syndromes, idioms of distress, and explanatory models or perceived causes
- Level of severity and meaning of the distressing experiences should be assessed in relation to the norms of the person's cultural reference groups
- Coping and help-seeking experiences including the use of professional as well as traditional, alternative, or complementary sources of care

III. Psychosocial stressors and cultural features of vulnerability and resilience

- Key stressors and supports in the individual's social environment (which may include both local and distant events)
- Experiences of racism and discrimination in the larger society
- Role of religion, family, and other social networks (e.g., friends, neighbors, co-workers) in providing emotional, instrumental, and informational support
- Cultural norms for family structure, developmental tasks, and community relationships
- Levels of functioning, disability, and resilience in relation to cultural norms and expectations for patient's gender, age, and social roles and status

IV. Cultural features of the relationship between the individual and the clinician

- Expectations for care and models and metaphors of helper or healer roles
- Differences in culture, language, and social status between a patient and clinician that may cause difficulties in communication and influence diagnosis and treatment
- Experiences of racism and discrimination in the larger society that may impede establishing trust and safety in the clinical diagnostic encounter
- Unrealistic expectations of the clinician by the patient and family

V. Overall cultural assessment

- Implications of the components of the cultural formulation identified in earlier sections of the outline for diagnostic assessment and treatment
- Other clinically relevant issues or problems as well as appropriate management and treatment intervention

Adapted from the CCS Handbook, Mezzich et al. (2009) and DSM-5 (2013)

Patients may use a variety of illness models to think about illness, including simple recollections of past experience, prototypes based on personal and popular examples, and explicit notions of causal mechanisms. Cultural models may be rooted in particular ontologies that include the role of spirits, ancestors, or other active agents in causing illness or promoting healing. These explanations or attributions influence help-seeking and expectations for care. Coping and help-seeking with persistent symptoms commonly involve the use of multiple resources including health care professionals as well as practitioners of traditional, alternative, or complementary medicine, religious and spiritual practices, and community organizations.

Psychosocial Stressors and Cultural Features of Vulnerability and Resilience

The third section of the cultural formulation identifies key stressors and supports in the individual's social environment (which may include local and distant events) and the role of religion, family, and other social networks (e.g., friends, neighbors, co-workers) in providing emotional, instrumental, and informational support. Social stressors and social supports reflect specific expectations and demands associated with culturally prescribed developmental tasks, family structure, and life cycle rituals. Levels of functioning, disability, and resilience should be assessed in light of the person's cultural reference groups and age- and gender-related norms.

Cultural Influences on the Relationship Between the Individual and the Clinician

This section of the cultural formulation addresses the impact of culture and context on the clinician–patient interaction. Consultant and patient each brings their identities in the larger social world into the consulting room, and their perceptions of each other influence the working alliance. Differences between patient and clinician in social status, ethnicity, religion, and racialized identity may cause difficulties in communication and impede establishing the trust and open communication needed for accurate diagnosis and effective treatment. Patients' views of the clinician may be influenced by past experiences with institutions and other health care systems, as well as cultural models of the appropriate role of a helper or healer.

Overall Cultural Assessment

The overall assessment summarizes the implications of the information collected in earlier sections of the outline for psychiatric diagnosis as well as a broader problem list of clinically relevant issues. The formulation includes considerations of how best to approach the patient, social implications of the illness, resources of healing and recovery, as well as appropriate management and treatment strategies. Examples of a brief and full formulation are presented in Appendices B and C.

Although it was introduced over 20 years ago, the cultural formulation has not become a routine aspect of psychiatric assessment and care in most settings. In part, this may be because it was presented as an outline with little indication of how to use it. To promote the use of the cultural formulation, DSM-5 has introduced a brief cultural formulation interview (CFI) with 16 questions that provide a simple way to begin this type of inquiry (American Psychiatric Association, 2013). There is also a version of the CFI designed to elicit similar information from a key informant or accompanying person. A series of supplementary modules explore dimensions of the cultural formulation in more depth, giving examples of ways to inquire in more detail about explanatory models of illness, levels of functioning, social networks, psychosocial stressors, religion and spirituality, cultural identity, coping and help-seeking, and the patient–clinician relationship. Three modules address specific populations, with versions for children and adolescents, the elderly, and immigrants and refugees. A final module is addressed to caregivers and aims to elicit their own concerns as well as pertinent information about the context of caregiving and social support for the patient.

CCS consultants contributed to the development of the CFI in DSM-5, incorporating elements of the interview methods used in conducting cultural consultations. In general, the aim of culturally oriented interviewing is to explore each dimension of cultural identity, background, illness experience, help-seeking, coping, and adaptation. While many patients appreciate clinicians' interest in their background and history, it may not be immediately obvious to patients why these contextual details are relevant to their care. When patients have experienced stigma or discrimination or seen negative portrayals of their ethnic group or collective identity in the media, they may view questions about their background as invasive and threatening. The clinician should be prepared to explain why a particular aspect of the patient's background is potentially important for clinical care.

Generally, it is best to begin the assessment with questions about the patient's presenting problems, concerns, and reasons for referral. Understanding this in detail will clarify the goals of the consultation, establish a common ground for further inquiry with the patient, and lead naturally to questions about the wider context. For example, exploring experiences of somatic symptoms or emotional distress leads naturally to questions about coping, the responses of others in the family or other social settings, past experiences with help-seeking and treatment, and concerns about the future. Furthermore, listening attentively to the patient's concerns, and displaying sincere interest and intention to help in a safe and confidential setting, establishes a trusting clinical alliance that can facilitate open discussion of sensitive topics.

The CCS inquiry aims to provide a clear picture of the patient's problems and potential solutions in social context. To that end, it is important that the clinician clarify unfamiliar or obscure details with the patient or others. This requires lines of questioning specific to each case, but the effort to clarify and understand must always be mindful of the patient's comfort and confidence in the clinician–patient relationship.

Areas of ambiguity usually remain, even after much inquiry, for reasons related to the clinician, the patient, and the context. The clinician may lack enough familiarity with the patient's background or lifeworld to know what questions to ask or may assume similarity or shared experience when there are actually differences. Intercultural work requires great patience and a high degree of tolerance for ambiguity and uncertainty. Clinicians may find this uncertainty threatening to their sense of competence and may push for clarity and closure before sufficient information has been collected. Finally, clinicians may find certain issues like racism or religious practices difficult to broach because of concern for patients' feelings or their own unexamined attitudes. All of these areas require training to attain a level of self-knowledge and skill needed to conduct the cultural assessment.

For their part, patients may find it difficult to clarify crucial elements of their cultural background and current context for similar reasons. They may not realize that the clinician does not share some of their experiences or that certain terms or concepts have different meanings across cultures. They may find certain lines of inquiry difficult to respond to because of strong emotions, fear of public exposure, and embarrassment or humiliation. Much cultural knowledge is tacit, so that patients may not be able to articulate the underlying conceptual models or values. Moreover, we are all embedded in social structures which may be hidden or taken for granted but that powerfully shape our experience. These structural dimensions are often crucial to understanding the social determinants of health. For example, hierarchies of power and inequities in health associated with racialized identities, caste, gender, and religious authority may all be viewed as simple facts about the world. Cultural ideologies may actually obscure rather than reveal these structural issues, since one function of culture is to normalize, legitimate, and maintain existing social arrangements. Adequate understanding of these structural dimensions of experience must then come from reflection by those who stand with one foot outside the system and can offer a self-critical perspective. For this reason, cultural consultation benefits from multiple perspectives and requires models of the determinants of health derived from research and critical analysis.

The third set of challenges in clarifying the nature of social and cultural issues in consultation stem from institutional constraints. Inquiry into social and cultural issues can be time consuming and resource intensive, requiring specific expertise and the use of interpreters, culture brokers, and others in multiple meetings with patients, their families, and service providers. Moreover, institutions may resist efforts to include attention to their own internal dynamics or position in the larger society as an essential component of the patient's predicament.

Preparing a Cultural Formulation

Cultural consultation aims to collect information needed to situate the patients' problems and concerns in social and cultural context. The cultural formulation brings this information together in a narrative with a summary that identifies key issues and implications for diagnosis, prognosis, and intervention. In routine care, the cultural formulation may be integrated into the text of standard medical reports with elements in the history of present illness; past medical history; developmental, family, and social histories; and the mental status examination. The relevant cultural issues can then be brought forward in the case formulation. At the CCS, this format is sometimes used by bilingual, bicultural consultants who do not need a culture broker and who weave the cultural information throughout their psychiatric evaluation.

More often, the CCS presents the cultural formulation as a separate report that accompanies a standard psychiatric evaluation. The report follows the outline for the cultural formulation (Table 3.2) and ends with the summary of key issues. During the clinical case conference, the formulation is integrated with findings from the general psychiatric evaluation to reach specific diagnostic impressions and treatment recommendations for the referring clinician.

The formulation is not simply a list of salient features of the patient's cultural background and current context but focuses on specific issues relevant to diagnosis, prognosis, and treatment. Some cultural information is important because it is central to patients' self-understanding and therefore plays an essential role in person-centered care (Mezzich et al., 2010). Acknowledging the patient's own models of illness and core cultural values and allegiances is essential to insure a sense of recognition and responsiveness in the clinical encounter and provide a basis for collaboration and negotiation of clinical goals. Consultation work also requires close attention to the concerns of the referring clinician. There may be aspects of culture that are issues for the clinician but not the patient. For example, clinicians may find the patient's behavior hard to understand, and the consultation aims to explain these by putting them in context (see Chapter 15).

However, the clinically relevant facets of culture and context include issues that are important not because of their salience for the patient or the referring clinician but because they may play a role in specific processes that contribute to psychopathology, disability, healing, and recovery. Although a sensitive clinician can elicit the patient's concerns, cultural formulation requires attention to a broad range of contextual issues, some of which may be outside of the patient's awareness. Recognizing which elements are relevant depends on knowledge of the role of social and cultural factors in psychopathology. This requires familiarity with the research literature on cultural psychiatry, which can be found in scientific journals and textbooks. To produce a clinically useful formulation, cultural information must be organized and interpreted in terms of models of psychopathology and healing. These may be framed in terms of developmental processes, the dynamics of family systems, narrative and discursive processes of self-fashioning, and social contextual factors that influence identity and adaptation. The cultural consultant uses knowledge of the relevance of specific social and cultural determinants of health to guide the clinical inquiry and to construct a problem list and formulation that relates the particulars of the patient's cultural background and current social context to their health problems and potential solutions.

The Case Conference

Almost all cases referred to the CCS are discussed at a weekly multidisciplinary case conference. In addition to the consultant, the meeting usually includes the culture broker and students or trainees from psychiatry, psychology, nursing, social work, and social sciences. The referring clinician and their team are invited but are not often able to attend. This meeting allows the consultant to obtain the perspectives of participants from different personal and professional backgrounds to refine the cultural formulation. When the referring clinician or members of the patient's treatment team are present, the meeting also serves as an opportunity for clarifying details about the case, more general knowledge exchange and learning about the referring clinicians' perspectives, addressing their concerns, and engaging them in developing a treatment plan.

The clinical director, or other senior consultant, chairs the CCS case conferences. The format of the meeting usually involves an introduction of people present. The referring clinician or representative of the clinical team, if present, may then be asked to outline the reasons for consultation. They may also add clinical updates about the patient since the last CCS evaluative session. When the referring clinician is not present, the CCS consultant presents the case following the usual format of a medical or psychiatric case history. The consultant or the culture broker then presents the findings of the cultural formulation. The referring clinician, if present, may ask questions or make clarifications throughout this process. The implications for diagnosis and the specific referral questions (e.g., understanding specific symptoms, improving the clinical alliance, or addressing obstacles to treatment adherence) are then discussed. The chair of the meeting then summarizes the main findings and conclusions and outlines the final diagnosis and recommendations to be sent to the referring clinician.

When the referring clinician is present, the meeting process is more complicated and has elements of an intervention. The chair of the meeting must pay close attention to the dynamics of the meeting, insuring that the referring clinician is engaged, their concerns elicited, and their questions addressed which being overwhelmed with extraneous detail or emotionally challenging material. Because the systemic analysis of cases often implicates interactional issues between clinician and patient or within the health care system, the referring clinician may feel challenged or even criticized. It is essential that any critique be presented in a respectful way so that the clinician feels empowered and enabled to respond adequately to the situation. The aim of the CCS is not to take over the care of patients but to enable the referring clinical team to provide culturally appropriate care and to increase their capacity to deal with similar cases in the future.

Although the CCS clinical director, a psychiatrist, chairs the meetings, the use of the cultural formulation as a framework for presenting infor-

mation and the focus of the CCS on social and cultural context gives a prominent place in the discussion to the perspectives of participants from other disciplines, like nursing and social work, that focus on experiential and social contextual issues (Dinh, Groleau, Kirmayer, Rodriguez, & Bibeau, 2012). The CCS case conference thus shifts the usual dominance of psychiatric perspectives toward a broader view that generates a clinical problem list that includes practical social issues and predicaments central to the patient's health and well-being. The cultural formulation provides a way to think about systemic issues in the health care system and encourages participants to identify gaps and issues that can be addressed through changes in policy and practice (see Chapter 16).

The CCS case conferences also serve an educational function for participants. We encourage students in health and social sciences to attend. Listening to the discussion helps them to understand clinical styles of reasoning and the challenges of applying social science perspectives to everyday clinical practice. Finally, the case conference meetings are audio-recorded (with the consent of all participants) and transcribed for ongoing research on cultural formulation (Adeponle, Thombs et al., 2012; Dinh et al., 2012).

Communicating with Referring Clinicians

Cultural consultation can be a lengthy process. To meet the needs of referring clinicians, CCS consultants prepare a brief preliminary report after the initial assessment of the patient (see Appendix B). This is usually less than one page in length and consists of key findings, preliminary diagnosis, and immediate recommendations. Giving this initial information to the referring clinician allows them to address urgent issues and sets the stage for the more detailed consultation that may follow weeks later (Appendix C).

As mentioned, referring clinicians are encouraged to participate in the CCS assessment interviews and the case conference. Taking part in the assessment interviews provides many benefits for the referring clinician. They can ask their own questions and clarify any issues that are unclear. They become more familiar with the use of interpreters and culture brokers and establish their own links with these resources. Finally, their presence signals engagement in the case and may allow the consultation process to strengthen the working alliance. Of course, the presence of the referring clinician also complicates the interaction, and the consultant must manage the multiple and sometimes conflicting agendas of members of the referring clinical team, the patient, and their entourage. When the clinician takes part in the assessment, the CCS consultant usually meets with them immediately before the evaluation to clarify the reason for referral and afterward for debriefing.

Referring clinicians are also encouraged to take part in the CCS case conference, and this also affords them an opportunity to raise further questions and concerns. Often the primary care physician involved in the case cannot attend because of other time pressures, but one or more representatives of the team working with the patient are present. This allows the CCS consultant a chance to further assess systemic and institutional issues during the case discussion. Throughout, the aim is to understand the patient's problems in context and support the frontline workers in developing more culturally appropriate care rather than to critique the work of community clinicians.

Follow-Up

Most often the CCS consultation process involves only a single encounter with the patient and their entourage or, when more extensive assessment is needed, a series of two to three meetings over a short period of time. The service does not have the mandate or resources to provide ongoing services. Rarely, however, the CCS may be involved in repeated consultations or short-term treatment. This occurs when there is a good fit between the consultant and patient (e.g., ethnocultural match), and no other resources are available. On some occasions, this has led to long-term treatment of complex cases (see, e.g., Chapters 7 and 8).

The CCS remains available to support the referring clinician. This usually involves brief telephone contacts to provide specific information or suggestions. The clinician may also arrange to attend a CCS case conference to present new information and discuss the implications. When there are significant changes in the patient's condition or an unsatisfactory outcome from the initial consultation, a follow-up consultation may be arranged to clarify the issues. In some cases, complicated problems persist, and a patient is referred multiple times for follow-up consultations. As a result, the CCS may stay involved with some cases for several years.

A major goal of the CCS is to improve the cultural competence of frontline clinicians, mental health practitioners, and institutions. To that end, the CCS provides in-service training and uses consultations as opportunities for knowledge exchange. When certain types of problems recur in a particular organization or institution setting, the CCS may offer or be asked to provide in-service training to address relevant issues. These consultations aim to support organizational cultural competence and cultural safety (Brascoupé & Waters, 2009; Fung, Lo, Srivastava, & Andermann, 2012).

Evaluation of clinical services is also an essential component of the work of the CCS as we strive to establish the utility of cultural consultation in terms of its impact on patient care, clinician and organizational cultural competence, and health outcomes. Chapter 2 presents the findings from the initial evaluation of the CCS. This work is ongoing and integrated into the protocols and procedures of the service.

Dilemmas in Cultural Consultation

Obtaining a consultation through the CCS can be a slow process, sometimes taking weeks to organize. Referring clinicians, family members, language interpreters, and culture experts must be identified, contacted, recruited (by explaining what the CCS does and the specific role they are being asked to play in the consultation), and offered a mutually convenient time to meet together. The setting of the evaluation may need to be negotiated according to the needs of the patient and the family. Along the way, treating clinicians may not see the utility of attending the consultation and may prefer that it takes place without them, or the patient may suddenly cancel the appointment at the last moment for reasons that are often unclear. Each disruption adds time to the already lengthy and sometimes frustrating procedure. Once the first evaluation takes place, further disruptions are common: patients or family members may arrive late, up to hours or even days after the scheduled time; patients may feel uncomfortable having interpreters or other members of the consultation team in attendance; or the patient's distress may be so overwhelming as to preclude meaningful assessment. After the evaluation begins, working through an interpreter may slow the clinical work down considerably, adding to the time of a regular evaluation (National Association of Community Health Centers, 2008). Often, after interviewing a patient the first time, it becomes clear that key family members or other informants are missing, thereby requiring a follow-up meeting and starting the whole process over again. All of these factors work against the model of routine psychiatric consultations that take place according to a predictable 50-minute hour.

While a basic cultural formulation should be part of routine clinical care, the cases seen by the CCS usually demand more in-depth work. The intensive nature of cultural consultation in terms of personnel, time, and resources and the high level of clinical skill needed to provide effective consultation are challenges to its implementation. Institutions may be reluctant to commit resources to clinical services perceived to be peripheral to the core tasks of mental health care. However, as illustrated in many of the clinical vignettes throughout this volume, the CCS works with very challenging cases where there are serious impasses. The time and effort required to understand the problem in context are well repaid when seemingly intractable problems are resolved and clinicians are empowered to respond more effectively to diversity.

Conclusion

We have outlined the process of cultural consultation in some detail to give a clear sense of what is involved. The approach we describe is pragmatic and can be adapted to a wide variety of settings based on demand and available resources. Other chapters in this book show how this process can give rise to new insights and reformulation of complex cases in ways that enhance clinicians' cultural competence, while improving the quality of care and clinical outcomes for patients.

Appendix A: CCS Intake Information

CCS

CULTURAL CONSULTATION SERVICE
NEW INTAKE FORM part 1 - Individuals

Type of case: # -

Date of referral(mm/dd/yy):	○ Urgent ○ Not urgent ○ ASAP

Referred by (Name & Institution)	Institution Type	Tel.
	Referrer 1 Type	
	Referrer 2 Type	Fax.

Principale Care Provider or Case Manager:	Tel.:
Others involved in Patient Care:	Tel.:

Patient's Family Name (Maiden Name)	First name

Address:	○ Male ○ Female ○ Other
Zip:	DOB(mm/dd/yy): Age:

Tel. (H): (W):	Marital Status:
Other Contact:	
	Med. No. Exp.
Immigrant Status:	

Country of origin:	Patient's Medical Insurance Coverage
Year of arrival (yyyy): Month (mm):	○ None ○ Private Plan
	○ Fed. Refugee Plan ○ DK
Ethnicity:	○ Prov. Gov. Plan ○ Other...

Mother tongue:	Education Level: Nb of years:
Speaks English? French?	

Other Languages Spoken	Empl. Status:
	Occupation:
	Religion:

Do you think the patient needs an interpreter?	○ NO ○ YES ○ DK	If yes, preferred language:
Have you been using an interpreter for this patient?	○ NO ○ YES ○ DK	If YES, language:

Why has an interpreter NOT been used? :	☐ Not Available ☐ Clinician acted as interpreter ☐ Not Needed ☐ Other...

Comments:

Appendix B: Example of a Brief Consultation Report

CCS Preliminary Recommendations	Name of Patient: SMITH, George Date of Birth: Medicare No.: CCS Case #:

Date of Referral:

Referred by: Dr. X, Psychiatrist, Hospital Y (Department Z)

Reason for Referral: Clarify contribution of cultural and religious beliefs to patient's symptoms and help-seeking behavior.

Impression:

Mr. Smith is a 31-year-old married, Haitian, Baptist man suffering from recently decreased sleep and an exacerbation of somatic and persecutory delusions, likely somatic illusions and/or hallucinations, and possible visual illusions.

There is a history of command auditory hallucinations although the patient denies auditory hallucinations today. He has been hospitalized twice previously, initially in 2012, with diagnoses including schizophreniform disorder, schizophrenia, schizoaffective disorder, and depression with psychotic features, with the most recent diagnosis being psychosis NOS. Previous chart notes indicate a limited functional capacity since the onset of illness, with abilities confined to caring for his home, and at least one illness exacerbation in the context of his children returning home from foster care.

Ms. Smith understands his problem as related to Vodou and believes the solutions available to him are prayer, Vodou-related treatments, and biomedicine. He describes his wife and their church in Montreal as identifying with a Baptist view of healing and says that they see his beliefs as evidence of mental illness, while family in Haiti seems to be more accepting of the idea that Vodou is contributing to his illness, although it is unclear to what extent they use that explanatory framework to understand all of the patient's symptoms.

Exacerbating factors may include a recent move, a change in his treatment team with less intensive follow-up, and possibly a change in medication. There may also be stress within the family, given the disagreements about the etiology of his symptoms and the appropriateness of various treatments.

It is important to note that Vodou in Haiti, while being tolerated to some degree by the Catholic Church, is eschewed as evil by most Protestant groups. This might be a source of family conflict and distress for the patient, exacerbating his symptoms.

The current working diagnosis is acute psychosis, due to exacerbation of paranoid schizophrenia.

Recommendations:

1. We will follow-up with the patient and his wife, to clarify her understanding of his illness, current functioning at home, premorbid functioning, their migration history, and whether he has any medical conditions that may need further medical attention.
2. Clarify current medication dosage (chart not available to us). We suggest increasing the dosage or switching to a different medication to control the patient's symptoms. He previously

responded to risperidone 3 mg, but this was discontinued due to hyperprolactinemia.

3. We recommend more intensive follow-up of the patient and his family by the referring team.

4. We will explore with the patient and her wife a possible renegotiation of illness explanatory frameworks and help-seeking behaviors, in order to ameliorate communication within the family and with the larger community and to facilitate coping.

Date of Consultation:

Consultant: (Signed) _____

Appendix C: Example of a Cultural Formulation

A. Cultural Identity

1. **Cultural reference group(s)**

   Mr. Smith self-identifies as a Haitian, Baptist. His mother converted from Catholicism to Protestantism following an illness, after which her children converted as well. Mr. Smith's wife, however, is Protestant from birth. Mr. Smith says that while his mother sometimes left Protestantism, she herself "never did."

2. **Language(s)**

   Mr. Smith speaks Haitian Creole and French; he has a secondary 3 equivalent education in Creole.

3. **Cultural factors in development**

   Mr. Smith immigrated to Canada in 2004. No other information available on developmental milestones or education.

4. **Involvement with culture of origin**

   a. **Contact with family or friends in country of origin**

   Mr. Smith has regular phone contact with his family of origin in Haiti. Friends, relatives, and members of their congregation visit the family frequently to help with his difficulties.

   Diaspora Haitians often interact closely with family members back home. Many have relatives living in high-income countries, and the diaspora sends more than US$800 million annually to family and friends in Haiti. Mr. Smith says he sends money back home, but, in his case, he does not feel this is an obligation.

   b. **Involvement with community organizations**

   Nil—see below

   c. **Does patient attend a group with peers of his culture of origin (e.g., religious organization or leisure setting)?**

   Mr. Smith participates actively in a Baptist Church, both religious services and some social activities. He has considerable contact with other congregants. The pastor calls on his home regularly to see how he is doing.

   d. **Does patient have friends from his culture of origin?**

   Mr. Smith mostly socializes with Haitians and has many acquaintances in the community; he does not have close friends.

   e. **Does patient socialize with extended family members?**

   He has a large extended family with whom he speaks with regularly and has aunts in a nearby city that he sees occasionally.

   f. **What is patient's perception of his culture of origin?**

   Mr. Smith appears to identify positively with being Haitian.

5. **Involvement with host culture**

   Besides attending hospital appointments and group therapy sessions, Mr. Smith does not interact in a sustained fashion with the host culture. These interactions are relatively superficial. Prior to his illness, he worked at a car wash, in a warehouse, and a convenience store, all of which include other employees from diverse backgrounds. There is no evidence of a negative perception or experiences with the host culture.

   The patient's wife is more extensively involved in the host culture. She has worked as a cashier and as a hairdresser.

Although there is racism against people of African descent in Quebec, there is also a fairly close relationship and affinity between Quebec and Haiti, based to some extent on a common language (French). Quebec has a relatively large Haitian population with about approximately 100,000 Haitians in Montreal (Lecomte & Raphaël, 2011, p. 4). There is also a fairly close relationship between Canada and Haiti: a former governor general of Canada (Michaëlle Jean) was born in Haiti, and Haiti is second after Afghanistan in the amount of development assistance received from Canada.

B. Cultural Explanations of the Illness

1. **Predominant idioms of distress and illness categories and perceived causes and explanatory models (mechanism, treatment)**

Mr. Smith's narrative is that "un mauvais esprit" has been waking him up at midnight, persecuting him, by walking around in his throat and stomach. He says she saw a cockroach—which is an embodiment of the evil spirit—coming out of his tongue as he was brushing it. Mr. Smith believes that a woman, with whom he used to be friends, wants him to die and made him mentally ill. Mr. Smith's problems seem to have been exacerbated by the fact that this friend lived with his family for a while. Mr. Smith says that he is fighting this but that the woman was jealous and acquired power over the patient by taking his clothes and letting his sweat touch her skin. In retrospect, the patient believes that during the period of time when this woman lived with him, she gave him potions to drink that made him ill and unable to gain weight from food. When the family went to Haiti together recently, Mr. Smith underwent *lavements* (cleansings) given by a Protestant group. These *lavements* helped him—he defecated bad things, an evil spirit, and the whole family believed he was healed. Mr. Smith believes he was victorious in his fight against the woman who had been harassing him, and therefore, he

had no persecution for 2 years. In 2010, there was a recurrence of persecution. He thinks the same woman as before took his "bon ange," wanted to make him a *zombie*. She moved the neurons in his head, making her mentally ill and provoking his first hospitalization. He says the medication helped to move away the evil spirits and replace her neurons when she was "ill in the head" in the hospital; however, they do not help in any other way. Currently, the spirits come every 3 h during the day and all night. He needs to rub salt or lemon on his skin to get the spirits to leave. He also rubs mayonnaise to soothe her skin—as per recommendations from family members in Haiti. He is praying with the Bible and other people are praying for her and telling her to pray (a pastor from Haiti, her father-in-law, her husband), but this is not sufficient. Healers may be helpful as well. However, she does not want to go to Haiti to find such healers because it would imply a lesser trust in God's powers. She believes this persecution will not kill her because she herself never harmed the other woman, even when she was living in the same house.

Mr. Smith uses various illness categories and explanatory frameworks: (1) Vodou in the religious sense and as referring to the common cultural beliefs in Haiti, (2) protestant belief in the power of God to heal, and (3) mental illness (mental health in Creole is "bien nan tèt" or being well in the head).

According to the literature, the belief in illness being "sent" is not limited to those who believe in Vodou, but is rather an overarching Haitian understanding of illness attribution: "Vodou is based on a vision of life in which individuals are given identity, strength and safety in a dangerous world through the thick fabric linking them together with other human beings, as well as spirits and ancestors. For this reason, disturbances in health or luck are a sign that relationships have been disrupted and may need to be mended. Vodou rituals heal individuals and groups by strengthening and mending relationships among the living, the dead, and the spirits" (Pierre et al., 2010).

Mental health problems are often attributed to supernatural forces. Mental illness, problems in daily functioning, and academic underachievement may all be seen as the consequences of a spell, a hex, or a curse transmitted by a jealous person. In such cases, people generally do not blame themselves for their illness or see themselves as defective. Indeed, the sense of self may even be enhanced as a curse is often aimed at a person deemed to be attractive, intelligent, and successful. Mental illness is also sometimes attributed to failure to please spirits (*lwa*s, *zanj*s, etc.), including those of deceased family members.

In Haiti, Vodou, while being tolerated to some degree by the Catholic Church, is eschewed as evil by most Protestant groups, although the language of Vodou may persist, even among Protestants, as seen above. Protestants that have emigrated may be more likely to look down upon traditional Vodou beliefs.

Mr. Smith believes that he needs to use a combination of treatment methods. This use of multiple sources is common in Haiti (as elsewhere) and in the Haitian community in Montreal. Some types of treatment methods are viewed more appropriate to certain circumstances. He has used Vodou spiritual healing, although he does not want his wife to know about this, because as a long-standing Protestant, she rejects this and would be angry with him if he knew. He uses folk "natural" healing methods like the *lavements* she received from the Church group and the ointments he uses on her skin. He also prays. In his belief system, God is the supreme healer. Finally, he also accepts biomedicine for mental illness, but his understanding of what mental illness is limited.

2. **Meaning and severity of symptoms in relation to cultural norms**
   a. **Of cultures of origin**
      Mr. Smith's beliefs about this other woman's powers and her persistent,
      preoccupied interpretation of his bodily symptoms are a delusional elaboration of Vodou beliefs, even according to Haitian beliefs, as confirmed by the culture broker.

      We were unable to speak with his family of origin to corroborate this information with them. They may be less aware of the severity of his symptoms given that they are in another country. However, his preoccupations are persistent, unlike the usual situation in illness caused by a spirit which presents as an acute crisis. Most people in his congregation understand his beliefs as related to mental illness. He is aware of this and states that the congregation members do not understand him and that friends tell him to "forget about the Vodou." The pastor "always prays" for him and has said that if she is "100 % with God," then the bad spirits will not be able to have power over him. According to Mr. Smith, his wife does not want to hear anything about evil spirits as she does not believe in them. She sometimes tells him it is "in your head." She believes medication and stress reduction, as well as prayer, will help him. Mr. Smith also says he has an aunt in Montreal who tells him to go to the hospital, take his medication, and pray.

   b. **Of host culture**
      Within the biomedical, North American host culture, Mr. Smith's beliefs are considered delusional. It is not clear to what extent his Haitian background was taken into account in previous treatment of his condition.

3. **Help-seeking experiences and plans**
   Mr. Smith's help-seeking reflects his own beliefs as well as his social networks. He goes to certain helpers because it is prescribed by doctors, people in authority like his pastor, his friends and extended family, and his wife. He avoids certain healers because it is proscribed (again, by her pastor, her husband), and finally he also finds ways to integrate her own beliefs about etiology and about what will be helpful.

a. **With the formal health care system**

Mr. Smith was hospitalized in psychiatry for the first time in Montreal. He is currently followed at a psychiatric outpatient department. He believes some of this health care system is helpful. However, he is using it mainly because he needs to keep the peace at home and also because it is something "to do... to keep me busy."

He believes the medications he takes are helpful only to improve sleep. He agrees that medication helped him when she was ill in hospital because his persecutor had made him mentally ill by affecting his brain ("a deplacé des neurones dans ma tête," lit. "moved the neurons in my head"). He does not believe that medication can help protect him from Vodou or help with the spirits. He has daytime sedation and a dry mouth and does not like the idea of increasing the dosage.

He comes to therapy groups because it is "something to do." At the groups, he is not introspective nor does he use them to better understand how mental illness affects him. This lack of self-reflection may partly reflect cultural values and style of coping that suggest it is not appropriate to dwell on one's ills but best to be active and to distract oneself.

b. **With traditional healers and alternative services**

Although the couple has different views about the appropriate use of traditional healers and other sources of help, they generally negotiate this without overt conflict.

Mrs. Smith states outright that, although prayer has a place in both their lives, the etiology of her husband's distress, and therefore the solution, is not solely religious, but is related to mental illness and is clearly exacerbated by stress. She therefore believes medications are the primary treatment he needs. She adds that most of the family and church community agree with her. Religion may help them to cope and

prayer may help to distract Mr. Smith, and he receives support through the pastor's regular telephone calls.

Her attitude is reflective of the tension between Protestant beliefs and Vodou beliefs, which are more tolerated by the Catholic Church, but that also persist as an idiom of distress (rather than as religious belief) among most Haitians. Her perception that Mr. Smith's symptoms are signs of mental illness may be also related to the psychoeducation sessions in Montreal after her husband became ill.

While Mr. Smith has used Vodou spiritual healing in the past, he does not talk to his wife about it. He uses folk "natural" healing methods, as recommended by family in Haiti and applied by his children. He refuses to go search out a healer in Haiti, as suggested by some family members, in part, because this would be a potential source of conflict with his wife.

His need to pray when he experiences "persecution" is consistent with his Baptist background, as is his belief that God is the supreme healer. His desire to use Vodou techniques and herbal remedies is also culturally appropriate, but he makes excessive use of these remedies and attributes more extensive powers to substances like lemon and garlic than commonly seen.

C. **Cultural Factors Related to Psychosocial Environment and Levels of Functioning**

1. **Social stressors**

None identified in country of origin. Stressors related to immigration and difficulty adjusting to host country include:
- Possible racism, although this has not been reported by the patient or his wife
- Concerns about finding adequate employment and feelings of embarrassment about his lack of self-sufficiency
- Financial stress

2. **Social supports**

For Mr. Smith, his wife and extended family in Haiti, as well as the pastor in his Church in Montreal, seem to be the most significant social supports.

3. **Levels of functioning and disability**

Mr. Smith is not able to work. He functions best at home, where he does some household chores. He is not able to do much childcare and relies on his wife to look after the children and provide discipline. He does participate in religious services but does not play other social roles.

It is not certain to what degree his functioning is limited as a result of acculturation difficulties, but it seems likely that a large component of his functional impairment is related to his mental illness. Further history is needed to be obtained to determine his functioning prior to the onset of the illness as well as regarding her functioning prior to the current exacerbation, in order to fully answer this question.

D. **Cultural Elements of the Clinician–Patient Relationship at Assessment**

1. **What is the clinician's ethnocultural background?**

The consultant in this case was a female psychiatrist who immigrated to Canada from Eastern Europe as a child. She has a personal appreciation of the challenges and hardships associated with immigration. The culture broker was a Haitian-Canadian graduate student in psychology. She has ambivalent feelings about Vodou as a healing practice, but she was able to reflect on her own attitudes and convey an attitude of interest and respect throughout the assessment. Mr. Smith clearly appreciated the opportunity to speak with the culture broker who he felt understood his background.

E. **Overall Cultural Assessment**

Mr. Smith is suffering from a paranoid psychotic disorder. However, part of Mr. Smith's difficulties can be conceptualized as a religious conflict within his family. He negotiates the divergent beliefs, which are common of Haiti, in ways that preserve family harmony. To some extent, his wife may discount his ideas about Vodou because she views him as mentally ill, and this may reduce the potential for conflict. Mr. Smith makes effective use of local religious resources as well as some support from extended family. Other sources of support are limited. Psychoeducation does not appear to be engaging Mr. Smith's main concerns or preferred mode of coping. He is more interested in participatory, social activities, preferably in the Haitian community. Such activities would be more appropriate for Mr. Smith and may be more therapeutic.

References

Adeponle, A., Thombs, B., Groleau, D., Jarvis, G.E. & Kirmayer, L. J. (2012). Using the cultural formulation to resolve uncertainty in diagnosis of psychosis among ethnoculturally diverse patients. *Psychiatric Services, 63*(2), 147–153.

American Psychiatric Association. (2000). *Diagnostic and statistical manual (4th ed.), text revision (DSM-IV-TR)*. Washington, DC: American Psychiatric Press.

American Psychiatric Association. (2013). *Diagnostic and statistical manual* (5th ed.). Washington, DC: American Psychiatric Press.

Brascoupé, S., & Waters, C. (2009). Cultural safety: Exploring the applicabiity of the concept of cultural safety to Aboriginal health and community wellness. *Journal of Aboriginal Health, 7*(1), 6–40.

Dinh, M. H., Groleau, D., Kirmayer, L. J., Rodriguez, C., & Bibeau, G. (2012). Influence of the DSM-IV outline for cultural formulation on multidisciplinary case conferences in mental health. *Anthropology & Medicine, 19*(2), 261–276.

Fung, K., Lo, H. T., Srivastava, R., & Andermann, L. (2012). Organizational cultural competence consultation to a mental health institution. *Transcultural Psychiatry, 49*(2), 165–184.

Kirmayer, L. J., Rousseau, C., Jarvis, G. E., & Guzder, J. (2008). The cultural context of clinical assessment. In A. Tasman, M. Maj, M. B. First, J. Kay, & J. Lieberman (Eds.), *Psychiatry* (3rd ed., pp. 54–66). New York, NY: John Wiley & Sons.

Lecomte, Y., & Raphaël, F. (Eds.). (2011). *Santé mentale en Haiti: La pensée critique en santé mentale*. Montreal, Quebec, Canada: Santé Mentale au Québec.

Mezzich, J. E., Caracci, G., Fabrega, H., Jr., & Kirmayer, L. J. (2009). Cultural formulation guidelines. *Transcultural Psychiatry, 46*(3), 383–405.

Mezzich, J. E., Salloum, I. M., Cloninger, C. R., Salvador-Carulla, L., Kirmayer, L. J., Banzato, C. E. M., et al. (2010). Person-centered integrative diagnosis: Conceptual basis and structural model. *Canadian Journal of Psychiatry, 55*(11), 701–708.

National Association of Community Health Centers. (2008). *Serving patients with limited English proficiency: Results of a community health center survey*. Bethesda, MD: National Health Law Program.

Pierre, A., Minn, P., Sterlin, C., Annoual, P. C., Jaimes, A., Raphaël, F., et al. (2010). Culture and mental health in Haiti: A literature review. *Santé Mentale en Haïti, 1*(1), 13–42.

Cultural Consultation in Child Psychiatry

Toby Measham, Felicia Heidenreich-Dutray,
Cécile Rousseau, and Lucie Nadeau

This chapter provides an overview of cultural consultation in child psychiatry. We will first outline the mental health needs of immigrant and refugee youth. Next, we will describe ways in which child psychiatric practice has been adapted to address the cultural context of children and families. We then describe two transcultural child psychiatry clinics in Montreal and Paris to illustrate how transcultural child psychiatry is practiced in different contexts with clinical examples exemplary of the work of each clinic. In addition to outlining practical strategies for consultation and intervention, our aim is to show how the work of these clinics depends on local cultures and resources as well as each country's history and attitudes towards immigration and minority ethnocultural groups. The chapter concludes with some reflections on how sociocultural context influences the practice of transcultural child psychiatry.

The Mental Health Needs of Immigrant and Refugee Youth

In Canada, the health of immigrants tends to be better than that of the general population in both sending and receiving countries, while over time, immigrants' health tends to worsen to match that of the general population (Kirmayer, Narasiah et al., 2011; McDonald & Kennedy, 2004). For children, a review of 20 international studies of immigrant children living in the Netherlands, Norway, Sweden, Greece, the UK, the USA, Canada, Australia and Israel found both higher and lower levels of problem behavior when compared to host-country youth (Stevens & Vollebergh, 2008). The authors noted that the development of problem behavior varied with the group studied, possibly due to differences in socioeconomic status, family stress and original culture between immigrant groups.

Refugee children have traditionally been considered at greater risk for mental health difficulties than immigrant youth, given the catastrophic life experiences that most have lived through. Difficulties include the development of posttraumatic stress disorder and depression (Attanayake

T. Measham, M.D., M.Sc. (✉)
CSSS de la Montagne (CLSC Parc Extension),
7085 Rue Hutchison, Salle 204.11, Montreal, QC,
Canada H3N 1Y9
e-mail: toby.measham@mcgill.ca

F. Heidenreich-Dutray, M.D.
Équipe mobile psychiatrie et précarité,
Centre hospitalier de Rouffach, 27, rue du 4ème RSM,
68250 Rouffach, France
e-mail: feliciadutray@gmail.com

C. Rousseau, M.D., M.Sc.
Centre de Recherche et de Formation,
CSSS de la Montagne, 7085 Hutchison, Local 204.2,
Montréal, QC, Canada H3N 1Y9
e-mail: cecile.rousseau@mcgill.ca

L. Nadeau, M.D., M.Sc.
CSSS de la Montagne (CLSC Parc Extension),
7085 Hutchison, Salle 204.10, Montreal, QC,
Canada H3N 1Y9
e-mail: lucie.nadeau@mcgill.ca

L.J. Kirmayer et al. (eds.), *Cultural Consultation: Encountering the Other in Mental Health Care,*
International and Cultural Psychology, DOI 10.1007/978-1-4614-7615-3_4,
© Springer Science+Business Media New York 2014

Table 4.1 Factors related to migration that affect children's mental health

Premigration	Migration	Postmigration
Age and developmental stage at migration	Separation from caregiver	Stresses related to family's adaptation
Disruption of education	Exposure to violence	Difficulties with education in new language
Separation from extended family and peer networks	Exposure to harsh living conditions (e.g., refugee camps)	Acculturation (e.g., ethnic and religious identity, gender role conflicts, intergenerational conflict within the family)
	Poor nutrition	Discrimination and social exclusion (at school or with peers)
	Uncertainty about future	

Adapted from Kirmayer, Narasiah et al. (2011)

Table 4.2 Factors influencing mental health outcomes in forcibly displaced children

Risk factors
 Exposure to premigration violence
 Female sex
 Unaccompanied
 Perceived discrimination
 Exposure to postmigration violence
 Several changes of residence in host country
 Parental exposure to violence
 Poor financial support
 Single parent
 Parental psychiatric problems

Protective factors
 High parental support
 Family cohesion
 High perceived peer support
 Positive school experiences

Adapted from Fazel, Reed et al. (2012)

et al., 2009). In addition, refugee children have been found to suffer from other internalizing and externalizing difficulties including adjustment disorders, sleep disturbances, nightmares, grief reactions, inattention, social withdrawal and somatization (Geltman, Grant-Knight, Ellis, & Landgraf, 2008; Lee, Shin, & Lim, 2012; Montgomery, 2011; Morgos, Worden, & Gupta, 2007).

Key risk and protective factors for immigrant and refugee children have recently been reviewed in the literature and are summarized in Tables 4.1 and 4.2 (Fazel, Reed, Panter-Brick, & Stein, 2012; Kirmayer, Narasiah et al., 2011).

Research conducted among children at high risk has nevertheless found that many are in good mental health. For example, a Quebec study of refugee children demonstrated positive mental health compared to Canadian-born peers, indicating that, despite exposure to stressors, there is much potential for well-being (Rousseau, Drapeau, & Platt, 2000). On the other hand, while it is often assumed that immigrant families have a lower rate of exposure to migration-related risk factors, this is not always the case. A study of mental health among immigrants in Montreal found that many families had faced organized violence prior to migration (Rousseau & Drapeau, 2004). Similarly, a study conducted in the USA among newly arrived immigrant school children found that a substantial proportion of youth had mental health difficulties such as posttraumatic stress disorder and depressive symptoms, with a number reporting exposure to premigration as well as postmigration violence (Jaycox et al., 2002).

The postmigration environment is increasingly found to be a key factor affecting the well-being of immigrant and refugee youth. For example, a longitudinal study of refugee youth in Denmark found that stresses experienced by young refugees during their exile and after their migration were more predictive of psychological problems than were the adverse experiences they had experienced before their arrival (Montgomery, 2008).

In summary, immigrant and refugee youth experience a variety of migratory trajectories, so that risk and protective factors experienced before, during and after migration affect their mental health in complex ways. The conclusion of Beiser, Dion, Gotowiec, Hyman, and Vu (1995) continues to hold true:

> Although migration and resettlement probably affect development, contingencies such as selection policies, premigration experiences and the interaction between migrant characteristics and the welcome

accorded by the host country determine whether or not immigration is followed by maladaptation or the realization of potential. (Beiser et al., 1995, p. 67)

Models of Mental Health Service for Immigrant and Refugee Children and Families

Mental health service underutilization is an issue for all children and a particular problem for immigrant and refugee children. Barriers to care including ethnic community factors, service system factors and societal factors all may impede youth's access to services. Different models of mental health service provision have emerged to address this, including ethnic-specific services and the delivery of more culturally responsive services in mainstream institutions (DeAntiss et al., 2009). Research conducted in the UK has shown that refugee children who receive culturally and linguistically adapted services in mainstream clinics are no more likely to drop out of treatment than host-country youth (Howard & Hodes, 2000). Children and families have also been offered preventive services and treatment in schools in the UK and Canada (Fazel, Doll, & Stein, 2009; Rousseau, Benoit, Lacroix, & Gauthier, 2009; Rousseau & Guzder, 2008).

Ecological models that take into account both social and mental health needs of refugee and minority families are increasingly employed. The Inter-Agency Standing Committee (IASC) recommends that emergency mental health and psychosocial support for refugee children should be implemented in a tiered manner; this can be visualized as a pyramid with universal provision of services at the base to ensure basic safety for all, and then allocation of services in a more targeted fashion, with interventions aimed at strengthening community and family supports, followed by the provision of focused nonspecialized support to a smaller number of people, and finally the provision of specialized mental health services to individuals with the greatest mental health needs forming the pyramid's top (Inter-Agency Standing Committee [IASC], 2007). All of these interventions are ideally implemented concurrently and with intersectorial collaboration.

The American Psychological Association has recently made recommendations for the provision of culturally competent multisectoral mental health services to refugee children in the USA (American Psychological Association [APA], 2010). School staff, primary care providers and community workers are often the first to learn of these children and their families' needs and thus represent a critical entry point for accessing services. Collaborative mental health care with community- and school-based services can provide key avenues for the delivery of culturally informed care for immigrant and refugee children and their families.

Transcultural Child Psychiatry Clinics in Montreal and Paris

Clinics have been set up by transcultural child psychiatric practitioners in Montreal, Canada and Paris, France to respond to the needs of minority and newcomer child and family patient populations. In Montreal, Cécile Rousseau and colleagues established the Transcultural Child Psychiatry Team in the outpatient child psychiatry department of the Montreal Children's Hospital (MCH). This clinic eventually moved out of the hospital to become a community-based, tiered collaborative care service operating out of primary health and social service community clinics in inner city neighborhoods. In Paris, Marie Rose Moro and colleagues organized an ethnopsychiatry clinic for children at the Avicenne Hospital in a northern suburb of the city. Each of these clinics emerged in a particular geographic and political context, and as a result each has developed assessment and treatment models that reflect the social and cultural circumstances of the countries, local communities and the health care systems in which they are based.

The McGill Transcultural Child Psychiatry Team

The development of the Transcultural Child Psychiatry Team of McGill University was influenced by the dual institutional foundations of McGill University's Division of Social and

Transcultural Psychiatry, first set up as a joint venture between the Departments of Psychiatry and Anthropology in 1955, and by its hospital base, the MCH, one of two pediatric tertiary care hospitals in Montreal that provides services to the city and its surrounding regions. The hospital had a well-established Multiculturalism Programme to address the needs of its diverse staff and patient population (Clarke, 1993), when the team was created, and this helped the team to develop a specialized hospital-based service for immigrant and refugee children and their families.

The MCH Multiculturalism Programme began in 1986 in response to a request from frontline staff who felt they needed to better understand the cultures of their patients. As a hospital with one of North America's busiest pediatric emergency rooms, the MCH serves a very large and diverse clientele. In 1986, about one-third of the hospital's patients spoke French at home, one-third spoke English and the remainder spoke other languages. The hospital's employees were equally diverse, coming from 45 different ethnic groups and speaking more than 50 languages and dialects. The objectives of the Multiculturalism Programme were to encourage understanding and respect for cultural values, beliefs and practices throughout the hospital community; to develop resources and educational programs to assist the hospital in meeting the needs of its culturally diverse community; to improve the liaison between the hospital and cultural communities by promoting hospital use of community resources and encouraging community participation in the hospital; and to promote cross-cultural sensitivity in other health and social service institutions. To achieve these goals, the program set up a number of services, including cross-cultural staff development programs; coordination of interpretation services within the hospital; an information, consultation and referral service; and a multimedia library specializing in cultures, cross-cultural health care issues and intercultural staff development. The program also organized activities for staff and the public with a focus on cultural communities.

The Transcultural Child Psychiatry Team was based at the MCH for an 8-year period, from 1999

Table 4.3 Referrals to the McGill Transcultural Child Psychiatry Team, 1996–2000

Referral source	%
School or community social worker or psychologist	26.8
MCH multicultural medical health clinic	21.3
Hospital-based psychiatrist or psychologist	15.5
Community health and social services for immigrants and refugees	9.6
Family physician or pediatrician	8.7
Family	5.4
Immigration services or immigration lawyer	2.5
Other	1.7
Unknown	8.4

to 2007. During that time, first- and second-generation immigrant and refugee children made up approximately 50 % of the school-aged population in Montreal (Sévigny, Viau, & Rabhi, 2002). In terms of the demography of recent immigrants to Montreal during the period spanning 1996–2001, the top ten countries of origin of the 114,180 newcomers were Algeria (9 %), China (8 %), France (7 %), Haiti (5 %), Morocco (5 %), India (4 %), Romania (4 %), Sri Lanka (3 %), the Philippines (3 %) and the Russian Federation (3 %) (Citizenship & Immigration Canada, 2005).

Children and youth who had experienced war or migration trauma were considered a priority for referral to the Transcultural Child Psychiatry Team. In addition, children who had experienced family separation and reunification as a result of the migration process, unaccompanied refugee minors and newly arrived children who were adjusting to a new schooling and social context were also seen at the clinic. Finally, the team welcomed referrals from families or service providers where assistance in elaborating cultural issues was identified as an important aspect of the medical or mental health diagnostic and treatment process.

A review of all 239 cases referred from 1996 through 2000 gives a picture of the work of the clinic (Measham et al., 2001). As seen in Table 4.3, the clinic responded to requests from diverse sources both within and outside the hospital. Clinic clientele were less likely to be self-referred, with only 5.4 % self-referring, than to be referred by a helping professional already involved with the family (86.2 %). The largest source of referrals to the clinic came from social workers and psychologists working in schools and in the city's community-based primary health care clinics, called Local Community Service Centers (in the French acronym, CLSC).

During those 4 years, the team provided services to children from over 70 countries. The vast majority of patients referred to the clinic were newcomers to Quebec. They came from a wide range of countries, the majority of which had recently experienced or were currently experiencing armed conflict. An exception was the children referred from Quebec's Cree community, members of Canada's First Nations communities in Quebec whose presence predates the colonization of Canada by Europeans.

Serious stressors and traumatic events occurred frequently in the histories of the clinic's clientele. Over half of the patients experienced separation from family members (56.1 %), largely as a result of the family's experience of armed conflict and/or the result of their migratory trajectory. Over half of the patients (52.7 %) had experienced organized violence. Finally, 6.7 % of the clinic's population experienced a refusal of their request for asylum. These numbers are all likely underestimates, as information was lacking for 15 % of patients referred to the clinic who did not attend their first appointment.

Children of all age groups were referred to the clinic. The mean age of children referred was 10, with equal numbers of children aged 5–9 and 10–14 being referred, at 32.2 % each, while 22.2 % of children referred were adolescents and 13.4 % were under the age of 4. More boys were referred than girls, with just under two-thirds of referrals being boys.

Children were seen in assessment and then provided services at the clinic. The initial assessment consisted of an evaluation of the presenting problem by the multidisciplinary team, which comprised professionals with diverse cultural identities and disciplines, including psychiatry, psychology and the creative arts therapies (Rousseau, 1998). The referring clinician, the patient and his or her family and other persons considered important

in their support network were invited to this initial evaluation. A professional interpreter was always offered to the family and invited with the family's permission. Interpreters assisted in the assessment in order to help understand both cultural and language issues.

The child and family psychiatric assessment took into account specific contextual and cultural issues. The team prioritized establishing a working alliance and a sense of safety in the clinical space prior to exploring topics that were considered particularly delicate such as traumatic issues, explanatory models of the illness and traditional healing practices. The presenting difficulty was explored from the vantage points of the child, his or her family members and the referring clinician, in order to take into account multiple viewpoints on how problems were perceived, understood and responded to and to acknowledge the fluidity of culture and acculturation processes within and across generations. Viewpoints explored included individual, collective, professional, spiritual, traditional and sociopolitical perspectives. The team inquired about these diverse perspectives on the assumption that families and individuals could hold multiple (and sometimes conflicting) views and have shifting identities. During the assessment process, team members reflected on the information being discussed with all parties present in order to help understand and find solutions to the problem at hand (Measham, Guzder, Rousseau, & Nadeau, 2010). Particular attention was paid to the negotiation and mediation of possible underlying tensions occurring in the therapeutic encounter (Measham, Rousseau, & Alain, 2003). Both assessment and treatment were conceptualized as offering a transitional space where therapeutic possibilities could be explored, allowing both ambivalence and uncertainty to be addressed as families negotiated their difficulties and found their own unique ways of healing.

Referring professionals often had difficulties evaluating whether children had a psychiatric disorder, with particular difficulty addressing cultural norms of child development and patient's explanatory models. Intergenerational differences, divergent methods of parenting and disciplining and questions about the applicability of DSM-IV diagnoses to their patients also led to requests for transcultural consultation. Questions for referral often were formulated in terms of specific concerns about the presence of posttraumatic stress disorder, attention-deficit/hyperactivity disorder and learning problems, as well as depression, suicidality, social withdrawal and aggressive behavior. Common concerns included the role of cultural issues in the evaluation of developmental delays and of medical symptoms, as well as referrals for the evaluation and treatment of psychotic symptoms. Finally, referrals were sometimes made after a professional involved with a family learned of the patient or their family member's experience of catastrophic events including genocide, whether or not the patient or family members themselves initially expressed a need for mental health services.

The evaluation involved an elaboration of the explanatory models of illness of the patient, family and institution (Kleinman, 1980; Kleinman, Eisenberg, & Good, 1978). This was complemented by a DSM-IV diagnosis and an integrated formulation and treatment plan addressing individual, family, social and cultural aspects of the child and family's well-being. Feedback was given to the patient, their family and the referrer at the time of the evaluation, with the referring party being included in the treatment planning.

The initial assessment meeting usually took about 3–4 h, particularly if an interpreter was present. At the start, team members would meet with the family and referring clinician together. Opportunities were provided to meet with identified patients and parents separately. The team paid particular attention to the role of trauma disclosure in the evaluation, taking note of the developmental status of the children and the readiness of the child and family to discuss issues related to their traumatic past, as well as individual and collective values around the perceived helpfulness of trauma disclosure (Measham & Rousseau, 2010). Following the assessment interview, the team took 15 min with the referring clinician to formulate their initial assessment and treatment recommendations. The diagnostic impression and treatment recommendations were then shared with the family and referring party as a point of departure to begin to co-create a treatment plan, and an agreement was then made for further appointments.

The type of follow-up offered to the family and referring party consisted of either liaison with primary care providers (collaborative care), the provision of open-ended individual or family therapy or brief crisis-oriented intervention with the possibility of ongoing care in the future as needed. Early efforts were made to link the family with nonprofit organizations in their communities and with their local community clinics to address psychosocial stressors and to increase social support. Families also frequently encountered barriers in accessing primary medical care, and the clinic worked collaboratively with the hospital's multicultural health clinic, which offers a specialized pediatric care clinic to newcomer children, as well as with a community-based clinic (CLSC) which offers medical services to newcomer youth and their families.

Conventional psychotherapy and pharmacotherapy were offered by the Transcultural Child Psychiatry Team to children and their families, as well as interventions that were specifically developed for the clinic's clientele. Treatment generally started with individual and family therapy with an initial focus on strengthening individual and family protective factors and resilience by exploring nontraumatic elements of the family's past and current functioning. For example, treatment might focus on exploring family traditions in their homelands, spiritual teachings and individual and family experiences of well-being. As treatment progressed, it could also include more direct exploration of traumatic issues.

Individual and family interventions that were frequently used included creative arts therapies and traditional storytelling therapy (Bagilishya, 2000; Heusch, 1998; LaCroix, 1998), as well as psychodynamically oriented individual psychotherapy and family therapy. Modifications of family therapy included the use of culture brokers and extended family councils, as well as the introduction of transnational social networks both in the imaginal space of therapeutic conversation and also, if desired and feasible, by letter, email or telephone conference. The inclusion of multiple team and family members in the therapy setting allowed the therapeutic space to represent and acknowledge multiple perspectives and worldviews relevant to understanding the meanings of children's difficulties and the actions needed to alleviate their distress.

The team directly addressed issues of social exclusion and discrimination and considered mediation and advocacy for patients' needs a crucial part of its mandate. In addition to working directly with children and their families, team members mediated and advocated with institutions, including schools, health and social service providers and immigration services with the family's consent. This could occur by having joint meetings with the family and the other professionals present or by offering meetings or phone calls to discuss psychosocial issues impacting on a child's care and well-being.

To support applications for asylum, the team provided letters describing a child's treatment with the service and their experience of war trauma. Requests were also made to have children abstain from participating in asylum hearings when participation was considered to be potentially damaging to their mental health (e.g., because of the risk of repeated exposure to their parents' retelling of traumatic experiences including rape and torture).

Where disagreements between families and host-country institutions appeared to be important contributors to a child's symptoms, the team would offer its services as a potential mediator to address these conflicts. Examples of disagreements with social service providers that the consultation team helped to mediate included divergent concepts of corporal punishment and physical abuse and definitions of children's social support networks, for example, recognizing the parental authority of kinship relatives when these relatives did not have legal rights in Canada as parental authorities. Meetings with medical services included negotiating concepts of illness and treatment recommendations, as well as concerns about treatment adherence.

These clinic meetings with social and medical services frequently improved trust and understanding among all parties, as previously confusing, disturbing or misunderstood symptoms and behaviors were reinterpreted in the light of the cultural background and traumatic migratory pathway of child and family. Schools, medical and social services frequently elaborated innovative plans to accommodate and support children and their families. Where interventions that were considered stigmatizing and unwanted by families were suggested, such as specialized educational instruction or the intervention of child protection services, the team attempted to provide a space for dialogue to address parental and professional concerns and identify areas of common ground centered on the best interests of children.

Outcome was judged by therapists in terms of a global rating of improvement in symptoms and functioning rated as good, moderate or poor. No outcome scores were available for 30 % of patients, who were either seen only once in consultation or lost to follow-up. For patients with follow-up, outcome was judged as good in 57 % of cases, moderate in 28 % and poor in 15 %. In general, cases with poor outcome shared a heavy burden of catastrophic stressors, with worsening of symptoms in the context of severe difficulties between families and host-country institutions in establishing a climate of trust and a shared vision of the child's best interests. In a number of these cases, the Transcultural Service failed in its attempts to act as mediator of divergent values between the family and the host-country institutions. A review of the cases referred to the service revealed that few treatments ended in a formal disengagement from therapy with a concomitant administrative "closure" of a file. In general, treatment and outcome were considered to be an ongoing and interlocking process, with the child's symptoms strongly influenced by the resolution of ongoing stressors including the reunification of families and the granting of asylum. The imposition of further stressors, including the rejection of requests for asylum, led to renewed treatment efforts as families attempted to cope with that event. Parallel to the process of treatment were the efforts of child and family to rebuild social ties during the resettlement process. To compensate for their ongoing tenuous circumstances, efforts were made to remain available to families for follow-up consultation and, when children turned 18, to insure referral to appropriate adult service providers.

Case Vignette 4-1

Tania was a 10-year-old newcomer to Quebec who attended a "welcoming class" in French public school in order to learn French. She was referred to the McGill Transcultural Child Psychiatry Team by her school because she was anxious and had extremely poor school attendance, as did her older sister. The family had migrated to Canada from the Balkan region, during the civil war. Prior to setting up the first appointment, the team offered to provide an interpreter, and Tania's mother asked for one interpreter who spoke the language of the dominant group in their country of origin rather than the language of the family's minority community. During a first family meeting, the children reported that they had a lot of anxiety symptoms whenever they left home. Tania's mother identified a treatment goal of decreasing her children's anxiety and improving their school performance and stated that she did not wish to discuss the family's past. An agreement was made to continue with a series of family meetings. Several sessions later, after some trust had been established, Tania's mother revealed that she had lost close relatives in her country's civil unrest and she found it unbearable to speak in her own mother tongue because it reminded her of her losses. She noted that her children were increasingly pressuring her to talk about their homeland and that she did not know how to manage this. She acknowledged both depressive and posttraumatic symptoms but initially refused any help for herself. The therapeutic work involved finding an aspect of the family's past that mother felt comfortable sharing that could provide some structure and meaning to the therapy and help support them during their current distress. Tania's mother began to talk about her own childhood and brought traditional sayings about child-rearing that her mother had shared with her in her own mother tongue, which she in turn shared with her daughters. Later in the course of her treatment, mother began to discuss the civil conflict that had led to the family's migration. A crisis presented late in the therapy, when mother reported suicidal ideation. A plan was made with child welfare services to accompany Tania's mother to the general hospital emergency room for psychiatric evaluation and to help her access mental health services. She began her own treatment for depression and posttraumatic symptoms, while family therapy continued with the Transcultural Child Psychiatry Team. The children's anxiety symptoms lessened, and their school attendance and performance improved dramatically.

This case illustrates the importance of addressing war trauma in a progressive way in a family context. Frequently, when children are referred for assessment and treatment, their parents are suffering equally, although they may not acknowledge this or wish for treatment. Family members need to address war trauma at their own pace, which may not be the same for different individuals within the family system. In this example, the children pressed for disclosure while their mother avoided it. The case also illustrates the complexity of ethnic matching as illustrated by the choice of interpreter. Mother asked for an interpreter from the dominant ethnic group, which she considered had persecuted her community. One might have thought that an interpreter from her own linguistic community would have been more appropriate. However, her maternal language represented too much proximity to her losses, and she was able to find a more manageable emotional distance at the beginning of therapy by using another language. Once an alliance had been established, mother began to talk about the civil unrest that had led to the family's migration.

Finally, the therapeutic space provided mother with an opportunity to bring elements of the family's history into the present, sharing comforting aspects of the past in the form of traditional sayings with her children. The case also illustrates the potential difficulty of providing mental health care in a specialized setting that does not offer mental health and social services for all family members. When mother required mental health services, it was necessary to refer her to the emergency room at another hospital in order to access services. Finally, while the Transcultural Child Psychiatry Team addressed the children's mental health symptoms, the family's social isolation remained prominent.

The Transcultural Child Psychiatry Team operated at the MCH for a decade, from 1996 until 2007. Its location within a university teaching hospital dedicated to the care of children allowed it to develop novel approaches to mental health care for immigrant and refugee youth. This was a particularly fecund period for the team's development, as students and researchers from many disciplines and clinicians were able to gather at one site, providing a rich environment for exchange. At the same time, the hospital-based model meant that referring professionals and families often had to travel long distances to the clinic, and the child's difficulties were addressed in a setting far removed from their local community.

To address this issue, the team began to offer more direct and indirect consultations and support to children and their families in proximity to their local neighborhoods. Preventive mental health services were also offered using creative arts techniques in some of Montreal's highly multiethnic schools, and direct consultations and indirect case discussions were held in community clinics, where practitioners from different environments (e.g., schools, child welfare centers, community clinics, and community groups) began to share their perspectives and collaborate in working with their clients (DePlaen et al., 2005; Rousseau & Alain, 2003).

The Transcultural Child Psychiatry Team was closed at the MCH in 2007, when service delivery at the hospital's department of psychiatry was organized into tertiary care specialty clinics, largely defined by diagnostic category (e.g., Autistic Spectrum Disorders and Anxiety Disorders). This change coincided with a provincial governmental reform of mental health service delivery, in which community-based health and social service institutions, called CSSSs (which incorporated previously established neighborhood-based Local Community Service Centers, or CLSCs) were designated as the entry point into the mental health system. The goals of this reform were to improve access to services and increase the capacity of primary care and social services to provide mental health care. The plan also included a role for consulting psychiatrists, or "psychiatres repondantes," to provide support to primary care providers in the community and help with referral to hospital-based tertiary care services when necessary.

The three child psychiatrists who worked at the McGill Transcultural Child Psychiatry Team shifted their work to a new community-based setting, the CSSS de la Montagne, located in one of the most multiethnic regions of Montreal. At the CSSS, the transcultural child psychiatrists work as consultants in a collaborative mental health care model with the CLSC's Youth Mental Health Teams (see Chapter 9), which in turn provide direct mental health care to children and families, and also support other teams in the community clinics that deliver general health and psychosocial care to families, schools, daycares and community groups in the CSSS's territory (Rousseau, Measham, & Nadeau, 2012). The catchment area of this CSSS had the largest number of newcomers arriving in Montreal between 2001 and 2006, as well as the largest number of persons who did not speak either English or French as their primary language (Agence de la santé et des services sociaux de Montréal, 2011). The three CLSCs in this CSSS's territory provide services to several inner city neighborhoods where 80 % of the children are either first (35 %) or second (45 %) generation immigrants or refugees.

Requests for consultation are welcomed from any practitioner in the CSSS, who acts as case manager for the child and family. The transcultural child psychiatrists and their trainees travel on a weekly basis to the different community clinics for consultations. The assessment team often consists of practitioners and families who have worked together for some time, with the transcultural child psychiatric consultant being a new addition to the group. A child and family evaluation proceeds with the treating professionals present and treatment recommendations can be directly conveyed. Treatment is provided by the community clinic health, mental health and social service personnel. The child psychiatry consultants are available in a shared care model, offering reassessment and case discussion as treatments are underway.

The strengths of this model are that service delivery is provided in the neighborhoods where children and their families live. This may increase the accessibility and availability of services and the impact of any consultation on subsequent care throughout the local system. In addition, because services are provided within local community clinics, families have greater access to the delivery of both primary health care and social service supports, which can be delivered in an integrated manner. The model relies on strengthening capacity at the primary care level, which requires team building, support and training, as well as the collaboration of the hospital psychiatry departments in the territories of the community clinics, which provide more specialized care and hospitalization when needed.

The second case example illustrates how community-based care has the potential to provide comprehensive care for a family experiencing multiple psychosocial stressors, particularly when both children and parents may have symptoms. It also illustrates how longer-term community-based collaborative care models can offer a venue to address the complexities surrounding both cultural and contextual factors that can contribute to a child's symptoms.

Case Vignette 4-2

Samantha, a 5-year-old visible minority English-speaking girl, was receiving services from a pediatrician, after presenting with a request for care for the ongoing treatment of attention-deficit/hyperactivity disorder. Following a move to the USA from West Africa with her mother as a toddler, she had been treated with speech therapy in English and started on stimulant medication. The family had been refused refugee status in the USA and had few social supports. Her pediatrician referred her to a specialized Autism Spectrum Disorders Clinic for evaluation. As the wait list for this specialized service was long and the child lived in the catchment area of the CSSS where the transcultural child psychiatry consultants worked in collaborative care, the referral was directed to community-based services and the CSSS was able to provide consultation within a few weeks.

Samantha spoke English but no French. However, she had just started elementary school in French, as is required for non-Canadian newcomers to Quebec. Samantha spoke little at her local school, had echolalia and was impulsive and hyperactive. She made little eye contact with her pediatrician during their appointments. These behaviors had prompted the concern that she might have an autistic spectrum disorder.

The consultant met with Samantha, her mother, a community-based social worker who shared mother's culture of origin and who had already been providing community-based social services to mother, as well as Samantha's school social worker, her French language speech therapist, and a community clinic childcare worker. Samantha's mother stated that she thought her daughter had a developmental problem and had begun to feel hopeless about whether her daughter would improve. She also began to discuss her fears that her struggles as a parent—though not her daughter's developmental issues—were due to a curse, which she had received in her country of origin.

On review with the school social workers and language therapist, Samantha did not

(continued)

present features typical of a child with pervasive developmental disorder. She was integrating well at school and did not have serious behavior problems there. Although she did appear to have a developmental delay, she had begun to speak a little and communicated well nonverbally, seeking out the attentions of her teachers. She had a prominent language difficulty, which appeared to be a major source of her frustration and difficult behavior. The family's social isolation, poverty and insecure migration status were important social stressors. There was also some question as to whether mother's concern about a curse was a culturally acceptable explanatory model for her own difficulties as a parent or reflected her own fragility or mental health problem.

Efforts were made with the community clinic to increase the family's local social support and to improve living conditions for both mother and child. Efforts were also made to increase contact with mother's wider social circle, including with her own relatives who lived in other countries. Feedback was given to the school to emphasize the positive effects that their structuring and supportive environment was having on Samantha's development and well-being. Home-based educator support was started to modify Samantha's difficult behaviors. Liaison with Samantha's pediatrician was made, and mother admitted that she was not regularly adherent with Samantha's ADHD treatment. Over time, Samantha's behavior improved and her relationship with her mother was strengthened. Samantha's mother fears about evil spirits lessened. The family later moved to another part of Montreal, where the local community clinic made contact with the family to offer continued support.

This case illustrates the complex relationship between challenging social circumstances, biological and cultural factors, parental mental health and psychosocial stressors and child development. The proximity-based care provided by the community services allowed mother and child to slowly build trust in their new environment, and this had a salutary effect on Samantha's development and mother's feelings of hope for her daughter. In addition, the community clinic team offered a space where mother could begin to discuss her family's story. In this case, while there were concerns for mother's mental health, the community clinic was able to provide support for mother and daughter as well as interventions that decreased ongoing psychosocial stressors. With intervention, mother's social isolation and fears lessened, and her strengthened alliance with her own social worker allowed her to accept support for her daughter.

This vignette also presents the possibility that proximity-based care, with close collaboration between families, schools and community health and social service providers, can help promote successful outcomes, particularly where there are issues of multiple differences such as race, ethnicity, culture and language. In this vignette, the school and community health clinic had strong working ties with their neighborhood and with each other, and this helped to create a working alliance with the family and a sense of welcome and belonging for them. This situation is in marked contrast with many cases seen by the Transcultural Child Psychiatry Team when it worked from its hospital base to try to provide cultural consultations to neighborhoods with which it did not have a previous working relationship with. In some of those cases, families and institutions were locked in intense conflict or impasses, and concerns about discrimination were raised. Strong advocacy for the families sometimes resulted in a paradoxical worsening of the family's situation, as the conflict between families and institutions escalated in response to the advocacy. This points to the need to build strong working alliances with institutions that can be mobilized to deal with challenging cases.

Ethnopsychiatric Consultation at Avicenne Hospital

Another approach to mental health services for first-, second- and third-generation immigrant children is provided by the Child and Adolescent Psychiatry Outpatient Clinic of the Avicenne Hospital in a northern suburb of Paris, France. The second author has worked at this clinic as well as the CCS in Montreal and this affords a comparative perspective on service models and practices.

The population served at the Avicenne clinic is referred from second- or third-line care by psychiatrists and other physicians, social workers, child protection services or sometimes at the request of families themselves. Among the reasons for referral are difficulties in clinical communication with the family. This includes issues of translation into the family's language or dialect as well as questions of comprehension of the family's explanatory models of illness. Moreover, facing diagnoses of severe and chronic mental illness, many families look for alternative explanations and draw upon cultural idioms of distress. This can cause difficulties in alliance building with caregivers and have effects on treatment adherence. In other cases, symptoms might be so saturated with cultural elements that in-depth assessment taking into account the migration history and the family's cultural origins becomes necessary. There is a growing need for culturally sensitive care and psychotherapy which takes into account the family's perspective on the illness. Many families are disappointed by mainstream services; they feel left out and poorly understood. The families' migration histories are varied; some have come to France as refugee claimants or through family reunification; others were born in France and have varying degrees of ongoing contact with their country of origin.

In France, the ethnopsychoanalytic approach of Devereux (1985) has been very influential. This approach emphasizes the complementarity of different disciplines, including psychoanalysis, anthropology, psychology, linguistics, history, systems theory and religious studies in social science research. For Devereux, all of these disciplines have clinical insights to offer, but owing to their different methodologies, they should not be used simultaneously but rather introduced separately and in a coordinated manner, thus offering different but complementary perspectives. Devereux's approach has been adapted to clinical situations with various modifications. For example, multiple methodologies may be used by different practitioners or by a single practitioner. In reality, patients frequently consult a mental health practitioner and a traditional healer at the same time (Kirmayer, Weinfeld et al., 2007). In transcultural consultation, this use of multiple sources of help may be made explicit, so that different approaches to healing can be addressed and discussed without idealizing or devaluing any particular tradition.

Building on Devereux's work, in the 1980s, psychologist Nathan (1986) developed an ethnopsychiatric group setting in which a culturally diverse team of therapists applies this complementarist method, working with a single family at a time (Corin, 1997; Streit, 1997). At Avicenne, Moro (1994; Sturm, Nadig, & Moro, 2011) adapted this approach to conduct therapy with children and their families, emphasizing that children belong not only to their parents' culture of origin but also to that of the host country's culture. Families come to see a multidisciplinary group of psychoanalytically trained psychiatrists, psychologists, social workers and nurses, most of whom are themselves immigrants or have lived in a culture different from their own. This group fulfills three functions. First, the identities of the therapists provide diverse representations of otherness (gender, ethnicity, migration status, profession). Second, the group provides psychological holding by working to maintain safety for the child and family. Third, the immigrant origins and institutional affiliations of the therapists themselves symbolize the migrant's necessary passage from one universe of experience to another. The team represents cultural diversity and functions as a "cultural frame" that facilitates the expression of traditional etiologies and access to representations of illness and therapeutics, both of which are considered central elements for appropriate diagnosis and treatment. Patients are invited to come with family or other persons close to them, and the referring professionals are encouraged to participate in order to share knowledge and to improve the continuity of care.

Therapists work systematically with interpreters who speak the patients' mother tongue and who are trained to work in the specific setting of the department. Interpreters translate what is said but also have the role of mediator between cultures (see Chapter 6). The analysis of illness representations from a linguistic point of view is an important part of the process, allowing for a better understanding of bodily metaphors and semantic networks of meaning through the exploration of literal translations and back-translations with native speakers and linguists (Moro & de Pury Toumi, 1994). Co-therapists may propose stories, metaphors or images as indirect interpretations of the psychic material and the resistances brought by the family. The aim is to access internal representations and affects by encouraging the family to use their own idioms and metaphors. This helps to build authentic narratives of both the parents and the children, which allow for a more complete view of the situation.

Therapists need to pay particular attention to the specific psychological vulnerabilities of children who have themselves migrated or whose parents have migrated. These children have a twofold challenge: their own, linked to the bicultural cleavage on which their identities are structured, and that of their parents, linked to migration. In order to assess the clinical situation of the patients and their families, Moro (1994) has proposed three intertwined levels of analysis of the cultural representations regarding the illness within the family. The first level of analysis concerns *ontological considerations* about the sick person. Not only is the question of who is sick in the family important, but even more so the qualities and the status of the sick person: "Who is this person, what is her essence, her nature?" The second level questions the *etiological explanations* given for the illness. It looks into the different causes of the illness and who advocates for them: "What has happened, what has been done or omitted?" The third level addresses the *therapeutic practices* that follow in a logical way from the propositions elaborated in the first two levels:

"What has to be done, who has to be involved?" Cultural practices are held to have potential protective effects and patients and their families are encouraged to engage in practices they believe to be helpful. In contrast to the practice of Nathan (1994), however, in Moro's approach clinicians do not meet with traditional healers or work with therapeutic rituals themselves because they believe that this role should be ascribed to a culturally authorized person.

Clinical work reveals the interactions between cultural frameworks of meaning and psychological frameworks. If illness representations are embedded in a larger family narrative, they can provide some meaning to the suffering experienced. Exploring cultural representations is not only a way of adding to the patient's history but also has therapeutic effects, just as the creation of a personal story does in narrative therapy. In some cases, cultural explanatory models seem to be rigid, are not very helpful in giving a meaning to the suffering of the family and stand in opposition to any kind of mainstream therapeutic intervention. In order to mobilize more flexible models, it is important to recognize and respect the families' positions and explore their capacity to invest in new visions of their difficulties. In an ethnographic description of this therapeutic setting, Sturm (2006) pointed out three axes which she found to be structuring transcultural therapeutic work: (1) on the basis of a strong *therapeutic alliance* between the family and the therapeutic group, (2) *mediation* between different explanatory models becomes possible and gives way to (3) *elaboration* (in a psychodynamic understanding) and "playing with cultural representations." The following case example illustrates these axes of transcultural work.

Case Vignette 4-3
Kevin, a 7-year-old boy whose parents had come to France from the Democratic Republic of Congo (DRC) 3 years prior to his birth, had been diagnosed with pervasive developmental disorder. The institution

(continued)

referring the case for ethnopsychiatric consultation found it very difficult to work with the parents, who steadfastly claimed that this disease did not exist in their home country. The parents did not agree to send their son to a day hospital programme, stating that all the other children there were very sick while their son was not. Instead, they sought help in their evangelical church community. The social worker involved in the case, who referred the family for consultation, feared that violent exorcism rituals would be performed on the boy.

At the first consultation interview, Kevin's parents presented a rigid explanatory model constructed around beliefs of sorcery coming from a maternal aunt in the DRC. Kevin's parents seemed depressed and in mourning for the ideal child they had hoped for. Conflicts between the maternal and paternal families were overt and nourished the ideas of sorcery. There was very poor contact with the family left behind in the DRC, who did not know about Kevin's illness. The social worker's fantasies of possible violence reflected her difficulties in understanding the inflexible position of the parents, which was sustained by the cultural idiom of sorcery.

Careful exploration of the couple's history, their migration and its causes, as well as increased use of the family's mother tongue, Lingala, through an interpreter allowed for the emergence of alternative cultural models explaining their son's illness. Co-therapists proposed explanatory models from other areas of the world, playing on similarities and differences in order to help the parents think about other explanations. Talking about idioms such as the transgression of taboos, the reincarnation of ancestral spirits and being a child with special gifts eventually led to a reconsideration of the boy's position within the family. The new narrative of the family and migration history allowed for renewal of contact with

family at home in the DRC from whom they asked for traditional and spiritual support. The family's social worker participated in the consultation, and this offered her a new vision of the family, making it easier for her to be empathic and caring towards them.

Conclusion

In some ways, cultural consultation in child psychiatry can be seen as simply good child- and family-centered care. However, close attention to the cultural dimensions and systemic contexts of illness and well-being challenges some of the taken-for-granted assumptions of standard practice and can address some of the blind spots of mainstream services. The comparison of two clinical models in this chapter shows how these specific settings and approaches enable clinicians to address issues associated with minority status or culture. In Montreal, the Transcultural Child Psychiatry clinic emphasized the importance of structural and political issues, addressing the systemic barriers which confronted patients and families. Although this stance of advocacy promoted innovative interventions, it also sometimes threatened institutions and increased clinicians' uncertainty and insecurity, as they faced the inadequacies of mainstream services and the dilemmas of social integration. While this uncertainty was stimulating and contributed to creative solutions, it also led to confrontations with mainstream institutions.

In immigrant receiving countries addressing the rights of minority children to effective prevention and treatment of psychopathology can be challenging because of limited resources and the slow process of institutional change. In addition, the increasing securitization of immigration policies, in particular since 9/11, has resulted in a deterioration of the rights of foreigners in host countries (Crépeau & Jimenez, 2004). Ensuring economic and social rights, including access to health care, is increasingly difficult as governments appeal to public anxieties about security and budget issues, which can result in a decrease in support for efforts to increase health care access and improve health care service delivery.

In Canada, the official policy of multiculturalism promotes the provision of support to ethnic communities and, as Beiser, Hou, Hyman, and Tousignant (2002) proposed, likely contributes to familial and social capital. At the same time, addressing discrimination directly in Canada is still difficult both because of political correctness which increases implicit forms of discrimination and because there has been little recognition or discussion in the mental health field of the country's history of racism and exclusion. The McGill Transcultural Child Psychiatry Team's focus on social, political and cultural contextual issues presented a challenge to institutional policies and routines. When the hospital outpatient model shifted its priorities to subspecialty clinics, the intercultural work was sidelined. The team adapted by moving to its current community clinic setting where it has been able to build stronger links with mainstream institutions. In part, this reflects the clinic mandate and emphasis which includes both social work and public health. In addition, the evolving shared care model with community workers has emphasized adapting interventions for their diverse clientele.

In Montreal, the move to a shared care or collaborative model in community settings has brought particular advantages. These include a greater ability to address children's difficulties through family systems approaches, as the health, social and mental health care needs of all family members are considered within the domain of the community clinic. This systemic, integrative view is in contrast to the segmented organization of care by age and specific types of illness that occurs in child and adult hospital settings in Canada. The community clinic also favors working with networks grounded in a child's community context and directly supports primary care personnel, as well as professionals working in community institutions such as children's schools. Finally, the stigma of consulting in psychiatry is lessened in a community clinic setting.

In France, the models of care for immigrant patients that have been developed reflect the "republican" ideal of the integration of immigrants into French society (Fassin & Rechtman, 2005). Cultural specificities and difficulties in adaptation to the new environment are considered to be part of the private sphere and the individual's affair. Thus the therapeutic setting at Avicenne Hospital does not propose a form of therapy that politicizes suffering or gives voice to the difficulties of everyday life in the host country, which include racism and discrimination. The emphasis is on the individual and family level of psychological processes with less attention to larger societal issues. By working in and with the patient's language, the Avicenne clinic's consultations take into account the local or emic point of view and individual narratives in a very respectful way. Most patients have previously experienced difficulties with the mainstream health care system and are very grateful for the experience of empathic and careful listening as well as the opportunity to relate their own explanatory models of illness. Working with culture as a therapeutic medium is an act of balancing the opening up of creative possibilities with the risk of reducing patients to their cultural identity. To maintain this balance in the therapeutic encounter, it is essential to take into account the complexity of hybrid identities, allowing patients to play with cultural representations and meanings. The group setting can provide an intermediate or transitional space that allows for this kind of therapeutic play.

On a pragmatic level, the group setting with multiple clinicians and interpreters present may be difficult to reproduce in other contexts. It is costly in terms of human resources and time. For training, however, the group setting offers unique advantages, giving trainees the opportunity to assist directly and to learn progressively how to design and introduce therapeutic interventions. Although the satisfaction of clients and referring practitioners is thought to be very high, there is little research on the effectiveness of this form of intervention.

In conclusion, there are limits to our current evidence base with regard to treatment interventions and service delivery models for minority youth. We have described two cultural consultation and treatment models in Montreal and Paris that have tried to address these limitations. These models are evolving works-in-progress; for example, the Montreal clinic's change to a collaborative care model of service delivery has increased accessibility to social support and heath care, and efforts are now underway to document the effectiveness of this new model. As transcultural practitioners, we look forward to the continued development of effective treatments and models of service delivery in child psychiatry in our rapidly globalizing world.

References

Agence de la santé et des services sociaux de Montréal. (2011). *Banque interrégionale d'interprètes 2010–2011.* Retrieved December 15, 2012, from http://publications. santemontreal.qc.ca/uploads/tx_asssmpublications/ isbn978-2-89510-624-1.pdf

American Psychological Association. (2010). *Resilience and recovery after war: Refugee children and families in the United States.* Retrieved September 2012, from, http://www.apa.org/pi/families/refugees.aspx

Attanayake, V., McKay, R., Joffres, M., Singh, S., Burkle, F., Jr., & Mills, E. (2009). Prevalence of mental disorders among children exposed to war: A systematic review of 7,920 children. *Medicine Conflict and Survival, 25,* 4–19.

Bagilishya, D. (2000). Mourning and recovery from trauma: In Rwanda, tears flow within. *Transcultural Psychiatry, 37*(3), 337–354.

Beiser, M., Dion, R., Gotowiec, A., Hyman, I., & Vu, N. (1995). Immigrant and refugee children in Canada. *Canadian Journal of Psychiatry, 40*(2), 67–72.

Beiser, M., Hou, F., Hyman, I., & Tousignant, M. (2002). Poverty, family process, and the mental health of immigrant children in Canada. *American Journal of Public Health, 92*(2), 220–227.

Citizenship and Immigration Canada. (2005). *Recent immigrants in metropolitan areas: Montreal—A comparative profile based on the 2001 census.* Retrieved December 15, 2012, from http://www.cic.gc.ca/english/ resources/research/census2001/montreal/partb.asp#b1

Clarke, H. (1993). The Montreal Children's Hospital: A hospital response to cultural diversity. In R. Masi, L. Mensah, & K. A. McLeod (Eds.), *Health and cultures: Exploring the relationships, policies, professional practice and education* (pp. 47–61). Oakville, Ontario, Canada: Mosaic Press.

Corin, E. (1997). Playing with limits: Tobie Nathan's evolving paradigm in ethnopsychiatry. *Transcultural Psychiatry, 34*(3), 345–358.

Crépeau, F., & Jimenez, E. (2004). Foreigners and the right to justice in the aftermath of 9/11. *International Journal of Law and Psychiatry, 27,* 609–626.

DeAntiss, H., Ziaian, T., Procter, N., et al. (2009). Help-seeking for mental health problems in young refugees: A review of the literature with implications for policy, practice and research. *Transcultural Psychiatry, 46,* 584–607.

DePlaen, S., Alain, N., Rousseau, C., Chiasson, M., Lynch, A., Elejalde, A., et al. (2005). Mieux travailler en situations cliniques complexes: L'expérience des séminaires transculturels institutionels. *Santé Mentale au Québec, 30*(2), 281–299.

Devereux, G. (1985). *Ethnopsychanalyse complementariste.* Paris, France: Flammarion.

Fassin, D., & Rechtman, R. (2005). An anthropological hybrid: The pragmatic arrangement of universalism and culturalism in French mental health. *Transcultural Psychiatry, 42*(3), 347–366.

Fazel, M., Doll, H., & Stein, A. (2009). A school-based mental health intervention for refugee children: An exploratory study. *Clinical Child Psychology and Psychiatry, 14,* 297–309.

Fazel, M., Reed, R. V., Panter-Brick, C., & Stein, A. (2012). Mental health of displaced and refugee children resettled in high-income countries: Risk and protective factors. *The Lancet, 379,* 266–282.

Geltman, P. L., Grant-Knight, W., Ellis, H., & Landgraf, J. M. (2008). The "lost boys" of Sudan: Use of health services and functional health outcomes of unaccompanied refugee minors resettled in the U.S. *Journal of Immigrant and Minority Health, 10,* 389–396.

Heusch, N. (1998). Cheminer en art-thérapie avec des immigrants d'origine russe. *PRISME, 8*(3), 160–182.

Howard, M., & Hodes, M. (2000). Psychopathology, adversity and service utilization of young refugees. *Journal of the American Academy of Child and Adolescent Psychiatry, 39,* 368–377.

Inter-Agency Standing Committee. (2007). *IASC guidelines on mental health and psychosocial support in emergency settings.* Retrieved September 2012, from http://www.humanitarian.info.org/iasc/

Jaycox, L. H., Stein, B. D., Kataoka, S. H., Wong, M., Fink, A., Escudero, P., et al. (2002). Violence exposure, posttraumatic stress disorder and depressive symptoms among recent immigrant schoolchildren. *Journal of the American Academy of Child and Adolescent Psychiatry, 41*(9), 1104–1110.

Kirmayer, L., Narasiah, L., Muñoz, M., Rashid, M., Ryder, A., Guzder, J., et al. (2011). Common mental health problems in immigrants and refugees: General approach to the patient in primary care. *Canadian Medical Association Journal, 183*(12), E959–E967.

Kirmayer, L. J., Weinfeld, M., Burgos, G., Galbaud du Fort, G., Lasry, J.-C., & Young, A. (2007). Use of health care services for psychological distress by immigrants in an urban multicultural milieu. *Canadian Journal of Psychiatry, 52*(4), 61–70.

Kleinman, A. M. (1980). *Patients and healers in the context of culture.* Berkeley, CA: University of California Press.

Kleinman, A., Eisenberg, L., & Good, B. (1978). Culture, illness, and care: Clinical lessons from anthropologic and cross-cultural research. *Annals of Internal Medicine, 88*(2), 251–258.

Lacroix, L. (1998). Revendication de l'identité chez une fillette sud-américaine adoptée: une démarche par l'art-thérapie. *PRISME, 8*(3), 150–159.

Lee, Y. M., Shin, O. J., & Lim, M. H. (2012). The psychological problems of North Korean adolescent refugees living in South Korea. *Psychiatry Investigation., 9*, 217–222.

McDonald, J. T., & Kennedy, S. (2004). Insights into the 'healthy immigrant effect': Health status and health service use of immigrants to Canada. *Social Science & Medicine, 59*(8), 1613–1627.

Measham, T., Guzder, J., Rousseau, C., & Nadeau, L. (2010). Cultural considerations in child and adolescent psychiatry. *Psychiatric Times*. Retrieved December 15, 2012, from http://www.psychiatrictimes.com/display/article/101681/1508374

Measham, T., Nadeau, L., Rousseau, C., Bagilishya, D., Foxen, P., Heusch, N., et al. (2001). The Montreal Children's Hospital's transcultural child psychiatry clinic: A unique clientele and a diversity of clinical interventions. In L. J. Kirmayer, C. Rousseau, E. Rosenberg, H. Clarke, J. Saucier, C. Sterlin, V. Jimenez, & E. Latimer (Eds.), *Culture and mental health research unit report no. 11, development and evaluation of a cultural consultation service in mental health* (pp. 1–10). Montreal, Quebec, Canada: Culture and Mental Health Research Unit, Jewish General Hospital. Appendix C1.

Measham, T., & Rousseau, C. (2010). Family disclosure of war trauma to children. *Traumatology, 16*(4), 85–96.

Measham, T., Rousseau, C., & Alain, N. (2003). La médiation: Articulation des espaces thérapeutique et politiques. In T. Baubet & M.-R. Moro (Eds.), *Psychiatrie et migrations* (pp. 195–202). Paris, France: Masson.

Montgomery, E. (2008). Long-term effects of organized violence on young middle eastern refugees' mental health. *Social Science & Medicine, 67*, 1596–1603.

Montgomery, E. (2011). Trauma, exile and mental health in young refugees. *Acta Psychiatrica Scandinavica Supplement, 440*, 1–46.

Morgos, D., Worden, J. W., & Gupta, L. (2007). Psychosocial effects of war experiences among displaced children in southern Darfur. *Omega, 56*, 229–253.

Moro, M. R. (1994). *Parents en exil. Psychopathologie et migrations (2002)*. Paris, France: PUF.

Moro, M. R., & De Pury Toumi, S. (1994). Essai d'analyse des processus interactifs de la traduction dans un entretien ethnopsychiatrique. *Nouvelle Revue d'Ethnopsychiatrie, 25*(26), 47–85.

Nathan, T. (1986). *La folie des autres. Traité d'ethnopsychiatrie clinique*. Paris, France: Dunod.

Nathan, T. (1994). *L'influence qui guérit*. Paris, France: Éditions Odile Jacob.

Rousseau, C. (1998). Se decéntrer pour cerner l'univers du possible: Penser de l'intervention en psychiatrie transculturelle. *PRISME, 8*(3), 20–36.

Rousseau, C., Benoit, M., Lacroix, L., & Gauthier, M. F. (2009). Evaluation of a sandplay program for preschoolers in a multiethnic neighborhood. *Journal of Clinical Child Psychology and Psychiatry, 50*, 743–750.

Rousseau, C. & Alain, N. (2003). Repenser la formation continue dans le réseau de la santé et des services sociaux: l''experiénce des seminaires interinstitutionnels en intervention transculturelle, Nouvelles Pratiques Sociales, 17(2):109–125.

Rousseau, C., & Drapeau, A. (2004). Premigration exposure to political violence among independent immigrants and its association with emotional distress. *The Journal of Nervous and Mental Disease, 192*(12), 852–856.

Rousseau, C., Drapeau, A., & Platt, R. (2000). Living conditions and emotional profiles of young Cambodians, Central Americans and Québécois youth. *Canadian Journal of Psychiatry, 45*, 905–911.

Rousseau, C., & Guzder, J. (2008). School-based prevention programs for refugee children. *Child and Adolescent Psychiatric Clinics of North America, 17*, 533–549.

Rousseau, C., Measham, T., & Nadeau, L. (2012). Addressing trauma in collaborative mental health care for refugee children. *Clinical Child Psychology and Psychiatry, 18*(1), 121–136.

Sévigny, D., Viau, A., & Rabhi, K. (2002). *Portrait socioculturelle des élèves inscrits dans les écoles publiques de l'Île de Montréal: Inscriptions au 31 Septembre 2001*. Montréal, Quebec, Canada: Conseil scolaire de l'Île de Montréal.

Stevens, W. J. M., & Vollebergh, W. A. M. (2008). Mental health in migrant children. *Journal of Child Psychology and Psychiatry, 49*(3), 276–294.

Streit, U. (1997). Nathan's ethnopsychoanalytic therapy: Characteristics, discoveries and challenges to western psychotherapy. *Transcultural Psychiatry, 34*(3), 321–343.

Sturm, G. (2006). Listening to the "other" in transcultural therapies: Worldviews, idiomatic expressions of illness and the use of cultural representations in transcultural communication. In V. Lasch, U. Sonntag, & W. Freitag (Eds.), *Gender, health and European cultures* (pp. 22–34). Kassel, Germany: Kassel University Press.

Sturm, G., Nadig, M., & Moro, M. R. (2011). Current developments in French ethnopsychoanalysis. *Transcultural Psychiatry, 48*(3), 205–227.

Working with Interpreters

Yvan Leanza, Alessandra Miklavcic, Isabelle Boivin, and Ellen Rosenberg

Working with interpreters is essential to the practice of cultural consultation. In mental health care, language remains the central vehicle for building an alliance; gathering information; conducting a mental status examination; gaining access to subjective experiences, emotions, and memories; and engaging in therapeutic interventions. Effective work with interpreters in clinical assessment and intervention requires consideration of ethical and pragmatic issues. Collaboration also requires an appreciation of the complex interactions of language, cognition, emotion, and expression. This chapter will provide an orientation to working with mental health interpreters, with a review of relevant research literature and theoretical models followed by guidelines and practical recommendations relevant to cultural consultation. For cultural consultation, knowledge of the sociocultural context of a patient's current and former life is crucial, and interpreters who only know the language in an academic way should be paired with a culture broker who knows the relevant social contexts. This broader role is discussed in Chapter 6.

Mental health interpreting has its own special characteristics which pertain to the need to deal with strong emotion and interpersonal conflict, to convey idiosyncratic features of the patient's style of expression in order to allow assessment of their mental state, and to track subtle shifts in experience that may be important both for maintaining rapport and intervening. This requires rethinking the dominant models of practice for interpreting which evolved in very different settings.

Y. Leanza, Ph.D. (✉)
Laboratoire Psychologie et Cultures,
École de psychologie, Université Laval, 2325 rue des Bibliothèques, Québec, QC, Canada G1V 0A6
e-mail: Yvan.Leanza@psy.ulaval.ca

A. Miklavcic, Ph.D.
Research Centre, St. Mary's Hospital, 3830 Lacombe Avenue, Montreal, QC, Canada H3T 1M5
e-mail: amiklavcic@gmail.com

I. Boivin, D. Ps.
Centre d'aide aux étudiants, Université Laval,
2305 rue de l'Université, Local 2121,
Québec, QC, Canada G1V 0A6
e-mail: isaboivin@gmail.com

E. Rosenberg, M.D.
Family Medicine, St. Mary's Hospital, 3830 Lacombe Avenue, Montreal, QC, Canada H3T 1M5
e-mail: ellen.rosenberg@mcgill.ca

Medical Interpreting as an Ethical Imperative

Verbal communication is central to the diagnostic and therapeutic tasks of all health professionals. In Canada, the codes of ethics that regulate the conduct of health and social service professions "stress the need for the provider to obtain informed consent, provide explanations, ensure confidentiality, and refrain from practicing the profession under conditions that may impair service quality" (Bowen, 2001, p. 20). Language barriers constitute a major impediment to health service delivery, and the failure to address them may constitute malpractice or, when they are institutionalized, an ethical, civil, or human rights violation (Blake, 2003).

According to the 2006 census, about 1.7 % of the population in Canada (i.e., about 520,380 people) knew neither of the two official languages, English and French (Statistics Canada, 2007a). Almost one in five (19.7 % or 6,147,840) of Canada's 31 million people have a mother tongue other than English or French (Statistics Canada, 2007b). For comparison, in 2000 in the United States, as many as 21,320,407 people (8.1 % of the population) spoke English less than "very well" (U.S. Census Bureau, 2000). In Australia in 2006, 561,413 people (3 % of the population) did not speak English well or not at all (Australian Bureau of Statistics, 2006). These statistics illustrate the magnitude of the challenge facing the health services in countries receiving large numbers of immigrants.

The scientific literature is replete with examples of poor-quality services due to the failure to address language differences. In some cases, this arises from barriers to access or biases in referral. For example, studies have found that non-English-speaking patients were less likely to be offered follow-up appointments after a visit to an emergency department in Los Angeles (Sarver & Baker, 2000) and women were less likely to receive preventive services for breast cancer in Ontario, Canada (Woloshin, Schwartz, Katz, & Welch, 1997). Language also influences the uptake of treatment interventions. Non-English-speaking patients visiting an ambulatory clinic in a teaching hospital in the USA have lower rates of adherence to treatment (David & Rhee, 1998). There is an ethical imperative to ensure equal access to health care services and equal quality of services; without successful communication, this cannot be achieved. Providing interpreter services in health institutions is a key means of meeting this ethical obligation. In recognition of this ethical and pragmatic issue, models of medical and community interpreting have been developing rapidly in several countries in recent years (Bancroft, 2005).

Medical and Community Interpreters and Culture Brokers

In addition to health services, interpreting occurs in many settings, including business, the military, the legal system, community services, and conferences. Most of the research on interpreting has been conducted in legal, community, or conference settings. Conference interpreting became a recognized profession after World War II and the Nuremberg trials, where for the first time simultaneous interpreting was available for a large audience and many languages. Professionalization occurred through the development of university level courses leading to degrees, the creation of national and international associations, and the establishment of codes of ethics.

Community interpreting—that is, "interpreting in institutional settings of a given society in which public service providers and individual clients do not speak the same language" (Pöchhacker, 2003 p. 126)—is fundamentally different from conference interpreting, both because it deals with conversations rather than monologues and especially because the interpreter is an integral part of the interaction, not simply an onlooker.

Culture brokering (also called *cross-cultural mediation*) can be defined as mediation between two culturally different realities for the purpose of reducing conflicts and/or producing a change between the two groups (Cohen-Emerique, 2003, 2004a, 2004b; Cohen-Emerique & Fayman, 2005). Culture brokering focuses on negotiating cultural differences and may or may not include linguistic dimensions. As such, community interpreting and culture brokering are distinct but overlapping. An interpreter can play many roles inside and outside the consultation room. Based on ethnographic research on medical interpreting in a paediatric hospital, Leanza (2005b) described four broad roles for interpreters: linguistic agent, system agent, community agent (also called a "lifeworld agent"), and integration agent. Acting as a linguistic agent, the interpreter attempts to remain impartial and does not add text or comments. In contrast, the three other categories imply that the interpreter enters the interaction as an active partner. As a system agent, the interpreter transmits the dominant discourse, i.e., biomedical information in health care, and cultural differences tend to be ignored. As a community agent or culture broker, the interpreter can be a mediator for both interlocutors, making additions that explain differences in values, address conflicts, or serve patient advocacy. As integration agents, interpreters may play roles outside the consultation setting, elsewhere in the health care system or in the community, helping the patient to find resources to better adapt to the society (e.g., accompanying a patient to the pharmacy). Research in health care settings indicates that these broader roles are not often employed by professional interpreters. In fact, in interactions when interpreters do add text, they most often act in the roles of system agent, giving biomedical advice (Davidson, 2000; Wadensjö, 1998). Health professionals rarely solicit the community agent roles even if they are aware of them (Leanza, 2005a, 2005b; Rosenberg, Leanza, & Seller, 2007).

Reflecting on the South African psychiatric system, Drennan and Swartz (1999) point out that asking the interpreter to play the role of a cultural informant carries the implicit assumption that culture is monolithic and can be summarized for easy consumption by mental health professionals. The cultural informant tends to be a one-sided role that does not include patient advocacy, which is a key aspect of culture brokering. The role of patient advocate requires great skill and self-confidence on the part of the interpreter who must be both an insider member of the health care team in order to be heard and an outsider, allied with the patient, in order to play the role of advocate. Working as an integral part of the treatment team may undermine this advocacy role which therefore requires explicit institutional recognition and support.

Neutrality: The Central Issue in Health Care Interpreting

With an environmental scan, Bancroft (2005) found that virtually all codes of ethics and standards of practice for health care interpreters emphasized three basic issues: confidentiality, accuracy or completeness, and impartiality or neutrality. Neutrality remains a controversial issue in mental health contexts. Examples of neutrality as an ethical principle can be found in the injunctions to *give no advice, allow no influence of feelings or beliefs on work,* and *insert no opinions even if asked.* This emphasis on neutrality is a direct effect of the ethics of conference interpreting in which interpreters must not add to the "official text" or change it in any way.

In psychiatry and psychotherapy, however, the neutral stance of the interpreter has been challenged by those who view neutrality as more or less impossible and who argue, instead, for the construction of a collaborative relationship between clinician and interpreter. Those who advocate neutrality in psychiatry are usually concerned with the potential for errors by interpreters with the resultant risk of poor quality of care (Demetriou, 1991; Farooq & Fear, 2003; Marcos, 1979). To reduce this risk, they may provide restrictive guidelines (Miletic et al., 2006) or even consider it impossible to offer effective psychological care through an interpreter (Yahyaoui, 1988). In collaborative care models, where a team may develop a more prolonged and complex interaction with patients, interpreters are sometimes integrated as team members (Bot, 2003, 2005; Raval, 2005; Raval & Maltby, 2005). This is usually the case in the Cultural Consultation Service, where a relationship develops with interpreters regularly used by the service.

Pioneering ethnographic research on medical interpreting by Kaufert and Koolage (1984) and later by Wadensjö (1998) made it clear that interpreters do not simply transmit information. Even when interpreters try to be neutral, research underscores the difficulty of attaining neutrality (Davidson, 2000; Hsieh, 2006a, 2007, 2009; Kaufert & Koolage, 1984; Leanza, 2005a, 2008; Pöchhacker, 2004; Rosenberg et al., 2007; Rosenberg, Seller, & Leanza, 2008). Indeed, from a pragmatic linguistic point of view, interpreters cannot avoid inserting some of their own knowledge and perspective into the clinical interaction both verbally and nonverbally (through the expression on their face, tone of voice, gestures, and timing). Interpreters are not invisible scribes but present as team members in the therapeutic setting, with their personal identities and social positions influencing the interaction. Moreover, interpreters' active involvement can be seen as an asset when both the interpreter and the health care professional share a patient-centered approach. What is essential for mental health consultation is the practitioner's ability to be sensitive to the interpreter's complex impact on the clinical interaction to ensure the process proceeds in a constructive way.

Case Vignette 5-1

The CCS saw a patient from an African country who was referred from the regional refugee clinic. He was seeking political asylum after having been tortured by police in his own country. He was very anxious with significant posttraumatic symptoms including flashbacks, sleep disorder, and depressed mood despite receiving high doses of medication from his primary care physician. The interpreter accompanying him identified with the patient's experience and began to intrude in the consultation with comments about his own police trauma and difficulties finding political asylum prior to his successful migration. He offered unsolicited advice on the legal options during the consultations despite the consultant's attempts to maintain boundaries and guide the process. A decision was made not to use this interpreter again for CCS consultations because his level of identification with patients was impairing his ability to function in this role.

As this case illustrates, although the interpreter's identity, personal experience, and perspective will inevitably have effects on the interaction, a basic level of professional neutrality is essential to be able to focus on the patient's needs and provide appropriate clinical service.

The Interpreter's Identity

Although interpreters are usually chosen on the basis of their linguistic skills, other characteristics including age, gender, socioeconomic status, education, ethnicity, and religion can be important issues in interpreted interactions. For example, in a study in a Swiss hospital, Sleptsova (2007) found that interpreters' socioeconomic status tended to be closer to that of health care professionals than patients. As a result, interpreters tended to align themselves with the physicians and nurses, and interpretation was biased in favor of the biomedical practitioner's perspective.

Interpreting in general has been a profession characterized by a larger proportion of women than men (Pöchhacker, 2003; Zeller, 1984). To our knowledge, only one study has directly addressed gender issues in interpreted medical consultations. Bischoff, Hudelson, and Bovier (2008) looked at patient–physician gender concordance and patient satisfaction about communication in professionally interpreted consultations compared to non-interpreted consultations. They found that the presence of a professional interpreter tended to reduce gender-related communication barriers in consultations. They suggest that professional interpreters who have training in cultural mediation are better able to manage complexities involving gender and facilitate the communication process within an ethical framework.

Language, geographic origin, ethnicity, religion, social class, education, and political orientation are all variables that can influence the interpreters position vis-à-vis the patient. Regional dialects, accents, and styles of speaking can convey a lot of information about social status and may facilitate rapport or create barriers. Discussing potential conflicts with the interpreter and being alert to them in the interaction can allow the clinician to optimize the match of interpreter and patient.

Case Vignette 5-2

A Rwanda Tutsi mother sought help for her 8-year-old son. The father was killed during the war, and the consultant felt that a Rwanda Hutu interpreter might be inappropriate. After inquiring, the mother disclosed that the boy's father was Hutu. They had a mixed marriage and that she believed that a Hutu interpreter would be more helpful than a Tutsi interpreter.

Despite efforts to identify an appropriate match, patients and interpreters may have unanticipated reactions to each other that must be negotiated in the clinical setting. This negotiation may be particularly complex in the case of small communities where interpreter and patient are likely to know each other or where they have other reasons to be especially concerned about potential breaches in confidentiality.

Case Vignette 5-3

An Eastern European immigrant family was interviewed by the CCS consultant with an interpreter whom they had previously seen at community gatherings. They were ambivalent about the mental health consultation because psychiatric services in their country of origin were associated with political persecution, stigma, and incarceration in asylums. When the consultant asked the interpreter to probe into issues related to criminal activity by a family member, the interpreter became very distressed and insisted that the consultation had to stop and a new interpreter found. He felt that his neutrality was compromized as the community was very small and he was known to the family. He shared the family's concerns about political abuses by psychiatrists in their native country and worried that the consultation might lead to problems for the family.

As these vignettes illustrate, the interpreter's identity may be an immediate issue, based on fears or projections, or become problematic as the interview unfolds. Flexibility in identifying and responding issues is essential to maintain trust and effective communication.

Trust is fundamental in any clinical encounter. Clinician, interpreter, and patient must all have a modicum of trust in each other. In an analysis of a set of health care practitioner and interpreter narratives on interpreted interventions, Robb and Greenhalgh (2006) drew on Greener's (2003) typology which distinguishes three forms of trust: *voluntary* ("based either on kinship-like bonds and continuity of the interpersonal relationship over time, or on confidence in the institution and professional role that the individual represents," p. 434), *coercive* ("where one person effectively has no choice but to trust the other," p. 434), and *hegemonic* ("where a person's propensity to trust, and awareness of alternatives, is shaped and constrained by the system so that people trust without knowing there is an alternative," p. 434). Only voluntary trust was associated with an openness to the patient's lifeworld and collaboration with the interpreter by the clinician. To enhance trust in the system, the patient may play a role in choosing an interpreter.

Organizational Issues in Working with Community Interpreters in Mental Health

Working effectively with community interpreters goes beyond the lists of technical tips focused on the interpreter–practitioner relationship commonly found in the literature (Bjorn, 2005; Hays, 2008; Jackson, Zatzick, Harris, & Gardiner, 2008; Prendes-Lintel & Peterson, 2008; Richie, 1964). Effective work requires changes at level of policy, health systems, institutions, and service organizations (Leanza, 2008). At present, community interpreters lack social recognition for their work. Attempts to make interpreters part of a routine health care practice are likely to fail without such recognition, which can only be

Table 5.1 Institutional guidelines for use of community interpreters

- Evaluate linguistic needs of institution, patient population and catchment area
- Establish language policies
- Develop working relationship with regional bank of professional interpreters
- Allocate resources to fulfil the linguistic needs
  - Adequate budget specifically earmarked for interpreters
  - Supervision time
  - Room for interpreters
  - Training for gatekeepers, health care practitioners and interpreters
- Insure adequate time in clinical services for work with interpreters
- Develop overall organizational cultural competence

achieved through policies, ethical guidelines, and legislation that support patients' right to have access to health care in a mastered and meaningful language. Policies must also address training and accreditation of interpreters, health care professionals, and gatekeepers.

Table 5.1 lists some of the resources needed at an institutional level to implement community mental health interpreters. Community interpreters are professionals, and as such, they require the resources and compensation associated with a profession: a decent salary, a formal place in the health care team, an office in the institution, continuing education, and supervision.

A major obstacle to the implementation of interpreting services in health care systems is financial expense. Hospital administrators tend to view interpreted interventions as only adding costs to health care without any clear clinical or economic benefits. However, a review of the literature by Bowen and Kaufert (2003) and subsequent studies (Hampers & McNulty, 2002; Jacobs, Shepard, Suaya, & Stone, 2004) demonstrated that the use of interpreting services may actually reduce costs and improve quality of care. Patients who are inadequately assessed and treated because of poor communication may go on to use additional health services in an effort to get appropriate care. Bowen and Kaufert insist that when assessing the cost-effectiveness of interpreting services, the benefits must be considered not just for a single institution but in terms of its impact on the entire health care system and society as a whole.

Interpreters need specific training in mental health issues as well as in the interaction of culture and psychopathology. Interpreters may find mental health interpreting particularly demanding or distressing and need specific training and support around affective issues. Interpreters who work with children and families need additional training in order to be able to address the child in an age-appropriate way and accurately convey information about the language and nonverbal communication skills of the child.

Mental health professionals also need specific training in how to work with interpreters. Health care training curricula need to include courses that sensitize students and future practitioners to issues of clinician–patient miscommunication and teach them how to work with an interpreter in different situations, as this is a specific competence. Working with an interpreter requires a shift from thinking in terms of a dyadic to a triadic interaction (Rosenberg et al., 2007). Training requires an investment of time and the opportunity to practice and apply skills under supervision. Research in continuing medical education shows that "one shot" formal didactic sessions do not improve practice and outcome; there is a need for an interactive training process or practice-based interventions (Davis et al., 1999; Davis, Thomson, Oxman, & Haynes, 1995). Hence, models and skills for working with interpreters should be included as basic curriculum in the undergraduate training of future practitioners as well as being included in the programs of postgraduate specialty training and maintenance of professional certification (Betancourt, Green, Carrillo, & Ananeh-Firempong, 2003). Language is only one aspect of culture, and working with interpreters should be integrated into broader models of cultural competence. This requires an approach that goes beyond viewing interpreting as simply a communication strategy to consider the wider social meaning of language and the social positioning of practitioners, interpreters, and patients. Positive outcomes depend on viewing the clinical encounter as a process of communication and negotiation in social context. This attention to social context will also enhance the professional recognition of the work of community interpreters and culture brokers.

Institutional Policies and Practices

The first step in establishing interpreter services is to evaluate the clinic's needs in terms of languages, frequency of use, specialized skills, and budget. This will determine the mix of in-house, on-call, and telephone interpreters best suited to meet local needs. Having a dedicated budget provides a structural incentive for health care practitioners to collaborate with interpreters. Interpreters must be adequately compensated to insure their stability and quality. Use of interpreters also requires organizational changes to allow the additional time and flexibility in scheduling and workload. A study conducted in Montreal by Battaglini et al. (2007) found that up to 40 % more time is required for medical consultations for immigrants who had been in Canada less than 10 years.

In Montreal, the regional health authority maintains a central bank of interpreters who are trained and available on call to visit clinics and hospitals. Unless there is an in-house interpreting service with its own office, however, on-call interpreters have no place to stay between interventions. In our own research in a comprehensive community health clinic Montreal, we found that interpreters in usually sat in the waiting room with patients (Rosenberg et al., 2008). Providing a physical space for interpreters is part of the institutional recognition of their activity and their integration in the health care team. This integration should also take the form of including interpreters in key clinical team meetings, such as case conferences. Providing supervision for interpreters, either alone or along with other health care practitioners, is essential for high-quality care.

Continuing education for both practitioners and interpreters should include all institutional staff who may function as gatekeepers, particularly receptionists and administrators. Learning to work together should be a priority in such institutional continuing education programs. The first barrier to employing interpreters is the inability of staff who act as gatekeepers to identify patients who need language services before they arrive at the hospital (Hasnain-Wynia, Yonek, Pierce, Kang, & Greising, 2006). Failure to provide access to interpreters has important legal implications in the areas of confidentiality, informed consent, and even the ability to carry out essential clinical tasks (e.g., the ability to assess suicidal risk).

Gatekeepers and Initial Assessment of the Need for an Interpreter

Gatekeepers may play a crucial role in inquiring about a patient's language, particularly in those clinical settings that do not have on-site interpreting services and therefore need to arrange these services in advance. A potential language barrier can be detected at the gatekeeper stage by asking questions such as: "Are you new in Canada?" "Would you like to have an interpreter?" Interpreters can be provided and longer appointments can be scheduled to provide time for translation, clarification, and explanation. Staff and administrators in primary care and other clinical settings should be sensitized as to how to interact with patients who have not mastered English or French or who are not familiar with the Canadian health care system. Reception staff should be prepared to provide help with the completion of any required forms and explain to patients the rationale for the questions asked.

At the CCS, it is the role of the clinical coordinator to inquire whether a patient needs an interpreter and clarify that family members should not assume the role of a professional interpreter. Sometimes the need for an interpreter can be ascertained by talking to the referring clinician, but often it requires discussion with the patient or family when setting up the consultation appointment. In some instances, the need for an interpreter does not become apparent until the initial consultation and a second interview must be arranged.

Selecting the Right Interpreter

In the choice of interpreter, awareness of social, cultural, and political issues is essential to gain and maintain patients' trust. Geography and identity, as well as past and present conflicts, must be considered when choosing an interpreter so that someone of the appropriate ethnicity, religion, political views, dialect, and gender is obtained. Patients' requests may sometimes seem arbitrary but, in our experience, are often well founded.

Vignette 5-4

A middle-aged Kurdish man from Turkey expressly demanded that his interpreter not be Turkish, suggesting as alternatives an Armenian or a Greek who spoke Turkish. Before the consultation began, he checked the ethnicity of the interpreter, and after he was reassured, he explained that he had been a victim of psychological and physical abuse by the Turkish military.

Vignette 5-5

A middle-aged couple from Bangladesh was referred to the CCS, for the assessment of the wife's chronic depression, which appeared to be exacerbated by tensions with her husband. A Bengali-speaking interpreter translated the questions the psychiatrist asked the couple, to which the husband responded exclusively. After a little while, the interpreter, who had noticed that the man did not speak Bengali fluently and had an accent, inquired from which part of the country they came, only to discover that the couple came from the same region as himself, where Chittagonian was spoken. The interpreter shifted languages, allowing the woman to understand and express herself, thus interacting directly. She exclaimed positively: "For 15 years I could not speak, finally I can!"

The following two examples show the complexity in selecting an appropriate interpreter and the unforeseen consequences of a mismatch.

This case illustrates both the difficulty of knowing precisely which language the patient is

most comfortable speaking and the benefit of finding a good match. Many countries have far more linguistic diversity than North America or Europe. An atlas of languages can be helpful at times (Asher & Moseley, 2007), but for many smaller groups, a precise match will not possible. Instead, a local common language (e.g., Arabic, Bahasa Indonesia, Swahili, Tagalog) may be the best that can be achieved. When family members differ in their skill with a language, assessment and interaction will have unavoidable biases that must be considered. Moreover, despite the appearance of using a common language, local variations may introduce important differences in meaning.

Vignette 5-6

An elderly Russian woman was referred to clarify her diagnosis. She was deaf and a sign language interpreter translated the interview. The patient provided information on her medical history, focusing on her cancer surgery, which had taken place many years earlier. For more than an hour, the interpreter kept repeating that the patient felt that cancer was coming out of her legs when suddenly she realized that it was not cancer but worms. The reason for the misunderstanding stemmed from the fact that the interpreter was trained in American Sign Language while the patient used Russian Sign Language and the two systems differed in important respects. The shift from worries about cancer to delusions about infestation with worms led to a change in diagnosis from hypochondriasis to psychosis.

If patients have concerns about confidentiality vis-à-vis other members of their linguistic community, they may perceive the presence of an interpreter/translator as threatening. Moreover, in small communities, there is a high likelihood that patients will know the interpreter. Each case, therefore, requires a specific assessment of the patient's needs and requirements for communication in their mother tongue or language in which they are most fluent.

Lack of confidentiality may also be an issue for the interpreter, who may feel burdened or exposed. On the other hand, an interpreter who has the requisite language skills but is obviously not part of the local community may be well situated to facilitate therapeutic exchange. For example, a Tamil man from Sri Lanka reacted positively to the presence of a culture broker who spoke Tamil but was not part of the Tamil community in Canada. Her status as both insider and outsider favored a therapeutic alliance by creating a space of trust.

Gender is another important variable in the construction of the triadic alliance required for clinical interpreting. Women from certain regions of the world may feel uncomfortable in the presence of a male interpreter. When feasible, it is helpful to ask patients if they have a preference for the gender of the interpreter. This is particularly important in cases of rape and violence. In these cases, female interpreters may be chosen by default as they are more likely to be acceptable to patients of either gender.

To foster a working alliance and continuity of care, it is good practice to work with the same interpreter for a given case whenever possible. Continuity is important to enhance the teamwork between clinicians and interpreters. For patients, changes in the therapeutic team can be stressful and disorienting. Patients develop alliances and attachments to the interpreter, and an abrupt switch can undermine trust and confidence.

In some cases, patients may become close to the interpreter, who may be seen as playing the role of a mother or older sister, mirroring the systemic transferences of family life and recreating safe relationships or networks within the clinical setting. For example, in several cases seen by the CCS, South Asian women who had recently married and migrated to Canada found the interpreter a person with whom they could identify but who represented a path of acculturation, providing an example of independence that was dissonant with their traditional role in the family but closer to their expectations of Canadian life (see Chapter 8).

The Use of Informal or Ad Hoc Interpreters

In many clinical settings, professional interpreters are not available or are not used because they are costly and difficult to arrange, or staff and administrators are not fully aware of their vital importance. Instead, family members, friends, or other clinical or support staff are recruited to serve as ad hoc interpreters. This practice, though widespread because of its low cost and convenience, is strongly discouraged because it has potentially serious negative clinical consequences. For example, a qualitative study of family medicine consultations (Leanza, Boivin, & Rosenberg, 2010) identified risks associated with having family members as interpreters. Family members often become the main interlocutors in the consultation, answering for the patient. They could decide not to convey patients' statements that they judged went beyond the expectations of a medical agenda and did not convey some of the physicians' statements in order to control patients' decisions.

When it is necessary to use "ad hoc" interpreters because of the lack of available professionals, it is important to recognize that their presence raises specific clinical issues (Hsieh, 2006a, 2006b). If the interpreter is a family member, there can be a range of different situations. Although such persons can play important, even vital roles in the diagnostic and treatment processes, they should not be the people responsible for ensuring the flow of information between the patient and the practitioner (Rosenberg et al., 2007).

In the case of a child interpreting for an adult (parent, grandparent, uncle, etc.), the clinician must avoid sensitive issues that would negatively affect the child or child–adult relationship. The child may also have limited capacity to translate complex issues. It is best to roughly evaluate what the problem is through the child and inform the patient of the need to find another interpreter in order to assure quality of translation and to avoid the child becoming further entangled in a difficult situation. Similar issues arise in the case of an adolescent interpreting for an adult. While the adolescent may have more capacity to understand complex issues, it remains important to be aware of sensitive issues that may be difficult to translate and to hear. If difficult issues such as sexuality, the diagnosis of a malignant disease, or war trauma are involved, the patient should be informed of the importance of including a professional interpreter to complete the consultation.

A growing body of literature looks at the role that children and adolescents may have as culture brokers and interpreters for their immigrant families (Jones & Trickett, 2005). Two opposing perspectives are found in the literature. The first perspective frame this interaction as a form of "parentification" or "role reversal" which undermines traditional power relations within the family and may expose children to major stressors (Trickett & Jones, 2007). In the medical literature, two studies suggest that involving children in the communication of sensitive issues (e.g., death, complex or life-threatening disease) can have traumatic effects on the child (Haffner, 1992; Jacobs, Kroll, Green, & David, 1995). An alternative view sees this role of the child as a common task and responsibility in migrant families that need not alter or disrupt family relations (Trickett & Jones, 2007). Indeed, Morales and Hanson (2005) review some research which suggests that children who function as language brokers "acquire higher cognitive and decision-making abilities due to their brokering experience" (p. 492). In some circumstances, the young interpreter may play a protective role as a family advocate, preventing physicians, employers, or others from embarrassing their relatives, and this successful advocacy may enhance self-esteem and self-efficacy (Free, Green, Bhavnani, & Newman, 2003; Green, Free, Bhavnani, & Newman, 2005).

In the case of adults (e.g., a husband interpreting for his wife (or vice versa) or an adult child interpreting for a parent), it may be tempting for the clinician to rely on this ad hoc interpreter. Although family members are often long-term caregivers and can be of invaluable help to understand the patients' reality, this is distinct from the task of working as an interpreter. In order to avoid misunderstandings on a long-term basis and also to have an outside perspective on the patient, it is important to employ a professional interpreter. In cases of possible maltreatment or domestic violence, it is crucial to avoid using family members as interpreters, as this may prevent the patient from disclosing issues of an interpersonal nature, including abuse.

The case of a parent interpreting for a child or adolescent is less common in migrant families, because children are among the first in the family to acquire facility in the new language, but this situation can occur, particularly with young children. It poses the dilemma that the child's perceptions are all filtered through the adult family member, and so areas of conflict or disagreement and nuances of emotional tone and meaning may be lost. Again, interpreting by a professional, even with the parent present for comfort, may improve the accuracy and completeness of the communication.

Bilingual health care staff may be able to interpret but require training for the task. It is important to first make certain the staff person is willing to perform this extra task, as not every bilingual person is comfortable interpreting. In any case, all of the rules previously discussed apply, namely, checking for concordance of gender, ethnicity, etc.; asking if both interpreter and patient agree to be matched; and reminding the interpreter of the importance of confidentiality. When professional interpreters are not available, it may be possible to train a pool of bilingual staff to act as interpreters and arrange institutional procedures that allow them to be on call when necessary.

Working with Interpreters in Cultural Consultation

The following suggestions (see Table 5.2) for working with interpreters are drawn from our work with the CCS, published guides for medical interviews with an interpreter (Bischoff & Loutan, 2008), and advice from Montreal's Inter-regional Interpreters Bank.[1] These suggestions are offered not as a prescriptive list of dos and don'ts but as

---

[1] The document can be downloaded at http://www.sante-montreal.qc.ca/

Table 5.2 Guidelines for working with interpreters in clinical settings

Prior to the interview

- Contact the interpreter before the consultation. Provide some general information regarding the patient and ask if he/she would be comfortable interpreting for the patient
- If the interpreter is not a trained or professional interpreter, determine his relation to the patient and remind him of the basic rules of interpreting
- Remind the interpreter that everything that is said in the consultation room must be kept confidential
- Ask the interpreter to translate everything that is said and to tell you when accurate translation is not possible
- Ask the interpreter to describe her impressions of the patient's feelings and emotions, making clear that you recognize the difficulty of this task
- Ask the interpreter to tell you when he/she is unsure of the meaning of the patient's verbal and/or nonverbal communication
- Arrange the interview setting so that patient and practitioner can see the interpreter and each other; placing three chairs in triangle is usually the best way to achieve this

During the interview

- Present yourself and the interpreter
- Ask the patient if he agrees to being interpreted by this interpreter
- Inform the patient that the interpreter will translate everything you and the patient say
- Inform the patient that the interpreter will respect confidentiality
- Look mainly at the patient and use first-person singular speech
- Use simple and short sentences
- Be aware of how your communicative style may be direct or indirect (e.g., the way you frame questions, you make comments, and the ways you interpret what the patient says)
- Summarize your understanding frequently, asking the patient to confirm or to correct you
- If the patient and interpreter have engaged in several exchanges without translation, interrupt them and ask the interpreter to translate

After the interview

- Ask the interpreter if she has something to add about the patient or the consultation process
- Check the interpreter's personal feelings about the content of the interview and offer sources of support for any distress uncovered
- Record the name of the interpreter and contact information in the patient's file for future reference

general principles to be applied flexibly, taking into account the particularities of the context, including the specific health issue, interpreter, time, and the type of consultation. These suggestions apply to interpretation for all kinds of health care. Those who interpret for mental health practitioners must have some additional training concerning mental illness and its treatment.

Preparing for the Consultation

When possible, the consultant should contact the interpreter before the consultation to provide some general information regarding the client and determine if he/she will be comfortable interpreting for the client. This initial contact can help uncover potential conflicts of interest, dual relationships, or errors in matching. If the interpreter is not a trained or professional interpreter, it is important to clarify his relation to the patient and to convey the basic rules of medical interpreting (i.e., the need for confidentiality, accuracy of translation, and the possibility of adding comments when necessary while clearly distinguishing these comments from the patient's actual statements).

The consultant should also briefly explain the patient's situation and the purpose of the consultation as well as the basic parameters, including the time available for the interview (which must be longer than usual as everything must be said twice). The consultant can also specify what the kind of translation needed; in general, this is the most complete and accurate possible, but if the interpreter can function as a cultural informant or culture broker, they may be able to supply additional cultural background information to the clinician and patient to improve the quality of communication (see Chapter 6 on culture brokers). Mental health interpreting requires close attention to feelings and emotions which may need to be described, in addition to translating the client's verbalizations. If the consultant has not worked with the interpreter before, it is worth clarifying how much experience the interpreter has had in mental health settings, and, if necessary, explaining the rationale for the specific interview methods including the formal mental status examination or any therapeutic interventions. It is important to record the name of the interpreter and context information in the patient's file for future reference.

Room layout also plays an important role in facilitating interpreting and the position of participants has both pragmatic and symbolic implications (Moss, 2008). The seating should be arranged so that patient and practitioner can both see the interpreter and each other; placing the three chairs in triangle is usually the best way to achieve this. When the interview is with a single patient, the interpreter usually sits near the patient. In situations where the consultation involves interviews with a group of people (e.g., family or members of the patient's social network), the interpreter may sit close to the practitioners with the group arranged in a circle or horseshoe configuration (Miletic et al., 2006). This arrangement is also used in French ethnopsychiatry consultations (Chapter 4).

All interpreted consultations are fundamentally cross-cultural encounters. As such, the most important issue is the practitioners' overall attitude to the encounter with the patient. The cross-cultural encounter may threaten the health care practitioner's personal and professional identity (Cohen-Emerique & Hohl, 2002; 2004). In order to avoid defensive reactions that can jeopardize communication or even abruptly end the encounter, Cohen-Emerique and Hohl suggest that practitioners go through a training process that includes the "discovery of self." Only when one is clear about the implicit rules and values in one's own cultural system can one understand the other and find ways, through negotiation and mediation, to offer culturally sensitive care.

During the Consultation

The first step in the actual consultation involves introducing the participants. The consultant should introduce the members of the team including the interpreter. If it has not already been determined, the patient should be asked if he or she agrees to have the interpreter and others present. During the interview, the consultant should look mainly at the patient and use first-person singular speech (i.e., "Did you feel sad?"); this direct speech will help keep the statement simple, avoid confusion as to who is speaking, and reinforce the relationship between the practitioner and the patient (Roat, Putsch, & Lucero, 1997). Interpretation takes time and requires close attention. The consultant can observe facial expression and paralanguage while waiting for the interpreter to complete the translation.

The quality of the communication process can be assessed during the interview by asking the interpreter for feedback at each step to be sure there is mutual understanding. It is useful to ask for brief summaries to ensure that all three parties have a mutual understanding of what has been discussed; this strategy is also called "back interpretation" (Hsieh, 2006b).

It is important to make efforts to insure that the patient feels comfortable. Most basically, this is achieved by one's attitude: showing an interest in the individual, valuing his/her background, and using a clear, nonspecialized vocabulary, free of jargon, that can be understood by both the patient and the interpreter (neither of whom are likely to have mastery over medical terminology).

Communication between immigrant and refugee patients and practitioners is often difficult because of linguistic barriers combined with misunderstandings that arise from different expectations of roles and outcomes and from different personal and cultural styles of communication or self-presentation (Gumperz & Roberts, 1991; Smith, DeVellis, Kalet, Roberts, & DeVellis, 2005). Humor, irony, and sarcasm can be sophisticated expressions of complex emotions, including mixtures of fear, anger, and criticism, and can easily be misunderstood in intercultural health care settings (Hartog, 2006).

One key issue during the consultation is control of the communication process. While some authors insist that the practitioner must stay in control of the process (Bischoff & Loutan, 2008), in practice it is rarely possible to maintain tight control at every moment as the interpreter may need to ask for clarification or respond spontaneously to maintain their human presence. Some loss of control is a normal part of a cross-cultural and cross-linguistic consultation. Control can be maintained over the overall structure of the interaction, while allowing some flexibility. Nevertheless, the clinician should have a clear sense of the ongoing process and content of communication and, if this is lost, should pause and ask the interpreter for clarification and re-establish the agenda and goals of the interview.

After the Consultation

After each interview, it is essential to have a "debriefing" conversation with the interpreter, to review the process of the interview and see if the interpreter has any observations to add about the patient or the consultation itself. It is also important to assess the interpreter's own feelings about the interview, which may have aroused emotions based on the content of the illness or various levels of identification with the patient and predicament (Loutan, Farinelli, & Pampallona, 1999; Valero-Garcés, 2005). In some cases, the interpreter may need follow-up to address emotional reactions or concerns. If exposed to traumatic stories, interpreters need to receive support similar to that available to therapists. A German study on the use of interpreters for refugees found a significant prevalence of PTSD among interpreters, most of whom were not trained and were refugees themselves or had experiences of child abuse and depression (Teegen & Gonnenwein, 2002).

A study conducted by Baistow (1999) in the UK examined the emotional and psychological effects experienced by community interpreters in public services. The majority (80 %) of interpreters surveyed reported feeling very positive about their work and found it fulfilling and rewarding. However, more than two-thirds reported feeling distressed sometimes by the material they had to interpret, and half reported that interpreting sometimes made them feel worried and anxious and experience mood or behavior changes. Baistow proposed several strategies to address

the emotional challenges of interpreting: (1) increased liaison between employers, service providers, and interpreter organizations (2) pre- and in-service training which addresses the emotional challenges of community interpreting work; (3) regular supervision for new or inexperienced interpreters; and (4) a referral service for one-on-one counselling of interpreters.

Working with Interpreters in Psychiatric Assessment

Psychiatric assessment has several goals: (1) identifying the patient's clinical complaints and concerns; (2) recognizing symptoms, behaviors and experiences that may indicate specific forms of psychopathology and make a clinical diagnosis; (3) gathering information about a patient's personal history and social context in order to understand their illness in the context of their biography and life circumstances; (4) identifying sources of strength and resilience that can be mobilized for helping interventions; and, most fundamentally, (5) developing and sustaining clinical empathy, rapport, and a working alliance. The central role of language in psychiatric assessment raises specific issues for mental health interpreting (Table 5.3).

Table 5.3 Key issues in mental health assessment with an interpreter

- Clinicians need to attend to both denotative and connotative meanings of language, styles of emotion expression, and linguistic idioms
- Interpreters need to be alert to regional accents, dialects, and implications of language for social status (both their own and that of the patient)
- Interpreters need to possess observational skills as well as knowledge of psychopathology so that they can help the clinician recognize specific symptoms (e.g., thought disorder)
- Switching language can convey important information about emotional meaning of specific memories and experiences as well as patient's efforts to position themselves in the clinical interaction
- Interpreters can provide information on cultural norms of expression that can assist in determining whether specific behaviors or experience are unusual

One key component of psychiatric assessment is the mental status examination, which gathers systematic information about symptoms, signs, and experiences needed to identify psychopathology. The formal mental status examination involves open-ended and semi-structured interviewing. In some instances, this may be supplemented by standardized tests, most often to assess cognitive status. In order to assist with this evaluation, the interpreter must understand the goals of the interview as well as the point of specific questions or tasks.

Case Vignette 5-7

An elderly Greek woman, who complained of being forgetful, was referred to the CCS for cognitive evaluation. The interview included administration of the Folstein Mini-Mental Status Examination (MMSE; Folstein, Folstein, & McHugh, 1975), a brief measure of cognitive functioning. She was asked to answer a few questions and to follow the instructions which were translated by the interpreter from the English version of the MMSE. As the interpreter presented the items, he was unaware of giving hints to the patient by making gestures and repeating phrases in ways that coached a positive response.

Language provides indications of mental status and neuropsychological functioning relevant to the patient's diagnosis (Jackson et al., 2008; Westermeyer & Janca, 1997). The voice may be monotonous or speech slow in cases of depression and disorganized or impoverished in schizophrenia. There are speech tics in Tourette syndrome and speech disorders which may have idiosyncratic presentations that can be mistaken for psychopathology. Deciphering these signs correctly may be crucial to adequately assess, diagnose, and treat mental health problems.

Any assessment or testing is made in reference to norms. In mental health assessment, this norm is often implicit, based on experience with individuals from the dominant cultural groups—most often middle-class, Euro-Americans

(Padilla, 2001). The sociocultural background and developmental experiences of patients influence their ways of thinking, expressing suffering, and presenting in clinical situations (Segall, Dasen, Berry, & Poortinga, 1999). All the areas assessed in the mental status examination are influenced by this background and current social and cultural contexts. Knowledge of the associated norms is therefore essential for identifying pathology.

The standard psychiatric mental status examination covers appearance, behavior (including attitude and relationship to the examiner), affect, mood, and cognition (including thought content and process, memory, insight, and judgement). For all of these areas, the interpreter can help the health care professional determine whether the expression is culturally normative or unusual. However, this often requires more cultural background knowledge and exploration with the patient and others in their entourage tasks that fall within the role of the culture broker (see Chapter 6).

Different styles of self-presentation by patients (Goffman, 1959) are a common cause of misunderstanding between physicians and migrants and often go unrecognized (Roberts, Moss, Mass, Sarangi, & Jones, 2005). These differences can include the degree of how personal or impersonal to be in addressing the other, how direct or indirect to be in self-presentation, what to emphasize and what to play down, how to sequence responses, choice of words and idioms, and a range of prosodic features, including intonation and rhythm that may convey irony, sarcasm, and other metalinguistic information (Roberts & Sarangi, 2005).

Nonverbal cues can easily be misinterpreted. Body posture is socioculturally coded, as is interpersonal distance (Hall, 1966). For example, a patient who does not look directly at the physician while talking and keeps her head down might be misinterpreted by the doctor as suffering from depression or domestic abuse. The socially appropriate degree of eye contact varies with gender, age, and authority according to cultural codes. In some cultures, there is a norm of not looking directly to at an elder, a male, and a person of authority, as a sign of respect and gender-appropriate behavior. There are many societies in which indirectness in communication is important for politeness, respect, and saving face in situations of potential conflict or disagreement. Directness and indirectness are also important clinically as ways to gain patients' adherence to treatment (Smith et al., 2005).

Structured Interviews and Psychological Testing

Structured interviews and psychological tests are important in research settings and can be useful supplements in clinical evaluation. While it may be tempting to have an interpreter informally translate tests' items "on the fly" during an assessment interview, there is evidence that such informal translation of tests is often neither reliable nor valid. As Vignette 5-2 presented earlier illustrates, it may be particularly difficult for an interpreter to translate specific items that involve unfamiliar or idiomatic expressions.

In addition to the difficulties such impromptu translation, psychological tests have generally been developed through research with specific populations and may not be valid when applied in other cultures or contexts. For a test to work across cultures, it is necessary to establish not only accurate linguistic translation but also meaning equivalence (Greenfield, 1997; Arnold & Matus, 2000).

In cross-cultural research, equivalence in meaning is achieved through a lengthy process involving several steps (Brislin, 1986; Westermeyer & Janca, 1997) (see Table 5.4). This procedure can be improved by insuring that the team of translators vary in age, sex, education, and social class and that the validation of the test is done on samples that also reflect the diversity within the culture (Sartorius & Janca, 1996).

Even if a psychometrically adequate test is available in the patient's language, the results must be viewed with caution. Cognitive testing results are strongly related to educational level (Carlat, 2005). Results are poor for those with less than 8 years of schooling even without any cognitive problems (Ainslie & Murden, 1993).

Table 5.4 Steps to establish the cross-cultural equivalence of psychological measures

Translation by a team of bilingual persons who have spent at least several years in each culture–language group

Back translation into the original language by one or more persons not familiar with ("blind to") the original version of the instrument

Revision of the translation on the basis of analysis of the three versions (i.e., original, translation, back translation) by a panel with expertise in the two languages, the assessment instrument, and the specific constructs or conditions under study

A *pilot study* in the target population to determine basic psychometric properties and identify problematic items or formats. This should include qualitative interviewing of subjects on the ways in which they understood the test and specific items

Revision of the translation on the basis of the pilot study data

Renorming the measure by administering it to general population samples

Revalidation of the measure by establishing its relationship to other "gold standard" measures of the construct

Cross-cultural research on cognitive development over the past few decades has shown that performance on cognitive tasks is highly dependent on enculturation and socialization (Dasen, 1975; Segall et al., 1999). Cognitive performance is oriented according to what is valued in a society and can be modified by training (Dasen, Lavallée, & Retschiski, 1979). Poor performance in an unfamiliar testing situation may not indicate a lack of competency in other more familiar settings. For example, Nunes, Schliemann, and Carraher (1993) found that street children in Recife (Brazil) performed very well in calculations about the price of the small items (candies, fruits) they sell, but underperformed when asked for the same calculation on a paper–pencil test in a classroom-like setting. It is not only the content of a test that may be confusing but the testing situation itself (Greenfield, 1997).

The interpreter can help the clinician understand the meaning of patients' answers to psychometric tests and give additional diagnostically useful information about how the patient is answering (e.g., with hesitancy or difficulty finding words). A skilled interpreter may recognize an inappropriate testing situation, i.e., a situation that would embarrass the patient or make him unable to answer. With instructions from the clinician, the interpreter can explain the testing or interview situation to the patient and facilitate the assessment process by providing appropriate clarification and reassurance.

The Complexity of Language in Mental Health

Ethnocultural identities and social position shape the language used to express experience. Every language has its own nuances of meaning tied to social predicaments, developmental experiences, and the structures of family and community life. These configure the language of subjective experience and emotion, which is a major focus for mental health assessment and intervention. Many people speak multiple languages, associated with different stages of development, education, migratory experiences, and periods in their life. Hybrid identities add additional complexity to the meaning and use of specific languages, which may be associated with specific aspects of identity or represent hybridity itself through creoles or patterns of switching (Harris & Rampton, 2002; Kirmayer, 2006).

Words have both denotative and connotative meanings. Denotation refers to the literal meaning of the word, while connotation involves the conventional associations that the word evokes. Connotations depend on social contexts, and even in the same linguistic or ethnocultural group, a word may have quite different connotations according to social class, educational level, and the context in which it is employed. Connotation can easily be lost if the interpreter translates word for word or does not have sufficient knowledge of the specific cultural contexts of the speaker and listener. A skilled interpreter works to find equivalent meanings, to convey not just the denotation but also some of the crucial connotations of specific words.

Capturing the meaning of words can be especially challenging in the domain of emotions.

Cross-cultural research reveals that certain emotions with a precise name in one language do not have close equivalents in other languages (Russell, 1991). Further, emotions that are distinct in one language may be blended or conflated in another. Although cross-cultural research on emotions has suggested the universality of a small set of basic emotions (Mesquita, Frijda, & Scherer, 1997), more complex emotion terms refer to social situations and predicaments that are shaped by culture (Kövecses, 2000). Translating emotional meaning therefore requires not simply finding a roughly equivalent term but explaining the social situations and events that engender the feelings and that call for specific emotional and behavioral responses.

Patients who come from small or homogenous communities may use compressed, condensed, or elliptical forms of language that reference shared experiences and events (Bernstein, 1966). To an outsider, this style of expression may seem laconic, opaque, or inarticulate. The language of symptom expression and emotion is closely bound to linguistic and cultural idioms. Patients may also use linguistic idioms that only a fluent speaker knows and that serve to convey subtle shades of meaning or attitudes. Such idioms can easily be misunderstood when interpreted concretely (Keesing, 1985). Idioms may vary with education, social class, and ethnicity so that even a fluent interpreter can miss local meanings.

The language that patients use in a health care setting may not be the one they use at home or the language in which they are most able to access memories, emotions, or use meaningful idioms of distress. Social context and efforts to portray oneself as linguistically competent may influence the willingness to use languages even when interpreters are available. Patients' decisions to use or avoid specific languages can provide important clinical information. Some patients may prefer to communicate in a second language because it affords them more distance from distressing feelings. For individuals who have acquired different languages at different developmental stages or life periods, memories may be stratified in terms of language. Switching from one language to another can be done deliberately in search of the right word or phrase, but it may also occur unconsciously as emotion intensifies or memories are accessed that are associated with a specific language, time, and place (Guttfreund, 1990; Westermeyer, 1989; Westermeyer & Janca, 1997). Language choice may be an adaptive strategy or ego syntonic defence and should not be discarded or ignored without appreciation of the patient's motives or intentions. Code switching may allow patients to move flexibly between social statuses and identifications, avoiding humiliation by agreeing to use the host culture language or denying affiliation with the maternal language to affirm a new identity.

To convey these nuances of language use, clinicians and interpreters must understand psychological dynamics, respect patients' modes of self-presentation, and attend to nonverbal communication. The consultant must discuss these issues with the interpreter before the interview and intervene for clarification when interaction around particular emotional states seems dissonant or unclear to avoid misdiagnosis or inappropriate intervention.

The Role of Interpreters in Treatment Interventions

Interpreters can be used to deliver psychotherapeutic interventions (Bolton, 2002; d'Ardenne, Ruaro, Cestari, Fakhoury, & Priebe, 2007). Various models of collaboration between interpreters and psychotherapists have been described in the literature (Baylav, 2002; Patel, 2002). Older models insist on the linguistic agent role of the interpreter as a neutral "translating machine" (Bradford & Munoz, 1993; Kline, Acosta, Austin, & Johnson, 1980; Price, 1975). Technical advice is given in order to overcome difficulties or risks associated with working with a third person in the consultation (Rack, 1982; Sabin, 1975). Unfortunately, the model of interpreter as a translating machine, or an invisible "nonperson" who does not have any influence on the interaction, ignores systemic interactional processes that may have major influence on the therapeutic process (Bot, 2005). More recent models emphasize that

Table 5.5 Key principles in providing CBT interventions with an interpreter

- Before beginning, brief interpreters on the logic behind interventions
- Unless interpreter is qualified to work as a co-therapist, encourage short renditions regularly translated to allow tracking process
- Neutrality of the interpreter should be maintained when possible
- Let the interpreter be a cultural informant providing additional background after the session

a skilled psychiatric interpreter should form a team with the psychiatrist (Westermeyer, 1989). After working together for a while, they will understand each other and know how to achieve therapeutic objectives together. The interpreter thus becomes a co-therapist, who is recognized as a full member of the team with psychotherapeutic skills (Mudarikiri, 2002; Westermeyer, 1989). At present, there is no clear evidence of the superiority of any one approach to working with interpreters in delivering psychotherapeutic or psychosocial interventions. The choice of a model therefore is dependent on practical and contextual factors, including the availability of interpreter services and other institutional resources, as well as interpreters' and practitioners' training, orientation, and cultural sensitivity.

Cognitive Behavioral Therapy

Each form of intervention raises specific challenges for the interpreter. For example, d'Ardenne, Farmer, Ruaro, and Priebe (2007) provide a detailed protocol for administering trauma-focused Cognitive Behavioral Therapy (CBT) through an interpreter (Table 5.5). This intervention raises specific issues because trauma-focused involves directing the client to recall and think about traumatic experiences they may have tried to suppress and forget. Interpreters must be briefed on the logic behind this approach in order not to find the intervention overly distressing or interfere with the treatment by attempting to protect clients. The imaginal exposure technique requires careful timing, with temporal proximity between what the clinician says and the patient exposure. For interpreters, this implies that they must translate short "chunks" and not pause for extended explanations of complex phrases or idioms. Comments on cultural meanings or ambiguities must be made after the consultation (d'Ardenne, Farmer et al., 2007, p. 316).

Family Therapy

Family therapists have long recognized culture as a crucial consideration in intervention (Falicov, 2003; McGoldrick, Giordano, & Pearce, 1996). The interpreter can play different roles in the therapeutic system that includes the consulting family members and the therapist, but there is agreement that, as part of an interactional system, the interpreter is always more than a translator. The interpreter can provide valuable information on cultural concepts of family and kinship and facilitate exchanges on sensitive topics like gender roles or hierarchy (Hémon, 2001; Macciocchi, 2005; Raval, 1996).

DiNicola (1986) underlines the informational and therapeutic richness of having two languages present in a family therapy setting. He recommends a close working relationship between therapist and interpreter to increase the reliability of the translation. Providing an interpreter can allow members of the family who might otherwise be marginalized to participate more actively in therapy. DiNicola discusses how the process of code switching, i.e., shifting from one language to another, can reveal important information about affective and cognitive states as well as interactional patterns. Because family members may not all share the same language proficiency, language switches can serve as boundary markers between the family members; for example, a family member can switch into the therapist's language in order to reveal something that he does not want to be heard by the rest of the family. But DiNicola warns that attention to language should not divert the therapist from tracking the pattern of interactions that is essential to family

assessment and intervention. Code switching is especially important to address intergenerational issues in migration because the emotional language of children and elders may differ and the use of language can highlight generational or dynamic issues crucial to understanding the family's conflicts or dilemmas.

In family therapy, the interpreter can help build common ground from which it is possible to do effective work even if expectations and beliefs are different (Macciocchi, 2005; Raval, 1996). Hémon (2001) describes how trained interpreters, with psychological knowledge, can function as "go-betweens" or culture brokers, adding necessary background information while providing the family with a reassuring presence as a compatriot who knows the health care institution and the therapeutic procedure. The third position is co-therapist. In Hémon's work, at the Centre Minkowska in Paris, the interpreter was usually a colleague or trainee mental health practitioner who speaks the family's language and who could, therefore, take an active role in the therapeutic process.

Group Therapy

Group therapy practitioners from several theoretical orientations have also produced research and reflections on working with interpreters. While Westermeyer (1989) cautions against group therapy with an interpreter, as it might impede group interaction, recent work suggests that a group led by a therapist who does not speak the same language as the participants working with an experienced interpreter can be therapeutic (Kennard, Elliott, Roberts, & Evans, 2002). A high level of mutual understanding can be reached, but this requires close attention to the dyad of group facilitator and interpreter. According to Kennard, Roberts, and Elliott (2002), the group facilitator should be involved in the selection and training of the interpreter who plays an ongoing role in the group. As in family therapy, patterns of language use and code switching in a group can reveal boundaries, alliances, and areas of affect or conflict (Röder &

Opalič, 1997). The process of interpreting during the session allows time for the therapist to observe verbal and nonverbal behavior in the group: choice of language, timing of language switches, and attitudes of the group toward the therapist (Wolman, 1970).

Psychodynamic Psychotherapy

Working with an interpreter in psychotherapy involves complex systemic interactions and emotional dynamics. Each of the three participants—patient, interpreter, and practitioner—will respond affectively, consciously or not, to the other two. This interplay of affective links is understood by psychodynamic therapists in terms of the concepts of transference and countertransference. Psychodynamic authors agree that these complex relations need to be clarified and integrated in the understanding of the patient's intrapsychic dynamics and responses in treatment.

When the interpreter is part of the therapeutic process, the patient may form two separate transferences, one with the practitioner and another with the interpreter. Due to the facility of communication and identification, the patient may develop a therapeutic alliance with the interpreter first (Westermeyer, 1993; Raval & Smith, 2003; Miller, Martell, Pazdirek, Caruth, & Lopez, 2005). The interpreter may be viewed in two opposing ways simultaneously. On the hand, the interpreter may be seen as an ally and a compatriot who shares a common language and has been through some of the same difficulties, with whom it is possible to identify. When interpreters themselves are migrants, this identification may include the impression that the interpreter occupies an intermediate and apparently successful position between two cultures (Aubert, 2008; Piret, 1991; Valero-Garcés, 2005; Westermeyer, 1989). At the same time, as a member of the same community, the interpreter may also represent a threat. Patients may fear a loss of confidentiality and exposure (Bot & Wadensjö, 2004), with the risk of being stigmatized in the community. Patients may feel ashamed having to disclose

mental health problems or conflicts in the presence of a compatriot. Finally, some patients may have migrated in part to get away from their cultures of origin. They may therefore want to free themselves from their mother tongue, which they associate with difficult attachments, oppression, or other conflicts (Aubert, 2008).

Writing about psychodynamic psychotherapy with refugees, Rechtman (1992) advises clinicians to take advantage of the time used by interpreter and patient in the second language to observe the patient–interpreter interaction in order to evaluate its emotional tenor. Sometimes this presence of the interpreter leads to splitting in which the interpreter and practitioner may become polarized as good and bad objects in the patient's representations (Aubert, 2008; Haenel, 1997). For example, the interpreter may be viewed as the bad object, someone who might denounce the patient's political views, and the therapist as the good object, an omnipotent rescuer who will protect the patient (Aubert, 2008; Haenel, 1997; Bot & Wadensjö, 2004).

Of course, interpreters have their own identifications and emotional reactions to the clinician and patient. For example, interpreters who strongly identify with specific patients may overprotect them (Haenel, 1997) or normalize their discourse because of feeling embarrassed by the patient's pathology (Westermeyer, 1993). In some instances, interpreters may feel threatened by the patients for objective reasons like differences in political position or ethnicity or religion that were associated with discrimination, violence, or genocide in their countries of origin. Interpreters' may also present feelings of admiration for the therapist while depreciating patients (Haenel, 1997). If recognized, these relational processes can be helpful in exploring patients' dynamics. If not addressed, however, they may lead to disruptions in communication or a loss of safety that jeopardizes the therapeutic process. Many of these responses are ordinary, expectable emotional reactions that should not be termed transference or countertransference (Spensley & Blacker, 1976). Other feelings may reflect distortions or fantasies based on personal issues. A third level represents the collective images or fantasies that patients and therapists have of each other in what has been termed ethno-cultural transference and countertransference (Comas-Diaz & Jacobsen, 1991). All of these types of emotional reaction need to be explored in regular post-consultation debriefings between the therapist and the interpreter (Rechtman, 1992). The interpreter may need support from the clinician in dealing with patients and situations that evoke intense reactions.

In addition to therapist's potential counter-transference toward the patient, a second coun-tertransference can arise toward the interpreter. This may be positive, as when the interpreter is seen as someone with whom to share the difficult life experiences of the patients—holding the patient's emotional world might be easier for two instead of one (Miller et al., 2005). But therapists often have strong feelings of exclusion, power-lessness, and loss of control in interpreted consultations (Raval, 1996; Raval & Smith, 2003; Miller et al., 2005). Such strong reactions can jeopardize the therapeutic process if not detected and worked through (Darling, 2004).

The psychodynamic concept of resistance can also be used to understand aspects of patient–interpreter–therapist dynamics. Patient's resis-tance may be expressed by attributing a slip of the tongue to the difficulties of translation, talk-ing only to the interpreter to avoid being more fully engaged in the therapeutic process (Piret, 1991), or using code switching to avoid the inten-sity of affect in the first language. Code switching can also be used intentionally by the therapist according to the effect wished, regulating emotional distance and sense of identification in order to overcome resistance, for example, using the patient's mother tongue to increase identifica-tion or decreasing the emotional intensity by using the therapist's language (Oquendo, 1996).

For psychodynamic psychotherapists, lan-guage is not only a medium for transmitting representations and affects but is it itself material to interpret in the therapeutic process. A choice of words, dialect, or language can represent both personal and collective issues of desire, regres-sion, power, and history (M'Barga, 1983). A patient's language reflects both pragmatics and

Table 5.6 Key principles for psychodynamic assessment and therapy with an interpreter

- Be aware of and address explicit and implicit transferential and countertransferential issues between the three protagonists
- Pay attention to and address particular forms of resistances that are likely to emerge in interpreted sessions
- Explore the implications of the choice of language
- Consider the interpretative nature of translations
- Use the interpreters' subjectivity as a valuable source of information

emotional dynamics (Rechtman, 1992). The word "interpreter" has a double meaning as someone who can translate from one language to another and someone who can grasp latent mean-ings within any action or experience (Darling, 2004; Kouassi, 2001; M'Barga, 1983). Some of these latent meanings are sedimented in language through metaphor or forgotten etymologies that may nonetheless influence thought and experi-ence. Translation then can be considered a form of psychoanalytic interpretation to the extent that it brings unconscious meaning to conscious awareness. Translation difficulties can be used as a therapeutic lever, as work by French ethnopsy-chiatrists has shown (de Pury, 1998; Goguikian Ratcliff & Changkakoti, 2004). In these situa-tions, the interpreter can function as a cultural informant explaining the significance of words in their social contexts to unpack the meaning of pathology, behavior or rituals.

Psychodynamic authors insist on the implica-tion of the interpreter in the therapeutic process. Above all, interpreters must be aware of their own biases and be engaged in the therapeutic work, reflecting on its language (Khelil, 1991). For Kouassi (2001), interpreters should acknowl-edge their own subjectivity as this can help patients build links between their experience and the social world, as well as between past and present. But this is not an easy task, and interpret-ers may feel a dissonance between the ideal of neutrality imposed by ethical codes and the emo-tional involvement asked by the therapist or demanded by the therapeutic situation (Goguikian Ratcliff & Suardi, 2006) (Table 5.6).

Conclusion: Building an Effective Partnership

The effectiveness of cultural consultation is due in large measure to the systematic employment of professional interpreters. The CCS works closely with professional interpreters, developing a collaboration based on mutual respect, dialogue, and repeated experiences over time with many cases. Interpreters are not only essential for accurate clinical communication in intercultural assessment but can contribute to the delivery of effective interventions (Chen Wu, Leventhal, Ortiz, Gonzalez, & Forsyth, 2006). In psychiatry and psychology, interpreters sometimes have been seen simply as translating "machines" but this view is misleading and potentially harmful for patients. We have shown that there is a wide range of possible roles for interpreters, from "informative translator," who can add some information about contexts and meanings to both patient and practitioner, to full co-therapist, whose subjectivity and insight can play an important part in patients' recovery.

Effective work with interpreters depends not only on interpersonal trust but also on clinical settings that allow the practitioner to make full use of the interpreter's knowledge and skills. This requires transforming institutional understandings of what interpreters do and of their place in the health care system. This transformation involves action at multiple levels of policy and practice: establishing guidelines that will influence training, clinical interventions, institutional practices, and social norms. There is also a need for continued research on mental health interpreting. The principles found in ethical codes for interpreters, which were largely derived from nonmedical contexts, need to be empirically studied and new practices implemented that address the various roles and functions of interpreters and culture brokers in mental health care.

The cultural consultation process requires professional interpreters with specific training in mental health. In addition to training, interpreters need personal qualities that enable them to be sensitive to psychological issues, aware of their own emotional responses and potential biases, and alert to the ways they are likely to be perceived by patients from different backgrounds. Clinicians can play an important role in training interpreters. In the CCS, this has occurred both formally by providing workshops for interpreters and informally by working together repeatedly on cases.

For interpreters to take their proper place as health professionals in the health care system, there must be national, regional, and institutional policies in place and an adequate budget allocated to interpreter services. Training needs to be provided to mental health professionals on how to collaborate with interpreters (Leanza, 2008). Quality assurance standards need to formally require the routine use of interpreters in mental health and to monitor and enforce these standards.

References

Ainslie, N. K., & Murden, R. A. (1993). Effect of education on the clock-drawing dementia screen in nondemented elderly persons. *Journal of the American Geriatric Society, 41*(3), 249–252.

Arnold, B., & Matus, Y. (2000). Test translation and cultural equivalence methodologies for use with diverse populations. In I. Cuéllar & F. Paniagua (Eds.), *Multicultural mental health* (pp. 121–136). San Diego, CA: Academic Press.

Asher, R. E., & Moseley, C. (Eds.). (2007). *Atlas of the world's languages* (2nd ed.). New York, NY: Routledge.

Aubert, A.-E. (2008). La transformation du côté du thérapeute comme préalable au changement du patient en situation transculturelle. *Pratiques Psychologiques, 14*, 67–78.

Australian Bureau of Statistics. (2006). *2006 Census data by location.* Retrieved May 20, 2009, from http://www.censusdata.abs.gov.au/ABSNavigation/prenav/PopularAreas?collection=census/period=2006

Baistow, K. (1999). *The emotional and psychological impact of community interpreting.* Paper presented at the First Babelea Conference on Community Interpreting, London, England.

Bancroft, M. (2005). *The interpreter's world tour: An environmental scan of standards of practice for interpreters.* Ellicott City, MD: National Council on Interpreting in Health Care.

Battaglini, A., Désy, M., Dorval, D., Poirier, L.-R., Fournier, M., & Camirand, H. (2007). *L'intervention de première ligne à Montréal auprès des personnes immigrantes: Estimé des ressources nécessaires pour une intervention adéquate*. Montréal, Quebec, Canada: Agence de la santé et des services sociaux de Montréal.

Baylav, A. (2002). Issues of language provision in health care services. In R. Tribe & H. Raval (Eds.), *Working with interpreters in mental health* (pp. 69–76). New York, NY: Brunner-Routledge.

Bernstein, B. (1966). Elaborated and restricted codes: An outline. *Sociological Inquiry, 36*(2), 254–261.

Betancourt, J. R., Green, A. R., Carrillo, J. E., & Ananeh-Firempong, O., II. (2003). Defining cultural competence: A practical framework for addressing racial/ethnic disparities in health and health care. *Public Health Reports, 118*(4), 293–302.

Bischoff, A., Hudelson, P., & Bovier, P. A. (2008). Doctor–patient gender concordance and patient satisfaction in interpreter-mediated consultations: An exploratory study. *Journal of Travel Medicine, 15*(1), 1–5.

Bischoff, A., & Loutan, L. (2008). *Other words, other meanings.* Genève, Switzerland: Hôpitaux Universitaires de Genève.

Bjorn, G. J. (2005). Ethics and interpreting in psychotherapy with refugee children and families. *Nordic Journal of Psychiatry, 59*(6), 516–521.

Blake, C. (2003, June). Ethical considerations in working with culturally diverse populations: The essential role of professional interpreters. *Bulletin of the Canadian Psychiatric Association,* 21–23.

Bolton, J. (2002). The third presence: A psychiatrist experience of working with non English speaking patients and interpreters. *Transcultural Psychiatry, 39*(1), 97–114.

Bot, H. (2003). The myth of the uninvolved interpreter interpreting in mental health and the development of a three-person psychology. In L. Brunette, G. Bastin, I. Hemlin, & H. Clarke (Eds.), *The critical link 3* (pp. 27–35). Amsterdam, Netherlands: John Benjamins Publishing Company.

Bot, H. (2005). *Dialogue interpreting in mental health.* Amsterdam, Netherlands: Rodopi.

Bot, H., & Wadensjö, C. (2004). The presence of a third party: A dialogical view on interpreter-assisted treatment. In J. Wilson & B. Drožđek (Eds.), *Broken spirits. The treatment of traumatized asylum seekers, refugees, war and torture victims* (pp. 355–378). New York, NY: Brunner-Routledge.

Bowen, S. (2001). *Language barriers in access to health care "certain circumstances": Equity in and responsiveness of the health care system to the needs of minority and marginalized populations* (pp. 145–160). Ottawa, Ontario, Canada: Health Canada.

Bowen, S., & Kaufert, J. M. (2003). Assessing the "costs" of health interpreter programs: The risks and the promise. In L. Brunette, G. Bastin, I. Hemlin, & H. Clarke (Eds.), *The critical link 3* (pp. 261–272). Amsterdam, Netherlands: John Benjamins.

Bradford, D. T., & Munoz, A. (1993). Translation in bilingual psychotherapy. *Professional Psychology: Research and Practice, 24*(1), 52–61.

Brislin, R. (1986). The wording and translation of research instruments. In J. Lonner & J. Berry (Eds.), *Field methods in cross-cultural research* (pp. 137–164). Beverly Hills, CA: Sage.

Carlat, D. J. (2005). *The psychiatric interview: A practical guide* (2nd ed.). Philadelphia, PA: Lippincott Williams & Wilkins.

Chen Wu, A., Leventhal, J. M., Ortiz, J., Gonzalez, E. E., & Forsyth, B. (2006). The interpreter as cultural educator of residents: Improving communication for Latino parents. *Archives of Pediatrics & Adolescent Medicine, 160*(11), 1145–1150.

Cohen-Emerique, M. (2003). La médiation interculturelle, les médiateurs et leur formation. In F. Remotti (Ed.), *Corpi, individuali e contesti interculturali* (pp. 58–87). Turin, Italy: L'Harmattan Italia Connessioni.

Cohen-Emerique, M. (2004a). Positionnement et compétences spécifiques des médiateurs. *Hommes et Migrations, 1249,* 36–52.

Cohen-Emerique, M. (2004b). Mediateurs interculturels dans le champ du travail social. *Agenda Interculturel, 221,* 14–23.

Cohen-Emerique, M., & Fayman, S. (2005). Mediateurs interculturels, passerelles d'identités. *Connexions, 83,* 169–190.

Cohen-Emerique, M., & Hohl, J. (2002). Menace à l'identité personnelle chez les professionnels en situation interculturelle. In C. Sabatier, H. Malewska-Peyre, & F. Tanon (Eds.), *Identités, acculturation et altérité* (pp. 199–228). Paris, France: L'Harmattan.

Cohen-Emerique, M., & Hohl, J. (2004). Les réactions défensives à la menace identitaire chez les professionnels en situations interculturelles. *Cahiers Internationaux de Psychologie Sociale, 61,* 21–34.

Comas-Diaz, L., & Jacobsen, F. M. (1991). Ethnocultural transference and countertransference in the therapeutic dyad. *The American Journal of Orthopsychiatry, 61*(3), 392–402.

d'Ardenne, P., Farmer, E., Ruaro, L., & Priebe, S. (2007). Not lost in translation: Protocols for interpreting trauma-focused CBT. *Behavioural and Cognitive Psychotherapy, 35*(3), 303–316.

d'Ardenne, P., Ruaro, L., Cestari, L., Fakhoury, W., & Priebe, S. (2007). Does interpreter-mediated CBT with traumatized refugee people work? A comparison of patient outcomes in East London. *Behavioural and Cognitive Psychotherapy, 35*(3), 293–301.

Darling, L. (2004). Psychoanalytically-informed work with interpreters. *Psychoanalytic Psychotherapy, 18*(3), 255–267.

Dasen, P. (1975). Concrete operational development in three cultures. *Journal of Cross-Cultural Psychology, 6*(2), 156–172.

Dasen, P., Lavallée, M., & Retschiski, J. (1979). Training conservation of quantity (liquids) in West African (Baoulé) children. *International Journal of Psychology, 14*(1), 57–68.

David, R. A., & Rhee, M. (1998). The impact of language as a barrier to effective health care in an underserved urban Hispanic community. *Mont Sinai Journal of Medicine, 65*(5–6), 393–397.

Davidson, B. (2000). The interpreter as institutional gatekeeper: The social-linguistic role of interpreters in Spanish-English medical discourse. *Journal of Sociolinguistics, 4*(3), 379–405.

Davis, D., O'Brien, M. A., Freemantle, N., Wolf, F. M., Mazmanian, P., & Taylor-Vaisey, A. (1999). Impact of formal continuing medical education: Do conferences, workshops, rounds, and other traditional continuing education activities change physician behavior or health care outcomes? *JAMA: The Journal of the American Medical Association, 282*(9), 867–874.

Davis, D., Thomson, M. A., Oxman, A. D., & Haynes, R. B. (1995). Changing physician performance. A systematic review of the effect of continuing medical education strategies. *JAMA: The Journal of the American Medical Association, 274*(9), 700–705.

de Pury, S. (1998). *Traité du malentendu. Théorie et pratique de la médiation interculturelle en situation clinique.* Le Plessis-Robinson, France: Institut Synthélabo.

Demetriou, S. (1991). Interpreters and psychiatry. In I. H. Minas (Ed.), *Cultural diversity and mental health* (pp. 65–69). Melbourne, Victoria, Australia: Royal Australian and New Zealand College of Psychiatrists and Victorian Transcultural Psychiatry Unit.

DiNicola, V. F. (1986). Beyond babel: Family therapy as cultural translation. *International Journal of Family Psychiatry, 7*(2), 179–191.

Drennan, G., & Swartz, L. (1999). A concept over-burdened: Institutional roles for psychiatric interpreters in post-apartheid South Africa. *Interpreting, 4*(2), 169.

Falicov, C. J. (2003). Culture in family therapy: New variations on a fundamental theme. In T. L. Sexton, G. R. Weeks, & M. S. Robbins (Eds.), *Handbook of family therapy: The science and practice of working with families and couples* (pp. 37–55). New York, NY: Brunner-Routledge.

Farooq, S., & Fear, C. (2003). Working through interpreters. *Advances in Psychiatric Treatment, 9*(2), 104–109.

Folstein, M. F., Folstein, S. E., & McHugh, P. F. (1975). "Mini-mental state": A practical method for grading the cognitive state of patients for the clinician. *Journal of Psychiatric Research, 12*, 189–199.

Free, C., Green, J., Bhavnani, V., & Newman, A. (2003). Bilingual young people's experiences of interpreting in primary care: A qualitative study. *British Journal of General Practice, 53*(492), 530–535.

Goffman, E. (1959). *The presentation of the self in everyday life.* London, England: Penguin Books.

Goguikian Ratcliff, B., & Changkakoti, N. (2004). Le rôle de l'interprète dans la construction de l'interculturalité dans un entretien ethnopsychiatrique. *L'autre, Cliniques, Cultures et Sociétés, 5*(2), 255–264.

Goguikian Ratcliff, B., & Suardi, F. (2006). L'interprète dans une consultation thérapeutique: Conceptions de son rôle et difficultés éprouvées. *Psychothérapies, 26*(1), 37–49.

Green, J., Free, C., Bhavnani, V., & Newman, A. (2005). Translators and mediators: Bilingual young people's accounts of their interpreting work in health care. *Social Science & Medicine, 60*, 2097–2110.

Greener, I. (2003). Patient choice in the NHS: The view from economic sociology. *Social Theory and Health, 1*, 72–89.

Greenfield, P. (1997). You can't take it with you. Why ability assessments don't cross cultures. *American Psychologist, 52*(10), 1115–1124.

Gumperz, J., & Roberts, C. (1991). Misunderstanding in intercultural encounters. In J. Blommaert & J. Verschueren (Eds.), *The pragmatics of intercultural communication* (pp. 51–90). Amsterdam, Netherlands: John Benjamins.

Guttfreund, D. (1990). Effects of language usage on the emotional experience of Spanish-English and English-Spanish bilinguals. *Journal of Consulting and Clinical Psychology, 58*(5), 604–607.

Haenel, F. (1997). Aspects and problems associated with the use of interpreters in psychotherapy of victims of torture. *Torture, 7*(3), 68–71.

Haffner, L. (1992). Translation is not enough. Interpreting in a medical setting. *Western Journal of Medicine, 157*(3), 255–259.

Hall, E. T. (1966). *The hidden dimension.* Garden City, NY: Doubleday.

Hampers, L. C., & McNulty, J. E. (2002). Professional interpreters and bilingual physicians in a pediatric emergency department: Effect on resource utilization. *Archives of Pediatrics & Adolescent Medicine, 156*(11), 1108–1113.

Harris, R., & Rampton, B. (2002). Creole metaphors in cultural analysis: The limits and possibilities of (socio-) linguistics. *Critique of Anthropology, 22*(1), 31–51.

Hartog, J. (2006). Beyond 'misunderstandings' and cultural stereotypes analysing intercultural communication. In K. Buhrig & J. D. T. Thije (Eds.), *Beyond misunderstanding* (pp. 175–188). Amsterdam, Netherlands: John Benjamins Publishing Company.

Hasnain-Wynia, R., Yonek, J., Pierce, D., Kang, R., & Greising, C. H. (2006). *Hospital language services for patients with limited English proficiency: Results from a national survey.* Chicago, IL: Health Research and Educational Trust.

Hays, P. A. (2008). *Addressing cultural complexities in practice: Assessment, diagnosis and therapy* (2nd ed.). Washington, DC: American Psychological Association.

Hémon, E. (2001). Le temps des migrants; les temps de l'exil. *Thérapie Familiale, 22*(2), 169–186.

Hsieh, E. (2006a). Conflicts in how interpreters manage their roles in provider-patient interactions. *Social Science & Medicine, 62*(3), 721–730.

Hsieh, E. (2006b). Understanding medical interpreters: Reconceptualizing bilingual health communication. *Health Communication, 20*(2), 177–186.

Hsieh, E. (2007). Interpreters as co-diagnosticians: Overlapping roles and services between providers and interpreters. *Social Science & Medicine, 64*(4), 924–937.

Hsieh, E. (2009). Provider-interpreter collaboration in bilingual health care: Competitions of control over interpreter-mediated interactions. *Patient Education and Counselling, 78*(2), 154–159.

Jackson, C., Zatzick, D., Harris, R., & Gardiner, L. (2008). Lost in translation. Considering the critical role of interpreters and language in psychiatric evaluation of non-English-speaking patients. In S. Loue & M. Sajatovic (Eds.), *Diversity issues in the diagnosis treatment and research of mood disorders* (pp. 135–163). New York, NY: Oxford.

Jacobs, B., Kroll, L., Green, J., & David, T. J. (1995). The hazards of using a child as an interpreter. *Journal of the Royal Society of Medicine, 88*(8), 474P–475P.

Jacobs, E., Shepard, D. S., Suaya, J. A., & Stone, E. L. (2004). Overcoming language barriers in health care: Costs and benefits of interpreter services. *American Journal of Public Health, 94*(5), 866–869.

Jones, C. J., & Trickett, E. J. (2005). Immigrant adolescents behaving as culture brokers: A study of families from the former Soviet Union. *Journal of Social Psychology, 145*(4), 405–427.

Kaufert, J. M., & Koolage, W. W. (1984). Role conflict among 'culture brokers': The experience of native Canadian medical interpreters. *Social Science & Medicine, 18*(3), 283–286.

Keesing, R. M. (1985). Conventional metaphors and anthropological metaphysics. *Journal of Anthropological Research, 41*(2), 201–218.

Kennard, D., Elliott, B., Roberts, J., & Evans, C. (2002). Group-analytic training conducted through a language interpreter: Is the experience therapeutic? Is it group-analytic? *Group Analysis, 35*(2), 237–250.

Kennard, D., Roberts, J., & Elliott, B. (2002). Group-analytic training conducted through a language interpreter: Are we understanding each other? *Group Analysis, 35*(2), 209–235.

Khelil, K. (1991). Des impasses de la traduction aux ouvertures de la psychothérapie. *Psychiatrie, Psychothérapie et Culture(s), 2*. Retrieved March 31, 2009, from http://www.p-s-f.com/psf/spip.php?article23

Kirmayer, L. J. (2006). Beyond the 'new cross-cultural psychiatry': Cultural biology, discursive psychology and the ironies of globalization. *Transcultural Psychiatry, 43*(1), 126–144.

Kline, F., Acosta, F. X., Austin, W., & Johnson, R. G., Jr. (1980). The misunderstood Spanish-speaking patient. *The American Journal of Psychiatry, 137*(12), 1530–1533.

Kouassi, K. (2001). Approche psychothérapique en clinique transculturelle. Triade thérapeuthe–Patient–Interprète. *Champ Psychosomatique, 23*, 137–143.

Kövecses, Z. (2000). *Metaphor and emotion: Language, culture, and body in human feeling.* Cambridge, England: Cambridge University Press.

Leanza, Y. (2005a). Roles of community interpreters in pediatrics as seen by interpreters, physicians and researchers. *Interpreting, 7*(2), 167–192.

Leanza, Y. (2005b). Le rapport à l'autre culturel en milieu médical: l'exemple de consultations pédiatriques de

prévention pour des familles migrantes. *Bulletin de l'ARIC, 41*, 8–27.

Leanza, Y. (2008). Community interpreter's power. The hazards of a disturbing attribute. *Curare, 31*(2+3), 211–220.

Leanza, Y., Boivin, I., & Rosenberg, E. (2010). Interruptions and resistance: A comparison of medical consultations with family and trained interpreters. *Social Science & Medicine, 70*(12), 1888–1895.

Loutan, L., Farinelli, T., & Pampallona, S. (1999). Medical interpreters have feelings too. *Médecine Sociale et Préventive, 44*(6), 280–282.

M'Barga, J.-P. (1983). Relation thérapeutique transculturelle: Interprétariat, interprétation. *Etudes Psychothérapiques, 54*(4), 292–300.

Macciocchi, A. (2005). Travailler avec les familles migrantes dans un contexte non volontaire: la question de la culture. *Thérapie Familiale, 26*(1), 77–86.

Marcos, L. R. (1979). Effects of interpreters on the evaluation of psychopathology in non-English-speaking patients. *The American Journal of Psychiatry, 136*(2), 171–174.

McGoldrick, M., Giordano, J., & Pearce, J. (Eds.). (1996). *Ethnicity and family therapy* (2nd ed.). New York, NY: The Guilford Press.

Mesquita, B., Frijda, N., & Scherer, K. (1997). Culture and emotion. In J. Berry, P. Dasen, & T. Saraswathi (Eds.), *Handbook of cross-cultural psychology* (Vol. 2: Basic processes and human development, pp. 255–296). Boston, MA: Allyn & Bacon.

Miletic, T., Piu, M., Minas, H., Stankovska, M., Stolk, Y., & Klimidis, S. (2006). Guidelines for working effectively with interpreters in mental health settings. Retrieved May 28, 2007, from http://www.vtpu.org.au/docs/interpreter/VTPU_GuidelinesBooklet.pdf

Miller, K. E., Martell, Z. L., Pazdirek, L., Caruth, M., & Lopez, D. (2005). The role of interpreters in psychotherapy with refugees: An exploratory study. *The American Journal of Orthopsychiatry, 75*(1), 27–39.

Morales, A., & Hanson, W. E. (2005). Language brokering: An integrative review of the literature. *Hispanic Journal of Behavioral Sciences, 27*(4), 471–503.

Moss, B. (2008). *Communication skills for health and social care.* London, England: Sage.

Mudarikiri, M. (2002). Working with the interpreter in adult mental health. In R. Tribe & H. Raval (Eds.), *Working with interpreters in mental health* (pp. 182–197). New York, NY: Brunner-Routledge.

Nunes, T., Schliemann, A., & Carraher, D. (1993). *Street mathematics and school mathematics.* Cambridge, England: Cambridge University Press.

Oquendo, M. A. (1996). Psychiatric evaluation and psychotherapy in the patient's second language. *Psychiatric Services, 47*(6), 614–618.

Padilla, A. (2001). Issues in culturally appropriate assessment. In L. Suzuki, G. Ponterotto, & P. Meller (Eds.), *Handbook of multicultural assessment* (2nd ed., pp. 5–27). San Francisco, CA: Jossey-Bass.

Patel, N. (2002). Speaking with the silent: Addressing issues of disempowerment when working with refugee people. In R. Tribe & H. Raval (Eds.), *Working with interpreters in mental health* (pp. 219–237). New York, NY: Brunner-Routledge.

Piret, B. (1991). La psychothérapie avec interprète est-elle possible? *Psychiatrie, Psychothérapie et Culture(s), 2*. Retrieved March 31, 2009, from http://www.p-s-f.com/psf/spip.php?article23

Pöchhacker, F. (2003). *Introducing interpreting studies*. London: Routledge.

Prendes-Lintel, M., & Peterson, F. (2008). Delivering quality mental health services to immigrants and refugees through an interpreter. In L. A. Suzuki & J. G. Ponterotto (Eds.), *Handbook of multicultural assessment: Clinical, psychological, and educational applications* (3rd ed., pp. 220–243). San Francisco, CA: Jossey Bass.

Price, J. (1975). Foreign language interpreting in psychiatric practice. *The Australian and New Zealand Journal of Psychiatry, 9*(4), 263–267.

Rack, P. (1982). Race, culture and mental disorder. In *Practical problems in providing a mental health service for ethnic minorities* (pp. 198–206). London, England: Tavistock.

Raval, H. (1996). A systemic perspective on working with interpreters. *Clinical Child Psychology and Psychiatry, 1*, 29–43.

Raval, H. (2005). Being heard and understood in the context of seeking asylum and refuge: Communicating with the help of bilingual co-workers. *Clinical Child Psychology and Psychiatry, 10*(2), 197–216.

Raval, H., & Maltby, M. (2005). *Not getting lost in translation: Establishing a working alliance with co-workers and interpreters. The space between experience, context, and process in the therapeutic relationship* (pp. 63–78). London, England: Karnac Books.

Raval, H., & Smith, J. A. (2003). Therapists' experiences of working with language interpreters. *International Journal of Mental Health, 32*(2), 6–31.

Rechtman, R. (1992). L'Intraduisible culturel en psychiatrie. *L'Évolution Psychiatrique, 57*(3), 347–365.

Richie, J. (1964). Using an interpreter effectively. A guide to avoiding mishaps and misunderstandings. *Nursing Outlook, 12*(12), 27–29.

Roat, C., Putsch, R., & Lucero, C. (1997). *Bridging the gap over phone: A basic training for telephone interpreters serving medical settings*. Seattle, WA: The Cross Culutral Health Care Program.

Robb, N., & Greenhalgh, T. (2006). "You have to cover up the words of the doctor": The mediation of trust in interpreted consultations in primary care. *Journal of Health Organization and Management, 20*(5), 434–455.

Roberts, C., Moss, B., Mass, V., Sarangi, S., & Jones, R. (2005). Misunderstandings: A qualitative study of primary care consultations in multilingual settings, and educational implications. *Medical Education, 39*, 465–475.

Roberts, C., & Sarangi, S. (2005). Theme-oriented discourse analysis of medical encounters. *Medical Education, 39*, 632–640.

Röder, F., & Opalič, P. (1997). A psychotherapy group for Turkish patients using an interpreter. *Group Analysis, 30*(2), 233–240.

Rosenberg, E., Leanza, Y., & Seller, R. (2007). Doctor-patient communication in primary care with an interpreter: Physician perceptions of professional and family interpreters. *Patient Education and Counseling, 67*(3), 286–292.

Rosenberg, E., Seller, R., & Leanza, Y. (2008). Through interpreters' eyes: Comparing roles of professional and family interpreters. *Patient Education and Counseling, 70*, 87–93.

Russell, J. (1991). Culture and the categorization of emotions. *Psychological Bulletin, 110*(3), 426–450.

Sabin, J. E. (1975). Translating despair. *The American Journal of Psychiatry, 132*(2), 197–199.

Sartorius, N., & Janca, A. (1996). Psychiatric assessment instruments developed by the World Health Organization. *Social Psychiatry and Psychiatric Epidemiology, 31*(2), 55–69.

Sarver, J., & Baker, D. W. (2000). Effect of language barriers on follow-up appointments after an emergency department visit. *Journal of General Internal Medicine, 15*(4), 256–264.

Segall, M., Dasen, P., Berry, J., & Poortinga, Y. (1999). *Human behavior in global perspective. An introduction to cross-cultural psychology*. Boston, MA: Allyn & Bacon.

Sleptsova, M. (2007). Wenn die vermittlung von informationen auf eine sprach-barriere trifft—zur zusammenarbeit mit übersetzern. *Therapeutische Umschau, 64*(10), 575–579.

Smith, V. A., DeVellis, B. M., Kalet, A., Roberts, J. C., & DeVellis, R. F. (2005). Encouraging patient adherence: Primary care physicians' use of verbal compliance-gaining strategies in medical interviews. *Patient Education and Counselling, 57*(1), 62–76.

Spensley, J., & Blacker, K. H. (1976). Feelings of the psychotherapist. *The American Journal of Orthopsychiatry, 46*(3), 542–545.

Statistics Canada. (2007a). *Population by knowledge of official language, by province and territory (2006 census)*. Retrieved March 30, 2008, from http://www40.statcan.ca/l01/cst01/demo15.htm

Statistics Canada. (2007b). *Population by mother tongue, by province and territory (2006 census)*. Retrieved March 30, 2008, from http://www40.statcan.ca/l01/cst01/demo11b.htm

Teegen, F., & Gonnenwein, C. (2002). Posttraumatic stress disorder of interpreters for refugees. *Verhaltenstherapie & Verhaltensmedizin, 23*(4), 419–436.

Trickett, E. J., & Jones, C. J. (2007). Adolescent culture brokering and family functioning: A study of families from Vietnam. *Cultural Diversity and Ethnic Minority Psychology, 13*(2), 143–150.

U.S. Census Bureau. (2000). *America speaks*. Retrieved March 30, 2008, from http://www.census.gov/population/www/socdemo/hh-fam/AmSpks.html

Valero-Garcés, C. (2005). Emotional and psychological effects on interpreters in public services: A critical factor to bear in mind. *Translation Journal, 9*(3). Retrieved May 2007, from http://www.accurapid.com/journal/33ips.htm

Wadensjö, C. (1998). *Interpreting as interaction*. Londres, England: Longman.

Westermeyer, J. (1989). *Psychiatric care of migrants: A clinical guide*. Washington, DC: American Psychiatric Press.

Westermeyer, J. (1993). Cross-cultural psychiatric assessment. In C. Gaw (Ed.), *Culture, ethnicity and mental illness* (pp. 125–144). Washington, DC: American Psychiatric Press.

Westermeyer, J., & Janca, A. (1997). Language, culture and psychopathology: Conceptual and methodological issues. *Transcultural Psychiatry, 34*(3), 291–311.

Wolman, C. (1970). Group therapy in two languages, English and Navajo. *American Journal of Psychotherapy, 24*(4), 677–685.

Woloshin, S., Schwartz, L. M., Katz, S. J., & Welch, H. G. (1997). Is language a barrier to the use of preventive services? *Journal of General Internal Medicine, 12*(8), 472–477.

Yahyaoui, A. (1988). Consultation familiale ethnopsychanalytique: le cadre interculturel. In A. Yahyaoui (Ed.), *Troubles du language et de la filiation chez le maghrebin de deuxième génération* (pp. 48–67). Grenoble, France: La pensée sauvage.

Zeller, C. M. (1984). *Ursachen und Auswirkungen der Feminisierung im Dolmetsch/Übersetzerstudium und Beruf*. Vienna, Austria: University of Vienna.

Culture Brokers, Clinically Applied Ethnography, and Cultural Mediation

6

Alessandra Miklavcic and Marie Nathalie LeBlanc

Cultural consultation frequently requires the use of resource people who can help interpret the cultural meaning of illness and healing. This task goes beyond linguistic interpreting and may be essential even when patient and clinician share a language. This chapter explores the multiple roles of culture brokers or mediators in health settings. In some settings, the task of cultural mediation is viewed as part of the cultural competence of health professionals, while in others, it is assigned to medical interpreters (who function as community interpreters) or involves a new type of practitioner. The professionalization of culture brokers (implying a definition of duties and conduct) has occurred in several national health care systems, with variations in status, roles, and practices.

A growing literature on this subject shows the timeliness of efforts to combine interpreting skills with an anthropological approach to mediation.

However, the literature is very scattered and comes largely from Europe where several models of cultural mediation have been developed. To date, there has been no systemic literature review of evaluation and implementation studies of culture brokers, including issues pertaining to policies, laws and regulations, formal and informal role definitions, recruitment and training methods for culture brokers, training for health professionals on how to work with brokers, quality assurance standards and mechanisms, and evaluations of process and outcome.

This chapter will look at the practice of cultural mediation and the role of culture broker in medical settings with a focus on the Cultural Consultation Service (CCS) of the Jewish General Hospital and ethnopsychiatric consultation in other settings. First, we examine the concept of culture broker in anthropology and its introduction in medical settings with underserved communities, especially Aboriginal communities and immigrants. Second, we discuss cultural mediation models that have emerged in the last 15 years in Europe, by providing a few examples of implementation and policies, mainly drawing on the models of cultural mediation used by ethnopsychiatric consultation clinics in France and Italy. Finally, we describe the cultural mediation practice of the CCS, providing vignettes that illustrate the roles of culture brokers, ethical issues relating to their participation in clinical settings, and the ways they contribute to cultural formulation and intervention.

A. Miklavcic, Ph.D. (✉)
Research Centre, St. Mary's Hospital Center, 3830,
Avenue Lacombe, Montreal, QC, Canada H3T 1M5
e-mail: amiklavcic@gmail.com

M.N. LeBlanc, Ph.D.
Département de Sociologie, Université du Québec à
Montréal, Case Postale 8888, Succursale Centre-
Ville, Montréal, QC, Canada H3C 3P8
e-mail: leblanc.marie-nathalie@uqam.ca

L.J. Kirmayer et al. (eds.), *Cultural Consultation: Encountering the Other in Mental Health Care,*
International and Cultural Psychology, DOI 10.1007/978-1-4614-7615-3_6,
© Springer Science+Business Media New York 2014

Current Anthropological Views of Culture

In recent years, multicultural governances in many parts of the world have increasingly recognized the fact that their diverse populations require specific services that are responsive to their "culture" (Gershon, 2006). The use of culture as a category to conceptualize citizenship rights and services carries both possibilities for recognition of diversity and improved social integration as well as the risk of creating essential identities and "othering" or institutionalized racism.

Since its inception as a discipline, anthropology has focused on culture as a key framework for analysis. Debates in anthropology over the past 25 years regarding the political and epistemological implications of the concept of culture have emphasized the fluidity of cultural entities and have encouraged an interest in hybridity, creolization, and métissage (Abu-Lughod, 1991; Appadurai, 1996; Bibeau, 1997; Clifford & Marcus, 1986; Hannerz, 1992; Marcus, 1992). These debates along with the forces of globalization have led to changes in the notion of culture with increased recognition of people who are situated "in-between" different cultural worldviews and who, therefore, function as cultural mediators or brokers. While earlier studies of culture brokers focused mainly on the analysis of the personal stresses experienced by people required to play the role of mediators, recent studies of tourism and mobile populations have highlighted the impact of culture brokers on cultural formations (Adams, 1997; Amit, 2007; Chambers, 2000).

While collaborations between clinical practitioners and medical anthropologists have increased in recent decades, the interactions between these two domains of knowledge are not without tension (Kleinman, 1987). When anthropological concepts of culture are deployed in clinical settings, they are often reformulated in the language of "cultural expertise," translated in easy-to-use "explanatory models," and hints on how to ensure compliance of specific ethnocultural groups (e.g., "the Sudanese," "the Sri Lankan") as if these were well-defined and homogeneous categories

(Kaufert, 1990; Kleinman & Benson, 2006; Taylor, 2003b).

In health care settings, "culture" may be treated as a fixed and unchangeable set of categories to be duly noted in the charts of patients from specific ethnic groups. This use of culture involves three basic assumptions that go against the thrust of current anthropological literature. The first assumption is that only immigrant patients are seen as culture bearers whose actions are ascribed to cultural beliefs that need to be "decoded," while health care providers are system bearers (Gershon, 2006), whose actions are rational, acultural, and based exclusively on medical evidence (Taylor, 2003a). The second assumption is that culture can be treated as a fixed characteristic or "factor" that can be applied in the same way to all people who belong to the same ethnic group (Taylor, 2003a, 2003b). Used in this way, culture becomes essentialized and medicalized (Santiago-Irizarry, 2001). The third assumption is that the word "culture" is useful as a less threatening term to stand in for the real problems of poverty, marginalization, and racism, which are more fundamental social causes of health disparities (Fernando, 2003; Gregg & Saha, 2006). The work of the CCS clearly shows the limitations of these three assumptions: medicine and health care practitioners are also shaped by their own personal and professional cultures; culture is not fixed but fluid and negotiable; and, in addition to justifying social regimes of marginalization and exclusion, culture can constitute important clinical problems in its own right. However, anthropological deconstruction of clinical realities, although providing much needed contextualization and critique, can provoke paralysis in clinicians because of their acute awareness of their biases and limitations, unless it also strives to provide a framework to guide necessary action under conditions of limited resources and continuity uncertainty.

Culture Brokers: Definitions in the Anthropological Literature

While the role of the culture broker has been discussed in health, education, business, museums, tourism, and justice, the concept became widespread in anthropology in the mid-1950s to describe processes of cultural contact in various contexts of domination, including trade, colonialism, nation-state building, and modernization. Eric Wolf (1956) pioneered the use of the notion of culture broker using the term to elucidate the beginning of the conflictual relationship between Spanish colonial rule and local peasant communities in Mexico. Culture brokers, in this context, are "nation-oriented individuals from the local communities" who "stand guard over the crucial junctures or synapses of relationships which connect the local system to the larger whole" (Wolf, 1956, p. 1075). Soon after, Clifford Geertz identified the Javanese *kijajis*, local Moslem teachers of Java, as the "most important cultural brokers" of post-revolutionary Indonesia (Geertz, 1960, p. 233).

In anthropology, culture brokers were initially defined as go-betweens who mediate and translate two culturally distinct realities or groups for the purpose of reducing conflict or producing a change in the quality of the relationship between them (Geertz, 1960; Jezewski, 1990; Paine, 1971; Press, 1969; Szasz, 1994; Wolf, 1956). Whether in negotiation between tradition and modernity (Geertz, 1960; Wolf, 1956), trade (Paine, 1971) or as a part of social networks in contexts of patronage (Barnes, 1954; Boissevain, 1974; Bott, 1957), the culture broker was depicted both as a mediator and an agent of change (Press, 1969). This initial conception of culture brokers shifted in the 1980s to take into account other categories of individuals or social roles that are "in-between" different social worlds and that are situated or position themselves as mediators and innovators, including tourist guides (Brown, 1992), children of migrants (Abu-Lughod, 1991), and native anthropologists (Narayan, 1993).

To be effective, Eric Wolf suggests that culture brokers must operate like Janus, facing both directions and able to cope with the tensions raised by the conflict of interests (Wolf, 1956). The ability to navigate between different cultural worldviews and social environments provides the culture broker with the possibility to acknowledge different perspectives and to adopt diverging, at times contradictory, behaviors, allowing for the creation of spaces for negotiation

between them. Innovations come about through the culture broker's attempts to bridge perspectives by circumventing sociocultural expectations and creating new possible ways of doing things.

In the field of ethnohistory, culture brokers appear mainly as individuals who mediated contacts between indigenous peoples and colonial administrations (Szasz, 1994). Culture brokers were those men and women, native and nonnative, missionaries, teachers, and so forth, who had good knowledge of both languages and who were usually related by birth or marriage to both indigenous and colonizing populations. The list of marginal individuals in more recent contexts includes migrant workers, foreigners, second-generation immigrants, persons of mixed ethnic origin, *parvenus* (upwardly mobile marginals), the *déclassés* (downwardly mobile marginals), migrants from country to city, and women in "nontraditional" roles (Turner, 1974). Of course, marginality alone does not equip an individual to be a culture broker. Culture brokers, as mediators and innovators, "must have their behavior sanctioned in some way by the host community and must maintain some sort of acceptable identity with the community of origin" (Brown, 1992, p. 369).

From Anthropological Concept to Actors in Health Care Settings

Across national settings, practices of culture brokering in health care differ greatly, in terms of background, roles, degree of institutional integration, and level of professional expertise. Categories of individuals who may act as culture brokers include the following: health practitioners, such as social workers, nurses, or psychologists, who can function as culture brokers by virtue of their bilingual/bicultural identity or direct knowledge of a specific community; social scientists, such as anthropologists or sociologists, who may be called upon to act as culture brokers because of their scientific knowledge; or individuals drawn from community groups such as voluntary organizations and religious institutions. Other terms used to refer to persons who are employed in health care institutions to mediate cultural differences include "patient advocate," "intercultural mediator," and "cultural interpreter."

The roles of culture brokers are defined by localized health care and social systems but are influenced by the dominant models of national integration and regimes of citizenship. For instance, culture brokers were introduced in North American health care settings in the late 1960s, following the recognition of serious inequalities in health care access for underserved ethnoracial groups and, subsequently, for new immigrants. The use of culture brokers needs to be situated in relation to the sociopolitical changes of the late 1960s, which marked a shift from an emphasis on assimilation to a diversity paradigm. Stemming from the battles of the civil rights movement, the diversity paradigm focuses on appreciating and valuing differences between individuals and groups. Multiculturalism policy in Canada is one reflection of this shift toward acknowledging diversity.

Culture brokers are often highly educated immigrant women, and the trajectories of migration have influenced the availability and role of culture brokers (Gentile & Caponio, 2006). For example, Gobbo (2004) provides a portrait of a Roma cultural mediator in Italy whose professional identity allowed her to capitalize on her marginal state of being "between communities." In an article on immigrant health services in France, Sargent and Larchanche (2009) described the different stages of the professionalization of culture brokers through the life history of a woman migrant who started as an interpreter in the mid-1980s. Despite the clear connection between life trajectories and professionalization among culture brokers, in the health care field, culture brokers have been conceptualized less in terms of the knowledge and skills acquired through the experience of migration than as a type of expertise that can be added to already established professions including nurses, social workers, and community interpreters—any of whom might function as a culture broker.

Culture brokers may also be professionals already engaged in health delivery. In the UK, the Nafsiyat model (Kareem, 1992) focused on the psychotherapist as a culture broker and integrated process-oriented supervision of the therapist on issues related to racism and discrimination. As culture broker, the clinician examines the impingements of ethnicity, racism, and the therapist's own ethnoracial identity on clinical assessment and psychotherapeutic process. Cultural mediation through the use of culture brokers has been recommended in the treatment of Black, minority, or ethnic (BME) patients in the UK to address issues of institutional racism (Fernando, 1995, 2002).

Defining the Position and Roles of Culture Brokers in Medical Settings

The ways in which institutions approach cultural difference largely determine the nature and function of culture brokers in health care services. For instance, within the cultural competence model of health care, which is now dominant in the USA, each health care provider must be able to mediate cultural meanings with their patient. This model requires training of practitioners on issues of cultural difference. In the cultural mediation model, more common in European settings, the culture broker is an "expert on culture," whose roles are to facilitate clinical encounters, prevent conflicts, and act as agent of social integration.

Bischoff (2006) distinguishes two approaches to culture brokering based on different ideologies of social integration and power relations. The first approach aims at assimilating the immigrant's point of view to that of the health care system as part of the larger society. The professional or institution decides when to include a culture broker, whose main role is to convey information to patients in order to enhance their adherence to treatment. In this approach, the patient's point of view is rarely taken into account. This one-directional approach often functions as a sort of institutional protection against possible legal repercussions, for example, insuring informed consent for diagnostic procedures or treatment. The second approach involves a more inclusive two-way exchange in which there is a significant level of trust and where the opportunity for each participant to understand something of the other's point of view is increased by providing real negotiation options and empowerment strategies. In practice, the position of culture brokers is usually situated between these two poles. At the level of working alliance, culture brokers tend to fluctuate between three basic roles: (1) as agents who work for public institutions and professionals, (2) as advocates who represent the interests of the ethnocultural and immigrant communities, and (3) as mediators who take a nonpartisan stance and strive to be "neutral" (Cohen-Emerique, 2004). Through these basic roles, culture brokers have proved to be useful participants in efforts to improve underserved communities' access to health care services and to build mutual trust between ethnocultural communities and health care institutions.

Countries with a longer history of multicultural practices such as the USA, Canada, Australia, United Kingdom, and New Zealand were the first to organize culture broker programs, specifically to reach indigenous groups in Canada and Australia and underserved groups such as Afro-Americans and Latinos in the USA. These interventions provided a way to ease some of the historical mistrust that many racially, ethnically, and culturally diverse minorities have in relation to health care institutions. The risk inherent in this approach is that culture brokers may be perceived as acting on behalf of the dominant culture and therefore falling into the paradigm of domination and marginality. For instance, in colonial and postcolonial settings, indigenous nurses have been trained in Western medical knowledge to act as culture brokers between the traditional healing system and the biomedical one. They have managed to mediate different understanding of illness, yet their professional affiliation pushes them to value the biomedical knowledge over the traditional healing system (Barbee, 1986; 1987; Kahn & Kelly, 2001; Marks, 1997), becoming an instrument of the colonial policy to replace the "indigenous health care systems." The role of culture broker is particular relevant in situations of conflict arising from divergent views of health and healing, which bring to the forefront the incommensurability of cultural values over issues such as informed consent and end-of-life decision making (Kaufert & Koolage, 1984; Kaufert & O'Neil, 1998; Kaufert, Putsch, & Lavallée, 1998).

The Training of Culture Brokers

While informal or ad hoc culture brokers are found in many different milieus, some countries facing persistent gaps in health service access and delivery have made efforts to develop and use formal culture brokers in their health care systems. This has especially been the case for indigenous populations in settler societies. In Australia, for example, Aboriginal health workers (AHWs) have been actively involved in community mental health (Soong, 1983; Trudgen, 2000; Willis, 1999). In remote and rural Aboriginal communities, Aboriginal paraprofessionals act as culture brokers and work in tandem with non-Aboriginal health professionals. Aboriginal community workers have received training through specific programs and certification to work in specific jurisdictions. For example, they may function as community health representatives, mental health workers, or alcohol and addiction program workers. The overarching purpose of the training is to produce paramedical professionals who can promote health education within their communities. Mental health workers, for instance, may be trained specifically to help community members with grieving and loss of relatives and friends through violent death or suicide. In Canada, Aboriginal medical interpreters have been trained to bridge both linguistic and cultural diversity and have received some official recognition (Burgess, Herring, & Young, 1995). Of course, the creation of a new type of paraprofessional raises issues for jurisdiction and collaboration; further, these interdisciplinary teams may fail to work effectively due to a lack of understanding of roles between non-Aboriginal health care professionals and Aboriginal paraprofessionals (Minore & Boone, 2002). This failure may occur because of a lack of preparation among professionals to work with interdisciplinary teams (especially with paraprofessionals) and a lack of clarity of the duties of the culture broker.

The culture broker approach has proved to be useful in other areas of health care, including nursing (Jezewski, 1990) and social work (Jackson, Graham, & Jackson, 1998 [1995]). Jackson describes the training of Interpreter Cultural Mediators (ICM), bilingual and bicultural people who are familiar both with biomedical practices and American societies and with the cultural practices of the minority group to which they belong. Their training includes basic knowledge of biomedical health care and institutions, with an emphasis on issues of prevention, child-rearing, and pregnancy. Through role-playing, they learn how to communicate with health practitioners and how to review cases. They work as part of a team composed of a nurse supervisor, community advisors, a program administrator, and medical directors, as well as other health and social services employees. Over a period of time, the ICM follows a family or a patient, visiting them at home to explore the family's needs, problems, and strengths, which are presented to the health providers to help develop a common strategy for care. The ICM thus combines cultural mediation with case management.

Culture Brokers in the Field of Mental Health

In mental health care, the term "culture broker" was introduced by medical anthropologist Hazel Weidman (1975) in the development of a community mental health program for the inner-city population in Miami, Florida. The goal of the program was to train participants to adopt a transcultural perspective in the delivery of health care to patients from multiethnic background. The term "culture broker" was adopted to describe an intermediary who worked with therapists from the mainstream culture and clients from a different culture; the broker's roles were to act as a facilitator of negotiation, understanding, and meaning-making. The culture brokers were anthropologists or social scientists who could clarify

the needs of the ethnic groups to health professionals and put them in contact with appropriate resources. The relationship between the ethnic group and the health care system was framed as symmetry or equivalence between two cultures. For Weidman, the practice of cultural brokering was an intervention strategy, combining research, training, and service; it substantially affected the service providers, who initiated a process of transformation geared to highlighting issues of cultural difference and health equity (Van Willigen, 2002).

In mental health settings, the key requirement for a culture broker is a thorough "knowledge of mental illness as conceived and perceived by the individual seeking the services as well as by the mainstream culture" (Singh, McKay, & Singh, 1999, p. 5). This requires the ability to understand patients' idioms of distress, as well as cultural dimensions of clinician–patient interaction, including nonverbal communication. The culture broker aims to sensitize the clinical practitioner to the patient's system of belief and also helps the patient understand and trust the health care system or institution. As a go-between, the culture broker makes explicit to both patient and clinician aspects of the cultures of both participants that are relevant to specific health care issues and helps patient and clinician negotiate the hybrid realities that characterize the lives of immigrants and other cultural minorities. Following this perspective, at the CCS, culture brokers often are asked to comment on how a patient's behavior would be perceived and understood and whether it would be considered usual or acceptable in his or her culture or community of origin.

Cultural Mediation in Europe

Although culture brokers are widely employed, they are not yet well integrated into mainstream health care in the USA or in Canada, where their profession remains informal and unregulated. In some European countries, however, culture brokers are increasingly recognized as professionals.

The *cultural/intercultural mediation model*[1] has been adopted in Europe to address the service needs of the growing migrant populations. This model emerged from a situation in which rapid changes in population caught service providers unprepared. Health practitioners soon realized that addressing linguistic barriers through interpreters was not sufficient in clinical situations which involved culture differences (Minervino & Martin, 2007). Culture brokers (or intercultural mediators) became a crucial resource to respond to the resultant "emergency." Starting in the early 1990s, cultural mediation services were set up in Spain and Italy and soon spread across the European Union. These services, which comprise both interpreters and intercultural mediators, are located either in hospitals (Belgium, Sweden, Switzerland) or in outpatient clinics (Italy).

Although there is a wide range of approaches to the implementation of intercultural mediation services across national contexts, there have been efforts within the EU to encourage collaboration and to organize pilot projects for exchange of methods and best practices and the setting of common standards of quality in relation to code of conduct and training (Bischoff, 2003; Molina, Gailly, Gimenez Romero, & Guest, 2001; Krajic et al., 2005). These processes of collaboration and exchange have encouraged the professionalization of cultural mediators, despite cross-national variations in training and curriculum (Pöchhacker, 2008).

Cultural mediators are often immigrants themselves who have a good grasp of the two systems of reference, but effective work as a culture broker requires training. A project entitled *T-learning to Improve Professional Skills for Intercultural Dialogue* in five European countries (Italy, France, Austria, Greece, Poland) developed training for cultural mediators using new information technologies (Halba, 2009). The curriculum included issues relating to multiculturalism and interculturalism, national and European policies in the field of immigration, and questions relating to the integration for migrants (housing, education and training, access to employment and health). Given the heterogeneity of European health care systems, however, translating good practices into common policy has been difficult.

In recent years, Belgium and Italy have been among the more active countries in the development and employment of cultural mediators in health care settings. In Belgium, implementation started in the field practice and became eventually a national policy program (Verrept, 2008). The government is taking an active role in developing a code of conduct for cultural mediators. In Italy, an immigration law was passed in 1996 in which the "auxiliary" profession of culture broker (*"mediatore culturale"*) was recognized in institutional settings (such as schools, hospitals, mental health services, police offices); as a profession, it is available to immigrants who have taken a vocational training course (Fiorucci, 2007). Despite this law, there is no national program for the participation of *mediatore culturale* in the national health care system. The employment of *mediatore culturale* remains very fragmented, with large variations across regions.

The literature on cultural mediators in Europe indicates that they are mainly employed in obstetrics and gynecology departments. In the general hospital of Liege, Belgium, the cultural mediator provides information and support before and after clinical encounters for the whole duration of the hospitalization (Fossi, 2004; Gentile & Caponio, 2006). A similar approach is taken at several hospitals in Italy. In Bologna, for instance,

---

[1] In communication studies and related disciplines, many terms have emerged to point to the process of communication between culturally diverse parties, including *cross-cultural*, *intercultural*, and *interdiscourse* communication. Although they often are used as synonyms, they imply distinct concepts of culture. Cross-cultural communication implies that there are distinct cultural groups and looks at their interaction comparatively. Intercultural communication starts from the assumption that there are distinct cultural groups but studies their communicative practices in interaction with each other. Finally, interdiscourse communication sets aside any a priori notion of group membership and identity to investigate how and in what circumstances concepts such as culture are produced. The interdiscourse perspective, therefore, looks at the context of communication and interaction as relational process.

the culture broker plays a central role at the Health Centre for Migrant Women and Their Children, founded in 1992 within the structure of the Santa Orsola Hospital. The consultation takes place in several stages. Female cultural mediators welcome the immigrant women, and in a preliminary talk, they elicit the reason for they visit. The mediators stay with the patient during the clinical examination intervening in case of linguistic/cultural misunderstanding. After the clinical encounter, the mediator discusses the visit alone with the patient, providing a space to express questions and concerns.

As an emerging profession, culture brokers face many of the problems encountered by community interpreters, including: difficulty in having their role adequately recognized by other professionals and administrators; the dilemmas of balancing "neutrality" with advocacy; the precariousness of their positions, which are seldom guaranteed continuity and consistent funding; and the lack of psychological support when dealing with challenging cases (Augusti-Panareda, 2006; Minervino & Martin, 2007).

Cultural mediation can contribute to a patient-centered approach in which culture is seen not as a fixed entity but as a process framed and negotiated in the context of the clinical encounter. However, because of power dynamics in the institutional settings that employ them, and often their own social vulnerability as recent migrants themselves, culture brokers tend to align themselves with the institution even when health practitioners may encourage them to align with the patient (Augusti-Panareda, 2006). Another risk is that culture brokers may tend to overemphasize the role of culture in the patient's point of view as a way to reinforce their role as experts on "the patient's culture." As Eric Wolf pointed out, culture brokers strategically use their knowledge and position of "in-between" in order to consolidate their expertise. Finally, the professionalization of the culture broker may mask policies of integration that sustain practices of "othering" by keeping newcomers with professional skills in this marginal role. Considering the immigrant by default, a "cultural other" tends to essentialize diversity and institutionalize racism.

Models of Ethnopsychiatric Consultation and Cultural Mediation

Several types of mental health consultations in Europe which follow an ethnopsychiatric or transcultural psychiatric approach employ cultural mediation as part of their therapeutic practice: in France, for example, at the Centre George Devereux and the Bobigny School at Avicenne Hospital, and in Italy, at the *Centro Frantz Fanon*. In these programs, mediation either may be viewed as a shared and diffused role within a multidisciplinary team group that co-constructs knowledge and practice or can be assigned to a particular person who takes the role of cultural expert; the two approaches can also coexist. The cultural mediation approach also extends outside the medical/therapeutic setting in that the culture broker acts as a liaison between different institutions and the patient and his or her family, in order to promote social and legal dimensions of the patient's well-being.

In the context of multidisciplinary team groups, the culture broker is generally a therapist who undergoes training in clinical psychology and anthropology or who belongs to a minority ethnic background. In these settings, culture is used as a therapeutic lever which, according to the specific consultation model, can be invoked and negotiated to create a space where the immigrant patient's suffering can be voiced and understood.

The Centre George Devereux

The Centre George Devereux was founded by psychologist Tobie Nathan in an attempt to bring together anthropological knowledge with clinical and psychoanalytic thinking (Freeman, 1997; Streit, 1997). Nathan introduced the concept of culture in healing practice, going against the grain of the French ideology of citizenship that is based on the republican value of universality and civic integration in which expressions of culture are downplayed in public and confined to the private sphere (Corin, 1997; Kirmayer & Minas, 2000).

Nathan approaches clinical consultations as moments of intercultural interaction that are played out in a symbolic intrapsychic space. His model has played an influential role in the development of ethnopsychiatry in France and abroad. Ethnopsychiatric consultations conducted by Nathan's team employ a model of large group settings comprised of the leading therapist, the interpreter, and the patient with family members as well as various co-therapists from diverse backgrounds (Nathan, 1994a, 1994b). In this particular setting, culture brokers are co-therapists, who may intervene by explaining how the patient's difficulties are viewed from their own particular cultural group (Zajde, 2011). Critiques of Nathan's work have noted the value of group settings for African immigrants and other groups, while raising questions about the extent to which this approach reifies culture and tradition in ways that may be inconsistent with migrants' experience of hybridity (e.g., Andoche, 2001; Corin, 1997; Fassin & Rechtman, 2005; Sargent & Larchanche, 2009).

At the Centre George Devereux, a group of expert therapists who are trained in anthropology have been called "ethno-clinical mediators." Ethno-clinical mediators are co-therapists who share a similar ethnic background with their patients and participate in the group therapy, taking the lead when needed by providing specific knowledge of a particular healing tradition. Besides his or her role in the group setting, the culture broker is given a proactive liaison role; that is, he or she can see the patient and family alone and may accompany the patient to different administrative and therapeutic appointments. Because the service is not fully covered by the National Health System, it is not accessible to individuals who do not have the means to assume the cost of the service.

covered by the National Health System. Its aim is to forge liaisons with social services of different kinds (schools, refugee agencies, child protection services, community, or work social services). Moro has integrated Nathan's model of ethnopsychiatry setting within a less prescriptive vision of culture, which considers *métissage* (hybridization) and identity as process-oriented and relational constructions (see Moro & Real, 2006; Sturm et al., 2008; Sturm, Nadig, & Moro, 2011). The consultation works with first- and second-generation immigrants; it offers individual and group setting therapies taking a psychodynamic approach in which the idea is not necessarily to "match" the patient's culture. Moro's approach emphasizes issues of positionality and power, namely, "who has the power to define the client's culture in therapy?" (Sturm et al., 2008). The patient is seen as the expert of his or her own culture. The concept of culture is applied in the therapeutic setting on two different levels: at a cultural-anthropological level in which the patient's emic view is elicited and at a psychoanalytic level through the notion of universal signs.

Therapists are trained in psychology, psychiatry, and anthropology. In the group setting, co-therapists present etiologies from different cultures in order to encourage patients to reflect on etiologies from their own cultural background and create a dynamic point of view. There is no need to have a "specialist" from the patient's culture; instead, the co-therapists play with universal logics of causation (jealousy, magic, sorcery, contagion, possession, etc.). There is always an interpreter in the patient's mother tongue, who may at times be asked to give some culture-specific inputs. Rather than resting on a prescriptive notion of culture, as is the case with Nathan's approach, "culture" becomes a tool that can be shared by the team with the input of all team members.

The Bobigny School at Avicenne Hospital

The Bobigny School, led by psychiatrist Marie Rose Moro, is a referral medical consultation at the Avicenne Hospital (Sturm, Heidenreich, & Moro, 2008; See also Chapter 4). The consultation is part of the health care system and therefore fully

The Centro Frantz Fanon

In Italy, the *Centro Frantz Fanon* in Turin, headed by Roberto Beneduce, was the first center in Italy to develop an ethnopsychotherapy intervention strategy based on cultural mediation and an ethnopsychiatric approach to mental illness

(Giordano, 2011). The *Centro* is a psychosocial and psychotherapeutic institute associated with the Turin Local National Health Service Zone and receives funding from diverse institutions (province, local government, European Union), which give social, psychological, and psychiatric assistance to immigrants. The center offers referral consultations and therapies to both regular and irregular (or "illegal") immigrants without distinction according to their status, as well as provides training courses for various health practitioners and social workers who work with immigrants. Specifically, the center aims to train cultural mediators, who in the Italian context are immigrants themselves. The center's therapeutic and political stance draws from three main influences: Tobie Nathan's French ethnopsychiatric tradition, Franz Fanon's critique of colonial relations and their entrenchment in identity formation, and the Italian tradition of social psychiatry linked to the deinstitutionalization movement of the 1970s (Giordano, 2006, 2011; Pandolfi & Bibeau, 2006). The *Psichiatria Democratica* (Democratic Psychiatry) Movement led by psychiatrist Franco Basaglia showed how social, economic, and political variables are intrinsic to the construction of the mentally ill and to their "confinement" within mental institutions. This movement focused on the subjective experience of the mentally ill and aimed to close mental institutions. It led to Law 180, passed in 1978, that sanctioned the closing down of the asylums and brought about the organization of community mental health services.

From its inception in 1996, the *Centro Frantz Fanon* had among its founders psychiatrists, psychologists, medical anthropologists, and culture mediators who had previously worked together in a project on migrants' health (Beneduce, Costa, & Favretto, 1994). The cultural mediation model is organized around a multidisciplinary group setting where diverse expertise, including that of the patient, is taken into account. Each participant in the therapeutic encounter is engaged in a form of mediation with therapeutic effect. In this setting, the role of the culture mediator is fundamental in translating from one etiological system to another. The center aims to provide a clinical space for mediation and therapy and acts as a liaison with other institutions outside the clinic.

Consultations take place in either individual or group settings. When appropriate from a linguistic and/or cultural perspective, cultural mediators participate in therapy sessions and are active in the consultation process. During the consultation, the cultural mediator is given room to freely engage with patients in order to elicit their life histories in a way that allows them to use to different vocabularies and etiologies, rather than conforming to the hegemonic discourse of psychiatric diagnostic criteria (Giordano, 2008). Further, the roles of cultural mediator extend beyond the clinical setting; there are instances in which the cultural mediator interacts on behalf of the patient with institutional services on matters of housing and immigration or plays a pedagogical role in cultural mediation training. In this work, the cultural mediator must translate between different cultural materials and work with the epistemological uncertainty and conflicts that characterize the immigrant experience. Cultural mediators must to be aware of their own migratory experience in order to grasp the stakes of intercultural communicative experiences. They must manage the difficult transference at play in the encounter with other immigrants and Italian mental health practitioners/or ethnopsychiatrists (Beneduce, 1999).

The Cultural Consultation Service Experience

In contrast with the European settings, in Canada, while professional associations for psychiatry and psychology have embraced the cultural competence model, there are no national guidelines for the use of culture brokers or mediators in mental health care settings. Clinicians who wish to work with culture brokers must draw them from immigrant or indigenous community members and professionals with expertise about specific patient cultures. There is no formal training for culture brokers. There also is a lack of policy, ethical guidelines, professional standards, or mechanisms for training, assessing, and monitoring the quality of culture brokers in Canada (Kirmayer, Groleau, Guzder, Blake, & Jarvis, 2003; Ng, Popova, Yau, & Sulman, 2007).

The CCS is one of several Canadian services where culture brokers are extensively used. The CCS has a pool of about 70 culture brokers who are employed on a case-by-case basis. They are often health professionals (mainly psychologists and social workers) who share a similar ethnic background with the patient or, less often, anthropologists with specialized knowledge of a particular geographic region or ethnic group. Culture brokers are identified by members of the CCS team. They are provided with a manual that outlines their tasks and provides an outline for the cultural formulation to organize their information gathering and reporting (Chapter 3).

About 50 % of cases seen by CCS employ a culture broker (see Chapter 2). In some instances, the consultant psychiatrist, who shares ethnocultural knowledge or background with the patient, plays this role. In other cases, the interpreter also acts as culture broker, while in about 15 % of cases, a separate culture broker is employed in addition to the interpreter. The CCS culture broker database contains a list of psychologists who are bilingual, psychiatrists, social workers, and community workers operating in the Greater Montreal area, as well as anthropologists and sociologists who are selected on the basis of their knowledge not only of migrants' cultures of origin but also of their local communities.

The CCS Process and Setting

A typical consultation at the CCS, involving a culture broker, takes place in three stages: initial intake when the need for a culture broker may be identified; one or more clinical interviews with the patient and their family which may include a CCS consultant psychiatrist, a culture broker, students, other clinicians, or case managers (social worker, psychologist, or family doctor); and a case conference during which the CSS team, including the culture broker, discusses the case to provide a response to the referring clinician's original requests and develop recommendations, treatment plan, or guidance for the patient's future care (see Chapter 3 for more detail).

Typically, the CCS clinician briefs the cultural broker prior to the first interview. Culture brokers may also consult the patient's medical file at the CCS office. This file includes the intake form with basic demographic information and reasons for referral as well as any medical reports that have been received and, in some cases, the patient's migration documents, such as the Personal Identification Form in which refugee claimants write up their story and the justification for their refugee claim (see Chapter 12).

Although the CCS clinician leads the interview, culture brokers have some freedom to intervene during the process. Most often, the culture broker will ask further questions or will pursue a line of questioning aimed at clarifying specific issues of culture and sociohistorical context. The culture broker's interventions in the interview process may also involve attempts to clarify the situation for patients and make them more comfortable. Similarly, interventions on the part of the cultural broker may also be oriented toward the bringing the CCS psychiatrist and the other case workers toward a better understanding of the patient's experience. For example, adolescent or young adult patients may use trendy urban expressions that may be misinterpreted as indicating pathology. In order to prevent or resolve miscommunication, the culture broker will verify the meaning of ambiguous expressions with the patient and then explain the meaning to the clinical team. Similarly, the culture broker may reframe questions that are likely to seem senseless to patients or suggest alternatives to address the basic clinical question. For example, instead of asking a depressed African single mother explicitly whether she is "able to care for her child," the culture broker may suggest an exploration assessment of other behavioral symptoms that may interfere with care giving such as difficulty sleeping, weakness, fatigue, or other somatic symptoms.

After each clinical interview with the patient, the CCS clinician debriefs the culture broker, discussing issues related both to relevant psychiatric conditions and sociocultural contexts. They discuss a tentative diagnosis, the stressors involved in the patient's situation, and issues that need to be verified or broached with the patient or others during additional clinical interviews. At this time, the culture broker may provide a first interpretation of the contextual elements that may be significant to understanding the patient's predicament. These elements may relate to political dynamics in the country of origin (including war, ethnic tensions, forms of public oppression, dictatorship); the history of colonization; the racialization of social relations in the country of origin and in the post-migration context of Montréal; religious beliefs and practices relevant to the country of origin; issues relating to gender, age, and social class; and so forth. Elements relating to the experience of migrants of similar origin may also be highlighted by the culture broker. The culture broker may offer a tentative analysis of the significance of the cultural idioms employed by the patient to express his or her predicament and distress. For instance, in some cases seen at the CCS involving patients of African origin, patients use idioms that refer to contemporary expressions of witchcraft, such as "feeling the wind pass," "having something eat at one's stomach," and "hearing the voice" of someone. The culture broker may raise these issues and suggest that they be explored further in a second interview. In the meantime, culture brokers, particularly those that are trained as social scientists, may review the relevant anthropological, sociological, or political literature, especially in cases where they are familiar with the region where the patient comes from but not with the exact ethnocultural group, village, or with recent political events.

The second clinical interview, when needed, follows a similar sequence to the first one. However, in some cases, the culture broker may take more of a lead in the interview process. The second interview may focus more on aspects of the patient's life trajectory that do not directly relate to the moment of migration, such as his or her life context before migration, plans for the future in Canada, as well as local and transnational family and social networks. In some instances, the culture broker may see a need for further interviewing to clarify specific issues, and this can be negotiated with the CCS clinician.

In the cultural consultation process, culture brokers may assume varying degrees of initiative: acting as silent observers, intervening in the interview process, or even conducting their own interviews. The appropriate role depends on the complexity of the clinical situation, the culture broker's relationship to the patient's culture of origin (as a professional expert or as someone with the same background), and the familiarity of the consultation team with the patient's sociocultural context.

Roles Played by Culture Brokers at the CCS

Many CCS clinical encounters use both interpreters and culture brokers; in some cases, the primary clinical consultant acts as a culture broker or interpreter (see Chapter 8); in still other cases, the culture broker also acts as an interpreter. However, the specific tasks of culture brokers are complementary to those of the medical interpreter. As opposed to the interpreter, who is present just for the clinical interviews, the culture broker usually is involved at several points in the assessment process and may come to know the case in depth. Thus, the culture broker may initiate questions directed to the patient, as well as to clinical case workers and family members, if present. If the patient is in the care of a multidisciplinary team, the culture broker acts as an advisor to the team members, the patient, and the family.

In addition to participating in the data collection phase of clinical assessment, the culture broker prepares a cultural formulation report, which informs the final clinical summary and recommendations given to the referring clinician. The culture broker also provides cultural input at the CCS clinical case conferences where relevant issues are discussed by members of the CCS and referring teams, who may pose additional questions to the culture broker.

The written report provided by the culture broker and presented during the case conference follows the outline for the cultural formulation developed originally for DSM-IV. The CCS uses an expanded version of the DSM-IV Outline for Cultural Formulation (Chapter 3). Although not all culture brokers at the CCS are initially familiar with the cultural formulation format, they are asked to follow it, and most find it provides an easy way to organize information that helps situate the patient in relation to both their cultures of origin and the host culture (Kirmayer, Rousseau & Lashley 2007). The cultural formulation includes attention to the clinician–patient relationship, which should include the culture broker's own relationship to clinician and patients. However, culture brokers tend not to write about the interpersonal and intercultural dynamics of the clinical encounters, perhaps because these require specific psychodynamic and systemic training to observe. Also, process observations may be awkward to document because they may pose challenges to the professionals involved (Dinh, Groleau, Kirmayer, Rodriguez, & Bibeau, 2012).

To a large extent, the mediating functions of culture brokers at the CCS involve three main tasks. First, culture brokers aim to make sense of the different narratives relevant to the patient's predicament in the context of the clinical interviews, during the case conference, and through their reports. These narratives include the stories told in the setting of the clinical interviews, which involve patients' illness experience, life trajectories, traumas, and migration history. Case workers or others present during the evaluation also supply narratives that require cultural interpretation, and there usually are also written narratives contained within official documents such as the PIF, medical records, and reports provided by the professionals. A second basic task of culture brokers is to clarify aspects of the health care system, migration process, work, and other social matters for patients and their family members. This may include administrative and practical issues. In some cases, for example, patients have difficulty navigating the administrative structures of government institutions or are confronted by challenges related to their migration status that require specific knowledge about the Quebec and Canadian context. Finally, culture brokers may be involved in negotiation of divergent viewpoints or conflicts between the patient and health care providers.

In many cases, this is framed as an opposition between a biomedical interpretation and particular cultural interpretations.

To illustrate the tasks performed by culture brokers at the CCS, we present several brief case vignettes. These cases illustrate the ways in which culture brokers can influence the clinical encounter to bring to the surface issues and dynamics not readily accessible to or easily understood by the clinician.

The process of making sense of the multiple narratives that surround a patient's predicament or ailment is often the first challenge for the CCS consultant. The case of a young woman from Nigeria, who had migrated to Canada on her own, illustrates clearly how the culture broker provided the patient's treatment team a radically different view of the patient's predicament.

Case Vignette 6-1

The CCS was called for an emergency consultation at an outpatient maternity clinic. The staff were seriously considering the separation of a newborn baby from her mother. Child protection services had been involved in the dossier. According to the treatment team and the woman's social worker, the woman did not show appropriate attachment to the baby, and they interpreted this as a response to the fact that the child was the result of a multiple rape in Nigeria. According to the maternity clinic staff, the first signs of "non-attachment" started to appear during prenatal care, when they found the patient was not adequately preparing for the arrival of her baby by purchasing baby clothes, furniture, and other items. As well, she missed many clinic appointments. After the child was born, they closely scrutinized her maternal behavior and found many problems, including that she was not following written instructions on how to take care of the baby and displayed aggressive behavior toward the staff. In one instance, they found the baby unattended and with a blanket over her head.

(continued)

(continued)

These and other signs of apparent neglect made them believe that the mother was not fit to keep her child. There was concern that the mother had an intellectual disability as well as possible psychotic symptoms. Before removing the infant from the mother, they called for an emergency CCS consult. The culture broker, an anthropologist with long research experience in West Africa, attended the consultation interview along with a CCS psychiatrist.

It was apparent from the beginning of the conversation that the young mother was not speaking standard English, but a West African Pidgin. This linguistic difference could account for her difficulty following instructions and her perceived lack of intelligence. As the interview proceeded, the woman disclosed for the first time that she was not able to read and was therefore unable to follow the instructions given to her. She also explained to the culture broker and the consultant psychiatrist that her baby was a gift from God. She had epilepsy and had been ostracized as a youth in Nigeria by both her family and the larger community. She thought that she would never marry, still less have a child. In this conversation, it became clear that her interpretation of her pregnancy was framed in relation to her experience of epilepsy, in contrast to the impression of the treatment team who saw it only in relation to the enduring trauma of the rape that resulted in her pregnancy.

The culture broker pointed out that the mother's aggressive behavior could be understood as a defensive strategy against the perceived threat of the staff. Moreover, for many Nigerian women, especially highly religious individuals like the patient, preparing a nursery and buying clothes and items for an unborn baby are considered to be "presumptuous" and potentially dangerous, as it is likely to bring about bad luck, even the death of the baby. Therefore, "nesting" in preparation for childbirth as it is commonly understood and practiced in North American contexts is to be avoided. The information provided by the culture broker was essential to avoid a potentially catastrophic intervention: separating mother and baby based on an incorrect assessment of her maternal capacity.

In the work of the CCS, both during clinical interviews and during case conference discussions, the culture broker provides insights into the clinical encounter by highlighting the macro-social dynamics of the patient's case, moving from the individual to interpersonal and sociocultural levels. The culture broker emphasizes social and historical dynamics that may help the clinician understand the patient's life trajectory and current predicament, such as the changing role of family dynamics, the patient's migration experiences, religion, and social, economic, and political contexts of the country of origin. Ideally, the culture broker also supplies cultural context for understanding "idioms of distress," to help differentiate normative cultural and linguistic modes of expressing distress from psychiatric signs or symptoms. This specific cultural knowledge adds clinically important information about the patient's lived experience that goes well beyond cultural stereotypes. This task requires a capacity to articulate the patient's shifting (sometimes inconsistent or conflicting) narratives while considering multiple, relevant frames of interpretation. This includes taking into account the impact of the different sites or settings where patients' narrate their experience. Successful culture brokering depends on the capacity to move beyond a culturalist perspective that tends to offer a stereotyped view of patients as exemplars of their "cultures of origin," while reducing the culture to a series of cultural traits. It also requires avoiding the trap of opposing cultural interpretations to a biomedical model. For many patients, these regimes of interpretation are not mutually exclusive.

A further case, in which the tension between cultural and biomedical idioms of distress played out differently, highlights the intricate tasks of cultural brokering.

Case Vignette 6-2

A young man from Rwanda was referred to the CCS by his social worker because the patient's claim for refugee status had been refused and he was entirely passive in proceeding to apply for legal status in Canada on humanitarian and compassionate grounds. In this case, the culture broker was an anthropologist with knowledge of contemporary African societies and the African migrant communities in Montreal.

At the time of the CCS assessment, the young man was living at a shelter for the homeless. However, he arrived for the interviews properly dressed and clean and was clear and articulate in his speech. Despite being homeless, he managed to organize his life by setting up a system to receive phone calls and renting locker space where he kept his belongings. The most striking aspect of his account was his emphasis on religion, more specifically his reliance on Jesus, to make sense of his situation. He stated that his will was being tested by Jesus. He had to accept this religious trial and wait for a sign from Jesus before taking steps to try to get work and complete the appropriate papers to advance his application for status in Canada on humanitarian grounds. This strong reliance on spiritual idioms and reasons for inaction was in tension with his legal and economic situation, which both demanded quick and decisive action.

After the first clinical interview, during a discussion of the case with the CCS consulting psychiatrist and the social worker, the culture broker proposed that, despite the high likelihood that there was a component of mental illness, with either a psychotic or post-traumatic syndrome, it might help the clinical alliance and the assessment process to accept the patient's worldview and to frame the interaction during the second interview in terms of the patient's religious interpretation. By doing so, the culture broker hoped to clarify whether the patient's homeless lifestyle and his strong spiritual beliefs (which, in themselves, were not so unusual for a young man from Rwanda) were culture-based ways of coping with the trauma of the Rwandan genocide and his current predicament in Canada or whether his passivity simply was due to psychiatric illness. In fact, in African cities, many young adults who are students at colleges or university, which had been the case of the patient, live in conditions that are similar to those at the homeless shelter: sharing a room with other students; not having private space to leave one's belonging; spending much time outside of one's room; needing to be autonomous to arrange for food, communication, and laundry; and so forth. Further, as is the case of a number of contemporary African societies, Rwanda has experienced a significant wave of religious revival over the past 30 years, with great impact on the religiosity of young Africans. The second interview, in which the culture broker played an active role, posing numerous questions and entering into direct dialogue with the patient, focused on the patient's capacity to project himself outside of his state of inertia by asking, for instance, what could constitute a sign from Jesus? Had Jesus given him a sign already? Could someone, such as a pastor, help Jesus give him the sign he needed to take action? In the course of this conversation, the delusional nature of the patient's thinking became more clearly apparent.

In this case, rather than reframing the patient's experience within the expected discourses of biomedicine and modernity, the culture broker validated the patient's frame of reference, hoping that this might find common ground for mutual understanding between the patient, the CCS psychiatrist, and the social worker. However, in this case, the cultural "acceptability" of the patient's established lifestyle and intense spiritual experience did not emerge in the discussion, and the patient's illness became more explicit.

Although the aim of culture brokering is to create shared understanding or a "fused horizon" in interpretive frames, the culture broker's interventions may also make the differences between actors' points of view more stark and obvious. The case of a young woman from Haiti illustrates how the culture broker may bring issues into the open in the clinical interview and, at times, "force" patients and others present to confront the potential contradictions between divergent accounts and interpretations that play a part in the patient's life situation.

Case Vignette 6-3

A migration lawyer, puzzled by the behavior of his client, a young Haitian woman who was facing deportation but refused any contacts with her family and any legal actions to prevent the deportation, contacted the CCS for a consultation. The patient did not seem to be aware of the gravity of her predicament. At the consultation, the psychiatrist soon recognized that the young woman suffered from psychosis, most likely schizophrenia, which had remained undetected for a long time both by the legal system and by her family. She was in need of further psychiatric assessment and care. However, the young woman was very resistant to her lawyer's request to contact her family. Both the psychiatrist and the lawyer hoped that the culture broker could encourage the patient to allow them to contact her family and to receive treatment.

The culture broker, a middle-aged woman from Haiti, tried to establish a rapport with the patient, by speaking Kreyol and asking a series of culturally appropriate questions, but the young woman did not speak Kreyol and did not respond to this effort. The culture broker creatively followed the cultural formulation template of the CCS inquiring about the patient's migration trajectories, her contacts with her host country, and whether she maintained links with Haitian culture.

She inquired about religion and Vodoun. However, the young woman did not provide any details on these matters, and as a consequence, the culture broker started to be visibly uneasy, as she failed to establish a connection by mentioning various cultural themes and practices.

At one point during the consultation, the culture broker got up, walked up to the client telling her to get up as well. Raising her voice, the culture broker reached out, shaking her hands at the level of the patient's shoulders, and spoke in an animated manner, almost shouting. There was a striking shift in register from modulated professional talk to a sort of colloquial and authoritarian speech. The culture broker started to speak in a style of French incorporating Haitian expressions, diction, and rhythm:

"We are not working for Canadian Immigration. Canada does not give a damn about you [*s'en fiche de toi*]," she said. "It is not important to us if you committed those crimes, but you need to allow us to help you. Do you know what Haiti does to criminals, my daughter?" she asked, closing her fists and moving both arms in a gesture of emphasis.

"No," replied the patient, staring at her.

"You will be put in prison. It is nothing like here. Prisons there are filthy, dark and crowded. You will sleep on the floor, no bed, and you cannot complain. They don't give you food. You need someone from outside who brings you food, and your family is here in Canada. And when they will eventually release you, no one will want anything to do with you, you will become a pariah. In their eyes, you had a chance to go to a rich country and you messed up. You could not regulate your own behavior...."

For a moment, the young woman seemed to have appreciated the seriousness of her situation. She asked for a lawyer, agreed to contact her family, and asked for a phone.

Through intonation, choice of words, and bodily posture, the culture broker enacted tacit knowledge (Gadamer, 1987) that she shared with the patient, despite the patient's long detachment from Haiti and her fragmented perception of reality. This conveyed the urgency of the situation, and the patient responded with more appropriate and adaptive behavior.

The culture broker herself was surprised by her action. As she later recounted, "I had the feeling I had to shake her. She was not there. I was not sure she was coming back to reality." In the first part of her intervention, she stated: "We are not working for Immigration Canada… we are here to help you." She marked her allegiance to her, in an attempt to create a space for trust. She then posed the heavily laden question: "Do you know what Haiti does to criminals, my daughter?" In asking this question, she referred to Haiti as powerful authority in relation to the highly stigmatized word "criminals," setting the context for the crude and frightening images that followed. At the same time, by adding the kin term "my daughter" at the end of the question, the culture broker invoked a frame of caring in which she identified her position as mother, which allowed her to adopt this scolding tone.

The literature on culture brokers in other contexts has shown how culture brokers very often act as normative agents of the hegemonic culture, reenacting essentialized traces of the "cultural other." The culture broker in this particular clinical encounter tried to appeal to this essentialized version of Haitian identity, only to realize that for the patient, the Canadian frame of reference was much stronger than that of her distant "home country." Yet, she was able to reach the patient, despite her fragmented reality, by invoking a style of communication and tacit cultural knowledge through a combination of body language, tone, choice of words, and images. While the lawyer and psychiatrist were constrained by an institutional morality and ethics of care rooted in their respective professional codes and discourses, the culture broker was able to provide a more intermediate or transitional space where communication could occur.

Despite such moments of successful communication, the task of mediating between differing and at times contradictory worldviews remains challenging. The success of brokering depends on the culture broker's capacity to render divergent regimes of interpretation meaningful and acceptable to the participants in the clinical encounter.

Case Vignette 6-4[2]

A 45-year-old man from a rural province of China was hospitalized for multiple self-inflicted injuries including an attempt to amputate his left hand. He explained his actions as the result of following instructions given by "celestial entities," who also demanded that he make food offerings to them, which he did by depriving himself of his own food. The patient, who did not respond to antipsychotic medication or electroconvulsive treatment, was referred to the CCS by the inpatient treatment staff who wondered whether the man's psychosis could be framed in the context of his culture of origin.

At the CCS clinical conference, which was attended by the inpatient treatment staff, the CCS psychiatrist, and the culture broker, marked differences in systems of knowledge about illness became apparent. After a short introduction and update on the state of the patient, who was still hospitalized and not responding to treatment by the inpatient staff, the culture broker, a Southeast Asian specialist, questioned out loud, "Could it be demonic possession? I am wondering whether an exorcism can help him?" The referring inpatient staff met these questions with stunned silence and the case conference came to an awkward end.

Here two different worldviews clashed, and communication could not resume. On one side was the culture broker, who did not provide a con-

---

[2] This case is discussed in further detail in Chapter 14 (Vignette 14-9).

text for his questions and did not clarify the meanings of possession in East Asian cultures. For the culture broker, spirit possession had a symbolic valence related to a wider set of meanings and practices, including the importance of maintaining good relations with the ancestors by food offerings. However, in introducing a point of view so different from the biomedical perspective, the culture broker did not appreciate the impact on the clinicians. For the inpatient treatment staff, the language of spirits and possession was far outside their usual conceptual frameworks and provoked defensiveness and withdrawal. The CCS consultation report which was sent afterward to the referring clinician provided a lengthy account of the missing context needed to frame the "spirit possession" interpretation and how it might be used as a strategy to work with the patient in negotiating his treatment. The offering of food to the spirits and ancestors is a common practice in Southeast Asia. If an ancestor was not properly buried and did not receive the appropriate offerings of clothing and incense and has no descendents taking care of their tomb, their spirit may become a "hungry ghost." This is the cultural context the culture broker failed to provide in her intervention. The CCS report suggested that the inpatient treatment staff negotiate with the patient to make an offering of food and investigate further whether the patient would like this offering to be "officiated" by a religious leader. This strategy was meant to engage with the patient in finding a way through which he could eventually reduce or eliminate the troubling voices.

In the case of a young woman from Morocco, the culture broker managed to bring two initially opposed sets of values together by herself typifying such an amalgamation.

Case Vignette 6-5

The young woman, who had recently immigrated to Canada from Morocco with her family, experienced a clash of cultural values between family and the new society. Her family firmly opposed her relationship with a boy she met at school. The conflict

between parents and daughter escalated, and she decided to move out from her parents' house and live with her boyfriend. Soon after the move, she started to have suicidal ideation and felt guilty about having betrayed her family and her own culture. In an attempt to address the conflict, a family meeting was scheduled at the CCS in which a culture broker took part.

The culture broker, a young North African woman, spent time with the family alone in order to identify their concerns and then with the young girl, voicing the reasons and fears of both sides. Through her behavior and interaction with the family, the culture broker managed to be perceived by both parties as a successful example of how it is possible to combine traditional values with adopted ones. In negotiating between the two parties, she cautiously introduced to the girl the importance of respecting the family hierarchy while helping the parents to adopt a more flexible position vis-à-vis the expectations they had for their daughter in a new society. As a successful example of bicultural identity, the culture broker's presence was reassuring to both the parents and daughter and allowed dialogue to be reestablished.

Strengths and Limits of the Culture Broker's Position

These cases illustrate some of the rich potential and complexities of the position of culture brokers in the clinical encounter. Culture brokers may be seen as sharing a common cultural identity with patients, as agents of the health care institution, or as external experts with specific status and affiliations in the ethnocultural community. Their identity and role raises sensitive issues around the power dynamics of the CCS and its cultural consultative process.

Earlier, we referred to Alexander Bischoff's (2006) classification, which highlights two distinct approaches to cultural brokering: an approach that aims to help the patient assimilate the health care provider's perspective and adapt to the dominant society and an alternative approach that aims for a more inclusive, two-way exchange, in which the cultural broker acts as a mediator and provides a framework for the construction of common ground. The cases discussed here show the ways in which the CCS cultural broker are encouraged to engage in two-way exchanges, which at times becomes a process of advocacy and, at times, a primary intervention. The cases of the young Haitian woman, the new mother from Nigeria, and the young man from Rwanda exemplify the inclusive process of two-way exchange.

To the extent that the culture broker is initiating interventions and changing the dynamics of the clinical interaction, these cases raise important ethical issues. At present, there are few professional guidelines governing this work, and the medicolegal responsibility for the quality of care rests with the treating clinician and the CCS psychiatrist. The CCS relies on a group of culture brokers who have been vetted and trained through the process of collaboration on the service. Over time, the skills, areas of competence, and limitations of specific brokers become clear to the CCS clinicians, and they may be given greater autonomy in the assessment process. New culture brokers, however, are monitored closely and sometimes are found to lack crucial skills or to express biases that impede the clinical process. All culture broker interventions are done with the approval and supervision of the CCS psychiatrist. The CCS consultant supervises the culture broker's work and intervenes whenever there is any question or concern about whether their actions are clinically appropriate and helpful.

This is illustrated by action of the consultant psychiatrist in a consultation with a family from Kosovo. A culture broker originally from the former Yugoslavia also acted as interpreter in a consultation with the family. At one point, in translating the psychiatrist's questions, the culture broker spoke at length in a harsh tone of voice. The psychiatrist felt on edge when he saw the family react with fearful expressions to the translation of his very neutral questions. He decided to intervene by continuing the consultation without the culture broker, using

French as medium, which the family members could partially master.

There are other instances in which the culture broker attempts to take over the role of the clinician. For example, a middle-aged man from Sri Lanka suffering from PTSD was referred to the CCS for an assessment in order to strengthen the therapeutic alliance with his physician. At the CCS, he was seen by a young female psychiatrist of South Asian origin along with a male culture broker who had practiced medicine in Sri Lanka but, on immigrating to Canada, could not get relicensed as a physician and became a medical technician. In the course of the CCS interview, the culture broker who shared with the patient's ethnic and religious background simply took over the consultation and silenced the psychiatrist. This behavior can be understood as an expression of the culture broker's own efforts to save face in front of his countryman because of the embarrassment of having a much younger female, professional in charge of the consultation. However, it had the effect of undermining the assessment process.

To some extent, all of the cases presented here raise issues of positionality at a second level in terms of the articulation between the roles of the culture broker and his or her own identity. The CCS employs two types of culture brokers who are called upon because of their cultural affinity with referred patients: (1) bilingual or bicultural clinicians who usually work in local medical or social service institutions; (2) non-health care professionals, including anthropologists or lay people from the community, who are recognized for their expertise on a specific sociocultural context, group or geographic region. Both types of culture brokers have strengths and weaknesses in their practice at the CCS. The differences between these two types of culture brokers are reminiscent of the debate in the 1980s and 1990s on "native anthropologists," that is, anthropologists studying their own people. These debates were structured around the epistemological advantages of "insider" and "outsider" anthropologists, where "native anthropologists" were often seen as having access to privileged knowledge due to their "natural" ties with the cultural context studied. This advantage seems to have been the case in the clinical encounter that involved the young Haitian patient and a culture broker of Haitian origin. While the culture broker assumed a shared Kreyol and Haitian cultural understanding that did not exist between her and the patient, they nevertheless found a common ground through using a culturally distinctive style of communication. On the other hand, in the cases involving the Kosovar family and the Sri Lankan patient, the apparent cultural proximity between the patient and the culture broker did not necessarily bring about a mediated understanding of the patient's predicament, albeit for different reasons. In fact, in these clinical encounters, the cultural proximity between the culture broker and the patients resulted in interpersonal dynamics that were not helpful to the cultural consultation process.

As these examples make clear, gender, education, social class, and other key markers of identity may emerge as crucial elements in the relationship between the culture broker and the patient. Indeed, an external culture broker who does not share an identity with the patient (e.g., a social scientist with knowledge of the culture) may have a more "objective" standpoint. However, the relevance of such a standpoint depends on the specific culture broker's personal style of communication and skill in the clinical encounter.

Clearly, successful culture brokering depends on brokers' critical awareness of their own culture and social positioning and sensitivity to interpersonal and social context. This may emerge out of a shared cultural background or from recognized expertise but requires the additional ability to recognize, tolerate, and mediate between diverging regimes of interpretation. As illustrated by the cases discussed here, successful cultural brokering is not built on cultural stereotypes. Grasping a patient's predicament requires more than an essentialized vision of his or her culture of origin; it implies that the patient's life trajectory be understood in the relevant historical, social, political, and economic frameworks.

Ultimately, the success of culture brokering may also depend on structural conditions that extend beyond the competences of individual culture brokers. While the clinical team at the CCS is concerned to integrate sociocultural context, biomedical and psychiatric knowledge remains central to the consultant's task. When there is uncertainty about a patient's medical and psychiatric condition, biomedical understanding of symptoms and illness experience is prioritized. In these cases, the initial clinical interview necessarily focuses on gathering information related to the patient's symptoms, mental status, medical and psychiatric history, and medication. Information related to the patient's legal situation in Canada, migration history, family history, and so forth are obtained next. Much of the work of culture brokers at the CCS is to convey information about relevant dynamics in patients' countries of origin or to provide a meaningful paraphrase of a patient's idioms of distress to the CCS clinical and treating teams. While in some cases, culture brokers establish some form of interpersonal tie with patients, the fact that the consultation usually is limited to two interviews limits culture brokers' capacity to play a more significant role in the patient's ongoing care.

Conclusion

Culture brokers are essential to the process of assessment and clinical negotiation at the CCS. The CCS experience in working with culture brokers has implications for their selection, training, evaluation, and regulation. In general, culture brokers must be carefully chosen for their interpersonal and communication skills. They should have a basic understanding of mental health issues in both sociocultural milieus (i.e., the patient's place of origin and the local context in which they currently live and receive care). Clinicians also need to learn work collaboratively with culture brokers. Before the first clinical interviews, a discussion between the CCS consulting psychiatrist (or the CCS resident) and the culture broker on the case is essential to establish common goals and plan a rough agenda and trajectory for the interview. It is important that culture brokers understand their own role within the clinical team.

While the culture broker should play an active part in the interview process, he or she should not take over the clinical encounter unless there is an explicit reason that warrants a more active role. In cases where the culture broker oversteps the bounds of their role, the clinician may need to intervene during the interview, especially when the culture broker's attitude or behavior is likely to jeopardize the clinical alliance.

Although the CCS currently recruits, trains, and evaluates culture brokers through ongoing consultation work, there is a need for formal training, assessment, and certification. Culture brokers should be trained systematically and evaluated periodically to maintain their certification. Training and assessment can build on the expertise of experienced cultural consultants, clinicians, and culture brokers who have managed to develop their skills through apprenticeship. In practice, it may be difficult to formally train a group of culture brokers adequate to address all clinical needs, because certain cultural knowledge and skills may be needed only occasionally, especially in settings with a great diversity of patients. Training clinicians to accept the expertise of culture broker and acknowledge their therapeutic role is also a challenge. Finally, there is a need for further research on effective mediation to inform the development of this essential adjunct to intercultural clinical work.

References

Abu-Lughod, L. (1991). Writing against culture. In R. G. Fox (Ed.), *Recapturing anthropology: Working in the present*. Santa Fe, NM: School of American Research Press.

Adams, K. M. (1997). Ethnic tourism and the renegotiation of tradition in Tana Toraja (Sulawesi, Indonesia). *Ethnology, 36*, 309–320.

Amit, V. (Ed.). (2007). *Going first class? New approaches towards privileged travel and movement*. London, England: Berghahn Press.

Andoche, J. (2001). Sante mentale et culture. Les avatars français de l'ethnopsychiatrie. In J. P. Dozon & D. Fassin (Eds.), *Critique de la santé publique*. Paris, France: Balland.

Appadurai, A. (1996). *Modernity at large: Cultural dimensions of globalization*. Minneapolis, MN: University of Minnesota Press.

Augusti-Panareda, J. (2006). Cross-culture brokering in the legal, institutional and normative domains: Intercultural mediators managing immigration in Catalonia. *Social and Legal Studies, 15*, 409–433.

Barbee, E. (1986). Biomedical resistance to ethnomedicine in Botswana. *Social Science Medicine, 22*, 75–80.

Barbee, E. (1987). Tensions in the brokerage role: Nurses in Botswana. *Western Journal of Nursing Research, 9*, 244–256.

Barnes, J. A. (1954). Class and committees in a Norwegian island parish. *Human Relations, 7*, 39–58.

Beneduce, R. (1999). Luoghi e strategie di un'etnopsichiatria critica. In POL. it.

Beneduce, R., Costa, G., & Favretto, A. R. (1994). *la salute straniera*. Napoli, Italy: Edizioni Scientifiche Italiane.

Bibeau, G. (1997). Cultural psychiatry in a creolizing world: Questions for a new research agenda. *Transcultural Psychiatry, 34*(1), 9–41.

Bischoff, A. (2003). *Caring for migrant and minority patients in European hospitals. A review of effective interventions*. Vienna, Austria: Ludwig Boltzmann Institute for the Sociology of Health and Medicine.

Bischoff, A. (2006). Intercultural mediation: Does it contribute to inclusion? Comparing policies and practices in the sectors of health, education, social and legal services: National Research Programme PNR 51: "Integration or Exclusion?" National Swiss Fond.

Boissevain, J. (1974). *Friends of friends: Networks, manipulators and coalitions*. Oxford, England: Blackwell.

Bott, E. (1957). *Family and social networks*. London, England: Tavistock.

Brown, N. (1992). Beachboys as culture brokers in Bakau town, the Gambia. *Community Development Journal, 27*, 361–370.

Burgess, W., Herring, J., & Young, T. K. (1995). *Aboriginal health in Canada: Historical, cultural, and epidemiological perspectives*. Toronto, Ontario, Canada: University of Toronto Press.

Chambers, E. (2000). *Native tours: The anthropology and travel and tourism*. Long Grove, IL: Waveland Press.

Clifford, J., & Marcus, G. E. (Eds.). (1986). *Writing culture: The poetics and politics of ethnography*. Berkeley, CA: California University Press.

Cohen-Emerique, M. (2004). Positionnement et compétences spécifiques des médiateurs. *Hommes et Migrations, 1249*, 36–52.

Corin, E. (1997). Playing with limits: Tobie Nathan's evolving paradigm in ethnopsychiatry. *Transcultural Psychiatry, 34*(3), 345–358.

Dinh, M. H., Groleau, D., Kirmayer, L. J., Rodriguez, C., & Bibeau, G. (2012). Influence of the DSM-IV outline for cultural formulation on multidisciplinary case conferences in mental health. *Anthropology & Medicine, 19*(2), 261–276.

Fassin, D., & Rechtman, R. (2005). An anthropological hybrid: The pragmatic arrangement of universalism and culturalism in French mental health. *Transcultural Psychiatry, 42*(3), 347–366.

Fernando, S. (Ed.). (1995). *Mental health in a multi-ethnic society: A multidisciplinary handbook.* New York, NY: Routledge.

Fernando, S. (2002). *Mental health, race and culture* (2nd ed.). New York, NY: Palgrave.

Fernando, S. (2003). *Cultural diversity, mental health and psychiatry: The struggle against racism.* New York, NY: Routledge.

Fiorucci, M. (2007). *Dossier: la Mediazione Interculturale e le sue Forme: Contesti, Esperienze e Proposte. Introduzione* [Intercultural mediation and its forms: Contexts, experiences and proposals. Introduction]. Rome, Italy: Studi Emigrazione, Centro Studi Emigrazione Morcelliana.

Fossi, A. (2004). La médiation interculturelle au milieu hospitalier, in: La médiation interculturelle au débat. *Les Cahiers du Carrefour Interculturel Wallon, 1,* 28–37.

Freeman, P. (1997). Ethnopsychiatry in France. *Transcultural Psychiatry, 34*(3), 313–319.

Gadamer, H. G. (1987). The problem of historical consciousness. In P. Rabinow & W. Sullivan (Eds.), *Interpretive social science: A second look.* Berkeley, CA: University of California Press.

Geertz, C. (1960). The Javanese Kijaji: The changing role of a culture broker. *Comparative Studies in Sociology and History, 2,* 228–249.

Gentile, E., & Caponio, T. (2006). Dossier mediazione. La mediazione interculturale nei servizi. Il caso della provincia di Bologna. *Osservatorio delle Immigrazioni, Special Issue,* 1–40.

Gershon, I. (2006). When culture is not a system: Why Samoan culture brokers can not do their job. *Ethnos, 71,* 533–558.

Giordano, C. (2006). *Translating the other: An ethnography of migrant encounters with the police, nuns, and ethno-psychiatrists in contemporary Italy.* Doctoral dissertation, University of California, Berkeley, CA.

Giordano, C. (2008). Practices of translation and the making of migrant subjectivities in contemporary Italy. *American Ethnologist, 35*(4), 588–606.

Giordano, C. (2011). Translating Fanon in the Italian context: Rethinking the ethics of treatment in psychiatry. *Transcultural Psychiatry, 48*(3).

Gobbo, F. (2004). Cultural intersections: The life story of a Roma cultural mediator. *European Educational Research Journal, 3,* 626–641.

Gregg, J., & Saha, S. (2006). Losing culture on the way to competence: The use and misuse of culture in medical education. *Academic Medicine, 81,* 542–547.

Halba, B. (2009). *T.I.P.S for intercultural dialogue: T-learning to improve professional skills for intercultural dialogue.* Paris, France: Institut de Recherche et d'Information sur le Volontariat (IRIV).

Hannerz, U. (1992). *Cultural complexity.* New York, NY: Columbia University Press.

Jackson, L., Graham, E., & Jackson, J. C. (1998 [1995]). *Beyond medical interpretation: The role of interpreter cultural mediators (ICMs) in building bridges between ethnic communities and health institutions.* Seattle, WA: Harborview Medical Center.

Jezewski, M. A. (1990). Culture brokering in migrant farmworker health care. *Western Journal of Nursing Research, 12,* 497–513.

Kahn, M., & Kelly, K. (2001). Cultural tensions in psychiatric nursing: Managing the interface between western mental health and the Xhosa traditional healing in South Africa. *Transcultural Psychiatry, 38,* 35–50.

Kareem, J. (1992). The Nafsiyat intercultural therapy centre: Ideas and experience in intercultural therapy. In J. Kareem & R. Littlewood (Eds.), *Intercultural therapy: Themes, interpretations and practice* (pp. 14–37). Oxford, England: Blackwell Scientific.

Kaufert, P. (1990). The 'boxification' of culture: The role of the social scientist. *Santé Culture Health, 7,* 139–148.

Kaufert, J. M., & Koolage, W. W. (1984). Role conflict among 'culture brokers': The experience of native Canadian medical interpreters. *Social Science & Medicine, 18*(3), 283–286.

Kaufert, J. M., & O'Neil, J. D. (1998). Culture, power and informed consent: The impact of Aboriginal health interpreters on decision-making. In D. Coburn, C. D'Arcy, P. New, & G. Torrance (Eds.), *Health and Canadian society: Sociological perspectives.* Toronto, Ontario, Canada: Univeristy of Toronto Press.

Kaufert, J. M., Putsch, R. W., & Lavallée, M. (1998). Experience of Aboriginal health interpreters in mediation of conflicting values in end-of-life decision making. *International Journal of Circumpolar Health, 57,* 43–48.

Kirmayer, L. J., Groleau, D., Guzder, J., Blake, C., & Jarvis, E. (2003). Cultural consultation: A model of mental health service for multicultural societies. *Canadian Journal of Psychiatry, 48*(2), 145–153.

Kirmayer, L. J., & Minas, H. (2000). The future of cultural psychiatry: An international perspective. *Cannadian Journal of Psychiatry, 45*(5), 438–446.

Kirmayer, L. J., Rousseau, C., & Lashley, M. (2007). The place of culture in forensic psychiatry. *The Journal of the American Academy of Psychiatry and the Law, 35*(1), 98–102.

Kleinman, A. (1987). Anthropology and psychiatry: The role of culture in cross-cultural research on illness. *The British Journal of Psychiatry, 151,* 447–454.

Kleinman, A., & Benson, P. (2006). Anthropology in the clinic: The problem of cultural competency and how to fix it. *PLoS Medicine, 3*(10), e294.

Krajic, K., Strassmayr, C., Karl-Trummer, U., Novak-Zezula, S., & Pelikan, J. (2005). Improving ethnocultural competence of hospital staff by trainwing: Experiences from the European 'Migrant-friendly Hospitals' project. *Diversity in Health and Social Care 2,* 279–290.

Marcus, G. E. (Ed.). (1992). *Rereading cultural anthropology.* Durham, England: Duke University Press.

Marks, S. (1997). The legacy of the history of nursing for post-apartheid South Africa. In A. Rafferty, J. Robinson, & R. Elkan (Eds.), *Nursing history and the politicsof welfare.* London, England: Routledge.

Minervino, S., & Martin, M. C. (2007). Cultural competence and cultural mediation: Diversity strategies and practices in health care. *Translocations: The Irish*

Migration, Race and Social Transformation Review, 1, 190–198.

Minore, B., & Boone, M. (2002). Realizing potential: Improving interdisciplinary professional/paraprofessional health care teams in Canada's northern Aboriginal communities through education. *Journal of Interprofessional Care, 16,* 139–147.

Molina, I., Gailly, A. G., Romero, C., & Guest, B. (Eds.). (2001). *Social linkworking and inter-cultural mediation in Europe. Pilot project TPL transnational partnership for linkworking, Sweden.* Stockholm, Sweden: Partnersap for Multietnisk Integration.

Moro, M. R., & Real, I. (2006). La consultation transculturelle d'Avicenne. In M. R. Moro & Y. Mouchenick (Eds.), *Manuel de psychiatrie transculturelle.* Grenoble, France: La Pensée Sauvage.

Narayan, K. (1993). How native is a "native" anthropologist? *American Anthropologist, 95*(3), 671–686.

Nathan, T. (1994a). *L'influence qui guérit.* Paris, France: Éditions Odile Jacob.

Nathan, T. (1994b). Les bienfaits des thérapies sauvages. Thérapie scientifique et thérapie sauvage. *Nouvelle Revue d'Ethnopsychiatrie, 27,* 37–54.

Ng, J., Popova, S., Yau, M., & Sulman, J. (2007). Do culturally sensitive services for Chinese in-patients make a difference? *Social Work in Health Care, 44,* 129–143.

Paine, R. (1971). Theory of patronage and brokerage. In R. Paine (Ed.), *Patrons and brokers in the East Arctic.* Toronto, Ontario, Canada: University of Toronto Press.

Pandolfi, M., & Bibeau, G. (2006). Suffering, politics, nation: A cartography of Italian medical anthropology. In F. Saillant & S. Genest (Eds.), *Medical anthropology: Regional perspectives and shared concerns.* London, England: Blackwell.

Pöchhacker, F. (2008). Interpreting as mediation. In C. Valero-Garces & A. Martin (Eds.), *Crossing borders in community interpreting definitions and dilemmas.* Philadelphia, PA: John Benjamins Publishing Company.

Press, I. (1969). Ambiguity and innovation: Implications for the genesis of the culture broker. *American Anthropologist, 71,* 205–217.

Santiago-Irizarry, V. (2001). *Medicalizing ethnicity: The construction of Latino identity in psychiatric settings.* Ithaca, NY: Cornell University Press.

Sargent, C., & Larchanche, S. (2009). The construction of "cultural difference" and its therapeutic significance in immigrant mental health services in France. *Culture, Medicine and Psychiatry, 33*(1), 2–20.

Singh, N. N., McKay, J. D., & Singh, A. N. (1999). The need for culture brokers in mental health services. *Journal of Child and Family Studies, 8,* 1–10.

Soong, F. S. (1983). The role of Aboriginal health workers as culture brokers: Some findings and their implications. *Australian Journal of Social Issues, 18,* 268–274.

Streit, U. (1997). Nathan's ethnopsychoanalytic therapy: Characteristics, discoveries and challenges to western psychotherapy. *Transcultural Psychiatry, 34*(3), 321–343.

Sturm, G., Heidenreich, F., & Moro, M. R. (2008). Transcultural clinical work with immigrants, asylum seekers and refugees at Avicenne Hospital, France. *International Journal of Migration, Health and Social Care, 4,* 33–40.

Sturm, G., Nadig, M., & Moro, M. R. (2011). Current developments in French ethnopsychoanalysis. *Transcultural Psychiatry, 48*(3), 205–227.

Szasz, M. C. (1994). Introduction. In M. C. Szasz (Ed.), *Between Indian and White worlds: The culture broker.* Norman, OK: University of Oklahoma Press.

Taylor, J. S. (2003a). The story catches you and you fall down: Tragedy, ethnography, and "cultural competence". *Medical Anthropology Quarterly, 17*(2), 159–181.

Taylor, J. S. (2003b). Confronting "culture" in medicine's culture of no culture. *Academic Medicine, 78,* 555–559.

Trudgen, R. (2000). *Why warriors lie down and die.* Darwin, NT: Aboriginal Resources and Development Services.

Turner, V. W. (1974). *Dramas, fields and metaphors: Symbolic actions in human society.* Ithaca, NY: Cornell University.

Van Willigen, J. (2002). *Applied anthropology. An introduction.* Westport, CT: Bergin & Garvey.

Verrept, H. (2008). Intercultural mediation: An answer to health care disparities? In C. Valero-Garcés & A. Martin (Eds.), *Crossing borders in community interpreting. Definitions and dilemmas.* Amsterdam, Netherlands: Benjamins.

Weidman, H. (1975). Concepts as strategies for change. *Psychiatric Annals, 5,* 312–314.

Willis, E. (1999). From culture brokers to shared care: The changing position of literacy for Aboriginal health workers in Central Australia. *Studies in Continuing Education, 21,* 163–175.

Wolf, E. (1956). Aspects of group relations in a complex society: Mexico. *American Anthropologist, 56,* 1065–1078.

Zajde, N. (2011). Psychotherapy with immigrant patients in France: An ethnopsychiatric perspective. *Transcultural Psychiatry, 48*(3), 187–204.

Family Systems in Cultural Consultation

Jaswant Guzder

> Just as family therapy…grew out of the myopia of the intrapsychic view and concluded that human behavior could not be understood in isolation from its family context, family behavior also makes sense only in the context in which it is embedded. (McGoldrick, Pearce, & Giordano, 1982, p. 4)

Systemic thinking is a cornerstone of the CCS model. The work of the CCS is based on a bio-psychosocial approach that examines the interaction of individual and systemic processes in the origin of problems and their resolution. This chapter will illustrate the application of systemic approaches drawn from family systems theory and therapy to the process of cultural consultation. The author and other members of the original CCS team were trained as family therapists and bring this systemic orientation to the work. Some of the cases referred to the CCS come from other individual and family therapists who are facing challenges or impasses in their work, and the consultant then works with them to devise strategies to move the therapy forward.

For the CCS, family systems are important in three main ways: (1) as a means to gain access to the social context of patients to understand their personal problems and resources for resilience and healing, (2) as a way to build working alliances with the patient and key family members to facilitate clinical engagement and treatment, and (3) as a way to identify family systems issues that may constitute core clinical problems in their own right. Comprehensive clinical assessment and systemic intervention require the input of the patient, the referring clinicians, interpreters, cultural brokers and other relevant systemic partners (e.g., family members, school, work, other health care workers). Many of the cases seen by the CCS involve dilemmas created in part by the structure of the health care system itself, and these structural problems also need to be considered from an interactional perspective. Finally, systemic thinking can be extended beyond the family and the health care system to understand patients' location in local communities as well as global networks.

The CCS model focuses on the consultant as a stranger to the system and on Otherness as a key element in structuring the problem-solving process. The consultation involves a process of inquiry that is equally attentive to the issues and concerns of the referring clinician and the patient.

J. Guzder, M.D. (✉)
Center for Child Development and Mental Health,
Institute of Community and Family Psychiatry,
Montreal, QC, Canada H3T 1E4
e-mail: jaswant@videotron.ca

In addition to the information obtained through interviews, the referring clinician is invited to a case conference formatted as a roundtable discussion with members of the consultation service. This allows exploration of referring clinicians' ideas about the case and some immediate response to their specific concerns.

Systemic understanding of individual or family coping and striving for wellbeing requires attention to the roles, power dynamics and authorizing myths which are often implicit in culture. Culture can be described as a system of beliefs or rules that govern social interaction (McGoldrick et al., 1982), but within the family the medium of culture is the emotional life of family members, which involves collective, intergenerational and individual identities. These identities are framed in terms of conventional life narratives according to cultural concepts of personhood (Kirmayer, 2007), but they may also reference collective cultural myths or ideologies. Cultural myths may hold repressed elements and justify taboos that shape the dynamics of the social world (Obeyesekere, 1990). Migrant families remain functional in the face of change by adapting or renegotiating their affective processes, structures and attachments to maintain agency and intimacy. Negotiations in the interpersonal spheres of family and community may involve changes in social and gender roles, distributions of power and developmental trajectories that may be perceived differently by each family member. Migrants may adopt novel, hybrid identities and new collective myths as they adapt and acculturate to new cultural contexts. Narrative reframing (Angus & Macleod, 2004), problem solving (Haley, 1976b; Watzlawick, Weakland, & Fisch, 2011) and memory work (Kidron, 2012) are all intrinsic to shifting family functioning and constructing hope and mobilizing resilience. These processes can occur at the level of the family as well as local and transnational communities (Kirmayer, Fung et al., 2012; Kirmayer, Sedhev, Whitley, Dandeneau, & Isaac, 2009; Ruiz-Casares, Guzder, Rousseau, & Kirmayer, 2013).

The family therapists Bowen (1978) and Carl Whitaker (Neill & Kniskern, 1982) emphasized that systemic thinking can be just as relevant as a framework for clinical work with individuals as it

is for work with couples or families. Cultural consultation, however, must also consider extra-familial systemic influences that have been less central in the family therapy literature, including racism, poverty, refugee status, immigration law and institutional agendas, as well as other social contexts and historical legacies (Aponte, 1994; Fernando, 1991; Hickling, 2005; Kareem, 1978). The "multicultural imagination" (Adams, 1996) highlights the biases of earlier family therapy work, which tended to focus on nuclear families (Nichols & Schwartz, 2006, p. 115) and ignore the wider social and cultural contexts of ethnocultural minorities or migrant families. Important systemic issues occur at the levels of the family, the community, the health care system and the institutions of the wider society. CCS assessments sometimes raise systemic issues in health care and other social institutions, including those of institutional racism (Boyd-Franklin, 2003; Fernando, 1991; James, 1996):

> Institutional racism is the collective failure of an organization to provide an appropriate and professional service to people because of their colour, culture or ethnic origin. It can be seen or detected in processes, attitudes and behaviours which amount to discrimination through unwitting prejudice, ignorance, thoughtlessness and racist stereotyping which disadvantages minority ethnic people. (Macpherson, 1999, p. 28)

Despite a society that is relatively tolerant and accepting, "visible minorities" and racialized groups in Canada may face considerable discrimination throughout the health care system and other institutions (Satzewich, 2011). Often, this prejudice is woven into institutional practices in ways that are tacit or implicit and, hence, difficult to name or discuss. Although issues of institutional racism or other types of bias may not be central in any given case, the consultant should remain alert to these larger social systemic processes which are always at play.

In the context of the CCS, the author's identity as a South Asian child psychiatrist, family therapist and psychoanalyst has allowed her to play a bridging role between host society and culture of origin in many of the referrals of South Asian patients (see Chapter 8). In several cases, the opportunity for ethnic or linguistic match led to longer therapeutic involvement as other resources in the community were limited. While this congruence was often helpful, it also sometimes posed strategic or countertransference challenges. Cultural consultants, like family therapists, must consider the impact of their personal and ethnic identities on the clinical alliance and therapeutic processes (Catherall & Pinsof, 1987; Kareem, 1992; Kaslow, 1987).

Systemic Discourse and Cultural Realities

While the dynamics of family systems and cultural contexts influence psychological processes, the dominant paradigms in mental health training, assessment and intervention have tended to minimize both cultural and systemic issues. Over the past 30 years, there have been a number of manuals presenting "recipe book" approaches to culture, which risk promoting stereotypic versions of ethnic identity. This work tends to approach culture in a static, essentialized way and fails to convey the subtlety and complexities of the interactional processes of acculturation, assimilation and identity post-migration. There are wide cultural variations within and between families, as well as complex intergenerational migration trajectories, and the consultant must remain alert to the clinical implications of hybrid identities. The consultation process is a dynamic investigation that needs to provide a safe space for the patient to explore their changing identity and position. Rather than prescribing fixed solutions or formulations based on ethnicity alone, we strive to remain open to the full range of social, cultural and political systemic issues that shape the lifeworld of the patient.

Referring clinicians seek a cultural consultation when they recognize that culture may be relevant to clinical questions or concerns. This recognition is influenced by many factors in clinicians' background and training, their contexts of practice and larger institutional structures and ideologies. Attention to culture may be raised by difficulties in case formulation or clinical engagement, a therapeutic impasse, the clinicians own uncertainty, frustration, discomfort with a patient or their ongoing interest and engagement in cultural diversity in their practice. Since much of the Euro-North American training of mental health professionals is grounded in idealized assumptions of universality and psychoanalytic positions on "neutrality," the subtle and complex psychosocial and cultural identities of patients, families and communities have been largely ignored in the clinical literature. Many clinicians have limited training or awareness of the systemic processes, power relations and cultural frames of reference that influence clinical encounters. As a result, for many clinicians, cultural dimensions of illness experience only become salient in exceptional circumstances. In postmodern contexts, the narrative school of family therapy has stressed the paradigm of "decentring" which involves the therapist's positioning to strive for a nonhierarchical and non-objectifying role in therapy with respectful awareness of the social embeddedness of both therapist and client (Kogan & Gale, 2004; White & Epston, 1990). Decentring, as a therapist position, promotes more objective listening to the local unfolding narrative and its embedding in larger cultural stories and guides the narrative process which uses techniques of objectifying or externalizing the problem, expansive questioning and rescripting favorite narratives to open options for emerging stories that promote coping and resilience (Angus & Macleod, 2004; Freedman & Coombs, 1996; Parry & Doan, 1994).

Claims of clinical neutrality or objectivity can also impede the recognition of cultural agendas at play in the clinical encounter. In family therapy, neutrality is a term that implies the therapist should not ally herself with any one member of the system to "unbalance" the alliance. The stance of neutrality also positions the therapist as a "curious, benevolent, unprejudiced" observer of the other. Neutrality, in classical psychoanalytic terms, however, directs the clinician to maintain an attitude of professional or affective neutrality in which:

> he must remain neutral in respect to religious, ethical and social values—that is to say he must not direct the treatment according to some ideal, abstain from counseling the patient,… not lend a special ear to particular parts of this discourse or read particular meanings into it, according to his theoretical preconceptions. (LaPlanche & Pontalis, 1973, p. 271)

Family therapists, like ethnographers and social scientists, have long recognized that this sort of neutrality is simply not possible (Selvini, Boscolo, Cecchin, & Prata, 1978). In "joining" a system, the therapist inevitably is changing the entity they are trying to observe. Hence, our very presence precludes the psychoanalytic version of neutrality in families where multiple alliances are necessary. The shift to systemic thinking and interviewing has implications not only for clinicians but also for interpreters, culture brokers and the other clinical partners and institutions implicated in cultural consultative work. In the past, psychoanalytic training along with many other schools of psychotherapy has tended to assume the universality of some psychological processes, implying that models of psychopathology and methods of intervention do not require adjustment in the face of cultural difference (Akhtar, 1995). This assumption of universality is congruent with clinicians' own concerns about fairness, appropriate roles and biases. Indeed, for many liberal-minded clinicians, even acknowledging difference is seen as a form of prejudice or discrimination: "A common assumption amongst therapists is that it is impolite to talk about race, and a color-blind approach to working with clients demonstrates the therapist's 'niceness' or 'goodness'" (Killian, 2001, p. 17).

However, far from being unbiased, neutral and accepting, such defensive color-blindness ignores salient dimensions of patients' experience and risks imposing unexamined ethnocentric norms and values on the clinical encounter. We therefore encourage ongoing supervision and internal reflection by clinicians and teams to maintain awareness of their own tacit values and assumptive worlds. This is challenging and requires a commitment to acknowledging one's own cultural biases and embedding in systems of power and privilege. Becoming aware of one's tacit cultural knowledge, attitudes and values can be facilitated by training in cultural psychiatry, intercultural experience and exposure to the comparative perspectives of anthropology and related social sciences:

> On a personal level, self-structures, reflecting cultural value systems, arise so early in life that they are pre-reflective, given, and difficult to break

away from… critical social sciences attempt to get a handle on these forces, on the personal and cultural levels, respectively, that constrain us, that are built into us. (Altman, 2006, p. 68)

Awareness of difference between individuals in the clinical encounter allows us to build bridges, but it does not dissolve the issue of culture, since we are all more or less invested in specific cultural frameworks as part of the scaffolding of individual and collective identity:

> Social categories of identity are integral to a deep sense of self, the experience of a true me. And if we accept this, then it follows that, in attaching to others, we are also, of necessity attaching to categories, however subliminal our sense of those might be… we cannot not attach, nor can we not belong… attachment and belonging are aspects of the same process (in a multicultural society). (Dalal, 2006, p. 148)

The work of cultural consultation therefore requires constant attention to the consultants' own embedding in the dynamics of local and global systems which have underpinnings in specific cultural models or paradigms, including those of science. Understanding these historical, cultural or mythic paradigms can be useful for joining with individuals or families and reframing their predicament through myths and metaphors drawn from their cultures of origin. While the stories of Abraham and Isaac, Mary and Joseph, Oedipus or Medea may be widely known as part of the Western historical legacy, in Asian and African traditions, there are quite different spiritual and religious myths that organize family maps and provide crucial foundations to moral worlds, life tasks, duties and obligations, developmental passages, identities and patterns of conflict resolution. Contemporary myths may also be accessed in the current vernacular of plays, films, art,

---

Case Vignette 7-1

Nalini, a 19-year-old college student with South Asian background, was referred to the CCS by her pediatrician after a poor response to antidepressants and 2 years of psychotherapy with a deteriorating outcome following a rape incident. Nalini was

(continued)

initially accompanied to the consultation by her mother, who would also phone-in during the session to check on her whereabouts. The father had refused to attend a family interview or give his wife permission to participate. At home, Nalini reported she was under virtual house arrest. Since the rape, her father had become increasingly paranoid and preoccupied with issues of racism and loss. Her mother, who was a second-generation North American migrant, was blamed for being too permissive because she had supported Nalini's taking a part-time job, and Nalini was raped en route home from work. Nalini's 9-year-old sister (who, like Nalini, was also an excellent student) had developed nightmares and enuresis, while Nalini was increasingly irritable and depressed. After the rape, she displaced her rage onto her mother and expressed longing to be a son to her father, identifying with her father's pervasive emotional power in the family. While Nalini ridiculed her mother for accepting her father's rigid oppression, she was anguished by his condemnation and verbal attacks in which he stated that she would never be "pure" again: "No one will ever want to marry you." We explored the impact of her ambivalent identification with her mother's legacy as a second-generation Asian woman and father's first-generation cultural ties as another process of locating herself in relation to traditional and mythic worlds and of negotiating her autonomy and power within a gendered hierarchy.

The rape had exposed the collision of cultures experienced by her parents as part of the South Asian diaspora in the West, while also reviving earlier traumas in the history of the couple and family. The CCS consultant was unable to engage the family as the father remained mistrustful and angry (at one point suggesting caste differences made it impossible for him to work with the consultant), and Nalini was referred to individual therapy. She felt very uncomfortable with the South Asian identity of the consultant "who would know about my parent's world" and sought out a therapist of Caribbean origin who would "understand racism issues…(and) look like me but not understand my (maternal) language." Conflicts over autonomy and the search for a representation of cultural hybridity were important in building the clinical alliance and deciding on an appropriate referral.

videogames or novels. The clinician may find mythic or contemporary cultural references useful vehicles for joining, empathic understanding, alliance building and validating patients' experience. Like linguistic fluency, understanding historical, ethnic and mythic paradigms provides access to the cultural imagination (Adams, 1996; Roland, 2007). Given the variability across generations and the unique hybrid identities that may be present in one family system, however, the clinician must be able to flexibly negotiate these borders of meaning to maintain a working alliance.

Case Vignette 7-2
A clinician treating a young man in long-term psychotherapy requested a consultation for his stepmother, an immigrant from Africa, who was his father's third partner. The referring clinician described the stepmother as "a psychotic wife" and reported that she had started a fire in the home. At the initial consultation, the patient, who was a well-groomed and dignified woman, remained silent and the consultant assumed that she did not speak any English. The consultant began to obtain a history by interviewing her husband in her presence. The husband presented himself as Canadian born with egalitarian values though he had

(continued)

had three arranged marriages. Citing her attempts to burn photos of his previous wife and children, the husband felt it was clear that she was ill and asked to have his wife medicated with neuroleptics. At this point the patient began to speak rapidly and with passionate intensity in a dialect of her natal language. She made it clear that she had felt victimized and oppressed within his extended family, disillusioned by her experiences in Canada, suppressed by her in-laws, blocked from travelling home to see her family when her father died, regularly beaten by her husband who was obsessed with having a son, and enraged that a therapist would assume that she could not understand English without asking her. The consultant realized he had been biased by the referring clinician's report characterizing the wife as psychotic, and so did not appreciate the structural implications of gender and power issues and had inadvertently colluded with the husband. The subsequent consultation process revealed family systems issues including serious marital conflict, domestic violence and unresolved mourning and trauma. The couple were referred for marital therapy at their request.

As this case illustrates, the clinician is located in particular social and cultural positions based on the patient's experience. The patient may be uncomfortable with too much proximity, so that ethnic match becomes an obstacle to the alliance. Neutrality, in systemic terms, involves working with this positioning to build an alliance and open up culturally acceptable options for intervention. The following clinical vignette illustrates how all participants in the consultation process are implicated in this rethinking of neutrality.

The systemic approach seeks to explore perceptions of power and powerlessness, agency and silencing and hierarchy and egalitarianism in the consulting process. Because language can be used strategically to create barriers and maintain power inequalities, it is essential to reserve time to speak to family members and interpreters about language translation needs and conditions. The consultation process can be experienced as a re-traumatization or revival of structural violence, as in this case vignette in which the wife was depicted as psychotic while, in fact, she had been victimized and was acting out within a closed family system that labelled her behavior as "mad" and "bad." The referring clinician was biased by seeing the system from the perspective of a stepchild and had not understood the complex dynamics or cultural agendas across the generations in this blended family system. Successful consultation depended on a respectful process that promoted cultural safety and allowed divergent perspectives to emerge.

The Systems Perspective: Theoretical Models and Therapeutic Agendas

While psychodynamic theory has approached symptoms as rooted in unconscious conflict, prompting a search for the hidden meanings to be brought to awareness, the family systems perspective seeks the meaning of symptoms and behaviors in their function as interpersonal communication or acts of positioning in interactional contexts (Boscolo & Bertrando, 1996; Epstein, Bishop, & Levin, 1980; Green & Framo, 1981; Haley, 1976a, 1976b; Hoffman, 1981; Wynne, McDaniel, & Weber, 1986). Psychodynamic models were the basis of early ethnopsychiatric theory (e.g., Devereux, 1970, 1978), and the application of family and systemic theories to ethno-psychiatry is a more recent endeavor (DiNicola, 1985a, 1985b, 1997; Falicov, 1983; Jasser, 2008; Knitzer, 1982; McGoldrick, 1998; Turner & Wieling, 2004). The work of anthropologist Gregory Bateson (Bateson, 1972; Bateson, Jackson, & Haley, 1956), along with others influenced by the perspectives of systems theory and cybernetics, contributed greatly to the interactional view of family process (Watzlawick & Weakland, 1977). Family therapists developed novel interviewing and interpretive strategies to understand the systemic origins and impacts of mental disorders on family members as well as the identified patient. From an interactional perspective, the child or other "identified patient" brings the family for treatment, and a key challenge of assessment is finding out who is "the real patient."

Strategic–systemic approaches in family therapy view the emergence of symptoms in a particular social and systemic context as part of the family's attempt to resolve problems (Andolfi, Angelo, & Menghi, 1983; Boscolo & Bertrando, 1996; Selvini & Weber, 1988). This perspective differs profoundly from the psychoanalytic preoccupation with personal meanings and insight in the confines of the therapeutic dyad (Dejong & Berg, 1998; Selvini, Boscolo, Cecchin, & Prata, 1980). Family therapists address pragmatic issues of transforming rigid or repetitive patterns that are embedded in systemic structures. These patterns are not captured by conventional psychiatric diagnoses. The goals of systemic work are largely focused on getting the patient or family not only to define the problem but also to decide on which problems they wish to resolve (Guzder, 2011). The clinical goal is the resolution of the problem not the achievement of insight. Hence, there is emphasis on achieving competence or optimal functioning rather than focusing on psychopathology. In systemic theory, problems often are attributed to failed attempts to arrive at a solution, which then become part of an emergent problem (Watzlawick, Weakland, & Fisch, 2011). As a result, the strategic–systemic therapist does not deal directly with resistances or underlying personality issues, which are central to psychoanalytic approaches but with ongoing social interactions which can be changed to shift the system towards better functioning. This orientation shifts the focus of assessment as well as intervention.

Minuchin's (1974) work on structural family therapy emphasized the universal need for functional hierarchical relationships between parents and children for healthy family functioning. He promoted key concepts in systemic thinking such as *enmeshment* (poorly defined or diffuse boundaries in a family system), *disengagement* (inappropriately rigid boundaries in a family), *joining* (the stranger therapist entering as a participant in the system) and *enactments* (embodied, interactional sequences which may be evoked by specific

contexts, for example, the use of family meals in the assessment and treatment of anorexia nervosa) (Minuchin & Fishman, 1981). This conceptual vocabulary and associated techniques, which grew out of Minuchin's work with teams at the Philadelphia Child Guidance Clinic, were widely adopted in family therapy. However, efforts to distinguish normal and pathological or functional and dysfunctional process in family therapy faced a challenge, as Euro-American paradigms were not always applicable across cultures. Although his own background gave him a flexible cultural repertoire, Minuchin recognized this challenge (Wynne et al., 1986, p. xii):

> A number of years ago I conducted a workshop in Israel, doing a number of consultations to seasoned family therapists who were stuck with some difficult families. The families, the therapists and I were satisfied with the consultations; and since I had no further feedback, I assumed that had been helpful. But when I did a follow-up a few years later, I learned that in a significant number of my consultations, I had failed to understand the context of the family. In effect, I had constructed and then proceeded to consult an ideal family in therapy with an ideal therapist, divorced from the social context (a psychiatric hospital, the Israeli mental health system or the kibbutz) that included these therapeutic systems. To work with a more expanded focus, I had to consult with my "consultees", since I was entering an arena with which they were more familiar. The consultant-consultee system then became more symmetrical, and also more helpful. I now try to include a feedback procedure in my consultations; never again can I be blissfully ignorant.
>
> I think that family therapy, as we teach it today, is trapped in the same ignorance. It's a one-way street. …(if) we abandon our provincialism, open our windows, learn something about the complexity and idiosyncrasy of systems, and soar to meta positions. Do we have the intellectual tools necessary for these explorations? Or will we have to admit that we need new tools?

Family assessment and therapy have been used to address many common predicaments such as adolescent separation from family (Haley, 1976a), domestic violence (Bograd, 1999; Greene & Bogo, 2002) and eating disorders (Minuchin & Fishman, 1981). However, although there are diverse theoretical models of family therapy (Boscolo & Bertrando, 1996), major contributors to the field generally have not distinguished between different cultural versions of these predicaments. Except for acknowledging their own position as outsiders in the family system, family therapists tended to ignore alternate cultural paradigms until the clinical realities of work with migrant families challenged generic theories built on the paradigm of the Euro-American nuclear family. The assimilationist, the "melting pot" ideology of the US society, gave way gradually to the acknowledgement of alternate histories and developmental trajectories. The recognition of cultural variations in structure, composition, developmental trajectories and mythic representations of families has also led to rethinking some of the assumptions of psychology rooted in Euro-American norms and values (Guzder, 2011). Uncritical use of these norms risks pathologizing families from other backgrounds as enmeshed, immature, primitive or dysfunctional (Kareem, 1978). At times, assumptions based on Euro-American cultural norms about what constitutes a healthy family have led to destructive views of minority and migrant families, minimizing their cohesiveness, resilience and strengths (Cohen & Timimi, 2008).

Family cultures can be broadly characterized as *collectivistic* or *individualistic* in orientation (Falicov, 1983). Collectivistic cultures arrange their interdependencies as central to meaningful identity, expressed in roles and obligations that shape early child socialization and are reworked over the life cycle. In contrast to the individualism of the dominant Euro-North American cultures, Asian and African families tend to emphasize collective identity, with structures that are shaped to varying degrees by intergenerational relationships, communal roles and status, membership in caste or clan and the veneration of ancestors. Anthropology has a long tradition of exploring the structure of family and kinship systems and work by psychological anthropologists, cultural psychiatrists and psychologists—including Doi (1973), Kakar (1978), Obeyesekere (1990), Roland (1988), and others—has laid the groundwork for understanding normal and pathological variations in family process and developmental agendas across cultures. However, much of this work has been heavily influenced by psychodynamic theories, which retain many cultural assumptions about

normal development and relationships. Sterlin (1989), for example, described *centripetal* and *centrifugal* family systems, which propelled children outwards to separate or inwards to remain close to their parents and extended family. As with most psychoanalytically informed writers, Sterlin used the ethnocentric nuclear model of individuation rather than acknowledging the alternate cultural norms of interdependent cultural familial matrices.

Consultants' assessment of familial distance or closeness depends in part on their own internalized norms and implicit models of autonomy and dependency. Understanding of family maps shifts with the clinicians' knowledge of culture and social context as they engage with the emotional processes of the family system. The capacity to join with many different kinds of systems by appreciating key elements of systemic organization is essential for the integration of psychodynamic, strategic and behavioral approaches in family assessment. Family systems approaches use several key cultural concepts in this work, including (1) intergenerational family processes involving gender, hierarchy and pre- and post-migration social contexts; (2) cultural memory and the socio-historical legacy of identifications of the family; (3) social networks of family, friends and institutions in both the adopted and origin countries; (4) the social, cultural and emotional place of spiritual or religious life; (5) the perceptions and roles of children towards the adults in their life and the influences of their peer group; (6) the family ethos which may emphasize autonomy (individualistic, egocentric model) or collective identity (collectivistic, sociocentric model); and (7) family maps of identity, roles and structure which influence patterns of interaction in the system (Akhtar, 2000; Boyd-Franklin, 2003; DiNicola, 1985a, 1985b; Hare-Mustin, 1987; Hays, 1996, 2008; McGoldrick, 1998; Perelberg, 2000; Sue & Sue, 1999; Turner & Wieling, 2004). The CCS model relies on culture brokers and a multicultural team to contribute knowledge of these dimensions of family systems to guide the assessment and case formulation.

Family systems approaches employ all the common strategies for building a therapeutic alliance including empathic listening, trust, holding and attention to narrative but have developed distinctive methods of interviewing, such as the use of *circular interviewing* (Tomm, 1985, 1989), which avoid the problems of direct confrontation when gathering information in closed systems or situations pervaded by secrets. Family interviews must deal with resistances but also must handle the risks associated with uncovering secrets such as incest, domestic violence, eating disorders or addictions. In circular interviewing, the clinician asks one family member to suggest what another member might be thinking or feeling, and this then guides the interviewer in generating questions. Another strategy of inquiry involves externalizing the problem—for example, viewing it simply as a pattern of behavior—in order to promote personal agency and problem solving within the family. Narrative therapy directs interviewing towards eliciting and creating family stories which become tools for change (Sluzki, 1992; White & Epston, 1990). Narratives are seen as rich with embedded meaning and a means to open families to self exploration for change. These methods are employed in systemic cultural consultation as ways to access meaning and devise interventions. The narratives that emerge in the consultation reference cultural myths, maps and agendas in ways that can clarify the systemic origins of problems and identify potential paths for change. These narratives can also be used to help the family recreate their own stories in ways that promote healing transformations.

Systemic Understanding of Symptoms and Presenting Problems

Current psychiatric diagnostic assessment largely focuses on discrete symptoms, syndromes and disorders, biomedical tests and psychological formulations. In the past, this diagnostic constructs were rooted in psychodynamic or psychoanalytic theory, but there are now more commonly based on models drawn from biological psychiatry or psychological approaches linked to cognitive behavior therapy. The contextual thinking central to systemic and cultural perspectives has remained largely at the margins of psychiatric practice

(Aponte, 1994; Kareem, 1988; Lewis-Fernandez, 1996; McGoldrick, 1998; Sue & Sue, 1999). The rich social science literature on non-Western cultural paradigms has also had minimal impact on mental health training (Akhtar, 2000; Greenberg & Witzum, 2001; Kakar, 1982; Kleinman, 1988; Obeyesekere, 1990). Clinically, the focus on DSM or ICD disorders is not sufficient to guide everyday practice. Families and individuals grapple not only with psychiatric disorders but with personal predicaments and other forms of distress that are rooted in the challenges of essential life tasks,

Case Vignette 7-3

Aaliya, a Pakistani mother with two sons, 10 and 5 years old, had been refused refugee status by the immigration board and was referred for cultural consultation by a community clinic while she awaited an appeal process. Her social worker had been concerned about her threats to suicide by jumping off a bridge with her children. In the assessment interview, Aaliya voiced her distress over her deportation order, alternately expressing rage and frustration and suicidal ideation in response to the refugee board's decision. She stated, "they don't believe me" and feared that she would be murdered if her ex-husband learned of her return to Pakistan. Aaliya had left her country of origin with her parents' help to escape an abusive marriage and the threat of gang violence. Her husband and his gang had harassed and beaten her parents after her departure. On arrival in Canada, she had become more isolated after two events. First, a leader in her community had stolen her money in a scam offering legal advice. Later, trying to build a network in her community, she confided her rape story to a close woman friend who then shunned her and revealed her confidences to others in the community. One of her sons, born in Canada, had developed symptoms of anorexia and depression with the news of deportation.

(continued)

During the long wait in Canada for determination of her refugee claim, her parents back in Pakistan had died. With the rejection of her claim for asylum, under the tenets of the "Third Country Rule" requiring deportation of refugees to the last country of transit, she would be returned to the site of her rape. This predicament precipitated a decompensation with recurrent flashbacks of her earlier abuse and rape. As a vulnerable single woman in a traditional community, she had been relatively isolated, with few social supports. She had renounced her religious beliefs after the traumatic events in Pakistan. During the first consultation interview, she related her predicament in a shrill, loud and tearful barrage reflecting her intense grief and rage.

Through the consultation exploring her family narrative, she was able to shift her threatening stance to one of calmer reflection. A safety plan was made with her social worker which included efforts to support her humanitarian appeal, limit the amount of antidepressant medication at her disposal to reduce the risk of overdose and provide respite care for her children in summer camp and day care. To further address her suicidal impulses, a narrative intervention was devised that asked her to imagine a conversation with her deceased parents and their responses to her suicide–homicide plans. This shifted her focus to unresolved mourning for the protective space of her lost family. We introduced a mourning ritual to link her with the protective memories of her parents, which had been suspended by the unresolved mourning of their deaths and her inability to be present at their funerals. As she put it, "it is as if they never died in my mind." Through this mourning ritual, she was able to regain a sense of connection with her parents and felt empowered to be able to show her gratitude to them through the rituals of prayer. Though she had been overtly angry with God for her predicament, the ritual offered a way to reconnect and addressed her guilt in renouncing care of her parents by leaving the country, which had left her feeling that "I killed them with worry about us." In the session, her dialogue with the invited "ghosts" of her parents enabled her to mobilize positive parental identifications and experiences of her secure attachment from childhood. The intervention worked with shifts in mentalization processes (Allen, Fonagy, & Bateman, 2008), moving from rage with dissociative states, to a more reflective state.

Her therapist reported that Aaliya's humanitarian appeal was ultimately successful 18 months later, with full remission of her suicidality and successful employment in the community. The success of this case was also based on the consultants' efforts to support the social worker by providing a safe space for Aaliya to work through her distress, offering instrumental help, instituting protective measures for her children, continuing medication, supporting a humanitarian appeal for refugee status and engaging in shared care with the local community clinic.

developmental passages, migration trajectories, uncertainties of citizenship status, racism, cultural conflicts, political upheaval and the broad matrix of what has been termed "social suffering" (Kleinman, Das, & Lock, 1997).

While there are many consultations where cultural aspects are significant or even crucial, there are other cases where they may be given exaggerated importance by the referring clinician or the patient. Though the referring clinician may be focused on discerning the cultural origins of suffering, cumulative trauma or emotional conflicts may be the main obstacles that impair the family's problem-solving capacity or strategies of resilience. At times, simply bearing witness to the patient's narrative in a period of difficulty and distress, such as enduring the uncertainty of refugee status or during a post-traumatic encounter, may be the most beneficial clinical intervention. Of course, whether cultural issues turn out to be

Case Vignette 7-4

Lakshmi, a married pregnant Nepali Hindu woman with two daughters 8 and 5 years old, was referred by a community clinic with "homesickness" and "treatment-resistant depression." Lakshmi had made several suicide attempts resulting in hospital admissions and had been repeatedly interviewed in an unsuccessful search for domestic violence to explain her persistent distress and failure to respond to numerous trials of antidepressant medication. At the CCS, she was seen initially alone with a Nepali Christian interpreter who had accompanied her regularly during 5 years of medical and psychiatric interventions at the community clinic.

On the second CCS visit, Lakshmi was seen only with her husband, as the couple stated that they spoke sufficient English to be seen without the interpreter. Her husband had given up his employment to care for Lakshmi, providing constant suicide watch through most of this third pregnancy. Lakshmi blamed her depression on her psychotic mother-in-law "who should be in your office but will never come." She was clear that she did not ever want to return to war-torn Nepal, as her family there had remained destitute. Since their marriage, her husband (whom she described as devoted and loving) had taken up the duties of an elder Hindu son looking after his unmarried sisters and widowed mother as his brother was banished for marrying a Christian girl. Lakshmi had been a devoted daughter-in-law until an episode when her mother-in-law, who had been exhibiting increasingly "bizarre" behavior, fed her infant daughter cologne to "cool her down" from a fever. Both Lakshmi and her husband agreed that his mother was psychotic,

with paranoid delusions, but the mother refused any psychiatric contact.

The cologne incident had resulted in a marital confrontation and worsening of her suicide behaviors. The interpreter had encouraged Lakshmi's subsequent conversion to Catholicism, Lakshmi began to regularly attend church with the interpreter, though her daughters continued to attend the Hindu temple with their grandmother and father. The interpreter became a key support for the patient, functioning like a sister-in-law, and was triangulated in the marital conflict supporting Lakshmi in defying her mother-in-law. Lakshmi felt this defiance of her mother-in-law would possibly force her husband to choose to live in a nuclear family in order to lessen the open conflict. In the CCS couple consult on the second visit, the consultant had excluded the interpreter and met the couple alone. The session reframed the husband's divided loyalties and devotion to his family, by making an explicit link with the mythic story of Ram, a revered Hindu incarnation of Vishnu in the epic *Ramayana* who was loyal to his widowed mother despite cruel and ill-advised parental behavior as he was taking the role of his father. This reframing suggested that Lakshmi had tried to be a devoted daughter-in-law and wife with a psychotic mother, but now the focus needed to be on her own children and their health. The narrative reframing shifted the focus from her disillusionment and fury at her husband's "choosing [his] mother over me." Lakshmi agreed that her husband was essentially kind to her and tolerant of her Christian faith, but she still felt responsible for his widowed mother and unmarried sisters.

Shortly after the first couple consultation interview, Lakshmi gave birth to a son, and a second CCS consult was requested by the obstetrical ward who noted her distress after the baby's birth. She was no longer suicidal but she remained at risk for

(continued)

postpartum depression. The consultant discussed her concerns about using antidepressants during breastfeeding. Lakshmi had previously taken antidepressants intermittently, had not understood the importance of consistent dosing and reverted to the use of holy water or other traditional remedies. A serious illness of her young daughter and the birth of a son occurred simultaneously and seemed to revive her maternal focus on family wellbeing. The couple was especially elated at having a first son, which culturally validated her stature within the family.

As part of a collaborative care model with the obstetrical and outpatient teams involved, the CCS consultant suggested a visiting nurse program and follow-up by the clinic to monitor the family. The interpreter was offered some supervision by the clinic and her agency to improve the flow of information to the health care team and maintain ethically appropriate boundaries in her practice.

central or peripheral to the patients' problem and its potential solutions, clarifying the cultural context can provide deeper understanding of symptoms or distress.

The community clinic that made the original referral was unaware of the cultural issues of the extended family, the interpreter's complex relationship with Lakshmi, and the boundary crossing that blurred her roles. The interpreter had become a "friend and therapist," and had been both a facilitator of Lakshmi's systemic protest and had promoted Lakshmi's efforts to separate from the enmeshed extended family system. The CCS consultant was able to work with the nurse physician team to help them appreciate the systemic predicament of Lakshmi and her husband, as well as their need for home care nursing for their baby and young daughter. A follow-up report indicated that Lakshmi and her husband had moved to a separate apartment and her depression had resolved. This vignette illustrates

the value of a system approach that includes understanding the cultural explanatory models of the interpreter and treatment teams, as well as family members.

The Familiar and the Unfamiliar: Encountering Cultural Frames in Family Systems

The family therapist seeks an understanding of the family system that identifies repetitive patterns of emotional communication or enactments that are central to family dynamics. Family stories or narratives employ metaphors or idioms of distress that may reference cultural myths and memories including deeply embedded histories of war, indenture or slavery. Accessing these myths and metaphors through a shared narrative may help to build bridges between systemic partners or generations within family systems. By eliciting, bearing witness to, and "holding" a narrative (Sluzki, 1992; White & Epston, 1990), the therapist can consolidate therapeutic alliances with family members. Empathic engagement depends on locating the individual's experience in cultural contexts, which can be understood, validated and integrated in the family assessment and intervention.

For families of refugees or others who have faced violence, bearing witness to a traumatic past during the consultation process sometimes promotes healing, while on other occasions it may be toxic, undermining fragile defences by provoking traumatic re-experiencing. At times exploring the family narrative can promote differentiation of family members and dissolve rigid positions or projections. However, the consultant must weigh the costs and benefits associated with uncovering stories of trauma especially if there is time-limited involvement or a lack of ongoing therapeutic holding.

The structural problems that Minuchin (1974) called "familial disorganization" and Aponte (1994) called "under-organized families," are common in chaotic systems overwhelmed by poverty or intergenerational struggles. In migrant families, these issues may surface along with the burdens of racial alienation, downward socioeconomic mobility, and war, trauma or devastating loss. The therapist enters territory where neutrality must be tempered by engagement with social, political and moral dilemmas before framing interpretations of family realities. Assessment of the family constellation must include everyone the family designates as a member rather than adhering to a narrow or nuclear definition of the family. In addition to extended family and transnational networks, the system may include ancestors or spirits. Recognizing the significance of ghosts, djinns or other spiritual entities in the family drama may require a shift in epistemological stance. As Witzum and Goodman (1999) note, the therapist does not determine the script but gains access to it by "suspending disbelief" to work within the mythic or religious belief systems of the family system. Ignoring these dimensions of family experience or even chastising patients for alien or "superstitious beliefs" is akin to refusing the gift of entry into their belief systems and can limit the opportunity to explore and

---

Case Vignette 7-5

The Wong family was sent by a school counsellor to consult about the suicidal threats of their 16-year-old son. However, Mrs. Wong appeared without her family and son as she wanted to see the consultant alone first, stating "I wasn't sure you would understand my Chinese family." The consultation involved a lengthy meeting with Mrs. Wong alone followed by a single family meeting.

Mrs. Wong was a married Chinese-Canadian woman, with four adolescent and young adult children. She and her husband had fled communist China overcoming many difficult obstacles. They lived together despite an "emotional divorce" for many years, during which time the husband was a good provider but had long hours of absence from the family. Mrs. Wong had dominated domestic decision-making for the family and children. She had converted to Jehovah's Witness after arriving in Canada, distancing herself from toxic

memories of her childhood and youth by religious conversion and avoidance of the local Chinese community. She pursued her religious activities without overt conflict until the arrival of her 90-year-old mother-in-law about 6 months prior to the consultation request. She said she was nervous about her son's suicide threats, which he related to the mother-in-law's presence. She reported that her son complained about his paternal grandmother that "she stinks of Chinese medicine and I hate it… I can't bring my friends here… I am so ashamed of the stink… I'm going to kill myself if you don't get rid of her." Mrs. Wong confided that she also detested her mother-in-law. She acknowledged she wished her mother-in-law was dead and constantly nagged her husband to send the mother-in-law to his elder brother "who should be looking after her." Since Mr. Wong's elder brother's wife had died by suicide in Vancouver, he had been devastated and unable to look after his ageing mother. Mrs. Wong also confided that she had a fear of the "wandering ghost" of her dead sister-in-law who "might take another victim with her." Her worry that the ghost might precipitate her son's suicide had brought the family to the consultation.

When a family meeting was convened, Mr. Wong heard out his children as they complained about his mother. With Mrs. Wong's silent, tacit approval, the children complained that the father's excessive loyalty to the grandmother was "ruining their home." Addressing the therapist rather than his wife, Mr. Wong stated he felt such sorrow in his heart that if he were to tell the depth of his pain, he would never rise from his chair. This metaphorical expression conveyed Mr. Wong's suffering, rage and shame at the impasse with his wife and children. The family meeting provided a place both to hear the family's anguish and reinforce father's position as the elder of the home with the authority to make a decision on his mother's care. The reflective space

(continued)

allowed the children to "hear" their father's pain and reframe his choices as the honorable duty of a Chinese son. The consultation supported the bicultural individuation of the children. Though the marital impasse was never directly addressed, the father's role in deciding about his mother's care was reinforced. The ghost of the sister-in-law reminded the family of the risks of continued escalation of the family conflict. Narrative and storytelling were used to bear witness with the mother in an individual session and to promote empathy and differentiate the family member's concerns during the family session.

The individual meeting with Mrs. Wong allowed the consultant to obtain the initial history, acknowledge her traumatic story, identify the "ghost" of the sister-in-law's suicide and reveal her mother-in-law's arrival as a disturbance of family homeostasis. The family meeting clarified the son's identification with the mother's distress. After this meeting, Mrs. Wong turned to her religious community for ongoing support, although her husband disapproved of her conversion, maintaining their emotional distance. The adolescent son was seen by his school counsellor who worked on his emotional separation and de-triangulation from the impasse in his parent's marriage. Mr. Wong decided to arrange for his mother to leave the home and move to another sibling's care. Mrs. Wong had endured considerable trauma and was only able to reconstitute her sense of identity by her religious conversion and participation in the Jehovah's Witness community, which embraced her and helped her to contain her traumatic memories by allowing her to avoid contact with her extended family and the local Chinese community. In addition, the integration of the cultural explanatory models related to suicide and unsettling family ghost stories put pressure on the parents to resolve the tensions which could

lead to the son's acting out of his suicide threat. His identification of the "strange smells" of his grandmother as toxic to the family was a useful metaphor for the generational conflicts triangulating children and elders, and the challenges of autonomy as his siblings and mother resolved to build identities outside traditional Chinese cultural norms.

elucidate traumatic, depressive or psychotic processes. The voices of magical beings or the metaphors based on these experiences may provide a crucial path to understanding the underlying dynamics of the family system (Guzder, 2007; Kakar, 1982).

Culture as Camouflage

For some families, attributing problems to cultural difference can serve as a way to avoid addressing areas of emotional conflict in relationships. Friedman (1982) suggested the term "cultural camouflage" to describe the failure to appreciate how emotional processes are at times masked by references to culture rather than determined by culture processes, enabling family members to blame their own background or those of others as the source of their discontent or inability to change. Cultural camouflage may allow family members to avoid taking personal responsibility for their own points of view. A focus on cultural issues by the therapist may engage the family in interminable discussions of background factors rather than uncovering core emotional issues and working towards meaningful changes in family

Case Vignette 7-6

Amina, a 42-year-old Middle Eastern woman with a well-documented 14-year history of schizophrenia, was referred to the CCS by her community clinic therapist.

(continued)

The therapist had requested the consultation around a question "Is there anything else I can do for this woman?" when she became aware that the husband planned to send Amina without her children back to her natal village. The therapist sympathized with the husband, who she described as a kind man burdened with the care of his four children and a psychotic wife. During Amina's long-term care and numerous hospital admissions for psychosis (some following miscarriages), professionals had never used interpreters as the husband had always spoken for her.

Amina arrived for the CCS interview accompanied by her community clinic therapist with her husband and three of her younger children, two sons aged 9 and 8 and a daughter aged 4 (who was not yet speaking). Her husband complained she was always restless and agitated, seldom did any housework, never went out to get groceries, left the home in filthy disarray, and neglected the children.

Addressed in her own language by the consultant, Amina stated she was ashamed to go out looking so unkempt and bring further shame to her children especially because her eldest 13-year-old son was so angry and abusive to her. He often said "I am embarrassed by you... I hate having a crazy mother like you."

The children were under a Youth Protection mandate originally because of concerns that they were being neglected. However, the Youth Protection worker rarely checked in since the 6-month assessment noted that "everything was stable and the father was seen to have good parenting capacity." When the older boy was expelled from his school a few months earlier, he was sent to an alternative school but was frequently truant. He had apparently joined a street gang and at times carried a knife, according to his younger brothers, and would wander the streets at night. None of these details were known to the father or the referring therapist prior to the consultation meeting.

When asked about the children's dirty clothes that smelled of urine, the father simply shrugged and said it was his wife's responsibility. It became clear that the father was seldom home because he had a young mistress and a new 18-month-old son. The mistress visited the household often and the children valued her presence because she was able to help them with their homework.

The father had arranged with Amina's brother (an immigrant in Australia) for Amina to be sent to live with her 90-year-old mother in their village. When asked what she felt about this plan, Amina begged not be separated from her children and asked if the CCS consultant could help her obtain a passport as "I don't want to be dumped in the village." She said that she did not mind if her husband took a second wife, but did not want to leave Canada.

The therapist privately shared with the consultant that she had read about "this culture which has no boundaries and lives in enmeshed systems... in an undifferentiated extended family." She was surprised that the mother had asserted her parental rights in the interview and requested a passport. She began to understand that her misinterpretation of descriptions of cultural norms had led her to dismiss clear evidence of neglect, absent parental authority, and to collude with the father's exclusion of the mother's voice in family decisions or health issues.

The cultural consultation focused on the need for interpreter services to assess the patient rather than using the father. The consultant explored the possibility that the therapist could help her obtain a passport, reinforcing the alliance with the clinic to assist her. The consultant diagnosed akathisia from excessive antipsychotic medication, which was reduced to treat the restlessness. Daycare arrangements and

(continued)

speech evaluation were arranged for the 4-year-old child with delays from under-stimulation and neglect. The Youth Protection had not been monitoring the family and had missed the conduct disorder of the 13-year-old boy, as well as the frequent absence of the father who was usually with his mistress and other child. The silencing of the patient was a kind of structural violence by both institutional and gendered hierarchies of the family, complicating the subaltern position of this immigrant mother with schizophrenia.

The therapist's formulation had been based on normalizing serious family dysfunction using cultural stereotypes. By evaluating family life in terms of these distorted norms, she had missed a more balanced view of the family's needs and issues. The CCS consultant found the clinic therapist open to revising her cultural stereotyping and misunderstanding of cultural boundaries and child-rearing norms in South Asia. She was also able to construct a new vision of her relationship with the patient who viewed her as an educated white professional who could understand the institutional context that had so disempowered her for years and speak out on her behalf.

functioning. Recognizing the potential for cultural camouflage allows us to consider whether specific cultural issues are important as mechanism of suffering, healing or resistance. Of course, both the clinician and the patient may engage in using culture as camouflage.

Cultural camouflage may be especially difficult to address when it involves cultural stereotypes and is embedded in institutional practices of cultural competence, as illustrated by Amina's case, or reflects issues of racism as seen in the following case of Shakeel. Understanding the unique migration histories and acculturation stresses of each member of the family are keys to uncovering the object relations and current cultural frames of reference that shape the family system and its interactions with host society institutions. Visible minority families, especially black families, frequently have suffered the impact of institutional racism, and culturally safe settings and methods of evaluation are essential to explore

Case Vignette 7-7

A cultural consultation was requested by a social worker for Shakeel, a 10-year-old Jamaican Canadian boy who had been expelled from school after attacking his principal and teacher. His social worker, also of Caribbean origin, formulated the problem as racism of the school personnel. The consultant met initially with the mother and son, and later with the network of social worker, community clinic, school and family including the maternal grandmother.

Shakeel had been born in Canada and raised by his single mother though she had sent him back to Jamaica from age two to four when she had been depressed and unable to cope with his hyperactivity. Shakeel's father had been absent since his birth, deported from Canada back to Jamaica for criminal activity. Though mother said he was rehabilitated, working, remarried and had younger children, grandmother maintained he was "bad news." Shakeel was very upset that his mother was now considering sending him back to his father in Jamaica. She felt he had been acting "like his father" so that he needed "to learn the hard way." Mother was also upset that Shakeel had been increasingly rude to her father fuelled by his grandmother's stories of their hostile divorce. Shakeel's mother had previously been estranged from her own mother until this family crisis, and she had relied on her father to parent Shakeel.

Shakeel was very bright and no sign of attention deficit or learning problems. He had difficulty accepting the authority of his mother after their family reunification at

(continued)

age four. Just prior to the CCS consultation meeting, he had an altercation with his mother which ended with police involvement and an emergency placement with his maternal grandmother. On exploring the family history, it emerged that Shakeel's mother had been abused by one of her brothers, who was favored by her mother. Shakeel's violent temper reminded her of this and other traumatic, abusive male relationships in her life. She had not recognized the attachment disruption as a factor in their parent–child relationship or Shakeel's intense "father hunger" and feelings of loss because of his father's absence; nor did she appreciate the impact on Shakeel of his father's history of criminality and her own depression.

underlying attachment issues or other psychodynamic issues (Boyd-Franklin, 2003; Fernando, 1991; Kareem, 1992; Krause, 2002; Whaley, 2011).

Shakeel's attacks on authority at school were initially framed as racism, externalizing complex family issues. In response to the CCS consultation, the social worker agreed that rather than projecting blame on the school, a more useful therapeutic plan for Shakeel would include working on limits, empowering his mother, fostering family attachments and securing his family life. After the consultation, the social worker who had much experience with difficult reunification issues in Caribbean families (Lashley, 2000; Rousseau, Hassan, et al. 2008; see also Chapter 13) began to recognize dysfunctional parent–child patterns rooted in disruptions of attachment across generations that could be addressed by strengthening the mother–son relationship, including re-establishing an appropriate generational hierarchy.

Building Bridges with Systems

Establishing a therapeutic alliance by joining the system remains the basic strategy for creating a safe space for working with families (Minuchin, 1974). This process of joining is complicated in cultural consultation not only because the referral may involve a complex pathway with multiple individuals and institutions involved but also because patients may have had experiences that make them mistrustful of health care providers, institutions or authorities. The routes of the referral process may have a significant impact on patients' comfort with the consultation process and with their view of the consultant and others involved, including the interpreter or culture broker. Patients may have developed issues of mistrust based on experiences of stigma, discrimination or marginalization. Systemic issues often determine the help-seeking behavior of patients and are inherent in negotiations with the patient to arrive at appropriate and acceptable interventions. Problems of institutional power and processes of labelling and exclusion may complicate the initial alliance.

Case Vignette 7-8

A Youth Protection worker asked for a single visit consultation for a 16-year-old Asian origin Muslim Canadian boy, Mehran, who was currently in placement. The worker was uncomfortable with Islamic cultural issues and unsure whether she could return Mehran to his family. Upon learning that he was found drunk at school, his father had slapped Mehran on the face cutting his lip, and his mother had hit him with a slipper leading to the involvement of Youth Protection after Mehran disclosed the incident at school.

Mehran and his youth worker came to the CCS interview along with his polite, articulate Bengali-speaking parents and 10-year-old brother. Mehran had been complaining for some months to his teachers about the high expectations of his parents, their traditional values, strict curfews at home, and especially his parents' disapproval of his wish to get a summer job or a cellphone. The parents explained that on

(continued)

learning of his provocative drinking behavior which violated Muslim tradition, both had slapped him, though previously they had never struck him. They were clearly devoted, highly educated parents and were devastated when both boys were immediately taken out of their home and placed. The school staff, on the other hand, had seldom met the parents and had built up an image of oppressive Islamic parents obstructing their son's potential for successful acculturation.

The youth worker admonished the parents for restricting Mehran's activity, though the parents lived in a neighborhood with rampant drug and gang activity. Father operated a business where he had watched the youth gangs in action on the streets. The worker reminded the parents that Quebec law allows 14-year-old youth the right to have abortion and to control many personal decisions and said that Mehran could chose permanent placement if his father did not relent and allow him to take a summer job. The father was outraged and declared this was a kind of blackmail, which he found racist. However, he was silenced by the threat of losing his son, while the mother looked on sadly. Mehran sat between his parents and complained that it was more difficult to negotiate his autonomy at home than for his Québecois peers with whom he identified. It appeared that he was closer to his mother and identified with her. She too was now negotiating more mobility in her adopted country and going to college with the support of his father, while Mehran's activity remained chaperoned and restricted. Both parents agreed they wanted Mehran home and wanted him to do well in school.

The CCS process was directed towards helping the youth worker to understand the collision of cultural values and Mehran's use of provocative behaviors to undermine parental authority and values. The parents felt the consultant gave them an empathic listening space and broadened their bicultural frame to understand Mehran's frustrations. The youth worker felt that she had minimized the health of the family system and reframed his behavior as adolescent provocation. She engaged a male colleague to work with his conduct and negotiation of autonomy within the family, recognizing that father-son issues were central to improving the home situation. Mehran quickly returned home and the worker supported the parents in contracting with him around autonomy issues.

In this case, the CCS consultant highlighted both the family's cultural transitions and their strengths in transmitting traditional values (Pillai et al., 2008). The family was able to work with the social service system to navigate Mehran's bicultural reality. The fact that the youth worker, a woman, held the institutional power in this situation posed additional difficulties for this patriarchal system. The potentially divisive and destructive shaming of the patriarch was averted by engaging a male worker for the family. Giving the couple a culturally safe place for discussion, and employing narrative therapy approaches with an interpreter present, allowed the parents to move towards a more flexible and creative problem solving, restructuring the family's approach to autonomy for their adolescent while respecting the realities of living in a high-risk neighborhood.

Ethno-racial minorities are often challenged by differences in child-rearing practices and the role of child protection services (reviewed in Chapter 13). South Asians, for example, may resist or mistrust child mental health or protective services or alternately express disappointment on the lack of such supports in their country of origin (Maiter & Stalker, 2011; Maiter, Stalker, & Alaggia, 2009). These responses must also be understood in systemic terms.

Case Vignette 7-9

Naz was a 17-year-old Pakistani Muslim adolescent who was referred by her school counsellor without her parents' knowledge. She had been seeing the counsellor for some months because of significant conflicts with her mother and looked on the counsellor as a kind father figure. She felt that her own father had been more loving than her mother, though there had been a long period of paternal absence from age 7 to 14 when he had come to Canada to establish landed immigrant status and find employment. She felt her mother was very envious of her father's affection towards her.

Although Naz was a good student, as the eldest daughter she carried a heavy burden of household responsibilities. She felt her mother was irritable and depressed having lost the warm surroundings of a familiar culture space, with servants and extended family, to land in the "deep freeze" of an isolated Montreal suburb. Mother had pressured Naz's father to marry Naz to a cousin in Pakistan on her graduation from high school. Naz had met this cousin once and was accepting of the arranged marriage. However, she wished to continue her education and she wanted to have his agreement on this condition.

The counsellor was very concerned about the human rights issue of forced marriages that seemed increasingly common in his South Asian Canadian adolescent caseload. He advised Naz that he would like to signal Youth Protection on her behalf as she had once reported that her mother had slapped her on the face over delays in doing housework. Naz was very upset by this suggestion, denying that she was being abused and said that his intervention would cause a terrible furor at home. She did not want to go into placement, nor would she consider independent living which "would break my family ties forever." The CCS consultant decided to inform Naz of her rights, offering to intervene with her family and informing her of the option of "independent living" arranged by social services. Naz, however, was adamant that she was close to her family and preferred to stay with them and negotiate an education after marriage by having her maternal aunts lobby on her behalf within the closed system of the extended family. She appreciated the neutral space of the therapy as a place to reflect on her life and options but did not want the counsellor to break her confidence. The counsellor felt anguished about her choice. Consistent with his perception of Canadian values, he perceived her as culturally oppressed by arranged marriage and patriarchy and he wanted to support her autonomy. The consultation process acknowledged the dissonance of cultural values and assumptions between therapist and patient then shifted to work with the counsellor focusing on the moral, cultural and ethical issues around his choice of Youth Protection versus confidential dialogue with this adolescent client. It remained difficult for him to accept Naz's insistence that her attachments within the extended families were protective factors while her maternal relationship was clearly troubled. The counsellor correctly was trying to distinguish between issues of forced marriage and arranged marriage, especially as he had been sensitized by recent incidents in Quebec of honor killings, which had been widely reported in the media.

The central role of schools and other community resources offering support to immigrants, increasingly raises complex issues of institutional, social and collective stereotyping (Rousseau & Guzder, 2008). The CCS consultant can operate in these cases as a supervisor, mediator and culture broker to create a safe space where teachers and professionals can look at some of the ethical, legal, systemic and psychodynamic issues that arise in intercultural encounters. As in other Western countries, children over fourteen in Quebec have rights for self advocacy and autonomy that are vastly different from many migrant families' cultures of origin. Negotiation of autonomy is complicated by legal, social and institutional norms and rules, as well as the fears and expectations that professionals and families bring as a result of stereotypes. In this case, the counsellor saw Naz as the victim of an oppressive system who needed his help to achieve emancipation. However, Naz insisted she was not a brown woman oppressed by her father but a person with considerable agency who simply needed a safe place to reflect on her dilemmas and work out strategies that would maintain crucial family ties and cultural values. Western psychotherapies and even social work have tended to put more emphasis on autonomy than belonging (Falck, 1988). Finding ways to help patients negotiate an adaptive balance between autonomy and interdependence requires careful exploration of the systemic dynamics of power, silencing, and culture change (Jack & Ali, 2010; Spivak, 2006). The aim is to support patients' voice and agency while respecting their need and desire to live life in and through family and community. The gaze of the dominant culture and the dissonances of cultural value systems are challenging for both therapist and client in this process. In most cases, the strain of acculturation can be resolved with the adoption of functional bicultural or hybrid identities. However, in some cases, these bicultural strains may increase the risk of domestic violence, child abuse or honour killing and require careful family and systemic assessment and intervention (Guzder & Krishna, 2005).

Conclusion

The cultural consultation model aims to provide a wider clinical lens to understand clinical problems in social and family context. Our clinical encounters with families and individuals help to reveal systemic processes. The consultant joins with the system to understand its dynamics but also to create a reflective space where family members can explore their diverse perspectives, strategies for problem solving, and sources of wellbeing. The consultation process works towards the co-construction of meaning across multiple frames of reference among participants in the clinical system, including family members, health and social services professionals, teachers and others actors implicated in the patient's problems. The consultation facilitates knowledge transfer to other mental health practitioners by linking cultural issues to more familiar systemic approaches. The focus in consultation is simultaneously on the patient and the therapist interacting with otherness—within themselves, with each other and in relation to larger social institutions and cultural frames. Cultural aspects of family and systemic processes provide the context of meaning that illuminates symptoms and behaviors pointing towards new possibilities for meaningful coherence and adaptive change.

Migration often necessitates the redrawing of family maps as families adapt to new places, spaces and contexts. The family's encounters with powerful institutional and political exigencies shape the interactional and emotional processes that generate or resolve distress in the system. Cultural consultation follows the lead of these affective and interactional processes to enter and engage or join with the family, while charting elements of the family's cultural maps to allow for the translation and reframing of symptoms and problems with the input of referring clinicians.

The consultant aims to engage families and therapists, bearing witness to their predicaments and distress and co-constructing narratives that can foster their resilience and assist them in problem solving, consensus building and finding ways to bridge the worlds of their origins and of their current challenges. Family therapy provides many tools to engage with systemic issues in vital dialogues that enrich the cultural consultation process. Though every culture has its own patterns, coherence, rules and structures, the flexibility of cultural paradigms and cultural imagination is often our best ally in achieving the goal of strengthening families and clinical alliances. In addition to exploring the central issues of each family, cultural consultation also engages with the therapists' own cultural background and the cultural assumptions that lie behind institutional practices to seek the most beneficial alternatives in intervention planning. Systemic thinking derived from family theory and therapy also can be applied to the dynamics of interactions within the clinical encounter itself. Understanding the systems of family, community, health care providers and institutions as well as local and transnational networks can lead to diagnostic revisions, shifts of clinical strategy or new solutions that might not be evident with an exclusive focus on the individual.

References

Adams, M. V. (1996). *The multicultural imagination: "Race", color, and the unconscious*. London, England: Routledge.

Akhtar, S. (1995). A third individuation: Immigration, identity, and the psychoanalytic process. *Journal of the American Psychoanalytic Association, 43*(4), 1051–1084.

Akhtar, S. (2000). *Freud along the Ganges*. New York, NY: Other Press.

Allen, J. G., Fonagy, P., & Bateman, A. W. (Eds.). (2008). *Mentalization in clinical practice*. Washington, DC: American Psychiatric Publishing.

Altman, N. (2006). Whiteness. *Psychoanalytic Quarterly, 75*(1), 45–72.

Andolfi, M., Angelo, C., & Menghi, P. (1983). *Behind the family mask: Therapeutic change in rigid family systems*. New York, NY: Brunner-Mazel.

Angus, L., & Macleod, J. (2004). *The handbook of narrative and psychotherapy: Practice, theory and research*. London, England: Sage.

Aponte, H. J. (1994). *Bread and spirit: Diversity of race, culture and values*. New York, NY: W.W. Norton.

Bateson, G. (1972). *Steps to an ecology of mind*. New York, NY: Ballantyne.

Bateson, G., Jackson, D. D., & Haley, J. (1956). Toward a theory of schizophrenia. *Behavioural Science, 1*, 251–264.

Bograd, M. (1999). Strengthening domestic violence theories: Intersections of race, class, sexual orientation and gender. *Journal of Martial and Family Therapy, 25*(3), 275–289.

Boscolo, L., & Bertrando, P. (1996). *Systemic therapy with individuals*. London, England: Karnac Books.

Bowen, M. (1978). *Family therapy in clinical practice*. New York, NY: Jason Aronson.

Boyd-Franklin, N. (2003). *Black families in therapy* (2nd ed.). New York, NY: Guilford.

Catherall, D. R., & Pinsof, W. M. (1987). The impact of the therapist's personal family life on the ability to establish viable therapeutic alliance in family and marital therapy. *Journal of Psychotherapy and the Family, 3*(2), 135–160.

Cohen, C. I., & Timimi, S. (Eds.). (2008). *Liberatory psychiatry: Philosophy, politics and mental health*. Cambridge, England: Cambridge University Press.

Dalal, F. (2006). Racism: Processes of detachment, dehumanization and hatred. *Journal of the American Psychoanalytic Association, 75*(1), 131–162.

Dejong, P., & Berg, I. (1998). *Interviewing for solutions*. Pacific Grove, CA: Brooks/Cole.

Devereux, G. (1970). *Essais d'ethnopsychiatrie générale*. Paris, France: Gallimard.

Devereux, G. (1978). *Ethnopsychoanalysis: Psychoanalysis and anthropology as complementary frames of reference*. Berkley, CA: University of California.

DiNicola, V. F. (1985a). Family therapy and transcultural psychiatry: An emerging synthesis. Part I: The conceptual basis. *Transcultural Psychiatric Research Review, 22*(2), 81–113.

DiNicola, V. F. (1985b). Family therapy and transcultural psychiatry: An emerging synthesis. Part II: Portability and culture change. *Transcultural Psychiatric Research Review, 22*(3), 151–179.

DiNicola, V. F. (1997). *A stranger in the family: Culture, families and therapy*. New York, NY: W.W. Norton.

Doi, T. (1973). *The anatomy of dependence*. Tokyo, Japan: Kodansha International.

Epstein, N. B., Bishop, D. S., & Levin, S. (1980). The McMaster model of family functioning. In J. G. Howells (Ed.), *Advances in family psychiatry* (pp. 73–89). New York, NY: International Universities Press.

Falck, H. S. (1988). *Social work: The membership perspective*. New York, NY: Springer Publishing Company.

Falicov, C. J. (1983). *Cultural perspectives in family therapy*. Rockville, MD: Aspen.

Fernando, S. (1991). *Mental health, race and culture*. London, England: MacMillan.

Freedman, J., & Coombs, G. (1996). *Narrative therapy: The social construction of preferred realities*. New York, NY: Norton.

Friedman, E. H. (1982). The myth of the shiksha. In M. McGoldrick, J. K. Pearce, & J. Giordano (Eds.), *Ethnicity and family therapy*. New York, NY: Guilford Press.

Green, R. J., & Framo, J. L. (1981). *Family therapy: Major contributions*. New York, NY: Internatonal Universities Press.

Greenberg, D., & Witzum, E. (2001). *Sanity and sanctity*. New Haven, CT: Yale University.

Greene, K., & Bogo, M. (2002). The different faces of intimate violence: Implications for assessment and treatment. *Journal of Marital and Family Therapy, 28*(4), 155–166.

Guzder, J. (2007). Fourteen djinns travel across the oceans. In B. Drozdek & J. Wilson (Eds.), *Voices of trauma*. New York, NY: Springer.

Guzder, J. (2011). Second skins: Family therapy agendas of migration, identity and cultural change. *Fokus: Pa Familien, 39*(3), 160–179.

Guzder, J., & Krishna, M. (2005). Sita-Shakti@cultural collision: Issues in the psychotherapy of diaspora Indian women. In S. Akhtar (Ed.), *Freud along the Ganges: Psychoanalytic reflections on the people and culture of India* (pp. 205–233). New York, NY: Other Press.

Haley, J. (1976a). *Leaving home*. New York, NY: Mcgraw-Hill.

Haley, J. (1976b). *Problem solving therapy*. New York, NY: Harper & Row.

Hare-Mustin, R. (1987). The problem of gender in family therapy theory. *Family Process, 26*(1), 15–27.

Hays, P. (1996). Addressing the complexities of culture and gender in counselling. *Journal of Counselling and Development, 74*(4), 332–338.

Hays, P. A. (2008). *Addressing cultural complexities in practice: Assessment, diagnosis and therapy* (2nd ed.). Washington, DC: American Psychological Association.

Hickling, F. W. (Ed.). (2005). *Images of psychiatry: The Caribbean*. Kingston, Jamaica: Stephenson.

Hoffman, L. (1981). *Foundations of family therapy: A conceptual framework for systems change*. New York, NY: Basic Books.

Jack, D. C., & Ali, A. (Eds.). (2010). *Silencing the self across cultures: Depression and gender in the social world*. Oxford, England: Oxford University Press.

James, C. (1996). Introduction: Proposing an anti-racism framework for change. In C. James (Ed.), *Perspectives on racism and the human services sector: A case for change*. Toronto, Ontario, Canada: University of Toronto Press.

Jasser, S. A. (2008). Islam and family structure. In S. Akhtar (Ed.), *The crescent and the couch*. New York, NY: Jason Aronson.

Kakar, S. (1978). *The inner world*. Delhi, India: Oxford University.

Kakar, S. (1982). *Shamans, mystics and doctors*. Delhi, India: Oxford University.

Kareem, J. (1978). Conflicting concepts of mental health in a multicultural society. *Psychiatrica Clinica, 11*, 90–95.

Kareem, J. (1988). Outside in–inside out: Some considerations in inter-cultural therapy. *Journal of Social Work Practice, 3*(3), 57–77.

Kareem, J. (1992). The Nafsiyat intercultural therapy centre: Ideas and experience in intercultural therapy. In J. Kareem & R. Littlewood (Eds.), *Intercultural therapy: Themes, interpretations and practice* (pp. 14–37). Oxford, England: Blackwell Scientific.

Kaslow, F. W. (Ed.). (1987). *The family life of psychotherapists: Clinical implications*. New York, NY: Hawthorne Press.

Kidron, C. A. (2012). Alterity and the particular limits of universalism: Comparing Jewish-Israeli and Canadian-Cambodian genocide legacies. *Current Anthropology, 53*(6), 723–754.

Killian, K. D. (2001). Reconstituting racial histories and identities: The narratives of interracial couples. *Journal of Marital and Family Therapy, 1*, 27–42.

Kirmayer, L. J. (2007). Psychotherapy and the cultural concept of the person. *Transcultural Psychiatry, 44*(2), 232–257.

Kirmayer, L. J., Fung, K., Rousseau, C., Lo, H. T., Menzies, P., Guzder, J., et al. (2012). Guidelines for training in cultural psychiatry. *Canadian Journal of Psychiatry, 57*(3), Insert 1–16.

Kirmayer, L. J., Sedhev, M., Whitley, R., Dandeneau, S., & Isaac, C. (2009). Community resilience: Models, metaphors and measures. *Journal of Aboriginal Health, 7*(1), 62–117.

Kleinman, A. (1988). *Rethinking psychiatry*. New York, NY: Free Press.

Kleinman, A., Das, V., & Lock, M. (Eds.). (1997). *Social suffering*. Berkeley, CA: University of California Press.

Knitzer, J. (1982). *Unclaimed children: The failure of public responsibility to children and adolescents in need of mental health services*. Washington, DC: Georgetown University Child Development Center. CASSP Technical Assistance Center.

Kogan, S. M., & Gale, J. E. (2004). Decentering therapy: Textual analysis of a narrative therapy session. *Family Process, 36*, 101–126.

Krause, I. B. (2002). *Culture and system in family therapy*. London, England: Karnac Books.

LaPlanche, J., & Pontalis, J.-B. (1973). *The language of psychoanalysis*. London, England: Karnac.

Lashley, M. (2000). The unrecognized social stressors of migration and reunification in Caribbean families. *Transcultural Psychiatry, 37*(2), 201–216.

Lewis-Fernandez, R. (1996). Cultural formulation of psychiatric diagnosis. *Culture, Medicine and Psychiatry, 20*, 133–144.

Macpherson, W. (1999). *The Stephen Lawrence inquiry*. London, England: Home Department.

Maiter, S., & Stalker, C. (2011). South Asian immigrants' experience of child protective services: Are we recognizing strengths and resilience? *Child and Family Social Work, 16*(2), 138–148.

Maiter, S., Stalker, C., & Alaggia, R. (2009). The experiences of minority immigrant families receiving child welfare services: Seeking to understand how to reduce risk and increase protective factors. *Families in Society, 90*(1), 28–36.

McGoldrick, M. (1998). *Re-visioning family therapy: Race, culture and gender in clinical practice*. New York, NY: Guilford Press.

McGoldrick, M., Pearce, J. K., & Giordano, J. (Eds.). (1982). *Ethnicity and family therapy*. New York, NY: Guilford Press.

Minuchin, S. (1974). *Families and family therapy*. Cambridge, England: Harvard University Press.

Minuchin, S., & Fishman, C. (1981). *Family therapy techniques*. Cambridge, England: Harvard University Press.

Neill, J. R., & Kniskern, D. P. (1982). *From psyche to system: The evolving therapy of Carl Whitaker*. New York, NY: Guilford Press.

Nichols, M. P., & Schwartz, R. C. (2006). *Family therapy: Concepts and methods* (7th ed.). Boston, MA: Pearson Education.

Obeyesekere, G. (1990). *The work of culture: Symbolic transformations in pychoanalysis and anthropology*. Chicago, IL: University of Chicago Press.

Parry, A., & Doan, R. E. (1994). *Story revisions: Narrative therapy in the postmodern world*. New York, NY: Guilford Press.

Perelberg, R. J. (2000). Familiar and unfamiliar types of family structure: Towards a conceptual framework. In J. Kareem & R. Littlewood (Eds.), *Intercultural therapy* (2nd ed.). London, England: Blackwell Science.

Pillai, A., Patel, V., Cardozo, P., Goodman, R., Weiss, H. A., & Andrew, G. (2008). Non-traditional lifestyles and prevalence of mental disorders in adolescents in Goa, India. *The British Journal of Psychiatry, 192*(1), 45–51.

Roland, A. (1988). *In search of self in India and Japan: Toward a cross-cultural psychology*. Princeton, NJ: Princeton University Press.

Roland, A. (2007). The uses (and misuses) of psychoanalysis in South Asian studies: Mysticism and child development. In K. Ramaswany, A. DeNicolas, & A. Banerjee (Eds.), *Invading the sacred*. Delhi, India: Rupa. Appendix 1.

Rousseau, C., & Guzder, J. (2008). School-based prevention programs for refugee children. *Child and Adolescent Psychiatric Clinics of North America, 17*, 533–549.

Rousseau, C., Hassan, G., Measham, T., & Lashley, M. (2008). Prevalence and correlates of conduct disorder and problem behavior in Caribbean and Filipino immigrant adolescents. *European Child & Adolescent Psychiatry, 17*(5), 264–273.

Ruiz-Casares, M., Guzder, J., Rousseau, C., & Kirmayer, L. J. (2013). Cultural roots of well-being and resilience in child mental health. In A. Ben Arieh, I. Frones, F. Casas, & J. Korbin (Eds.), *Handbook of child well-being*. New York, NY: Springer.

Satzewich, V. (2011). *Racism in Canada*. Don Mills, Toronto, Canada: Oxford University Press.

Selvini, M. P., Boscolo, L., Cecchin, G., & Prata, G. (1978). *Paradox and counterparadox*. New York, NY: Jason Aronson.

Selvini, M. P., Boscolo, L., Cecchin, G., & Prata, G. (1980). Hypothesizing-circularity-neutrality: Three guidelines for the conductor of the session. *Family Process, 19*(1), 3–12.

Selvini, M., & Weber, G. (Eds.). (1988). *The work of Maria Selvini Palazzoli*. London, England: Jason Aronson.

Sluzki, C. E. (1992). Transformations: A blueprint for narrative changes in therapy. *Family Process, 31*(3), 217–230.

Spivak, G. C. (2006). *In other worlds: Essays on cultural politics*. New York, NY: Routledge.

Sterlin, H. (1989). *Unlocking the family door*. New York, NY: Brunner-Mazel.

Sue, D. W., & Sue, D. (1999). *Counselling the culturally different: Theory and practice* (3rd ed.). New York, NY: John Wiley.

Tomm, K. (1985). Circular interviewing: A multifaceted clinical tool. In D. Campbell & R. Draper (Eds.), *Applications of systemic therapy: The Milan approach*. London, England: Grune & Stratton.

Tomm, K. (1989). Externalizing the problem and internalizing personal agency. *Journal of Strategic and Systemic Therapies, 8*(1), 54–59.

Turner, W. L., & Wieling, E. (2004). Developing culturally effective family-based research programs: Implications for family therapists. *Journal of Marital and Family Therapy, 30*(3), 257–270.

Watzlawick, P., & Weakland, J. H. (Eds.). (1977). *The interactional view: Studies at the mental research institute, Palo Alto, 1965–1974*. New York, NY: Norton.

Watzlawick, P., Weakland, J. H., & Fisch, R. (2011). *Change: Principles of problem formation and problem resolution*. New York, NY: W.W. Norton.

Whaley, A. L. (2011). Clinicians' competence in assessing cultural mistrust amongst African American psychiatric patients. *Journal of Black Psychology, 37*(4), 387–406.

White, M., & Epston, D. (1990). *Narrative means to therapeutic ends*. New York, NY: W. W. Norton.

Witzum, E., & Goodman, Y. (1999). Narrative construction of distress and therapy: A model based on work with ultra-orthodox Jews. *Transcultural Psychiatry, 36*(4), 403–436.

Wynne, L. C., McDaniel, S. H., & Weber, T. T. (1986). *Systems consultations: A new perspective for family therapy*. New York, NY: Guilford Press.

Gender, Power and Ethnicity in Cultural Consultation

8

Jaswant Guzder, Radhika Santhanam-Martin, and Cécile Rousseau

The young women with amber skin, hair and brows of black
as crows' wings, eyes of lionesses in heat,
dressed in silks of delirious hues...
they wander through foreign rooms in the last daylight of the century
painting their eyes...
somewhere out of them, alive or dead I have sprung
yet no one seems to recognize me.

From: "Ancestors" by Rishma Dunlop (2004, p. 31)

Introduction

Gender, power and ethnicity are universal factors in structuring clinical work, influencing the therapeutic alliance, transference, countertransference

J. Guzder, M.D. (✉)
Center for Child Development and Mental Health,
Institute of Community and Family Psychiatry,
4335 Cote St. Catherine Road, Montreal, QC,
Canada H3T 1E4
e-mail: jaswant@videotron.ca

R. Santhanam-Martin, Ph.D.
Victorian Transcultural Psychiatry Unit, Level 2,
Bolte Wing, St. Vincent's Hospital, Nicholson Street,
Fitzroy, VIC 3065, Australia
e-mail: radhisanthanam@gmail.com

C. Rousseau, M.D., M.Sc.
Centre de recherche et de formation, CSSS de la
Montagne, 7085 Hutchison, Local 204.2, Montréal,
QC, Canada H3N 1Y9
e-mail: cecile.rousseau@mcgill.ca

and the processes of assessment and intervention. In any clinical encounter, the identity of the clinician influences the process, but these issues are thrown into relief when the clinician comes from a visible minority or racialized group (Fernando, 1991; Pinderhughes, 1989; Tummala-Narra, 2004, 2005). While clinicians' personal backgrounds, including the dynamics of their family of origin, are always relevant in clinical work (Catherall & Pinsof, 1987), this dimension is especially important for consultants from minority backgrounds, whether working individually or as members of multicultural teams.

To illustrate the interplay of gender, power and ethnocultural identities in clinical work, this chapter will present CCS cases seen by two South Asian origin consultants and a French-Québecois child psychiatrist (CR) trained in Canada with extensive South American and European experience. The South Asian therapists were a third-generation Indian origin, Canadian-trained

L.J. Kirmayer et al. (eds.), *Cultural Consultation: Encountering the Other in Mental Health Care*, International and Cultural Psychology, DOI 10.1007/978-1-4614-7615-3_8, © Springer Science+Business Media New York 2014

child psychiatrist (JG) with clinical experience in Canada and India and a first-generation immigrant to Australia (RSM), with training and clinical experience in India, Australia and Canada as a child and family clinical psychologist. The cases we present were chosen because they show how the ethnicity and gender of the minority clinician can evoke a range of systemic, cultural and dynamic issues in work with a heterogeneous South Asian clinical population. In addition to the consultants' reflections, these issues were further analyzed and discussed at the weekly CCS case conferences where the consultants, referring clinicians, colleagues and students all contributed to case formulation. These interdisciplinary case conferences played an important role in highlighting systemic factors and understanding the dimensions of power, ethnicity and gender. As the case material will illustrate, the South Asian clinicians embodied the host country's institutional power and its deficiencies, and yet the fact that they also shared background and identity with patients allowed them to represent or mirror the shifting experiences of vulnerability and strength of patients and their families at intrapsychic, intra-familial and sociopolitical levels.

Contextualizing Clinician Identity and Training

The seminal work of Fanon (1961, 1967) drew attention to the power of gaze of the Other as a mediator of racism and to the cultural scotomas that blind participants to this destructive power. Fanon's reflections on his experience as a Black psychiatrist treating both the White colonist and the colonized subaltern provided the first in-depth analysis of the impact of colonialism on the clinician's own identity. His reflections also propelled subsequent work in postcolonial studies, addressing the social meanings and power dynamics of race, class, gender, ethnicity, nationality and language (e.g., Davar, 2009; Gilroy, 2004; Nandy, 1980; Said, 2003a, 2003b; Spivak, 2006). This literature is particularly relevant to minority clinicians,

who themselves are part of diasporic peoples and must regularly negotiate expressions of power, prejudice, identity and cultural dissonance that reflect this colonial history (Akhtar, 1995; Hickling, 2007; Fernando, 1995, 2002; Kareem, 1992; Maiter & Stalker, 2011; Young-Bruehl, 1996).

Earlier work on the racially or culturally different clinician has identified multiple ways in which these socially constructed identities influence clinical work, including racial bias, cultural countertransference, as well as culturally or historically rooted phantasy (Adams, 1996; Akhtar, 1999; Holmes, 1992; Kareem, 1992; Tummala-Narra, 2007; Young-Bruehl, 1996). Effective cultural consultation requires an awareness of the constraints of these factors on clinicians' agency, engagement and positioning as well as on clients' responses (Bhui & Bhugra, 2002; Kareem, 1992; Maiter, Stalker, & Allagia, 2009). The process of cultural consultation strives to create conditions that promote cultural safety (Kirmayer, 2012; Williams, 1999). The clinician's identity is integral to the process of creating cultural safety by bringing other perspectives to clinical assessment and intervention. Though an initial positive alliance may be strengthened by language, gender or ethnic match of therapist and clients, these same factors can also disqualify or disempower the clinician. In this chapter, we will use clinical vignettes from the work of the CCS to illustrate this process in the work of South Asian female consultants. The need to protect confidentiality limits our discussion of how the cases are complicated by the unique heterogeneity and hybridity of South Asian diasporic communities and families, but the cases reveal some of the common predicaments associated with migration and acculturation (Bhugra, 2004; Guzder, 2011; Fernando & Keating, 2009; Akhtar, 2005). Despite the apparent ethnic matching, clinician and client may be similar only in skin color or limited shared cultural knowledge, and the consultation often requires the presence of interpreters and culture brokers to bridge gaps in communication and mutual understanding. The superficial appearance of similarity can result in an initial positive alliance, as well as resistances that undermine cultural safety. In addition, the female consultant may face power issues embedded in traditional South Asian-gendered hierarchies that mirror patients' individual or family predicaments in the North American context.

While mainstream Euro-North American culture has integrated a variety of psychotherapy approaches to deal with mental health problems, South Asian societies tend to deal with distress and conflict through culturally embedded frameworks that include familial and religious strategies (Kakar, 1982; Chaudhry, 2008; Rahman et al., 2009). Cultural consultation aims to understand these frameworks and integrate them into clinical work with migrant families and individuals (Akhtar, 2005; Comas-Diaz & Greene, 1994; Malat, van Ryn, & Purcell, 2006; Tummala-Narra, 2004).

Diverse pathways of migration, generational differences, sociopolitical histories, religious and faith-based practices, caste hierarchies and familial and community dynamics all impact on the integration and assimilation patterns of the South Asian diaspora. Since each family member may acculturate in markedly different ways, they may view the consultant in different ways through processes of cultural transference that reflect these different realities and phantasies. The conflicts, resonances and dissonances that surface in cultural consultations challenge clinicians' professional training which is rooted in mainstream Eurocentric models of developmental psychology and psychotherapy. Though the South Asian clinicians brought culturally informed understandings of these families, as well as linguistic competence in several languages of the Indian subcontinent (Tamil, Gujarati, Hindi, Urdu and Punjabi), the consultations demanded rethinking their own sociopolitical and historical positioning as well as some of the assumptions of standard mental health theory and modifying practice to include the use of interpreters or culture brokers from the community.

The clinical literature documents the ways in which migration and culture change lead South Asians to experience shifts in roles or power, as well as problems of institutional and familial dissonances (Abbasi, 2008; Bhugra, 2004; Davar, 1999;

Guzder & Krishna, 2005; Maiter & Stalker, 2011; Maitra, 2006; Singla, 2005; Tummala-Narra, 2007). There is also a substantial interdisciplinary literature exploring historical, cultural, caste, political and legal dimensions of South Asian subaltern and female identity (Guha & Spivak, 1988; Lau, 1995; Thapan, 1997; Uberoi, 1999). Gender and power emerge in this literature as critical issues which often silence subalterns, women and children (Jack & Ali, 2010; Spivak, 2006). Silencing of women within the gendered hierarchy inhibits their self-expression, agency and power but secures the homeostasis of the family system or social group by avoiding potential escalation of conflicts, with retaliation, loss or injury to other family group or community members. By integrating aspects of attachment theories, relational theories and cognitive theories of depression, the "Silencing the Self" model (Jack & Ali, 2010, p. 7) can help explain the increased vulnerability to depression and suicide found among South Asian women in some contexts (Guzder, 2011).

Negotiating Gender and Power in South Asian Immigrant Families

South Asia has enormous cultural diversity, yet there are commonalties in traditional norms not only with regard to collective value systems that contrast with the emphasis on individualism in the West (Bhugra, 2004; Fernando, 2003; Kakar, 1997; Roland, 1991) but also with regard to women's roles both within and outside the family (Eilberg-Schwartz & Doniger, 1995, 1996; Guzder & Krishna, 1991; Thapan, 1997; Trawick, 1990; Uberoi, 1999). Traditional structures of caste or religious affiliation, which provide a sense of continuity, meaning and identity, may contribute to social or systemic stability and protect families and individuals from some of the destructive effects of poverty, caste, war or other adversities. Compared to women, South Asian men traditionally inherit a familial status that confers more privilege and power. Women often negotiate power more indirectly within the family, accumulating power within gendered hierarchies based on the status of their natal family, motherhood, the birth of sons and the accrued respect of age (Guzder & Krishna, 2005). There is a split in the cultural roles of women in these societies who may be idealized and revered as matriarchs and yet, in reality, may remain devalued and undermined within the patriarchy (Kakar, 1990; Guzder & Krishna, 1991). Though feminine status seems to be promoted by the mythical status of the goddesses, the revered position of religious renunciants, the popular admiration of Bollywood stars or limited numbers with prominent roles in political and economic elites, in reality, most women in traditional South Asian families continue to struggle with issues of voice, agency and power. Tensions between cultural idealization and devaluation of the feminine may emerge in migratory contexts and are complicated by social class, caste and other divisions of power. As a group, South Asian women are also vulnerable to social injustices including foeticide, dowry death, physical abuse and rape (Guzder & Krishna, 1991, 2005). These injustices are maintained by gendered hierarchies, as well as unequal legal status and socio-economic standing. Kakar (1989) and Obeyesekere (1990) have suggested these inequities are also psychologically maintained by issues of sexual ambivalence and intrusive dependence (Kakar, 1989). Women's identities are organized around mythical and cultural ideals enacted in laws, moral codes and ritual practices which strive to maintain cohesion and homeostasis of family hierarchies. Boundaries of sexual purity or restraint versus impurity or transgression (Doniger, 1999; Douglas, 1966; Spivak, 2006; Thapan, 1997) are often constructed in terms of the honor (*izzat*) of family, clan or menfolk (Guzder & Krishna, 1991). *Izzat* (a Hindi, Urdu and Farsi term) refers to a code of honor prevalent in the northern Indian subcontinent regions. The concept of *izzat* not only maintains perceptions and codes of social conduct but also is tied to the reciprocity of families or groups who must strive to settle social debts after violations of honor codes, including, in some instance, seeking revenge through "honor killing" (Coomaraswamy, 2005; Jafri, 2003; Penn & Nardos, 2003). This cultural

embedding encompasses sexual purity, social conduct and honor. These agendas are challenged by migration and modern lifestyles, which may increase options for autonomy and identity differentiation for women and children in urban, cosmopolitan places, expanding their capacity to resist devaluation or abuse. Contemporary social realities of the Indian subcontinent offer increasing options for women as evolving cultural, social and political contexts have opened new possibilities for identity, gender roles and agency. Despite these changes, a 2007 research report prepared by the Indian Government on child abuse indicated that a majority of girl children wished they had been born male (Kacker, Mohsin, Dixit, Varadan, & Kumar, 2007).

In the past 20 years, migration of South Asian families to Canada has increased and included more families escaping pre-migratory trauma such as civil unrest, war or torture in parts of Sri Lanka, Bangladesh, India, Nepal and Bhutan. Some families bring preexisting fragility while others transplant frames of reference such as enduring caste conflict or honor codes. In the Quebec context, social changes since the 1970s have emphasized gender equality and displaced traditional Catholic attitudes to marriage and women's roles in favor of more flexible definitions of family and couple relationships. The political expectation for immigrants and their children has been on rapid acculturation to Quebec values and language. Quebec society has focussed on its own vulnerability as a francophone society trying to maintain its language and culture in the predominately English-speaking North American context. This has led to a shift in political language from the multiculturalism embraced in the rest of Canada to the notion of *interculturalism*, which acknowledges Quebec as a distinctive culture interacting with the traditions of newcomers. The diversity of the metropole of Montreal and the increasing proportion of non-European immigrants to Quebec have stimulated debate on "reasonable accommodation" around the extent to which mainstream institutions should be altered to meet the needs of newcomers (Bouchard & Taylor, 2008). Although Quebec has both French and English public school systems, with the passage of the Charter of French Language in 1977 (Bill 101), all immigrant children, including those for whom English was their previous language of instruction, must attend a *class d'acceuil* (welcome class) to prepare them for integration into French schools. As a result, in most of the case histories we present below, the children speak French, English and multiple Indian dialects to varying degrees, while their parents and the South Asian origin consultants often spoke English and Indian dialects. In many cases, therefore, the adults have less mastery of French than the children, further complicating processes of identification and acculturation.

Local host culture tensions sometimes compel immigrant families to redefine or reorient their structure and functioning by shifting developmental positions and assigning new roles to members. With shifts from extended to nuclear family, each generation and gender may encounter new and unexpected pressures and predicaments (Akhtar, 1999). Studies in India of culture change with urbanization and shifts in traditional family structure indicate that both adolescents and women are particularly vulnerable to increased mental disorders due to the way these changes affect family life (Carstairs & Kapur, 1976; Goodman, Patel, & Leon, 2008). Atif Rahman and colleagues (2009) have shown that the risk of depression among young Pakistani women increases with marriage and disturbed family relationships. In a large sample of Goan adolescents, Pillai et al. (2008) found that families adhering to traditional constraints or values had adolescents with very low rates of mental disorders, while families living in the metropoles that offered more autonomy choices experienced rates comparable to those of Euro-North Americans.

Migration can bring both successes and losses for South Asian men who may experience unanticipated upheavals in their personal and family identity with social dislocations and an increase in some mental disorders (Bhui & Bhugra, 2002). The loss of male peers and role models, shifting positions in the extended family system, challenges to the entitlements of patriarchal power and loss of culturally sanctioned mediators, such as trusted extended family members, are some of the factors that may undermine previously adap-

tive identities and coping strategies. While some men respond to the challenges of migration with resilience, others may experience intense resistance to change, and the stresses of acculturation may result in substance abuse, gambling, domestic violence or other mental health problems. Some of these men perceive little compensation for their losses after migration to Western societies, especially if their roles as providers, positions of power and self-esteem are undermined. For men, the changes in status associated with migration may intensify issues of shame or dishonor and increase the risk of violence related to perceived threats to family or group honor (Guzder & Krishna, 1991; Ghosh, 1994).

In contrast, South Asian women, although affected by changes in family networks, support, mediators and role models (Uberoi, 1999), may find themselves in a host society which affords them new options for negotiating power and economic possibilities that allow greater independence or autonomy for themselves and their children. Legal rights, including the option of leaving abusive spouses, divorcing and retaining child custody rights, are new possibilities for these women. Those who choose the path of separation or divorce may be distressed by the loss of support from the extended family even if they are relieved to escape from oppressive family situations (Guzder & Krishna, 1991).

Both men and women may be compelled in varying degrees to undertake a transformation of values and renegotiate their marital relationships as they adapt to new realities post-migration. Research documents the increased socioeconomic status of second-generation Canadian South Asian immigrant women, who surpass their male counterparts (Ghosh, 1994). These women face fewer social obstacles to economic advancement post-migration than they encountered in their societies of origin.

Encountering a female South Asian therapist in a clinical setting inevitably raises issues about the rescripting of gender norms with migration. The female clinician may be viewed ambivalently as a substitute for traditional cultural mediators, who usually are elders, religious figures, members of the wider extended family circle or a cohesive community. She may also be seen as a mediator with the host country, a position which can be perceived either as helpful or as a betrayal. These complex and often simultaneous role attributions play a key role in the therapeutic process, especially when the therapists' gender and power attributes are dissonant with traditional constructions of identity.

Gender in Cultural Consultation

Although there is some evidence that immigrants access medical services at the same rates as those born in Canada (Kirmayer, 2008), most South Asian families do not voluntarily seek medical help for mental health problems. They may feel reluctant to seek a consultation and have considerable apprehension related to stigma and the dangers of institutional power, since mental health issues are traditionally resolved in the privacy of the family (Kakar, 1982; Timimi & Maitra, 2005). In addition, when these families enter treatment with a South Asian woman consultant, the clinician's position of power may directly challenge and threaten to destabilize the traditional gender hierarchy. The clinical encounter then may intensify existing vulnerabilities of masculine identity. While therapy is intended to provide a space to reframe issues of power and role dissonances, this opportunity may be welcome by some family members but resisted by others. In the clinical vignettes below, we explore the paradoxical dynamics of having a South Asian woman therapist for migrants who reside in the traditional structural rubric of power and gender.

As a clinician, the female family therapist implicitly borrows the power of the host society's health care institutions. Since migrant South Asian families, particularly men within these families, already feel systemically disempowered by the host culture, the reversal of the traditional gender hierarchy in the clinical encounter becomes a double disempowerment. This may then lead to individual or family resistances to the consultation or intervention process because the therapist is affectively situated in an ambivalent oppressor role. At the same time, as a South Asian woman, the clinician may evoke positively invested gender norms associated with

matriarchy, of respect, submission and obedience. Her position of power within the therapeutic space then is paradoxically both a reminder of gender role reversal and a reproduction of familiar gender interactions which were possible in the pre-migratory period. These dialectical positions create the possibility of using a transitional space (Winnicott, 1966) for considering options, reframing, individuation and therapeutic work. As Fruggeri (1992) points out, power need not be celebrated nor demonized "Rather, the therapist should take responsibility for his or her power construction within the constraints of the relational/social domain." Thus, "power negotiation" is a critical tool available to the therapist who may need to invalidate her position of power to empower the family.

Case Vignette 8-1

Begum was a 32-year-old Bangladeshi Muslim woman who had made multiple suicide attempts. She had been raped in the detention center of another country en route to Canada where she had claimed refugee status and given birth to this child shortly after her arrival. She was referred to the CCS from the regional refugee service for advice on the treatment of her depression. During the initial CCS interview with a male psychiatrist, she remained essentially mute and wept. A second consultation was arranged with a South Asian female consultant, where Begum openly expressed her outrage at the subservient position of women in her country of origin, recounted her own history of domestic violence and the circumstances of her rape. She explained her silence during the initial interview as reflecting her association of the male consultant with the patriarchy of her culture of origin, as well as Canadian immigration authorities and institutional power hierarchies.

Since the CCS work is done within university hospitals, consultants are endowed with the power of both health institutions and academia.

Although women increasingly dominate the helping professions in South Asia, often without occupying power positions equivalent to men, their presence in the therapeutic context is likely to reflect the possibility of shifts in power. The culture of institutions both idealizes and devalues female professionals. The South Asian consultant working within these institutions must be aware of their own possible over-identification with the family's struggle to deal with dominant institutions such as refugee boards, youth protection or schools. In the family's struggle with power both within the family and also in the broader context of host society institutions, the female South Asian consultant may be identified as a matriarchal resource with strong positive transference overriding the family's anxieties about institutional power and this may facilitate assessment and treatment. In this case, however, the consultant may be idealized and viewed as having exaggerated power. She may be asked to advocate on behalf of the family or transgress institutional constraints. Alternatively, the consultant may be seen in a persecutory light as an extension of the host society's obstacles to validation or acceptance. These responses may be obstacles to assessment or may help to uncover underlying clinical issues.

Case Vignette 8-2

A South Asian psychiatrist (JG) was asked to consult on an inpatient unit for a 14-year-old boy from Pakistan who had spent months out of school at home with his anxious mother. Shortly after the consultation, the mother shared with the referring treatment team that the South Asian consultant had put microphones in restaurants and was sending persecutory messages to her. After months of her son and husband not disclosing her delusions and hallucinations, her paranoid delusional response to the therapist's name and ethnicity helped the team clarify the diagnosis and explain the school phobic behaviors. The shared ethnicity of the consultant was a clear factor in this disclosure.

An understanding of cultural and intrapsychic themes related to gender helps the consultant navigate the shifts in power and position from validating to invalidating and closeness to distancing during the consultation. CCS consultants work with their own subjectivity regarding the cultural underpinnings of gender and power, by listening to their internal discomfort and anxieties that arise in response to their positioning as both insider and outsider. Since ethnic match often creates an initial positive working alliance (Malat & Hamilton, 2006), the consultant and the institutional setting may be perceived as less "strange" or "estranged." Initially, the fear of being among strangers may be mitigated by sharing a common language and heritage, while issues of gender may become clearer as family conflicts or other power issues emerge. Anxieties about strangers may also be projected onto others involved in the consultation, including professional interpreters hired from the regional health care interpreter service. Attitudes toward interpreters may include concerns about confidentiality and the potential for indiscretion or leaking secrets to the community and mask fears of the clinician or institutional setting. The fears of disclosure may take on a persecutory quality. However, the presence of interpreters usually increases safety and alliance. In some instances, interpreters and clinician may be "adopted" as fictive family members (i.e., aunt, sister) or may be called for help in crisis situations. The CCS consultants aim for a position between these extremes, as close but not intimate. In this process, gender is sometimes a disqualifying element ("you are turning my wife against me") or a necessity for alliance ("I will only see you as you are a woman").

Social and political realities, including events such as the terrorist attacks of 9/11, have heightened public anxieties about certain ethnoracial groups (Tummala-Narra, 2005) and have had an impact on levels of persecutory anxiety, cultural difference or mistrust experienced by minorities in the clinical encounter. For effective consultation, these anxieties about cultural difference must be acknowledged as they may also arise in the referring team or the consultant. A similar response of validating rather than denying differences that impact on the clinician–patient relationship is advocated by Holmes (1992) using the situation of a Black female clinician working with White clients. Holmes notes that working across difference can be difficult or at times impossible when the therapist's own equilibrium is disrupted, for example, when the patient's focus remains on difference and mistrust and this prevents the establishment of basic trust and a working alliance with the consultant. A focus on "racial enactments" or other forms of cultural difference can be useful to the clinical process. The recognition of difference need not impede progress, though "racial enactments typically implicate the very issues— idealization, envy, jealousy and devaluation—likely to upset one's narcissistic equilibrium" (Leary, 2006, p. 650). Blindness to the basis of cultural differences in values, developmental experiences, rituals, maturational markers and goals and aspirations limits the options for clinical rapport and intervention. As Tummala-Narra (2005) and Apfel and Simon (2000) point out, most clinicians are not familiar with analyzing their political positions when confronted with racial or ethnic conflicts and may defensively resort to detachment, isolation, hyper-professionalism (Dunayevich & Puget, 1989) or fall into over-identification with the minority patient with whom they share ethnicity.

Gender, Color, Ethnicity and Loyalty: Cultural Consultation Deconstructed

The cases described below were seen at the JGH CCS (Chapter 3) or the MCH Transcultural Child Psychiatry Team (Chapter 4). The consultants worked with the referring clinicians, sometimes alone or with their teams, who were generally present for initial consultations along with interpreters. The MCH service usually used a reflecting team in a group including the family but respected the wishes of patients, if they preferred to be seen with several members of the team. Though the CCS usually provides limited consultations, some of the case vignettes reflect more extended interventions undertaken with individuals or families due to their complexity. A team consultation was offered to the referring agency or

case manager if the patient refuses direct contact with the CCS team.

The next case illustrates how ethnolinguistic matching may allow improved communication and a positive identification with the female consultant by reframing gender and power issues in ways that promote resolution of conflict between a migrant family and host society institutions.

Case Vignette 8-3

A consultation was requested by an inpatient team for the family of Sevaanan, a 10-year-old boy from Sri Lanka hospitalized for several months for suicide threats and severe anorexia. Sevaanan had a history of oppositional behaviors and had recently disclosed abuse by his father to his school. The initial assessment by a South Asian CCS consultant and a Canadian child psychiatrist (CR) was followed by several family sessions with the South Asian consultant (RS) which took place in the hospital.

The family had migrated to Canada 15 years earlier from Sri Lanka during the upheaval of civil war in a context of severe hardship. The couple had managed to cope with parenting and marital issues during their first 9 years in Canada until their second child, a daughter, was diagnosed with autism. Despite their previous capacity to cope, the couple experienced a crisis, with the father progressively removing himself emotionally from the family and accumulating gambling debts. A youth protection investigation had not been able to validate the boy's allegations of physical abuse by his father, while the parents were mainly concerned that he was losing weight. Though the family had been seen by a series of professionals, the history remained unclear. The parents had said they understood English and had not insisted on an interpreter because Sevaanan was fiercely opposed to it, and they did not dare oppose him fearing his anorexia would worsen. The inpatient unit had relied on Sevaanan for interpreting.

(continued)

As an initial step, the consultation addressed the linguistic barriers as a power issue and obstruction to a therapeutic alliance with the parents. Sevaanan tried to boycott the use of Tamil during the assessment, but the alliance between the South Asian consultant and the child psychiatrist persuaded the parents not to give in and to acknowledge their need to use Tamil in therapy. By introducing a South Asian female clinician who spoke Tamil, a positive alliance was quickly established between the couple and the team. The consultant asked the parents "How was it for you when you were not able to speak to the team and Sevaanan was doing all the talking?" The mother responded that she had not thought that the team would listen to the distorted picture Sevaanan had related because "he is just a young boy." The parents had been deeply shamed by the boy's allegations, which had brought their family under a youth protection mandate. They had no youth protection system in Sri Lanka and did not understand that a child could accuse his parent and be taken seriously. The parents' sense of being heard, understood and empowered by the South Asian consultant, who represented both host and culture of origin societies, was a significant turning point in the consultation. For almost a year, Sevaanan had triangulated his parents, diminishing his father's role to that of "abuser, gambler and failure." The triangulation made the marital strain more explicit as Sevaanan appeared to champion his mother. This powerful family position contributed to his strong resistance to the introduction of the female South Asian consultant who displaced his central role as mediator of all communication with the family. Once the language barriers were addressed, the process of parental re-empowerment and team building was identified as a priority and allowed the team to begin addressing the marital schism and family losses.

There were several ways in which the father perceived himself as powerless and a failure: he had failed in his role as an eldest son to look after his parents, renouncing his filial duties and abandoning them in Sri Lanka during war time; he was powerless to protect his daughter from a serious disabling illness; and, because of gambling, he had failed to provide for his family. His position as "bad, abusive father," rather than an effective parent who could be productive in the family, had been reinforced by trauma as well as underlying distress, guilt and shame.

It was possible to re-empower the father because both parents positively identified with the female consultant at a collective ethnocultural level and recognized the institutional power that enhanced her position. Alliance building included listening to their discussions of numerology and Hindu explanatory frames of reference. As a way to construct hope for the father, the therapist introduced the story of Prince Yudhisthira from the *Mahābhārata*, a hero who falls from grace due to gambling but redeems himself with honesty and family loyalty (Smith, 2009). These shared stories from Hindu mythology provided a vehicle for the family's co-construction of a narrative that renewed the father's power (Briggs, 1996) and created momentum for change in the family. At a deeper level, the mythological story reduced the dissonance between the host society and culture of origin by encouraging the couple to assert their parental power by negotiating within the institutional frame. Once child abuse accusations were withdrawn, Sevaanan shifted his position progressively to a less dominant, less victimized identity and was less emotionally burdened by his role in the family. His parents worked on strengthening their parental functioning. When the son expressed his resentment of the female consultant, disparaging her interventions with open hostility, both parents were able to mobilize a joint

(continued)

response to his defiant stance, identifying with the consultant as a respected matriarchal figure. Reframing the father's position and emphasizing the son's need for the parenting team's authority helped them to mobilize a structural shift to reassert appropriate parental boundaries. Further couple sessions explored marital strain, difficulties coping with the younger child's diagnosis of autism and the impact on mother of the father's previous losses, while family sessions focussed on the developmental needs of both children.

In this case, the female South Asian consultant was a bridge between the family and the treatment team. She engaged the parents and particularly the father in ways that helped them regain their sense of agency and power in part by validating his loss and grief. The consultant's language skills and cultural knowledge were relevant not only to facilitate communication but to make use of mythic paradigms and stories that are part of oral tradition to convey the potential for reconciliation to loss and failure and the possibility of resilience and renewal. While the son initially resented the female therapist and actively disparaged her interventions, both parents were able to identify with her as a respected professional figure. The child psychiatrist consultant's "in-between" position helped to move beyond the splits or polarities of South Asian family versus Canadian hospital team. Modelling authority and mobilizing a structural shift to assert a need for parental boundaries were two critical steps that allowed therapeutic progress.

The next vignette involves similar configurations of power and gender but this time with an adult patriarch who discounts the consultant. It illustrates how a strategic reframing allows the female consultant to join with a father, who initially challenges her authority, allowing him to feel less threatened and to shift to accepting help from a professional who comes to embody the role of an elder matriarch, despite her youth.

Case Vignette 8-4

A cultural consultation was requested by the outpatient team of a children's hospital for Mala, an adolescent girl with first-episode psychosis and mild mental retardation. Mala's family, from Bangladesh, was struggling to come to terms with their youngest daughter's illness. Six months into treatment, her father remained fiercely overprotective and kept her home from school. Her mother tried to reintegrate the girl into normal activities, insisting her daughter begin with simple household chores, but this approach was resisted by father who felt that mother should be a caretaker because their daughter was "fragile" and "sick."

The cultural consultant, who was a South Asian woman in her thirties, agreed to follow the family for a few joint therapy sessions with the Canadian child psychiatrist. During one of the family therapy sessions as parental conflict was being clarified, the mother said: "It has always been difficult, as he never supports my decisions when it comes to the ways of disciplining our children." When the therapist asked the father to respond to what the mother had just said, he replied by addressing the therapist, "You are quite thin. Is your health all right?" This apparently tangential remark questioned the therapist's physical strength and, by analogy, her ability to deal with the family's difficulties. Of note, the father never made this type of personal remarks to the Canadian clinicians. The South Asian therapist's first reaction was to receive this as direct disqualification of her as a professional and a deliberate attempt to derail her line of inquiry. In effect, an older South Asian man was responding in a patronizing way to a much younger South Asian woman who had trespassed boundaries and challenged him, albeit gently, to respond to his wife's perception of his lack of support. The remark could be seen as his defensive

(continued)

response to having his paternal role disqualified, by disqualifying the therapist's role, in turn. It could also be understood as an indirect expression of his powerlessness in the hospital interactions dominated by White female clinicians. Realizing this, the therapist responded by saying, "You feel like looking after everybody, especially the women. You want to take care of your daughter and your wife. You even worry about my health." This positive reframing moved the focus from his defensive stance to his positive efforts to be a caretaker and benevolent provider. He received this reframing as a reassurance of his valued position in the family hierarchy. Feeling less threatened, he proceeded to express his helplessness and impotence in dealing with the crisis of his daughter's psychosis. The discussion of vulnerability allowed realignment of parental positions and the common theme of powerlessness that joined the parenting couple. This strategic therapist response was cognisant of gender and power attributes by the client and made it possible for the couple to process other themes of dependence, silencing, control and autonomy related to their fears and advocacy for a vulnerable adolescent with a first-episode psychosis.

During family therapy sessions with South Asian families, it is not uncommon for the female therapist to feel disqualified, as described in the two preceding vignettes. Although the challenge from the family may be expressed more directly if the therapist is of South Asian origin, the power position of the mainstream female clinician may also be resented and contested. Reframing the disqualification of the South Asian clinician allowed the clinician to join with the family's feelings of being disqualified in relation to host society institutions. These interventions consolidated the therapeutic alliance and allowed the consultant to explore the broader implications of each family member's

experience of being rendered powerless or silenced whether by the larger society, cultural community or internal family dynamics. The use of gender- and hierarchy-based challenges to the clinician's authority is similar to the defensive manoeuvres of cultural camouflage discussed in Chapter 7 (see also Friedman, 1982), where underlying psychodynamic or systemic issues are camouflaged by invoking cultural norms and motifs. To circumvent this potential use of culture as camouflage, the cultural consultant must remain attentive not only to the obvious cultural themes and issues but also to significant issues of family process, structure and affect. The consultant strives to establish a systemic position as mediator (Messent, 1992). The mediator's empathic understanding of family and collective values provides an opening for identifying cultural strengths. In the cases above, substituting a Western model of individual voice or interpreting the father's response as simply a diminution of matriarchal influence might have closed the possibility of validating cultural strategies to strengthen the common ground of the parenting couple. Silencing is a common issue in gendered hierarchies (Jack & Ali, 2010). In clinical assessment and intervention, silencing has the effect of segregating women's experience, limiting the possibilities for dialogue and an inclusive negotiation of the position of both genders. The systemic approaches of narrative therapy and the strategy of circular questioning which asks family members to reflect on each other's responses deliberately work to include marginalized and silenced voices and introduce new options for dialogue guided by the therapist.

Women in South Asian societies learn to claim their power and position through modelling the behaviors of their older counterparts in the extended family who negotiate power by diplomatic shuttles between men, and sometimes between senior women, in the hierarchy. This modelling of instrumental effectiveness and tacit power is not available in the nuclear family of migrants, who also must contend with radically different notions of gendered power in the new host culture. However, while women's position and power may change profoundly with migration, at the same time, they represent and are expected to maintain continuity with the lost world for the family as a whole and, in particular, for the men. The tensions between the new opportunities for power and agency that come with migration and the obligation and desire to maintain cultural continuity may apply both to the women in the family and to the "other" South Asian women who encounter the family as consultants.

As in the case of other migrant communities, South Asian couples and families must renegotiate their roles to meet new demands of the Canadian milieu. For example, as Sluzki (1979) has suggested, migrant families may initially negotiate or develop splits between instrumental and affective roles with a key member, usually the male provider, functioning in a present-oriented provider or "survivor" mode, while another family member, often a woman, "holds" the past intact. The parenting couple thus preserves family stability until the emergent role of individuating children at adolescence or other events often destabilize this strategy. Pregnancy can be an especially critical time for immigrant women who may be more vulnerable to depression owing to a lack of extended family and community supports or other stresses associated with migration (Zelkowitz et al., 2004). Families may achieve a precarious balance that hides male role dislocations or downward social mobility, until the occurrence of unexpected stressful events such as the diagnosis of developmental disorders in a child, behavioral or mental health problems in an adolescent, serious medical conditions of a parent or the loss of a job by a breadwinner. The following case vignette illustrates issues of gender and power exposed by a postpartum crisis.

Case Vignette 8-5

Ajanta, a 22-year-old Muslim woman, who had emigrated from Pakistan 3 years earlier, was referred for cultural consultation by a community clinic for postpartum depression, anorexia and somatic complaints unresponsive to multiple consultations. She was seen initially with her husband, her French Canadian therapist, an interpreter (who had been refused by her husband but requested by the patient) and the caretaker of her children, who remained in the waiting area with her 18-month-old twin girls. The interpreter was an older Pakistani woman who had been in Canada for more than 20 years, had children and a career, who introduced, through her own self-disclosure in the later sessions, another layer of complexity and identification to the therapeutic encounter.

Ajanta had been unable or unwilling to wean the twins. She adamantly refused to put them in day care, because she equated this step with acquiescing to her husband's plans that she was "not returning home." The couple was at an impasse in their conflict over the husband's wish that his wife and the twins remain in Canada rather than moving back to her country of origin or even going for a brief visit to renew her links with her parents. The husband agreed that young mothers usually return to their natal families especially after a first childbirth as part of the nurturing of the young mother and support of her child care skills. Ajanta had been determined to go home to her natal village where she longed to be cared for by her parents and also to complete her mourning for a recently deceased uncle to whom she had been strongly attached in childhood. Her husband strongly resisted her plans to visit to Pakistan, insisting that the twins might be kidnapped or fall ill. He showed little empathy for his wife, who was a maternal cousin, and wanted to be present for the consultation "to supervise" the intervention rather than involving himself as part of the process of problem solving. The couple were seen for four sessions alternately together and alone.

Though diagnosed in primary care with postpartum depression, Ajanta had rejected antidepressant medications. She was afraid of the limitation on breast feeding when taking medication. Additionally, she felt that

(continued)

"depression" was highly stigmatized because it implied she was "mad" and further disempowered her voice and agency in negotiations within the family. She appeared to be appeasing her husband who had labelled her depression as "weakness and laziness," though in individual therapy sessions, she attributed her lack of direct assertion of her motives to the powerful patriarchal position of her husband and his family. He was angry that she had not adapted well in Canada ("so many people want to come here… she is so fortunate and ungrateful"). He wanted her to get a job and accept Canada as her home. Her passive strategies of resisting acculturation, symptoms of anorexia and refusal to wean the twins appeared to limit the husband's sense of control and undermined the hierarchy.

Ajanta felt that, as a South Asian woman, the consultant could both mediate the marital strain and understand her extended family pressures which she had not shared with the referring therapists ("they don't understand"). She attributed enhanced power to the therapist as a matriarch who could counter the husband and his close alliance with his mother and sister. When seen individually, she discussed her ambivalence about married life both in Canada and Pakistan. She insisted that her husband was not physically abusive, though clearly he was extremely controlling. She emphasised that she appreciated her husband as a good provider and father. Additionally, she felt she could not explicitly reveal her marital unhappiness to him or to their relatives in the extended family, especially as this was a cousin marriage. She explained that direct confrontation would cause great "family problems," including raising problems of dishonor (loss of *izzat* or honor) and bringing shame on her father. After voicing her frustration with her husband's family, especially his loyalty to his mother and sisters, who had advised him not to send her

home, she began to focus in the sessions on options for her autonomy in Canada.

Identification with the therapist helped Ajanta in building bicultural frames of reference. She proceeded to wean the babies and agreed to put them in day care. However, she resisted her husband's push for her to return to work prematurely by using the support of the clinic therapist who she felt was "outside the culture and could shame him." But resisted her husband's push for her to work prematurely by using the support of the clinic therapist who was "outside the culture and could shame him." She felt relieved that her voice was heard in the marital and individual sessions though she was disappointed that the consultant had not been able "to force my husband to send me home". She stated she had seen the consultant as an elder matriarch who appeared to have considerable institutional and social power from her husband's perspective.

Both members of the couple were grappling with losses and cultural shifts which were the focus of this intervention. The husband needed to be seen as a strong caretaker who nevertheless masked his deep sense of powerlessness and struggles of divided loyalty between his family matriarchs and his young wife. Despite his apparent dominance and continual assertion of patriarchal authority, the referring therapist pointed out that the husband was unable to change his wife's feelings and his coercive strategies were viewed negatively by the clinic.

In the course of the consultation, the husband was seen briefly individually, and it emerged that he had been intimidated by a Pakistani gang in Montreal and felt he could not relate the resultant shame and fears to his wife. In fact, he had gone to the police in Canada without telling his wife, but he was more concerned about the gang's threats to his family's safety should they return to his country of origin. Disclosing this predicament to the consultant elicited

(continued)

feelings of shame and discomfort but then allowed him to relate these issues to the other professionals involved and later to his wife. He stated that he felt tremendous relief that he could speak safely about his vulnerabilities with a South Asian clinician. However, he remained ambivalent and suspicious of the consultant, mentioning later to the referring clinician that if the consultant continued to see his wife, she might become less obedient. In the last joint session, he left saying, "If you ask me to change I will become more depressed than my wife, then who will look after us?"

In this case, the South Asian consultant provided a transitional space to reconsider the diagnosis of depression, revisit role shifts and cultural adjustments and support the couple's move from a symbiotic relationship with the twins to an appropriate stage of differentiation and gradual autonomy. During the individual session with Ajanta, the interpreter had offered additional support to the young wife through her own self-disclosure as a South Asian woman who had moved back and forth between Pakistan and Canada, offering another model of identification and validating future possibilities of integration. The interpreter had also asserted herself when the husband dismissed a need for her interpreting skills during the intense discussion in the therapy sessions, reinforcing the need for the young wife's "voice" to be heard and directly opposing the husband's silencing strategies.

The referring clinic felt that a hospitalization for an anorexic crisis in the wife had been averted by the consultation, because the wife began to eat as the marital tension remitted and the couple's functioning improved. The clinic staff had taken a position of advising rapid assimilation, emphasizing to the couple the need to adopt local or "Quebec" values rather than exploring the couple's own cultural frames of reference. However, the couple's strain and impasse suggested their issues were embedded in the dislocation of family paradigms, traditional roles, external issues (threats from a local gang), dynamics of cousin marriage and the loss of the usual cultural supports with a first child. Ambivalence over the demands of acculturation was experienced by both partners in the couple but was framed in terms of gender and power agendas.

In cultural consultation, the institutional context interacts with issues of gender and power and sometimes reveals forms of institutional racism (Fernando, 2002). These patterns of discrimination can be quite subtle and difficult to expose because they are associated with strong cultural norms and ideologies. The CCS and MCH teams were located within university hospitals that represent the power of health institutions and academia, which are rooted in the values of the dominant culture. Parts of the world where institutional values reflect familial patriarchal entitlements may be perceived by North American mental health practitioners as disempowering and oppressing women. This same attitude may be extended to the perception of the consultant from a minority background, complicating her interventions with colleagues.

Case Vignette 8-6

A South Asian woman who was about to be deported while actively suicidal and threatening to kill her children was evaluated by the CCS, and a report was prepared for a humanitarian appeal to the immigration board. A psychiatric consultant for the government agency called the South Asian CCS consultant to question her "overly" sympathetic report and asked if the consultant was favouring migration of South Asian woman due to her own ethnicity.

While the potential for over-identification is certainly possible in any clinical interaction when countertransferential issues are raised, in this case the desperate situation of the patient was discounted by the government consultant who questioned the CCS consultant's "objectivity", with little substantive basis to his speculation. In addition to a general scepticism about the claims of refugees, it is likely that gender bias contributed to this attempt to dismiss the consultant's report. This type of disqualification by professionals can be difficult to manage. The existence of a service like the CCS can provide an institutional and academic base from which to respond to such biases. Political, legal, ethical and institutional racism issues or realities may also arise that require a discussion with the referring and consulting team.

Of course, strong identification with patients can occur and make the consultation process particularly difficult as illustrated in the following vignette.

diminish her in her husband's eyes and permanently undermine their marital relationship. This narrative was very distressing for the consultant who was bound by confidentiality not to disclose the events but sought legal advice on how to guide the patient toward appropriate legal recourse.

Again, in cases like this, a high level of identification between consultant and patient may make disclosure of some kinds of difficult material more possible, but it also poses difficulties for the consultant who will benefit from team or peer supervision to manage the potential personal and professional issues. Additionally, the issues of refugee rights and advocacy in legal processes raise other dimensions of power which are realities in cultural consultation work.

Case Vignette 8-7

A South Asian married woman refugee reported being raped during police interrogation in her country of origin. She wanted to see the South Asian consultant to share her feelings of despair after being raped by her immigration consultant in Quebec who had directed her to her lawyer. She was terrified to see him alone or to reveal these rapes to her husband as she would be considered irremediably impure. She also feared the agent had contacts back in her home country who could hurt her children left behind. She wanted to share these issues with the consultant but did not want to disclose them more widely. She said that God could hear her despair better now, and she prayed that her sons would someday avenge her. She named her sons as part of the patriarchy who would be outraged by the rape and uphold her communal and personal honor. However, she explained that she feared that disclosure of the rape would

Case Vignette 8-8

Ayad, a 24-year-old South Asian male refugee claimant, was referred by a community care facility where he was being carefully monitored and medicated after discharge from a hospitalization for several suicide attempts. He was awaiting an appeal of his application for refugee status, and the cultural consultation was requested by a male staff member of the facility who had developed a close alliance with the patient and accompanied him for a single consultation visit. Trials of many different medications and consultations with other mental health professionals had led to no improvement in Ayad's self-harm behaviors.

Ayad was homosexual and had had a relationship across caste lines with the son of a prominent politician in his place of birth in South Asia. He had been kidnapped for ransom and the father of his companion had made death threats to his family. His mother secretly sold some family land to pay the ransom, contravening his father's

(continued)

decision to refuse to accede to the coercion. After his mother paid the ransom and obtained his release, Ayad broke his promise to his mother to end the affair and returned to his former partner. The relationship finally ended when the partner's father sent his son away to get married. Ayad's father was devastated by both the public exposure of his son's homosexuality and his violation of caste boundaries in the relationship. His father was furious when he discovered that his wife had taken money for the ransom from their dowry and retirement savings.

Ayad was devastated when his lover's father issued death threats. He had attempted suicide in India, telling his family he was still in love with this young man. His father had then "excommunicated" him from the family. His mother, however, had raised enough funds to send him to Canada "to be safe." His affair became common knowledge in his urban setting and led to the disruption of his sister's arranged marriage, which further exacerbated his guilt. He had made suicide attempts in Canada both out of "lovesickness" and guilt. When his father had received news of the last suicide attempt, he wrote to Ayad and advised him to "be a man and complete the suicide as his mother was in a deep depression" so that "the family could be rid of his bad influence in order to marry his sisters." However, Ayad's mother begged him not to suicide and believed he should make a new life in Canada.

The referring treatment team held more egalitarian views on his right to homosexuality and to grieve his lost partner, joining with him to validate the injustice he had endured as a victim and expressing outrage on his behalf in response to his father's advice to suicide. While they were supportive and protective of the patient, their strategies had not had a positive impact, and, in fact, his distress, suicide threats and acts of self-harm escalated. The therapists at the care facility partly blamed Ayad's problem on the impact of the "primitive cultural taboos" and prejudice of his family and South Asian culture. They understood the patient's guilt at being unable to resolve hopeless family issues and his attachment to his lover. They felt they were empowering Ayad, by discussing the potential to allow himself opportunities for gay life in Canada as major incentives for wellness, provided the uncertainty of his refugee status was resolved. The staff identified Ayad's resilience in his ability to work, and he was seen as having good potential for social integration, but they did not understand why his suicide ideation and attempts continued despite their active support.

As Ayad related his story to the South Asian female consultant, his main focus was his feelings of outrage at his father's lack of support and his response of acting out the father's message. He minimized the impact of his actions on his relationship with his mother, his sisters and family. It appeared that his mother was also now depressed and possibly suicidal. Ayad had a sense of entitlement to his mother's resources and showed little gratitude or respect for his mother's efforts to save him and get him to Canada. Ayad's preoccupation with his love affair had blinded him to the advocacy and courage of his mother in getting funds to pay the ransom for his release and allow his flight.

Ayad's suicide gestures were considered in the light of the gender, legal and structural violence inherent in his family situation. The consultation focussed on broadening his sense of choice and agency to allow him to consider alternate identifications and pathways to conflict resolution. He had not recognized how his feelings about his parents played a significant role in his suicide behaviors. While the female therapist, joined with his male care facility staff,

(continued)

could be supportive of his romantic attachment, the intervention focussed on parental and systemic aspects of the suicide behaviors and his feminized position of agency with respect to his father.

Kakar (1997, 1981) has explored the maternal feminine identifications and bisexuality of identity formation in South Asian context. Despite some recent increase in acceptance of open homosexuality in large urban centers, in most of South Asia, homosexuality remains discrete and hidden. The emergent gay discourse in India has not mitigated the tensions of a social space where homosexuality, bisexuality and other variations in sexuality or gender identity evoke phobic responses and A (Bose & Battacharya, 2007). In traditional families, homosexuality is often countered by forced marriage in an attempt to change the sexual orientation and normalize the situation with a social façade of acceptable heterosexuality as illustrated in this clinical vignette by the family's solution for Ayad's partner.

In this case, over-identification with host country perceptions of tolerance of homosexuality may have inadvertently reinforced the father–son conflict as the referring treatment team colluded in exacerbating the patient's acting out, without eliciting a more inclusive picture of the family's predicament. The referring clinicians' acknowledged that they had not considered the impact of the patient's behavior on the female members of the family nor had they understood the parental dynamics, issues of caste privilege, gender hierarchy, impact on arranged marriage, socio-economic or political context. The client felt the cultural consultation opened a renewed opportunity to show gratitude to his mother, and his suicide attempts stopped despite his anguish.

Conclusion

The cases we have presented illustrate how, in considering issues of gender, ethnicity and power, the cultural consultant must reach beyond the dominant

paradigms of mental health training to allow multiple voices and perspectives to emerge. Working with the cultural contexts of collective values and gendered hierarchies inherent to South Asia families broadens the horizon of clinical conversations and the construction of solutions. Cultural parameters must be recognized to understand the divergent perspectives of the patient, family and the institution. Acknowledging these elements provides the basis for a reflective process of inquiry, but even with ethnic matching, deliberate efforts to identify blind spots and attempts to adapt perspectives, confusion and uncertainty may remain.

Cultural consultation requires an understanding that power relations in host societies and institutions interact in complex ways with the social fabric of gender and family structures from non-Western cultures. Creating secure transitional spaces within therapeutic settings allows families or individuals to rethink and renegotiate their agency, position and power in contexts of cultural change and the destabilization or hybridity of cultural norms that comes with migration. These power negotiations involve deeply embedded identifications, structural issues including political and social issues, changes in hierarchical strategies and increasing tolerance for the options and confusion of values related to cultural change. Clearly, the changing dynamics of gender, race, ethnicity and culture cannot be captured through generalizations. These dynamics must be constantly reassessed not only for each patient but also over the course of treatment. As we have seen in the clinical examples, the process of empowering individuals within systems can have unexpected, destabilizing and harmful repercussions or provide openings for positive and creative solutions. Through his or her gender and ethnicity, the consultant may embody specific identities that can be threatening or validating positions for different generations of family members of either gender.

Following Foucault (1967), we would argue that power can be thought of more as a strategy than a possession—as ways of configuring relationships that emerge from cultural narratives and discursive practices, that circulate within local and transnational communities and that are revised in new contexts. As therapists, we are constantly revisiting our blind spots and striving to acknowledge hidden power relations by searching for projections, implicit or hidden meanings, listening to silence, working with confusion, identifying institutional agendas and tracking affective responses in the clinical encounter. We seek to unmask power to understand the underlying agendas and intentions in both social and familial interactions. Since medical encounters usually subordinate the patient's voice to that of the physician (Addilakha, 2008), we often fail to hear the suppressed narratives of patients and their families. These blind spots become particularly hazardous in the context of intercultural work, where misunderstandings or missed understandings are even more likely.

Migration and cultural hybridization are part of lifelong developmental processes of individuation that may suppress or validate various identifications and strategies in the ongoing flux of life events and change (Akhtar, 1999). Using examples of work with South Asian families, we have tried to show how consultants' personal characteristics, especially gender and ethnicity, whether they work alone or within a hybrid team, can provide entry points for clinical dialogue and possibilities for therapeutic intervention. We emphasize that clinical work cannot be separated from wider agendas of power that are embedded in host country institutions and cultural frameworks. The cultural consultation process constructs a collage from the diverse perspectives of referring clinicians, patients, families and consultants. In this process the diversity of identities among clinicians and sometimes consultant may facilitate the representation of the relations among genders, across generations and between minority and majority groups. This *bricolage* allows us to look at intersecting frameworks rather than rooting our work in a single model drawn from the dominant ethnocentric discourses of biomedicine, psychiatry, mental health or social services. Power and gender, language and ethnicity and sameness and difference are dimensions of clinical work which must acknowledge the multiple dialectics, diverse realities and complex transformations of identity inherent to migration experience.

References

Abbasi, A. (2008). Whose side are you on? Muslim psychoanalysts treating non-Muslim patients. In S. Akhtar (Ed.), *The crescent and the couch: Cross-currents between Islam and psychoanalysis*. New York, NY: Jason Aronson.

Adams, M. V. (1996). *The multicultural imagination: "Race", color, and the unconscious*. London, England: Routledge.

Addlakha, R. (2008). *Deconstructing mental illness: An ethnography of psychiatry, women and the family*. New Delhi, India: Zubaan.

Akhtar, S. (1995). A third individuation: Immigration, identity, and the psychoanalytic process. *Journal of the American Psychoanalytic Association, 43*(4), 1051–1084.

Akhtar, S. (1999). *Immigration and identity: Turmoil, treatment, and transformation*. Northvale, NJ: Jason Aronson.

Akhtar, S. (Ed.) (2005). Freud Along The Ganges. New York: Other Press.

Apfel, R. J., & Simon, B. (2000). Mitigating discontents with children and war. In A. Robben & M. Suarez-Orozco (Eds.), *Cultures under siege: Collective violence and trauma* (pp. 102–130). New York, NY: Cambridge University Press.

Bhugra, D. (2004). Migration, distress and cultural identity. *British Medical Bulletin, 69*(1), 129–141.

Bhui, K., & Bhugra, D. (2002). Mental illness in Black and Asian ethnic minorities: Pathways to care and outcomes. *Advances in Psychiatric Treatment, 8*, 26–33.

Bose, B., & Bhattacharya, S. (Eds.). (2007). *The phobic and the erotic: The politics of sexualties in contemporary India*. Calcutta, India: Seagull Book.

Bouchard, G., & Taylor, C. (2008). *Building the future: A time for reconciliation (abridged report)*. Quebec, Canada: Commission de consultation sur les pratiques d'accommodement relies aux differences cultural, Gouvernment du Quebec.

Briggs, C. (Ed.). (1996). *Disorderly discourse: Narrative, conflict and inequality*. New York, NY: Oxford University Press.

Carstairs, G. M., & Kapur, R. L. (1976). *The great universe of kota: Stress, change and mental disorder in an indian village*. Berkley, CA: University of California.

Catherall, D. R., & Pinsof, W. M. (1987). The impact of the therapist's personal family life on the ability to establish viable therapeutic alliance in family and marital therapy. *Journal of Psychotherapy and the Family, 3*(2), 135–160.

Chaudhry, H. R. (2008). Psychiatry care in Asia: Spirituality and religious connotations. *International Review of Psychiatry, 20*(5), 477–483.

Comas-Diaz, L., & Greene, B. (Eds.). (1994). *Women of colour: Integrating ethnic and gender identities in psychotherapy*. New York, NY: Guilford Press.

Coomaraswamy, R. (2005). Preface: Violence against women and 'crimes of honour'. In S. Hossain & L. Welchman (Eds.), *'Honour': Crimes, paradigms and violence against women* (pp. xi–xiv). London, England: Zed Books.

Davar, B. V. (1999). Indian psychoanalysis, patriarchy and Hinduism. *Anthropology & Medicine, 6,* 173–194.

Davar, B. V. (Ed.). (2009). *Mental health from a gender perspective.* New Delhi, India: Sage.

Doniger, W. (1984). *Dreams, illusions and other realities.* Chicago, IL: University of Chicago Press.

Doniger, W. (1999). *Splitting the difference: Gender and myth in ancient Greece and India.* Chicago, IL: University of Chicago Press.

Douglas, M. (1966). *Purity and danger: An analysis of concepts of pollution and taboo.* London, England: Routledge & Kegan Paul.

Dunayevich, J. B., & Puget, J. (1989). State terrorism and psychoanalysis. *International Journal of Mental Health, 18*(2), 98–112.

Dunlop, R. (2004). Ancestors. In R. Dunlop & P. Uppal (Eds.), *Red silk: An anthology of South Asian Canadian women poets* (p. 31). Toronto, Ontario, Canada: Mansfield.

Eilberg-Schwartz, H., & Doniger, W. (Eds.). (1995). *Off with her head!: the denial of women's identity in myth, religion, and culture.* Berkeley: University of California Press.

Fanon, F. (1961). *The wretched of the earth.* New York, NY: Grove Press.

Fanon, F. (1967). *Black skin, white masks.* New York, NY: Grove Press.

Fernando, S. (1991). *Mental health, race and culture.* London, England: MacMillan.

Fernando, S. (Ed.). (1995). *Mental health in a multi-ethnic society: A multidisciplinary handbook.* New York, NY: Routledge.

Fernando, S. (2002). *Mental health, race and culture* (2nd ed.). New York, NY: Palgrave.

Fernando, S. (2003). *Cultural diversity, mental health and psychiatry: The struggle against racism.* New York, NY: Routledge.

Fernando, S., & Keating, F. (2009). *Mental health in a multi-ethnic society: A multidisciplinary handbook* (2nd ed.). London, England: Routledge.

Foucault, M. (1967). *Madness and civilization: A history of insanity in the age of reason.* London, England: Tavistock.

Friedman, E. H. (1982). The myth of the shiksha. In M. McGoldrick, J. K. Pearce, & J. Giordano (Eds.), *Ethnicity and family therapy.* New York, NY: Guilford Press.

Fruggeri, L. (1992). Therapeutic process as the social construction of change. In S. McNamee & F. J. Gergen (Eds.), *Therapy as social construction* (pp. 40–53). San Diego, CA: Newbury Park.

Ghosh, R. (1994). Multicultural policy and social integration: South Asian Canadian women. *International Journal of Gender Studies, 1*(1), 49–68.

Gilroy, P. (2004). *Postcolonial melancholia.* New York, NY: Columbia University Press.

Goodman, A., Patel, V., & Leon, D. A. (2008). Child mental health differences amongst ethnic groups in Britain: A systematic review. *BMC Public Health, 8,* 258.

Guha, R., & Spivak, G. C. (Eds.). (1988). *Selected subaltern studies.* Oxford, England: Oxford University Press.

Guzder, J. (2011). Second skins: Family therapy agendas of migration, identity and cultural change. *Fokus: Pa Familien, 39*(3), 160–179.

Guzder, J., & Krishna, M. (1991). Sita-Shakti: Cultural paradigms for Indian women. *Transcultural Psychiatric Research Review, 28,* 257–301.

Guzder, J., & Krishna, M. (2005). Sita-Shakti@cultural collision: Issues in the psychotherapy of diaspora Indian women. In S. Akhtar (Ed.), *Freud along the Ganges: Psychoanalytic reflections on the people and culture of India* (pp. 205–233). New York, NY: Other Press.

Hickling, F. W. (2007). *Psychohistoriography: A postcolonial psychoanalytic and psychotherapeutic model.* Mona, UT: UWI Carimensa.

Holmes, D. E. (1992). Race and transference in psychoanalysis and psychotherapy. *The International Journal of Psychoanalysis, 73,* 1–11.

Jack, D. C., & Ali, A. (Eds.). (2010). *Silencing the self across cultures: Depression and gender in the social world.* Oxford, England: Oxford University Press.

Jafri, A. H. (2003). *Honour killing: Dilemma, ritual, understanding.* Karachi, Pakistan: Oxford University Press.

Kacker, L., Mohsin, N., Dixit, A., Varadan, S., & Kumar, P. (2007). *Study on child abuse: India, 2007.* New Delhi, India: Ministry of Women and Child Development, Government of India.

Kakar, S. (1982). *Shamans, mystics and doctors.* Delhi, India: Oxford University.

Kakar, S. (1989). The maternal-feminine in Indian psychoanalysis. *International Review of Psychoanalysis, 16*(3), 355–365.

Kakar, S. (1990). *Intimate relations: Exploring Indian sexuality.* New Delhi, India: Penguin Books.

Kakar, S. (1997). *Culture and the psyche.* New Delhi, India: Oxford University Press.

Kareem, J. (1992). The Nafsiyat intercultural therapy centre: Ideas and experience in intercultural therapy. In J. Kareem & R. Littlewood (Eds.), *Intercultural therapy: Themes, interpretations and practice* (pp. 14–37). Oxford, England: Blackwell Scientific.

Kirmayer, L. J. (2008). Empathy and alterity in cultural psychiatry. *Ethos, 38*(4), 457–474.

Kirmayer, L. J. (2012). Rethinking cultural competence. *Transcultural Psychiatry, 49*(2), 149–164.

Lau, A. (1995). Gender, power and relationships: Ethnocultural and religious issues. In C. Burke & B. Speed (Eds.), *Gender, power and relationships* (pp. 120–135). London, England: Routledge.

Leary, K. (2006). How race is lived in the consulting room. In K. White (Ed.), *Unmasking race, culture, and attachment in the psychoanalytic space.* London, England: Karnac.

Maiter, S., & Stalker, C. (2011). South Asian immigrants' experience of child protective services: Are we recognizing strengths and resilience? *Child and Family Social Work, 16*(2), 138–148.

Maiter, S., Stalker, C., & Alaggia, R. (2009). The experiences of minority immigrant families receiving child welfare services: Seeking to understand how to reduce risk and increase protective factors. *Families in Society, 90*(1), 28–36.

Maitra, B. (2006). Culture and the mental health of children. In S. Timimi & B. Maitra (Eds.), *Critical voices in child and adolescent mental health.* London, England: Free Associations Books.

Malat, J. R., van Ryn, M., & Purcell, D. (2006). Race, socioeconomic status, and the perceived importance of positive self-presentation in health care. *Social Science & Medicine, 62*(10), 2479–2488.

Malat, J., & Hamilton, M. A. (2006). Preference for same-race health care providers and perceptions of interpersonal discrimination in health care. *Journal of Heath and Social Behavior, 47*(2), 173–187.

Messent, P. (1992). Working with Bangladeshi families in the east end of London. *Journal of Family Therapy, 14*, 287–304.

Nandy, A. (1980). *At the edge of psychology: Essays on politics and culture.* Delhi, India: Oxford University.

Obeyesekere, G. (1990). *The work of culture: Symbolic transformations in pychoanalysis and anthropology.* Chicago, IL: University of Chicago Press.

Penn, M. L., & Nardos, R. (2003). Culture, traditional practices, and gender-based violence. In R. Nardos, M. K. Radpour, W. S. Hatcher, & M. L. Penn (Eds.), *Overcoming violence against women and girls: The international campaign to eradicate a worldwide problem.* New York, NY: Rowman & Littlefield.

Pillai, A., Patel, V., Cardozo, P., Goodman, R., Weiss, H. A., & Andrew, G. (2008). Non-traditional lifestyles and prevalence of mental disorders in adolescents in Goa, India. *The British Journal of Psychiatry, 192*(1), 45–51.

Pinderhughes, E. (1989). *Understanding race, ethnicity, and power: The key to efficacy in clinical practice.* New York, NY: Free Press.

Rahman, A., Ahmed, M., Sikander, S., Malik, A., Tomenson, B., & Creed, F. (2009). Young, single and not depressed: Prevalence of depressive disorder among young women in rural Pakistan. *Journal of Affective Disorders, 117*(1/2), 42–47.

Roland, A. (1991). *In search of self in India and Japan: Toward a cross-cultural psychology.* Princeton, NJ: Princeton University Press.

Said, E. (2003a). *Reflections on exile and other essays.* Cambridge, England: Harvard University Press.

Said, E. (2003b). *Freud and the non-European.* London, England: Verso.

Singla, R. (2005). South Asian youth in Scandinavia: Inter-ethnic and intergenerational relationships. *Psychology and Developing Societies, 17*, 217–235.

Sluzki, C. E. (1979). Migration and family conflict. *Family Process, 18*, 379–380.

Smith, J. D. (2009). *The mahabharata.* New Delhi, India: Penguin.

Spivak, G. C. (2006). *In other worlds: Essays on cultural politics.* New York, NY: Routledge.

Thapan, M. (1997). *Embodiment: Essays on gender and identity.* Calcutta, India: Oxford University Press.

Timimi, S., & Maitra, B. (2005). *Critical voices in child and adolescent mental health.* London, England: Free Associations Press.

Trawick, M. (1990). *Notes on love in a Tamil family.* Berkley, CA: University of California Press.

Tummala-Narra, P. (2004). Dynamics of race and culture in the supervisory encounter. *Psychoanalytic Psychotherapy, 21*(2), 300–311.

Tummala-Narra, P. (2005). Addressing political and racial terror in the therapeutic relationship. *The American Journal of Orthopsychiatry, 75*(1), 19–26.

Tummala-Narra, P. (2007). Skin colour and the therapeutic relationship. *Psychoanalytic Psychology, 24*(2), 255–270.

Uberoi, P. (1999). *Families, kinship and marriage in India.* Delhi, India: Oxford Press.

Williams, R. (1999). Cultural safety. *Australia and New Zealand Journal of Public Health, 23*(2), 213–214.

Winnicott, D. W. (1966). The location of cultural experience. *The International Journal of Psychoanalysis, 48*, 368–372.

Young-Bruehl, E. (1996). *The anatomy of prejudice.* Cambridge, England: Harvard University Press.

Zelkowitz, P., Schinazi, J., Katofsky, L., Saucier, J. F., Valenzuela, M., Westreich, R., et al. (2004). Factors associated with depression in pregnant immigrant women. *Transcultural Psychiatry, 41*(4), 445–464.

Community Consultation and Mediation with Racialized and Marginalized Minorities

Shirlette Wint

This chapter documents the process of mediation with ethnocultural communities in public and private spaces. It examines how communities construct and use community and institutional networks to support their social identities and cope with crises in individuals or within the group. I will describe the salient concepts that inform and shape my community consultation and mediation practice and present strategies for successful mediation work with ethnic communities that protect and support cultural heritage. The consultation approach is illustrated with examples of communities effectively negotiating both "non-dominant" and "dominant" cultural resources in their interactions with mainstream sites of services. I will also draw from my collaboration in research studies of the experience of racialized minorities and my work as a culture broker for the CCS.

The last 30 years have been taxing for community activism in North America, with severe cutbacks in social programs and increased poverty among the urban poor. Within this landscape of social disparity, I have worked towards developing tools in clinical practice that can assist individuals and groups with a history of marginalization in self-development and solidifying their often contested identities. The modern and postmodern struggles of marginalized groups have largely coalesced around economic issues, and equal service and representation in the public spheres of government, health, and politics. Moreover, in Canada, there has been a shift in ethnic community development, from a focus on social class and economy to a focus on *multiculturalism* and *cultural competency*. Unfortunately, this shift has occurred at a time when ethnocultural communities are being pressured to assume more of the responsibility to address social problems within their communities, with local and federal governments holding them accountable to resolve these issues on their own with minimal intervention and support.

Though my practice is not limited to one particular group, a large proportion concerns itself with finding ways to bring about collective and individual transformation among marginalized individuals and groups in Montreal's metropolitan region. Often these group and individuals—be they Indigenous, Afro-Canadians, immigrants, gays and lesbians, single parents, or sex trade workers—are struggling with the futility of trying to compel governments and social institutions to recognize them as whole and authentic. As a psychotherapist and cultural consultant for the last 20 years, I have employed a wide range of experiences in the fields of social work, elementary education, community mental health, and community action research to evaluate and find creative solutions to complex social problems.

The underlying principle behind this work is the belief that fundamentally, each individual has

S. Wint, M.S.W. (✉)
88 Rue Charlotte #1108, Montreal, QC,
Canada H2X 4E2
e-mail: swint67@hotmail.com

L.J. Kirmayer et al. (eds.), *Cultural Consultation: Encountering the Other in Mental Health Care,*
International and Cultural Psychology, DOI 10.1007/978-1-4614-7615-3_9,
© Springer Science+Business Media New York 2014

an innate need and desire to experience a sense of belonging in the society in which they live and that when this need and desire goes unfulfilled, the individual or group is left with a sense of marginalization and emotional distress. It follows then that those who find themselves marginalized may need assistance to achieve better social integration and a sense of belonging in civic society (Merton, 1978; Taylor, 1994). In this approach to clinical practice, the client may be an individual, family, or community. Healing or transformation is achieved in a variety of ways, through group workshops, individual consultations, and working collectively with other community organizations, churches, or government agencies. The collaborative work with other community systems during the treatment process is designed to result in a transformative experience for both individual and group. In several instances, there has been a trickle down or spillover of therapeutic benefits to the larger society, particularly when art and culture are used as vehicles of communication in psychosocial interventions in community settings.

Often the first step in working with the marginalized is to convince the individual or group that they must become visible to themselves regardless of whether the dominant structures of the society recognize them as such. Concrete ways of accomplishing this task are through assisting the client in seeing the abundance of riches of knowledge, history, and tradition that exist in their own cultural group and helping them recognize how their community has contributed to the larger society. When community interventions are successful, the group is able to embrace the past, see progress, and view the future with optimism and agency rather than seeing themselves only as voiceless victims. This last point is essential: the majority of youth and adults who experience identity crises and who are seen in community organizations for mental health problems come from families where clarity about the internal and external forces of oppression is significantly lacking in their everyday interactions with family and other close relations. Knowing that they are constantly under the gaze of the dominant society impacts on how Blacks or other racialized minorities go about developing aspirations, how they formulate their

hopes and expectations, and how they conform to or reject specific social norms. Consciousness of always being under the gaze of the other also impacts on marginalized individuals' capacity to take a critical distance from their lived experiences (Frankenberg, 1997). In therapeutic work, it is evident that consciousness of oppression sometimes limits the individual's ability to express feelings and develop effective strategies for living including the use of irony, conceptual experimentation, and creative transgression.

Regardless of the setting and the problem, a common goal in most clinical work with marginalized minority communities is that participants will benefit from a transformative process that leaves them feeling that they belong to a larger community, the human community, which encourages them to reach beyond the borders of their own cultures of origin when searching for solutions in times of crisis.

This approach to community consultation and mediation might be termed *transculturality*. This term is an apt metaphor for my practice since it evokes the movement from one social position and worldview to another that is the focus of cultural consultation. The consultant also embodies movement in that professional itinerancy is intrinsic to working with marginalized communities who often do not have the infrastructure or budget to hire full time professionals. More importantly, movement often begins with the client's migration from one country to another, from a small rural region to a big city, from a homogeneous community to one with a diversity of cultures, or from a poor heterogeneous inner-city neighborhood to a more homogeneous suburban community. Although the majority of migrations are successful, when coupled with social adaptation difficulties, the experience can be extremely difficult for some groups and individuals.

In most contemporary urban centers, individuals have experiences with cultural difference and diversity on a daily basis, on public transportation on the way to work, at the grocery store, in interactions with their children's caretakers, at the bank, in church, and so on. Similarly, nearly everyone is inhabited by multiple cultural beliefs and practices, some from their own cultural background, others from the diverse cultures that they negotiate and transact with every day and which they use more or less unconsciously when appropriate. Whatever its developmental roots, one's identity is constructed over a lifetime and is not fixed or stagnant but renegotiated and transformed as difference is encountered. Although these encounters are determined largely by social forces beyond the individual, the texture and outcome of such encounters remain the responsibility of each individual as an active participant in a pluralistic society.

Through acculturation, the individual and group embody cultural responses that become second nature and that can be sources of strength and support during times of crisis. The aim of community consultation and mediation in mental health is to recognize and exploit this cultural capital to address mental health problems. Of course, in everyday life, many marginalized groups do this very well and deal with common mental health problems on their own or with resources of the family and community. They consult mainstream systems for diagnosis and treatment when they have especially puzzling or serious health problems or when ordinary remedies and solutions prove inadequate and the problem persists. As a result, by the time people arrive for consultation in the mental health system, they have their own ideas of what may be wrong and what is likely to be helpful. Sometimes, the mental health practitioner's diagnosis is contested because the client has a different interpretation of the problem or they have multiple concerns and feel that the issue that the mainstream system has identified as the focus of treatment is not the primary problem or priority. This is illustrated by work with a mothers' group in an inner-city neighborhood in Montreal.

Case Vignette 10-1

I was contracted by a community center for women to provide individual and group consultation to 12 mothers with an average age of 28, the oldest being 42 and the youngest 14 years old. Most of the mothers were without partners. Several had histories of violent, abusive relationships with the fathers of their children. The meetings were held at the center twice per week, with one day devoted to a 2-h group meeting and the second day for individual consultation. The goal was to help strengthen participants' life skills through group and individual counselling. The group selected topics of interest, which included overcoming poor self-image, clarifying needs and wants, becoming assertive, anger management control, conflict resolution, and healing emotional wounds. Most of the mothers were born in the Caribbean or South Asia. A few had early African-Canadian ancestry, tracing their history to the first slaves brought to Canada rather than more recent migration from the Caribbean.

When I had been working with the mothers for about 6 months providing group and individual consultations, one of the mothers, a 42-year-old woman of Caribbean origin and mother of 4 went through a very difficult period with her ex-partner who had tried to strangle her. During my individual and group work with her, it became apparent that she was experiencing some cognitive difficulties which had led to other problems related to housing, finances, and parenting. Her distress was apparent to the other group participants who tried to support her by normalizing her feelings and encouraging her to talk about her situation. Working closely with the client and the workers of the community organization, we tried unsuccessfully to get the client to recognize that she was showing signs of cognitive dysfunction. While the client accepted the support and accompaniment regarding her physical health, she seemed indifferent to our concern regarding her mental health. We concluded that because the client perceived herself as occupying an already marginalized role in her family, she did not want to add the stigma of a mental disorder to an already very long list of problems. While she smiled and listened to

(continued)

our concerns, she showed no desire to follow-up with an evaluation with a psychiatrist. Eventually the client was successfully treated for a gynecological problem, but staff at the community center continued to have concerns for her mental health. She had mentioned to several workers that she was afraid to take money from the automatic bank machine for fear that she was being followed. As a result, she often did not have enough money to buy groceries to adequately feed her four children. Knowing that her ex-partner had followed her in the past, we did not entirely dismiss her fears. However, when the complaints began to intensify, the director consulted with the client's sister who confirmed that the client had a history of odd behavior but stated that it was "nothing to worry about". The client had no history of alcohol or substance abuse. She had not finished high school but had no intellectual disability.

I worked with the director of the center to devise an intervention plan that provided necessary support to the client in a way that did not stigmatize or alienate her. The plan recognized the client's strength, notably her care and attentiveness for the well-being of her children. Even on very cold and wet days, she travelled across town to bring her 2-year-old son to his play group and participate in the center's group for mothers. The intervention plan consisted of a worker from the center accompanying the client to the bank once a month to ensure that she withdrew enough money to buy a month's groceries for her family. (Monies from Social Welfare were deposited into the client's account once per month.) The support of the local community health center (CLSC) was also enlisted to monitor the client's progress through home visits. The home visits helped to structure the client in how she carried out parental tasks and eventually helped to decrease symptoms of anxiety and paranoia.

In community consultations, it is in the area of mental illness that ambivalence or resistance to treatment is most apparent. The most common problems involve adjustment disorders accompanied by somatic symptoms that may be difficult to diagnose or treat. Historically marginalized groups, including women and immigrants, may shield emotional distress behind undiagnosed and complex physical ailments (Leccia, 2008; Ton & Lim, 2006; Whitley, Kirmayer, & Groleau, 2006a, 2006b). Dissatisfied by the response of the medical system, they look to alternative sources for healing. In African, Caribbean, and Indigenous cultures, nearly every form of food is thought to have medicinal value. Until recently, in urban settings, special efforts were needed to obtain the "natural" medicines needed for self-treatment. In today's global culture, health food stores with a range of food, herbal, and other remedies can be found in nearly every neighborhood in North America communities. While the diagnosis determined by biomedical practitioners may not be contested, for many people, there is comfort in the "creolization" of treatment, combining elements from different traditions in new ways. Multiple treatments may be used at the same time reflecting what makes most sense and seems to be most helpful for the patient (Lim, 2006). The cultural consultation work at the CCS supports this approach, as illustrated by this excerpt from one of cases in which I acted as a culture broker.

Case Vignette 10-2

Ms. Brown was a 44-year-old Black woman of Caribbean origin who was a refugee claimant, referred to the CCS by her treating physician. She also had a young son who had been placed in foster care by Youth Protection during her hospitalization and treatment and having her son return home depended on her getting well. She had been previously hospitalized and diagnosed with a psychotic disorder. At the time of hospitalization she was delusional and aggressive with auditory hallucinations. During the CCS interview, Ms. Brown

(continued)

expressed concern about the appropriateness of her past treatment. She did not see how the medication that her doctor had prescribed could really help her. She thought that it might alleviate some of her stress but did not believe it would cure an illness that had been caused by someone "working Voodoo" on her. She felt that only a spiritual healer could provide effective treatment by confronting the person responsible for making her ill. Her ideas that healers can manipulate the forces of nature and influence ordinary outcomes in everyday life were consistent with her cultural background. She had clear ideas about what would be necessary for her treatment, including structured fasting, meditation, and prayer officiated by someone who had understood the process of counterbalancing the workings of evil with good. Ms. Brown described how her mother had recovered from a similar situation with similar strategies.

Before coming up with a cultural model that met the needs of the patient, the CCS team and I, as the culture broker, worked closely with Ms. Brown to develop an appropriate treatment plan that included the resources she identified as potentially helpful for her healing. That included reaching out to the pastor of her church. As she began to feel more secure, I suggested that she be linked to community resources to provide her with a supportive social network by connecting her to a women's group that had several members of Caribbean origin. The community organization also provided her with a place to have supervised visits and reconnect with her son who had been placed in foster care by a Youth Protection mandate while she was hospitalized.

This vignette underlines some recurring factors in working with individuals from marginalized groups: the need to maintain control (hence the

efforts to involve Ms. Brown in her treatment plan) and a reluctance to discuss past trauma with a preference to focus on concrete ideas and current tasks. Given appropriate and consistent support, many clients prefer to solve problems on their own. In this particular case, however, my knowledge of community resources enabled me to help the CCS team identify a community group that was the right match for the patient's needs. In addition, my sharing some cultural symbols of identity with the patient such as race, ethnicity, gender, and being a fellow immigrant likely facilitated a therapeutic alliance and encouraged the patient's investment in treatment and healing.

Immigrants and refugees migrate from their places of origin with spiritual and religious beliefs that can be a source of support during periods of stress as well as providing a language through which they articulate their concerns. In this case, Ms. Brown referred to "Voodoo", a term that has become common across Caribbean Canadian communities for referencing any kind of magical belief. Ms. Brown knew that the culture broker would understand her use of this term, which served to convey her desire for spiritual or religious treatment. In revealing to the team how she wanted to be treated, Ms. Brown also was indicating that she had inner resources that could be tapped to develop a treatment plan that included conventional psychiatric treatment. The consultation team made it clear to Ms. Brown that they respected her cultural competence and knowledge about her illness and came to an agreement with her that allowed her to use both conventional and nontraditional modalities, sometimes simultaneously. Ms. Brown acknowledged the benefits of having her symptoms of psychosis reduced with medication, but she also cited the benefits of having individual prayer sessions with her pastor.

Marginalization, Cultural Identity, and Choice of Adaptive Strategies

Two decades of working first with Africans of the Diaspora, first in New York City and then in Montreal, have led me to believe that many of the mental health disorders that trouble this group are rooted in their response to racism and can be defined by what Frantz Fanon (1967), more than 40 years ago, termed a condition of 'wounded consciousness'. Fanon suggested that Blacks, as a social group, are at risk for difficulties in social adaptation which can lead to mental illness unless they free themselves from the subjugation of their identity by images provided by the colonizers, and reinvent more satisfactory images for themselves. Fanon wrote that Blacks exhibited a "neurotic personality" and attributed this to a collective awareness of a common experience of oppression and a shared history of colonization and slavery. Healing was possible through a collective catharsis in which collective aggression could be channelled. Though Fanon's thesis was grounded in the experience of marginalization of Blacks of the Diaspora, elements of this predicament fit the experience of other ethnocultural minorities and racialized groups in Canadian society. Taylor (1994), for example, argued that other cultural minorities struggle and succeed in Canadian society despite "an image of inferiority" perpetuated by the dominant culture which maintains a paternalistic relationship with cultural minorities.

Some of the ways that the phenomenon of "wounded consciousness" plays out in contemporary Canadian society are illustrated in the reflections of Dawn, an immigrant from the USA, who I interviewed for a study on the subjective well-being of Black Canadians. At the time of the study, Dawn was working as a physician at a Montreal hospital. Based on the discriminatory treatment she received from her peers and subordinates, she was convinced that racism flourished in her hospital because of institutional collusion. She was dissatisfied with her work arrangements but believed that she had to continue putting in 6-day work weeks because if she stopped, her White colleagues would consider her lazy. Over time she had become so discouraged with her experience of unequal treatment that she decided to distance herself from the subordinated identity associated with "Blackness". She commented:

> I cannot imagine the day when any society will not promote fair over dark. Yeah that's right. I don't know how it started but if we look in fairytales the princess was White, the witch was Black. I don't know how that started but I don't think that it will ever stop. I am reluctant to label myself as Black — why be associated with a negative stereotype? (Wint, 2000, p. 82)

Dawn's response to racism and exclusion involved knowing how to "play the game" and fit into the dominant mainstream culture. She was able to pursue this solution because of her professional accomplishments. For others, however, fitting in may not be an option because they lack the appropriate background or social status. Bourdieu (1977) suggests that a lack of "cultural capital" accounts for why some Blacks and other marginalized groups who do not come from "high status origins" do poorly in school and the work place. Some immigrant children and minorities from disadvantaged backgrounds may not have the "sophisticated vocabularies and precise information about how school [and mainstream society] work" (Plaza, 1996, p. 246) that Dawn used to navigate through university and professional training.

> When I was in university, I socialized with mainstream White students, and asked questions of professors. I banked on them remembering me for having made extra effort when it came time to distribute grades. Other Black students remained aloof and did not ask professors to clarify concepts they did not understand for fear of being labeled ignorant by what they perceived to be racist professors. Also, they did not mix with other White students but studied among themselves. In my view, they contributed to their own limitations by not increasing the pool of students with different strengths in their study group. Consequently, they did not always do well on exams. When you get to higher levels of education, all the concepts you need to learn are not written in books. The way you gather the information is by associating with your peers. A lot of times, I didn't get the answers, but you don't develop your ideas in isolation. You develop your ideas through interaction. (Wint, 2000, p. 53)

Dawn's strategies attempted to address some of the psychological challenges that come from prevalent stereotypes of Black and other racialized minority groups (Steele, 2010).

Although Africans of the Diaspora face similar challenges to identity formation as a result of racism and resultant social exclusion, their attitudes to this predicament and coping strategies are diverse. They also differ in the emphasis they place on racial affiliation as an aspect of their identity. However, most share a collective history of "enforced subordination and oppression" (Eyerman, 2004). For these reasons, clinical assessment and treatment must consider the level and degree to which particular forms of marginalization are currently affecting the well-being of the individual or group.

The pervasive experiences of racism in everyday life and their effects on identity influence help-seeking and treatment expectations. Many individuals in Montreal's Black communities do not perceive themselves as having ready access to tools or resources that could enhance their overall well-being. As a result, they expect that their personal goals and aspirations will likely not be met and their happiness not achieved. The need to have these basic expectations recognized and understood is one reason that patients may desire ethnic-specific treatment when possible (Wint, 2000).

The struggle for emotional integration and social belonging is as much a preoccupation for the group as it is for the individual. In Montreal, focus group research with parents and youths aged 14–18 of both genders from Caribbean and Filipino origins examined how their perspectives changed over time through their participation in groups that explored problem solving, building community alliance, strengthening school and group alliances, and developing a sense of connectedness to the dominant host culture. The focus groups took place in community centers and churches in Montreal. The study concluded that participants expressed pessimism and a reluctance to use mainstream sites of services to facilitate their integration into Quebec society (Measham & Wint, 2007). Participants could not envision a "harmonious integration" (Diener, 1984) or fulfillment of their life goals in Quebec society. Youth participants in particular, described severe marginalization and expected to confront further obstacles. Consequently, they tended to suppress their goals and desires, diminishing their chances to achieve well-being (Diener, 1984). While lowering their goals and expectations might be interpreted as an adaptive strategy, protecting youth from disappointment, if continued into adult-hood, the result is a widening of the gap between immigrant youth and their counterparts in mainstream society. Rather than contributing to well-being, therefore, this self-handicapping creates more opportunities for disappointment, frustration, and failures for the individual and the marginalized group.

In community consultation, many of the clients that I encounter share similar backgrounds associated with lowered expectations and self-exclusion from mainstream society that aggravate their social marginalization and economic poverty. Research suggests that some ethnic minorities that have experienced racial discrimination may choose to underachieve academically because they do not perceive themselves as having equal access to the dominant forms of social capital needed for success (Carter, 2003). Thus, "many African American students may lower their academic aspirations, believing that high achievement will only benefit 'White', middle class students" (Carter, 2003, p. 137). The negative impact of common stereotypes may also function as cognitive biases outside of awareness (Steele, 2010).

Similar patterns of avoidance and self-defeat may occur in other domains. For example, young adults needing psychological support may hesitate to approach mainstream service providers in schools, clinics, or hospitals, worried that they will not receive a culturally sensitive response. In these cases, the individual or group is so immersed in their chosen or imposed identity associated with marginalization that they are unable to reach out for necessary treatment and support. In *The Nature of Prejudice* (1954/1979), psychologist Gordon Allport argued that individuals and groups prefer to confirm their prejudices about others who are different from them rather than revise their thinking. This conservatism applies to the targets of prejudice as well as to those who practice racist discrimination. This tendency to find evidence to confirm our prejudices persists even when the group disproves the stereotype. Allport maintained that, in the end, it does not matter how many times the individual or group dispels a commonly held perception of themselves, the assumptions about the devalued group remain intact. Toni Morrison wrote that "among

Europeans and the Europeanized, this shared process of exclusion—of assigning designation and value—has led to the popular and academic notion that racism is a 'natural', if irritating phenomena" (Morrison, 1992, p. 7).

While Allport was primarily looking at the damaging effects of prejudice on African-Americans, a similar process may affect other marginalized groups' perception of mainstream individuals and institutions, including health services. Groups that have experienced repeated exclusion tend to view dominant systems as intractable, and this may prevent them from benefiting from needed care when it is available. Stereotyping at its worst robs the individual and the group of their identities and reinforces false beliefs that can have costly and detrimental consequences for the group (Steele, 2010).

One might ask if groups find mainstream cultural institution so lacking in sensitivity, why do they not simply seek out the services in their own cultural communities? Unfortunately, the demand for culturally sensitive service far outweighs the supply of health institutions with well-developed programs addressing the needs of cultural minorities. In addition, there are not enough trained mental health professionals from marginalized cultural communities to serve and outreach to these minority groups. In general, stereotypes continue to dominate in health and other major institutions even after they have been reduced in academia, religious, political, and economic institutions that have been complicit or silent about the perpetuation of racism in the past. By networking and creating alliances with community organizations, churches, and some medical clinics in ethnic diverse neighborhoods, practitioners can mitigate the impact of marginalization.

The ambivalence of marginalized communities towards using mainstream services to treat their psychic distress is due mostly to concerns that they may not be received and treated with sufficient care and respect. They may believe that someone who looks like them is more likely to understand their everyday experience and address their clinical problems or predicaments. They may also fear that if they open themselves up to influences of the dominant culture they will be assimilated or absorbed into that more powerful group and lose their collective identity. Though Canadian society in the twenty-first century is becoming less ethnocentric and more pluralistic, marginalized ethnic minorities may still feel great apprehension about their ability to preserve individual and collective self-determination (Kymlicka, 1998; Leonard, 1997; Taylor, 1994).

Having worked both in marginalized and mainstream community settings, it is clear to me that the reluctance of some cultural minorities to use mainstream institutions is not due to a lack of awareness of available services. Rather, their infrequent and selective use of mainstream services reflects deeply held concerns about how they will be dealt with. When they have the opportunity to voice their feelings in a safe setting, many express the fear that they will be treated in a racist manner. Formal and informal discussions with community leaders in the Caribbean, Haitian, and Filipino communities support this impression. These leaders have also expressed a great deal of frustration and anger at being further disempowered when they protest about unequal treatment to agents of the dominant institutions and find that their complaints are dismissed or they are accused of being "overly sensitive" or, still worse, "playing the race card". Encounters such as these produce an intercultural impasse, exacerbating current myths, stereotypes, and biases, segregating groups and rendering the process of coping with mental illness or other psychic distress more difficult. It is particularly difficult to raise issues of racism and inequality when they are embedded in institutional practices. Referring to such institutionalized racism, Elliot and Fleras (1992, p. 336) write: "this type of racism is impersonal, unconscious, unintentional, and covert… and is the consequence of seemingly neutral rules, policies, or procedures that establish its distinctive character." Ruth Frankenberg (1997, p. 3) notes that such institutional dominance typically is "rationalized, legitimized, and made ostensibly normal and natural."

Recognizing structural and systemic forms of racism requires an awareness of larger social processes. When perceptions of inequality and injustice are dismissed as evidence of hypersensitivity or a "culture of victimization", it becomes difficult for individuals and groups to identify and talk about their experiences of structural violence and everyday micro-aggression (Sue et al., 2007). Not being able to define and name racist and discriminatory acts when they are recurrent intensifies the psychological marginalization of minorities and makes it more difficult to develop productive and positive strategies for opposing social exclusion. In Western countries, the groups most often silenced by such dismissal are peoples of African descent, Indigenous peoples, gays and lesbians, and the poor.

Resolving racially charged situations when integration is the only imagined outcome presents seemingly insurmountable challenges, particularly when integration is defined as a one-sided process of submission to the dominant "White" culture. "What integration has meant for many Whites is that Blacks [and other non-Whites] had to interact with them on their own terms. Not only do many [Whites] not want to participate in other cultures, but they feel theirs is *the* culture" (Wein, 1992, p. 92). This is the current state of affairs in many North American urban cities and describes the climate in which many marginalized groups are trying to find place and space for themselves in mainstream societies.

In an interview for a study on the links between racism and the subjective well-being of Black Canadians, Joan a Caribbean-born, middle-class mother and business woman described her understanding and difficulty identifying racism when it appears.

> …because racism when it is presented, it is in such a covert way, it is something you feel and sometimes you question your feelings…I think people hesitate because others might think that it is your crutch to getting that advancement on the job. I think Blacks have a tendency to second guess themselves and ask "Am I really seeing what I am seeing? Am I really feeling what I'm feeling? Am I being paranoid? Let's give it another chance." That's probably why [Black] people don't come out and say "*racism*". (Wint, 2000, pp. 67–68)

In this climate of ethnic and cultural divides, it is imperative that mainstream institutions rise to the challenge of meeting the community health care and other service needs of our diverse population. It is important that these institutions are successful in their endeavours because it is often within these settings that people from different cultures meet for the first time, with a common concern and seriousness of purpose. Hospitals, community medical clinics, schools, and social service settings provide opportunities for people to enter into dialogue and construct new paradigms based on authentic expression and exchange of their experiences. The outcome of these first encounters may determine whether or not an individual or group will feel excluded or work towards integration into the larger Canadian society.

Negotiating Community Relationships: The Consultant as Insider and Outsider

Though my field of practice includes diverse marginalized groups, the position from which I practice is influenced by my racialized identity, ethnicity, class, gender, and political values—all of which make me sensitive or less responsive to specific issues that may come up during community consultation and mediation. As an Afro-Caribbean professional consulting with a wide range of individuals from Montreal's Afro-Canadian communities, I am mindful of the need for critical self-reflection in my work. In contemporary society, ideas, allegiances, and identities are influenced by immigration and globalization of economies and cultures. As a result, one cannot always recognize the extent to which one's cultural identity is the product of individual efforts at self-fashioning or reflects wider currents. When working with Black clients who interpret and make meaning of their social worlds in racial terms, there is an acute awareness that I too am governed by White dominance which impacts on the very language I speak and the clinical concepts I use. Unlike many of my clients, however, I look for meaning not in racialized constructs but in the emerging process of creolization that is shaping the global framework (Bibeau, 1997). This perspective allows me to seek out best practice models and to confront my own biases and hesitations regarding assumptions about racialized identities and transactions insofar as they influence cultural models for interpreting the lived experiences or the experience of collective trauma of marginalized groups.

Mental health interveners do not enter the therapeutic space with a tabula rasa. Moreover, each encounter presents potential barriers and opportunities for a successful alliance that will promote the well-being of the individual or the group. Generally, sharing the same background and cultural affiliation as clients helps the processes of building an alliance, assessment, and subsequent mediation and resolution of personal or group conflict. However, there are times when clients have experienced so many traumas that they have become deeply suspicious of outsiders and resist efforts to explore areas that they feel are the private domain of the group. Additional time and care should be taken during evaluation of these clients, knowing that they may be reluctant to provide information about occupation, place of employment, or the nature of their illness experience or past medical treatment. Frequently, the reluctance to divulge personal information is related to fear about confidentiality despite reassurance. At other times, this reticence is simply normal behavior for the individual who is a member of a cultural community where secrets are considered necessary for survival and maintained through harsh social sanctions from one generation to the next. The sanctions against disclosure of collective secrets or private knowledge can go as far as ostracism from family and group. This practice creates an "us and them" relationship with the consultant, host country, and to some extent even with other ethnic minorities that share racial affiliation. There is an implicit agreement in some minority groups that they can never entirely trust the Other. This has been particularly evident in my work with clients from Haitian and Indigenous communities, who may be unwilling to name names or places, evading inquiry or providing vague responses. A member of the Haitian community who has travelled and lived in many urban communities commented, "as soon as you unmask a Haitian person another mask takes its place". Evidence of distrust similarly restricts the helping process when working as a cultural broker within the CCS process. At such times

because of the initial wariness of the patient, the fact that the cultural broker shares a common background with the patient does not always break down barriers of resistance to what the patient may perceive as intrusive and unsolicited relationships. These barriers are easier to address in one-to-one interviews with the patient than when working with a multidisciplinary team or group consultation. In the one-to-one interview, patients also may be more likely to use cultural terms or colloquialisms to describe their experiences and concerns. With a team, on the other hand, there may be greater opportunity to pay close attention to body language and it may be easier to ask the patient for clarification.

While secrecy and distrust are understandable survival strategies and must be negotiated during the period of building the therapeutic alliance, they become especially challenging when treatment depends on individuals' capacity to examine painful collective experiences that remain difficult to articulate or "taboo" in their cultural communities. In the case of Africans of the Diaspora, where the public portrayal of the individual's cultural group often has been negative and they feel they have been unfairly judged, there may be great reluctance to risk repeating the experience in therapy even when the therapist is Black. This is a daunting position for second-generation Afro-Canadian immigrants who cannot even claim to have directly experienced a traumatic event, even though they manifest the symptoms of trauma, which DeGruy-Leary (2005) has come to describe as "post traumatic slave syndrome" among African-Americans. Slavery and colonization are no longer active institutions in North American but they continue to inform collective identity. However, these experiences are different for different individuals and groups within the African Diaspora.

Self-disclosure may be problematic for marginalized individuals who suffer from social isolation and do not habitually share their inner thoughts and feelings with anyone. When lack of self-disclosure impedes the clinical relationship, rather than viewing the client as uncooperative, the professional often can move the process forward by reevaluating with the individual, family, or group their therapeutic goals and treatment.

For example, when a young Haitian client declined to divulge information about her community, this posture brought to mind the conflicts within and between Afro-Canadian communities, divided by geographic location, cultural practice, religion, and language. Although these groups share a similar history of slavery, their contemporary experiences, including their migration trajectories and subsequent reception, have been different. A White consultant may not know about the tensions between Francophone Haitians and Anglophone Caribbean Blacks and may not recognize the nuances that go into building trust and forming alliances between these groups. Some theorists have invoked the concept of internalized oppression to explain why members of an oppressed group may come to have negative views of others like themselves (Freire, 1973). If these issues are not openly discussed, they can become major obstacles to sharing scarce resources and working together to achieve some level of empowerment and critical consciousness.

Given the segregated social spaces and experiences in North American communities, a White professional may have little knowledge of Black culture and may therefore tend to view the Black client in terms of mass-media stereotypes. To date, working through the issues of racism remains underdeveloped in the training of most mental health professionals. As a result, stereotypes in the clinical context often go unchallenged. This is especially so for psychotherapists and psychoanalysts in private practice, where the prevailing attitude seems to be "that an individual pays for a service and is free to choose to leave, or to remain, depending on the way they view the quality of the service" (Thomas, 1999, p. 146).

Defensiveness is almost always a part of the therapeutic relationship with marginalized individuals who perceive their problems as stemming from external sources. The resistance encountered in the clinical encounter is often greater when working with vulnerable groups than with the general population. There is more of a tendency to externalize and blame problems on the external world, "the system" "institutional racism", and so on. There is also an inclination to be reactive and quick to defend the individual and the group against what is perceived as general rejection

from dominant institutions. In such situations, the consultant must be ready to absorb the hostility and suspicion that clients may direct towards them. I can usually tell from a client's body language that they do not expect me to support them in their interpretation of the problem. It is as if the clinician is being placed on trial and will most definitely be found guilty. At such moments, the interaction can be helped along if the professional can bring attitudes of humility, respect, empathy, and compassion to the encounter. An effective response from the professional validates the client's feelings while firmly but gently reminding the client of his or her therapeutic goals, which are usually to learn more effective coping strategies even when faced with events that are largely beyond their control.

Pride occupies a huge place when working with clients of Caribbean, Haitian, and African heritage, especially first- and second-generation immigrants. As a result, some individuals may present clinically as reserved, closed, or passive. Many middle-aged Caribbean women show a kind of stoicism as if they take pride in not showing any vulnerability. They may reveal that no one really knows them and what they are really feeling. Often these individuals have suffered a great deal of loss, including failed relationships, those left behind in the migration process, and the unmet expectations of full integration into Canadian society. These issues are common among immigrants from different backgrounds and may be reinforced by particular cultural or religious values. Thus, in reference to working with Vietnamese families, Axelson (1999, p. 449) writes that:

> restraint of personal feelings and unwillingness to disclose personal problems or to reveal emotions will work against traditional counselling goals of self-disclosure. Therefore, openness as a basis of understanding and talking out problems in a traditional counselling process will not be possible to the same degree as with most culturally assimilated Americans.

For this reason, it may be very difficult to get these individuals to participate in group therapy due to their fear of verbalizing feelings and confronting others. Successful interventions rely heavily on the consultant's ability to help individuals reinterpret their history in ways that give them a more positive view of past experiences and future prospects. This must be done in parallel with efforts to help them deal with psychic pain, while attending to other situational stressors such as finding jobs, improving academic performance, obtaining health care, and building relationships with others that will improve their quality of life.

External social determinants should be acknowledged as probable causes of clients' difficulties, but if these are the only contributors recognized, then an impasse may rapidly develop. Individuals must be encouraged to explore other contributors to their difficulties. If the consultant stays stuck in generalities, the client will likely follow suit. This holds true for the CCS model of intervention, which involves time-limited consultation with one or two encounters with the patient. Generally the approach that works best in this situation explicitly asks the patient for their collaboration in an effort to understand the clinical problem and assist them in finding appropriate resources to address their own specific issues and concerns.

While racial or cultural differences between client and consultant can influence the process of assessment and intervention outcome, so can other social dimensions such as class, gender, and sexual orientation. The following three vignettes illustrate diverse roles that culture plays in the consulting and mediation process.

Case Vignette 10-3

James was a 21-year-old Black male of Caribbean origin. During the 5 years he had lived in Canada, he has suffered cruel treatment repeatedly from a relative who had helped him to settle in Canada. Despite the abusive treatment received by the patient from his relative, he spoke of her as someone towards whom he bore "no ill will". He was not evasive but he did not show any eagerness to reveal information about the relative that had treated him badly. It was clear that he felt a certain loyalty to her.

In some patterns of migration, immigrants may be received initially by a "hub household", which provides shelter and support while they get their footing in the new society. As Bashi (1997) has described, however, some immigrants have ambivalent feelings towards the hub household (or host family) while feeling indebted to the larger hub network as a whole. This sense of indebtedness may prevent the patient from voicing anger towards the hub household. Bashi also noted that receiving immigrants sometimes exerts pressure on a new immigrant; the newcomer will comply with unreasonable requests because they do not want to be perceived as ungrateful back home. As a result, they will be reluctant to "betray" the hub household even when that relative is cruel and makes unreasonable demands that threaten their well-being.

Case Vignette 10-4

Mary was a middle-class, middle-aged Black woman of West Indian origin who was referred by her treating psychiatrist. Her presenting problems were physical and emotional difficulties related to her marriage. She described preferring a Black therapist in private practice as opposed to using the public mental health systems fearing that workers in those systems would apply stereotypical generalizations, labels, and prescriptions. After several sessions, Mary mentioned that her husband was under a "spell" put on him by his mistress. She did not elaborate but admitted to having consulted someone who "knew about these things" before coming to see me. I did not pressure her for further clarification because I knew that individuals of West Indian origin, particularly first-generation immigrants, often look for magical explanation in times of crisis or mental disorganization; usually this type of explanation is considered in parallel with an ongoing search for other explanations and sources of help. I allowed Mary to determine how much to explore this magical explanation for what had happened

(continued)

to her. As it turned out, she was more interested in developing a deeper understanding of the complexities of her marriage and how she had come to view herself as victimized and powerless.

Being able to recognize to what extent the client shares the traditional cultural values of the group and where there is acceptance of dominant society values can be key to successful interventions and engagement between individual and professional. A clinician more interested in the exotic might have placed an unnecessary focus on Mary's nontraditional and non-Western belief systems. The resultant intervention would have approached Mary's problems as being due to external forces, and this might have reinforced her sense of disempowerment and prevented her from working through the issues she was facing in her marriage.

Insider/Outsider: Black Therapist/ Black Client

Since I work in the area of cultural and community mediation, I expect and welcome Black clients who seek a Black psychotherapist. The process of working through presupposes that the professional is able to face the challenge of resisting the powerful countertransference issues that arise when a Black patient expresses self-hatred, without becoming either overly nurturing or rejecting (Kareem & Littlewood, 2000). Some Black patients, when they discover the professional is Black, may unconsciously expect unprofessional and inferior treatment, which can create tension in the first encounter. This negative expectation may be revealed in expressions of surprise when the encounter unfolds in a professional manner as indicated by comments like: "I didn't know what to expect" and "you're so professional." Although the process of building trust and rapport may be accelerated when client and consultant share the same cultural heritage, ethnicity, or racialized identity, individuals may still anticipate that because of the power differential

in the relationship, the consultant will treat them with the same paternalism and condescension they expect from members of the dominant cultural group.

Other pitfalls that occur when the consultant shares the same ethnicity as the client are related to the unexamined values and shared assumptions that the professional may not question. For this reason, it is critical that consultants carefully consider their own values, the values of the larger society, and their professional values as they are expressed in the norms and goals of clinical work (Axelson, 1999, p. 47).

A climate of trust can be encouraged if professionals acknowledge that specific aspects of the individual's difficulties might be an outcome of how that individual's ethnocultural or racialized group has been impacted by socioeconomic or political marginalization and exclusion or other forms of structural violence. However, while such externalizing explanations can be a legitimate defence against racist practices of the dominant society, when they serve as the core of collective identity, they can undermine the strength of the group and the individual. Unfortunately, this remains a common framework which many Africans of the Diaspora use to construct their identities, despite evidence that the large majority of Blacks are "informed, advanced, self-reliant, and capable of [resisting] institutional racism and discrimination" (Smith, 1996a, 1996b, p. 6). The following case example illustrates one individual's struggle to create and sustain a social identity that is based on frameworks other than race:

Case Vignette 10-5
Jean is a 25-year-old Canadian-born Black male of Haitian origin. He was referred for anger management by his Employment Assistant Program, because he specifically asked for a Black therapist. During the first consultation, he described more than ten incidents of racial discrimination at work. This included derogatory comments made about him, being asked to do work that was

(continued)

not in his job description, being asked to do dangerous work that was against company protocol, and having his pay withheld or being fired when he brought the problem to the attention of supervisors. Jean also described many troubling symptoms, including difficulty sleeping, anxiety, dizziness, sadness, involuntary movements in his legs, and an obsessive tendency to scratch himself. He spoke of how angry he was and that he needed help coping with financial and other stressors. Finally, he described never having had access to positive role models in his immediate environment. He had few satisfactory social relationships and his only outlet was weight training and boxing after working 8–12 h per day.

Jean was allotted 8 h of counselling by his employer. I saw Jean a total of 7 times over a period of 3 months. Most consultations went on for 75–90 min. Community consultations are different from traditional therapy sessions in that they often last longer than the usual 50 min and the interval between consultations may be 3–4 weeks. Consultations with Jean were more systematic because he was in a crisis situation. Over the 3-month period that I saw Jean, he became unemployed and changed jobs twice and was often extremely distressed. He had two distinct stances: part of him was optimistic and looked forward to a better and brighter future in Canadian society; hence, he refused to accept being treated as "inferior" and wanted to see the good in some of the very people he described as rejecting him. At the same time, he also rejected Quebec society and talked of moving out of Quebec to what he hoped would be a less "hostile" environment in the neighboring province of Ontario. However, Jean's dominant experience, expressed in the therapeutic space, was that of a hurt individual who had a hard time understanding why his White Québécois friends with the same level of education and vocational training, and the

same background of poverty, were doing better than him. He described having no support from family, noting that his mother was "in another reality" and his brothers were indifferent to his situation.

The intervention focused on providing Jean with emotional support and a great deal of discussion about the complex social relations that resulted from his being from a cultural and ethnic minority. Efforts were made to reinforce his self-confidence by having him draw upon personal experiences of previous successes and reminding him that prior successes could be repeated in the future. This also served to restructure his negative expectations as well as providing him with strategies for coping with the fear that he would become aggressive each time he encountered an obstacle.

By providing Jean with the tools to restructure his perception of his present situation and the social condition and status he aspires to, or feels entitled to, he was able to transform his overall level of satisfaction and greatly improved his capacity to advocate socially and professionally on his own behalf (Campbell, 1981). Jean was given specific tasks and oriented towards social activities that eventually broke a cycle of social isolation and widened his social supports. He was also directed towards other community resources for legal counselling on discrimination and labor rights. A follow-up phone discussion with Jean showed him grappling with some of the same issues; he had a job that he hoped to keep, he was sleeping better and felt more hopeful. He still had plans to leave Quebec.

This vignette illustrates some of the contradictory experiences of marginalized racial and cultural minorities. They may feel vulnerable, yet come to the consultation bringing feelings of resentment and may be confrontational. They may present themselves as victims who seek recognition and reparation for past wrongs, while remaining steadfast in the belief that they should be self-sufficient and only seek outside support when situations reach crisis proportions. In most cases, marginalized individuals do not hold their employers accountable for discriminatory treatment. However, they may gain a sense of empowerment just by knowing that this recourse is open to them. As Plaza suggests, regarding Africans of the Diaspora, they "carry within their psyche a certain core arsenal of mobility strategies and philosophies to help them avoid disappointment and to realize a sense of achievement in whatever circumstances they might be in" (Plaza, 1996, p. 268). These coping mechanisms are used whenever unpredictable situations are encountered.

Jean's protests against discrimination in the workplace occurred as individual acts, not as part of a larger political movement. In the Black and Caribbean communities with which I am most familiar, the forms of expression and the ways to manage psychological distress have changed over the last few decades, with more mediation taking place in the private sphere than in public settings such as was common during the struggle for civil rights during the 1960s. During the fight for civil liberties, Blacks customarily fought together, gained strength, and took comfort from their shared struggle. In contemporary Canadian society, the emphasis is on individuals' efforts to achieve success, and it is more difficult to conceive of a collective identity and a sense of belonging within a global culture that has abandoned more socially conscious politics in favor of a superficial political correctness that satisfies neither dominant nor minority culture. Several quality-of-life studies support the belief that Blacks as a group have been experiencing a collective post-Civil Rights disenchantment and inertia (Diener, 1984; Hughes & Thomas, 1998; Thomas & Holmes, 1992). Hunt (1996, p. 279) notes that Blacks are nearly as materialistic as Whites, yet even when successful, they tend to cultivate an identification with "the perception of the general condition of [the] group rather than [the individuals] own socio-economic status." This phenomenon of passivity is often encountered in the initial CCS consultation. Fortunately, within the Black and Caribbean patients, the personal characteristics of pride and an all encompassing need to avoid becoming dependent on others serve as motivating factors in getting patients to exercise individual agency.

Best Practices in Community Consultation with Marginalized Groups

Marginalized individuals and communities usually perceive their life chances and opportunities as being less than that of the dominant majority. Hence, their expectations, values, interpretations, and definitions of fulfilment and success in life may differ from those of the majority. These communities tend to be sceptical of consultation and mediation processes that promise them positive outcomes despite obviously unequal power relationships. From the start, the consultants' role in these unequal encounters is to work towards cultural safety by providing emotional support to groups or individuals who may be more acquainted with exclusion and rejection than with recognition and acceptance. Because of the general distrust of outside intervention, an initial period of relationship building is a crucial part of any consultation. There is no place in this process for the consultant who has a clinical attitude of non-engagement and emotional distance. It is not enough to provide vulnerable individuals with a name and phone number for help. They need to be assured that sites of referrals will be welcoming or they will not follow through on referrals or will wait until their situation becomes critical before they act. Marginalized individuals need to have access to culture brokers, mediators, guides, or advocates who can help them negotiate potential conflicts that may impede their treatment when hospitals, clinics, or social service institutions are dismissive or resentful of requests for cultural accommodation. Whether in public or private settings, marginalized individuals may require assistance to decode the bureaucratic systems that can address their needs. A first contact telephone call with a medical or other social institution may have to be made from the consultant's office. Follow-up is also essential for success; these hard-to-reach clients are easily discouraged and therefore difficult to motivate. Often, however, all they need is one success in negotiating the diverse service systems to make the transition from dependency to autonomy. The importance of this outreach has been clearly demonstrated in integrated care for depression with low-income minority women in the USA (Miranda et al., 2006).

The more marginalized the group or individual, the more difficult it may be to gain their trust and build a therapeutic alliance, especially if the consultant discounts or ignores concrete and practical concerns, hence the importance of ensuring that the issues worked on are those identified by the client and not only those chosen by the consultant or the referring clinician. Even when they are very distressed, many immigrant and marginalized clients may want to solve practical problems before they agree to explore underlying causes to their difficulties, which may be rooted in early psychic traumas. In the setting of the community organization or church, tangible and sometimes material resources must first be provided along with abundant emotional support in order to create a favorable environment for the individual or group that can facilitate the use of available services. Practical interventions may include getting someone from a community center to accompany an individual to medical appointments to help clarify confusing diagnoses, assisting with writing letters for college applications, providing babysitting resources, directing individuals towards mutual support groups, finding a general practitioner, or obtaining free legal advice.

Capacity Building

Often marginalized individuals and groups present a defensive or angry exterior because they lack self-confidence. They live in a society in which they have few opportunities to see themselves reflected in a positive way. As a result, they have difficulty developing trusting relationships with others outside of their families and geographic communities. The consultant's task is to convince clients that they have the ability to learn the necessary skills to direct their lives onto a course that will bring them a greater sense of focus and fulfilment as well as lessen psychic conflicts with society. This may involve a shift from helping individuals to reconfigure their own ego functioning or ways of coping to understanding the social context and dynamics of their cultural group and the political processes of marginalization in relation to the dominant society. At such times, the writings of Paulo Freire (1973) appear more relevant than those of Freud or other psychodynamic theorists. Freire's teachings about anti-oppressive practice and its link to psychic liberation provide a crucial underpinning for community consultation practice. Freire's work leads to an emphasis on dialogue founded on respect in which the professional works in partnership with the patient to find viable solutions to the problem at hand. This approach can often successfully engage disadvantaged and resistant clients. In community consultation and mediation, much work must be done to expose and demystify the complex relationships between dominant social systems and the diverse responses of clients who are subjugated by those systems. This "pedagogy of the oppressed" can contribute to strengthening internal resources and building social capital which will allow individuals and communities to advocate for themselves as they discover alternative ways to regain their mental and physical equilibrium.

Consistent validation of marginalized clients' experience fosters trust and builds the therapeutic alliance. While initial trust and rapport are facilitated when the consultant and the client share cultural background or ethnicity, their subsequent development depend on the consultant's skill in communication (Axelson, 1999, p. 430). The communication style used during the consultation process with marginalized individuals is central to creating a professional relationship that will be therapeutic for the individual and leads to greater collaboration between client and consultant. In contrast to the open-ended style promoted by psychodynamic psychotherapy, in community settings, many individuals may prefer more directive communication styles that focus on concrete suggestions, plans, and explicit encouragement.

The cultural consultant is not an expert on the client's experience or lifeworld. The individual's or the group's thoughts and feelings must be elicited and explored throughout the process of assessment and intervention. One aim of consultation is to assist individuals in their search for explanations of their difficulties and help them develop alternative ways to understand and address their dilemmas. Providing individuals with concrete information about their background and collective history can help them to determine where their own experience fits with these larger social forces and cultural paradigms. The consultant does not impose ready-made meanings but helps prepare a canvas on which the client can begin to sketch a healthier version of themselves.

Marginalized individuals may be uncertain of their place in their communities of origin and the larger society and may need confirmation or validation of their feelings especially when they are unaware of the historical factors that have shaped their cultural group. Even when they know the history, they may have never given themselves permission to examine the wounded parts of themselves and they may be afraid to do this without guidance.

> Rejection of primary culture is likely to lead to the confusion and self-doubt that is found in a marginalized existence. Consultants who seek to assist in the resolution of a state of marginality need to understand the client's psychodynamics, the two cultures, and a process that will facilitate movement toward desired goals. (Axelson, 1999, p. 431)

The cultural consultant thus must work with both the individual psychodynamic processes of defensiveness and vulnerability and the collective social and political processes that undermine the sense of power and well-being of both groups and individuals.

Conclusion

After more than 25 years working with marginalized groups in private and public settings, it is clear that much remains to be done to make mental health services safe and sensitive to difference. Despite gains over the years, mainstream institutions still compel individuals to fit into treatment models in which they do not recognize themselves. Professionals are not encouraged to create and explore alternative treatment approaches that are responsive to culture and context. Openness to diverse practice models would surely provide much food for thought and move the idea of integration to a level beyond the restrictive dichotomies of professional versus traditional, conventional versus alternative, and, implicitly, "us versus them."

Regardless of the domain of practice, the marginalization and exclusion of certain groups is a serious challenge for a liberal democratic society like Canada (Taylor, 1994). Addressing this disparity is not only the responsibility of government and policymakers, local mental health administrators and professionals can also take a stance on issues related to unequal service delivery and discrimination. There is a need for a dialogical process that reflects Canada's diverse cultures (Leonard, 1997)—one that recognizes the value for pluralistic societies and credits diverse cultures with their own knowledge and prescriptions for well-being.

The development of culturally safe mental health practice models is crucial to the Canadian vision of a multicultural and pluralistic society in which government is ethically and legally bound to take the lead since culturally marginalized individuals and groups may not have the capacity to form effective movements of resistance around issues based on race, ethnicity, religion, sexual orientation, and class.

As more and more social movements are formed around culture and ethnic identity with a focus on cultural politics rather than on broader issues of class and racial inequalities, health professionals will need to be both culturally competent and politically aware so that they can make the links between their clients' individual situations and larger social structural issues afflicting society. If health professionals are to be good advocates for their clients, this social, cultural, and political awareness must be an essential feature of mental health practice. Together with their clients, culturally competent professionals should be able to deconstruct the themes of identity, cultural difference, and intercultural misunderstandings and learn how to work as partners to develop effective treatment plans. Interactions that are rooted in the principles of humility, respect, and openness to the other can help individuals develop positive visions of themselves including a shared collective identity and cultural solidarity with the dominant society, focused on hope for the future. Such strategies would allow each cultural group to find some measure of identification with the dominant culture without concern for loss of cultural or ethnic identity.

In a social climate of continuing racial, ethnic, cultural, and linguistic divisions within Canada's multicultural society, the ability of health care professionals and cultural brokers to respect the uniqueness of each group including that of the "host" country is an opportunity to contribute to positive social change, for the benefit of both the individual and the larger society. From a structural perspective, there needs to be ongoing dialogue between the institutions that provide services and the communities they serve. This dialogue can help heal some of the wounds of misunderstanding and mistrust that have developed over a long period of time. Overcoming structural inequalities at institutional levels will also require an admission that the process of decolonization is incomplete and continues to be a formidable task for both colonizer and colonized. Here we can draw on the experience of Blacks, feminists, and Indigenous peoples who continue to struggle to find their space and place in a Eurocentric and often male-dominated social and economic world. Unanimously, these groups have cited consciousness raising, critical thinking, and critical education as being essential to achieving social equality for members of minority cultures.

As professionals striving to work in ways that are in harmony with the needs of a culturally diverse population, it is important that we enter into a dialogical relationship with our clients. This should include inviting clients to share their knowledge about us and to reflect on what they believe health care services can and should do for them. This form of "empowerment" is a reasonable starting place for a relationship based on respect, trust, and genuine interest in the other. This is not an abstract political ideal—the truth is,

systemic and structural oppression affect us all and eventually erode our sense of well-being. Respect for cultural diversity in mental health services is an opportunity for all concerned to renew their commitment to the values of racial, ethnic, and cultural diversity that are part of multiculturalism.

References

Allport, G. W. (1979). *The Nature of Human Prejudice.* Basic books. (Original work published 1954).

Axelson, J. A. (1999). *Counseling and development in a multicultural society* (3rd ed.). Toronto, Ontario, Canada: Brooks/Cole Publishing Company.

Bashi, V. (1997). *Survival of the knitted: The social networks of West Indian immigrants.* Unpublished doctoral dissertation, University of Wisconsin-Madison, Madison, WI.

Bibeau, G. (1997). Cultural psychiatry in a creolizing world: Questions for a new research agenda. *Transcultural Psychiatry, 34*(1), 9–41.

Bourdieu, P. (1977). Cultural reproduction and social reproduction. In J. Karabel & A. H. Halsey (Eds.), *Power and ideology in education* (pp. 487–511). New York, NY: Oxford University Press.

Campbell, A. (1981). *The sense of well-being in America.* New York, NY: McGraw-Hill.

Carter, P. L. (2003). "Black" cultural capital, status positioning, and schooling conflicts for low-income African American youth. *Society for the Study of Social Problems, 50*(1), 136–155.

DeGruy-Leary, J. (2005). *Post traumatic slave syndrome; America's legacy of enduring injury and healing.* Portland, OR: Uptone Press.

Diener, E. (1984). Subjective well-being. *Psychological Bulletin, 95*(3), 542–575.

Elliot, J. L., & Fleras, A. (1992). *Unequal relations: An introduction to race and ethnic dynamics in Canada.* Toronto, Ontario, Canada: Prentice Hall.

Eyerman, R. (2004). Slavery and the formation of African American identity. In J. C. Alexander (Ed.), *Cultural trauma and collective identity* (pp. 61–111). Berkeley, CA: University of California Press.

Fanon, F. (1967). *Black skin, white masks.* New York, NY: Grove Press.

Frankenberg, R. (1997). Local whiteness, localizing whiteness. In R. Frankenberg (Ed.), *Displacing whiteness: Essays in social and cultural criticism* (pp. 1–33). London, England: Duke University Press.

Freire, P. (1973). *Education for critical consciousness.* New York, NY: The Continuum Publishing Company.

Hughes, M., & Thomas, M. (1998). The continuing significance of race revisited: A study of race, class, and quality of life in America, 1972 to 1996. *American Sociological Review, 63,* 785–795.

Hunt, M. (1996). The individual, society, or both? A comparison of Black, Latino, and White beliefs about the causes of poverty. *Social Forces, 75*(1), 293–322.

Kareem, J., & Littlewood, R. (Eds.). (2000). *Intercultural therapy* (2nd ed.). London, England: Blackwell Science.

Kymlicka, W. (1998). *Finding our way: Rethinking ethnocultural relations in Canada*. Toronto: Oxford University Press.

Leccia, J. (2008). *Culture as a clinical discriminant*. Unpublished paper presented at the 42nd Annual Conference of the Medical Association of Psychiatrist of Quebec. Quebec, Canada: Gatineau.

Leonard, P. (1997). *Postmodern welfare: Reconstructing an emancipatory project*. London, England: Sage.

Lim, R. F. (Ed.). (2006). *Clinical manual of cultural psychiatry*. Washington, DC: American Psychiatric Publishing.

Measham, T., & Wint, S. (2007). Cultural capital: A protective factor. *Afro Canadian Art Foundation Annual Art & Culture Review*. Montreal, Canada. Lovell Litho & Publications Inc.

Merton, T. (1978). *No man is an island*. New York, NY: Harcourt Press.

Miranda, J., Green, B. L., Krupnick, J. L., Chung, J., Siddique, J., Belin, T., et al. (2006). One-year outcomes of a randomized clinical trial treating depression in low-income minority women. *Journal of Consulting and Clinical Psychology, 74*(1), 99–111.

Morrison, T. (1992). *Black matters: Playing in the dark: Whiteness and the literary imagination*. Cambridge, England: Harvard University Press.

Plaza, D. E. (1996). *The strategies and strategizing of university educated black Caribbean-born men in Toronto: A study of occupation and income achievement*. Unpublished doctoral dissertation, York University, Toronto, Ontario, Canada.

Smith, H. Y. (1996a). Building on the strength of black families: Self-help and empowerment. In S. Logan (Ed.), *The Black family: Strengths, self-help and positive change*. Boulder, CO: Westview Press.

Smith, R. T. (1996b). *The matrifocal family: Power, pluralism and politics*. London, England: Routledge.

Steele, C. M. (2010). *Whistling Vivaldi And other clues to how stereotypes affect us*. New York, NY: W.W. Norton.

Sue, D. W., Capodilupo, C. M., Torino, G. C., Bucceri, J. M., Holder, A. M. B., Nadal, K. L., et al. (2007). Racial microaggressions in everyday life: Implications for clinical practice. *American Psychologist, 62*(4), 271–286.

Taylor, C. (1994). *Multiculturalism*. Princeton, NJ: Princeton University Press.

Thomas, L. (1999). Racism and psychotherapy: Working with racism in the consulting room: An analytical view. In J. Kareem & R. Littlewood (Eds.), *Intercultural therapy* (2nd ed., pp. 146–160). Oxford, England: Blackwell Science Ltd.

Thomas, M., & Holmes, B. (1992). Determinants of satisfaction for blacks and whites. *The Sociological Quarterly, 33*(3), 459–472.

Ton, H., & Lim, R. (2006). The assessment of culturally diverse individuals. In R. F. Lim (Ed.), *Clinical manual of cultural psychiatry* (pp. 5–31). Washington, DC: American Psychiatric Publishing.

Wein, B. (1992, March). The roots of racism. *New Woman, 22*, 89–96.

Whitley, R., Kirmayer, L. J., & Groleau, D. (2006a). Understanding immigrants' reluctance to use mental health services: A qualitative study from Montreal. *Canadian Journal of Psychiatry, 51*(4), 205–209.

Whitley, R., Kirmayer, L. J., & Groleau, D. (2006b). Public pressure, private protest: Illness narratives of West Indian immigrants in Montreal with medically unexplained symptoms. *Anthropology & Medicine, 13*(3), 193–205.

Wint, S. (2000). *Race and the subjective well-being of Black Canadians*. Unpublished masters thesis, McGill University, Montreal, Quebec, Canada.

Addressing Cultural Diversity Through Collaborative Care

10

Lucie Nadeau, Cécile Rousseau, and Toby Measham

Introduction

In the last decade, collaborative mental health care has become a widely recognized approach to improve accessibility to mental health care and provide efficient and cost-effective patient-centered care (Kates et al., 2011). Collaborative care is based on strong partnerships between primary care and mental health professionals, with the goal of establishing a comprehensive network providing a full spectrum of care in mental health. A recent reform of mental health services in Quebec, the "Plan d'action en santé mentale" (*PASM*, Mental Health Action Plan), implements collaborative care as the central component of mental health delivery. This shift in service organization provides new avenues to deliver culturally sensitive mental health care. This chapter describes how collaborative care can be a useful model of service delivery for culturally diverse populations and how it can address specific needs of communities facing multiple forms of social structural disadvantage, precarity and exclusion.

In the following sections, we first consider the scope of the challenge of accessibility in mental health care. We then present general principles of collaborative care between primary care professionals and mental health specialists, before expanding on two key avenues identified by the Canadian Collaborative Mental Health Initiative (CCMHI) as ways to adapt collaborative care to the needs of culturally diverse populations: (1) partnership with communities, which includes working with interpreters, and (2) awareness of historical and cultural specificities in the collaborative care model. The chapter continues with an outline of training methods to support collaborative care projects for culturally diverse populations. We use case examples of work with children and families drawn from our own project on the implementation of a collaborative mental health care for youth in a community setting in Montreal with many recent immigrants. The chapter illustrates a key message from the report of the World Health Organization (WHO) and the World Organization of National Colleges, Academies and Academic Associations of General Practitioners/Family Physicians (WONCA) on mental health in primary care (WHO & WONCA, 2008), namely, that "there is no single best practice model that can be followed by all countries. Rather, successes have been achieved through sensible local application of broad principles" (p. 1).

L. Nadeau, M.D., M.Sc., F.R.C.P. (C) (✉)
C. Rousseau, M.D., M.Sc.
T. Measham, M.D., M.Sc., F.R.C.P. (C)
CSSS de la Montagne (CLSC Parc Extension),
7085 Hutchison, Montreal, QC,
Canada H3N 1Y9
e-mail: lucie.nadeau@mcgill.ca;
cecile.rousseau@mcgill.ca; toby.measham@mcgill.ca

L.J. Kirmayer et al. (eds.), *Cultural Consultation: Encountering the Other in Mental Health Care,* International and Cultural Psychology, DOI 10.1007/978-1-4614-7615-3_10,
© Springer Science+Business Media New York 2014

Collaborative Care to Improve the Accessibility of Services

Access to mental health services is a major public health concern in Canada as in many other parts of the world (WHO & WONCA, 2008). In Canada, estimates are that one-in-five adults may have a mental health problem, while only half of those in need of mental health services actually consult a health professional (Lesage et al., 2006). Children, who are reported to have a 10–20 % prevalence of mental health problems both locally and internationally (Brauner & Stephen, 2006; Costello, Swendsen, Rose, & Dierker, 2008; Patel, Flisher, Hetrick, & McGory, 2007; Verhulst, VanderEnde, Ferdinand, & Kasius, 1997), also have difficulty accessing mental health care in Canada (Ministère de la santé et des services sociaux, 2005; Spenser, Gilles, & Maysenhoelder, 2009; Waddell et al., 2005) and in other countries (Hickie et al., 2007; Leckman & Leventhal, 2008). Recent data in Canada suggest that children have more difficulty than adults accessing services (Benigeri, Bluteau, Roberge, Provencher, & Nadeau, 2007; Spenser et al., 2009). For immigrants, refugees and ethnocultural minority groups, the barriers to care may be still more severe. Lack of resources, the stigma associated with mental illness, structural inequalities and cultural differences all contribute to the inaccessibility of mental health care to specific ethnocultural groups or communities.

Primary care has long been recognized as the de facto mental health care system in North America (Regier et al., 1993). Children and families who do receive treatment most often access it through primary care settings (Burns et al., 1995; Leaf et al., 1996; Lesage et al., 2006; Rushton, Bruckman, & Kelleher, 2002). In medium- and high-income countries, mental health care is mostly provided by primary care physicians, whereas in low-income countries most professional care is provided by nurses. These facts support the need for innovative ways to increase the capacity of primary care mental health systems to provide services and to support primary care providers already involved in mental health care.

Principles of Collaborative Care

Collaborative mental health care involves mental health experts working with first-line care providers in the delivery of mental health promotion, illness prevention, the detection and treatment of mental illnesses, as well as rehabilitation and recovery support. Current collaborative care models emphasize a patient-centered approach in which service users are considered part of the collaborative team and actively engaged in treatment decision making (Kates et al., 2011). By definition, collaborative care involves diverse service providers, aiming to build trusting working relationships between partners whose roles and contributions are recognized and adapted to the local context and culture of care and are flexible enough to follow the patient's changing needs. For collaborative initiatives to achieve success, some further conditions must be fulfilled: they must be integrated within the services planning, use effective practices based on both evidence and experience, include a care coordinator and provide ready access to psychiatric consultations. Marginalized groups with poor access to care, including members of Indigenous communities and migrants, should be prioritized in collaborative care initiatives with respect to their complex needs. The recent strategy of the Mental Health Commission of Canada (2012) advocates for the broad use of collaborative care models, which also allow physical and mental health issues to be addressed together.

The changing language used to describe the forms of collaboration between general health and mental health professionals illustrates how actors in the field have gradually questioned the power imbalance between health and other service providers in current service systems models. In Canada, the CCMHI first used the term "shared care" to describe the kind of collaborative mental health care they advocated. However, this term tended to be associated with the sharing of care among physicians (mostly general practitioners and psychiatrists), thus leaving out the knowledge, skills and collaborations occurring with other professionals, as well as the importance of dialogue with communities and patients. The term "collaborative care" is now preferred by the CCMHI and is seen as encompassing this larger sense of collaboration (Kates, 2008). This shift in the conceptualization of "shared-care" with an empowerment of all actors is represented in recent conferences, where multidisciplinary teams present together and where many different actors in the collaborative care arena have opportunities to be heard.

Unfortunately, the published literature suggests this shift toward multidisciplinary collaboration has not yet been fully embraced in practice. A recent inventory of 90 Canadian collaborative mental health care initiatives found that most used an approach based on consultations requested by family physicians to either psychiatrists, psychologists or other members of a mental health team, often nurses (Pauzé, Gagné, & Pautler, 2005). The collaboration between medical and mental health professionals in community-based care enriches the practice of mental health care and allows for adequate consideration of medical and developmental aspects. This approach though centers on medical aspects of mental health care and thus emphasizes diagnostic and psychopharmacological issues. As a result, it runs the risk of minimizing the sociocultural dimensions of mental health care, as this knowledge is less dominant in the medical model. Broader collaborative care models recognize that medical staff often need the support and knowledge of nonmedical professionals to provide integrated care that is sensitive to the cultural and social specificities of a given population and acknowledges the essential contributions of these nonmedical partners.

A growing literature on interprofessional collaboration seeks to identify the particularities of multidisciplinary work and to identify the key elements needed to build efficacious and sustainable collaborations. Collaborating among professionals from different disciplines requires revisiting issues of power (D'Amours, 2005; Rousseau, Ammara, Baillargeon, Lenoir, & Roy, 2007). Elements of a workable interprofessional relationships include forming partnerships around common goals and values grounded in respect for collegiality, building on each other's professional knowledge and experience, and sharing responsibilities for

decision making and planning interventions (Houle, unpublished report, 2007).

Effective partnerships demand that partners identify, develop and share a common project. Bilodeau, Lapierre, and Marchand (2003) described four phases to this process: (1) *formulation of the problem* (the promoters of the project start a movement to identify the actors concerned with the project, their interests and the issues linking them together), (2) *sensitization* (the strategies of the different actors are combined to gather actors around a shared objective and negotiate roles), (3) *involvement* (the actual taking of roles by the actors) and (4) *mobilization* (participation of a critical mass of actors within the project in order for innovation to become pertinent, useful and indispensable). This description of the process emphasizes that partnership is built over time within a care system through ongoing dialogue and liaison between partners rather than simply with punctual or one-off consultations. Collaborative care models are compatible with systemic approaches and are likely to improve shared decision making and responsibility among providers (Chenven, 2010). For Dewar (2000), collaboration implies accountability and recognition of all collaborators in their respective roles within a bottom-up perspective.

Adapting Collaborative Care to Address the Cultural Specificities of Communities

The movement promoting collaborative care has also emphasized the local adaptation of services and, in particular, the adaptations needed to provide services to marginalized communities. Collaborative care advocates a community-based approach which allows for a reconsideration of macro-level issues about mental health care delivery in general and more specific consideration of majority-minority group issues. Migrant and refugee communities have been recognized as having difficulties accessing mental health services in Canada (Bowen, 2001; Canadian Mental Health Association, 2003; Chen, Kazanjian, Wong, & Goldner, 2010; Fenta, Hyman, & Noh, 2006; Hyman, 2004; Sadavoy, Meier, & Ong, 2004).

Table 10.1 Key issues for collaborative care with ethnoculturally diverse populations

Accessibility of services

Accessibility needs to be improved by building partnerships with patients and communities. These partnerships should be founded on trust, power-sharing and engagement of the community in the governance of community health care. Accessibility requires that services:

- Are appropriately located
- Are linguistically appropriate, with access to professional interpreters competent in mental health and providing health information in accessible language
- Are culturally appropriate, with culturally competent and socially informed service providers
- Include a diversity of professionals: physicians, settlement workers, advocates, religious and community groups, nurses, physiotherapists, occupational therapists, psychologists, clinical counsellors, health brokers, interpreters, psychiatrists, lawyers, mental health workers, dietitians, addiction counsellors, pharmacists, educators, and community liaisons
- Implement a diversity coordinator in community health centers who can link with resources in the community
- Make use of paraprofessional health care providers or culture brokers who help patients navigate the health care system, improving access and quality of care

Cultural competence

Cultural competence and safety are needed at the level of professionals and institutions. Delivery of services must be tailored to the unique needs of the ethnocultural community. Primary health care providers need increased awareness of cultural issues including:

- Specific needs and appropriate manner in which to serve ethnocultural groups, including religious, cultural and spiritual traditions, differences in roles and family relationships and dietary and other lifestyle choices
- Recognition that mental health issues may be expressed through somatic complaints and may coexist with and aggravate common medical conditions
- Ways that poverty, racism and discrimination and structural disadvantage may affect health and services
- Policies and legislation that affect ethnocultural populations
- Dynamics of migration and resettlement dynamics
- Ways of working in culturally specific or specialized services that may address the needs of multiple ethnicities and cultures in one setting or specific to a particular cultural group or ethnicity

Training

- There is a need to develop formal cultural competence training in professional programs and to follow this up with accreditation of programs and maintenance of skills by professionals.
- Training is also needed for culture brokers and paraprofessional health care workers.
- Strategies are needed to facilitate foreign-trained mental health professionals' accreditation and entry into the workforce.

Funding

- Funding should be secured to provide culturally appropriate services and materials.
- Immigrant agencies should be included as partners in federal, provincial and municipal funding structures.

Research

- There is a need of longitudinal outcome research with culturally valid measurement or evaluation tools applicable to immigrant and refugees.
- Research should encourage "bottom-up," collaborative and participatory action methods.

Among the obstacles to care for immigrants and refugees are fear of stigmatization, mistrust of an unfamiliar health care system, communication difficulties, concern about being misunderstood and experiences of discrimination (Kirmayer et al., 2011). Overcoming these barriers may be especially challenging in urban settings where poverty and high levels of ethnic diversity coexist.

This CCMHI developed toolkits addressing collaborative mental health care for particular populations. The toolkits were developed by expert panels that reviewed the literature and consulted key stakeholders including health care and social service providers and consumers, settlement organizations, interpreters and community representatives. One of these toolkits outlines key elements to address the problems of underutilization and stigma in culturally diverse populations (Canadian Collaborative Mental Health Initiative 2006) (Table 10.1).

In 2010, the Canadian Collaboration for Immigrant and Refugee Health (CCIRH) published a series of evidence-based guidelines for primary care health promotion among newly arrived immigrants and refugees to Canada (i.e. within the first 5 years of resettlement) (Pottie et al., 2010, 2011). The guidelines focused on 25 conditions identified by family physicians as priorities through a Delphi procedure, which included five mental health problems: depression, PTSD and torture-related trauma, acculturation issues, domestic violence and child maltreatment (Swinkels, Pottie, Tugwell, Rashid, & Narasiah, 2011). An overview paper underlined the crucial role of primary care as a site for mental health promotion and access to mental health care and described the clinical relationship with the primary care provider as pivotal in the detection and treatment of common mental health problems (Kirmayer et al., 2011). The guidelines recommend that clinicians in primary care focus on clinical utility in establishing mental health care priorities. For example, screening for depression is recommended only if it is part of an integrated treatment system, with "systematic patient education, availability of allied health professionals to support continuity of care, frequent follow-up, a caseload registry to track patients, caseload supervision by a psychiatrist if indicated, stepped care and a plan for preventing relapse" (Katon & Seelig, 2008). Clinicians are encouraged to be alert to signs of PTSD but not to implement routine screening for traumatic events because disclosure of trauma in well-functioning individuals, without appropriate therapeutic support, may lead to re-traumatization. In accord with the CICMH Toolkit, the CCIRH guidelines recommend:

- Attention to the social and cultural context of patients' illness experience, including variations in the expression, interpretation and reactions to symptoms and illness, patterns of coping and seeking help, styles of communication and expression of emotions and sources of help sought outside the biomedical health care system
- The use of professional interpreters and culture brokers

- Inquiry about the family system and social network and inclusion of family members in the assessment process and treatment plan
- Consultation and collaboration with community organizations which can act as support systems, provide resources and information during the period of resettlement and integration into the host society and create a culturally safe space for integrated care.

There is growing evidence that collaborative mental health care can increase access to mental health services in context of multiethnic populations. In a study in Boston, USA, co-location of primary care and mental health services and trainings seminars increased referrals to mental health and engagement of Chinese-American consumers (Yeung et al., 2004). Collaborative care models including clinics, schools and community organizations can be particularly helpful when servicing refugee patients, considering the privileged position of these partners to detect problems given their proximity to families' living environment, and the capacity of psychiatric consultants to assist primary care clinicians help families holding trauma narratives by organizing a safe environment around the family (Rousseau, Measham, & Nadeau, 2012). In settings where trauma focused psychotherapy is not available, committed primary care professionals and community workers can provide adequate psychosocial support and empathic listening bringing relief to a family.

Building Partnerships with Communities

Collaborative mental health care can give patients a stronger voice and sense of agency in health care decision making, by shifting from hierarchical models of care centered on professional expertise to one that works in partnership with patients and their families (Kates, 2008). Collaborative mental health care also favors working closely with communities, which can be consulted on how services should be configured and implemented. In contrast with "community-placed" initiatives, in which external organizations implement an initiative without the active participation of the community (Trickett, 2009), collaborative care aims at *community-based* initiatives in which communities take an active role in both planning and capacity building (Pautler & Gagné, 2005). As envisioned by the CCMHI, collaborative care can go beyond organizational modifications to address the social implications of the ways in which mental health care is provided.

This community approach can highlight existing differences in perspective between majority and minority groups. As such, it challenges the knowledge and power imbalance that exists between health care providers and the populations they serve. The collaborative care arena is moving toward greater recognition of the experience and knowledge of ethnocultural communities. Although community organizations are increasingly recognized for their role in giving a voice to users of the mental health system, they still play a relatively minor role in service organizations which are dominated by mainstream institutions. The exercise of power in these institutions can occur in ways that are particularly threatening to minorities. The notion of *cultural safety*, developed in a Maori context by nurses in New Zealand (Koptie, 2009; Papps & Ramsden, 1996), emphasises that addressing the power disparities in health care institutions is essential to provide an ethical foundation for collaborative care (Brascoupé & Waters, 2009; Smye, Josewski, & Kendall, 2010). Although framed originally in terms of the predicament of Indigenous peoples in settler societies who have endured colonialism, marginalization and oppression, cultural safety provides a useful construct to address the relations between immigrants and other ethnocultural minority groups and the mainstream mental health services. Indeed, many of these groups have a historical legacy of colonialism and ongoing experiences of racism and discrimination that can make encounters with mainstream institutions threatening.

Effective collaborative care also requires attention to the interaction of individual and collective identities of providers and patients. Attention to context in mental health care implies an openness to learning about individuals' experiences and worldviews, as opposed to stereotyping patients and families based on preconceived notions of ethnic, racial or religious groups. In practice, clinicians need knowledge, skills and attitudes that facilitate dialogue with different family members and the heterogeneous members of cultural communities (Nadeau, 2007). For example, transformations of traditional roles with migration and acculturation are often at the root of family crises. Clinicians can assist with the renegotiation of family roles and relationships, but particular skills are needed to mediate the issues that may arise when migration results in divergent experiences for youth and their parents or men and women encountering new gender roles and configurations of relationship (see Chapter 7). Community organizations can be both partners and actors in this transformation.

The worldviews of migrant youth typically borrow from both their culture of origin and the host culture, and as such they have access to multiple cultural models to build their identities and make sense of their experience. Some studies suggest that youth who have a bicultural identity may thrive and have better mental health than their peers who adhere exclusively to culture of origin or host culture (Berry, 1998; Bibeau, 1998; LaFromboise, Coleman, & Gerton, 1993; Schwartz, Unger, Zamboanga, & Szapocznik, 2010). Bicultural youth are able to maintain a nourishing link to their culture of origin while simultaneously investing in the host society. As they grow, they construct relationships between these two worlds. They inhabit an in-between space (Ang & Van Dyne, 2008), which may be a source of rich knowledge and opportunities, but can also challenge existing values. In collaborative care, the wish to recognize the voice of these youth must be balanced with the need to include their parents' models of intergenerational relationships, including traditional patterns of decision making within families. Frequently, host country professionals differ about the best way to address youth responsibilities and rights while taking into account their need to belong to their families and their culture of origin. Professionals need to avoid aggravating these tensions as they mediate between these divergent perspectives. The following vignette illustrates how collaborative care can help resolve service providers' divergent interpretations of intergenerational family conflict.

Case Vignette 9-1

Yasmine, a 13-year-old girl who came to Canada from Algeria at the age of 8, was aggressive toward peers, challenging of authority figures and oppositional at home. She also had sleep disturbance and academic difficulties. Yasmine wanted to cut ties with her extended family because she attributed all the conflicts in her family to her uncle's authority which she felt was illegitimate. She rejected the extended family model which she associated with strict limit setting and many rules and wanted a nuclear family model, similar to that of her friends' families, which she thought would give her more power. Her parents hesitated to change the traditional organization of the family and to introduce more distance in their relationship with the uncle. The primary care providers from the school and the clinic disagreed on the potential solutions to this conflict. Some thought the youth should be allowed to focus on nuclear family activities, while others expressed discomfort at the way that Yasmine framed her difficulties and felt they were being pressured to choose between two legitimate positions expressed by the youth and her family. The child psychiatry consultation with the family included all partners and aim to facilitate a discussion of the diverging views. The dreams of the parents for their child were discussed and reframed as an "in-between" position that gave importance to both the nuclear and extended family models, making it possible to belong to the host community while preserving links with the culture of origin. Through the consultation, it became apparent that the parents themselves felt uncomfortable having to choose between these two models. The consultation allowed both the youth and her parents to feel supported and helped the primary care providers to overcome their split and continue their ongoing support.

Giving voice to women is another challenging issue in collaborative mental health care with migrants. Some families from communities with traditional gender roles may perceive community organizations and mental health professionals in societies that emphasise gender equality as overly encouraging of the independence of women. At the same time, many women have experienced transformation of traditional roles during the migratory process. They may, for example, have had to adopt the role of provider for the family while separated from their husband, or they may have already questioned traditional gender roles in their country of origin but have become able to express their concerns more freely in the host country. These shifts in gender roles also must be negotiated with awareness of alternative value systems and perspectives.

Training in Cultural Competence for Collaborative Care

As outlined in the introduction to this volume, providing mental health care to populations with high levels of diversity may require cultural adaptation of services. The cultural backgrounds of professionals, patients and families influence the conceptual frameworks used to interpret signs of difficulty or affliction as illnesses, understand the meanings of illness and identify appropriate action (Corin, Uchoa, Bibeau, & Koumare, 1992). Cultural competence implies being alert to factors such as communication style, power, role, gender and age that vary with culture and social status (Gorman, 2001). Cultural and contextual issues may mediate access and barriers to care (Sue, 2001). Cultural competence includes the capacity of the mental health professionals to be aware of their own cultural identity and presentation to the other, mobilizing different aspects of a complex self-identity to fit the needs of the situation (Ewing, 1990).

Cultural competence cannot involve simply acquiring a fixed body of knowledge about a culture, because culture by its very nature is an evolving system or meanings, subject to constant revision and transformation by its members as well as external influences (Bibeau, Chan-Yip, Lock, & Rousseau, 1992). Promoting cultural awareness among mental health care providers therefore requires training programs that include both reflexive and clinical skills. This can be incorporated into continuing education through various pedagogical approaches including in-service conferences for case discussion or performing joint clinical work, in which primary care providers can observe and participate in the process of exploring cultural aspects during a specific consultation (De Plaen et al., 2005; Rousseau, Alain, De Plaen, Chiasson-Lavoie, et al. 2005).

Because collaborative care projects regularly involve many collaborators, training of the participants is a complex enterprise. Each collaborator has his or her own knowledge and awareness of cultural diversity and experiences of otherness. In general, the health care system provides few opportunities for workers to discuss their personal and clinical experiences related to culture and to integrate social and cultural issues into their professional knowledge and skills.

Awareness of the social and historical experiences of individuals and communities is at the heart of collaborative mental health care in transcultural contexts. This approach favors the identification, recognition and acknowledgement of a multiplicity of individual and collective factors that impact on a particular clinical situation. Illness narratives bring their share of uncertainty and diagnostic challenge, even more so when they involve many interacting sociocultural elements. This may lead to the misattribution of symptoms, for example, when a child's hypervigilance and agitation are interpreted as signs of attention-deficit hyperactivity disorder because there is no recognition that the child experienced major trauma (such as organized violence or abuse) leaving him with persistent fears. Many clinical situations are the result of the complex dynamics between personal (constitutional-temperamental), familial and social issues. Culturally sensitive assessment and care can allow for pertinent contributing factors to surface in due time.

Only this more detailed contextual information can clarify the diagnosis in complex, ambiguous clinical situations. For example, the suspicious attitude of a refugee teenager may be the result of post traumatic stress disorder, mistrust of a still unfamiliar host society, a coping strategy in the face of discrimination or a sign of an emerging psychotic disorder. A migrant child presenting with conflictual relationships with the mother might have attachment disorder given that she was separated from the mother early in life without benefitting from consistent caring figures or might be expressing a combined mother and child depression when family reunification after many years of separation during the migration process brings ambivalence, anger and guilt while they struggle with poverty. A 10-year-old boy having difficulty in school may be mentally challenged or have major communication difficulties due to language barriers that were never properly assessed.

A major challenge for collaborative care is how to provide a holding space for patients and their families where the multiple meanings of symptoms can be explored and where doubts, disagreements and uncertainty can also be heard while insuring that the clinical process does not become a new venue for conflict. Multidisciplinary input and the engagement of interpreters and culture brokers help identify different contributing factors in complex clinical cases. Each partner in clinical care has his or her own knowledge and experience to contribute. The primary care professionals involved may have known the patient and family for some time and can provide a longitudinal history of the illness, increasing the likelihood of an accurate diagnostic and treatment plan. Families have often developed trust and a working alliance with these care providers, who may have helped them in very concrete ways in addition to offering psychosocial support. Thus, the consultation starts within a somewhat familiar setting in the company of their primary care providers for these families.

A Youth Mental Health Care Project in a Multiethnic Neighborhood

About half of Montreal's school-aged children are first- or second-generation immigrants (Sévigny, Viau, & Rabhi, 2002). Over the last decade, we have been involved in implementing a collaborative mental health care program in a community-based health and social services institution in Montreal, Canada, the Centre de santé et de services sociaux de la Montagne (CSSS DLM). The CSSS includes community clinics in three multiethnic neighborhoods of Montreal, which are among the most culturally diverse areas of the city. According to the 2006 Canadian census, 52 % of the population in the catchment area of the CSSS are either immigrants (45.7 %) or nonpermanent residents (6.3 %), and 45.8 % have neither French nor English as a mother tongue, but one of many other languages (Paquin, 2008).

The collaborative care project developed through a 10-year partnership between the CSSS and the transcultural child psychiatry team of the Montreal Children's Hospital lead by the second author. The goal of the project was to provide youth mental health services to newcomer migrant families who were experiencing mental health difficulties related to resettlement or to a previous exposure to organized violence. Partners included frontline professionals involved in the psychosocial care of children and adolescents, as well as others specialized in the care of refugee claimants.

During the first phase, indirect consultations to mental health care workers and direct consultations to children and their families were provided at the hospital, and joint case discussion seminars between the hospital outpatient team and community mental health care providers took place in the local community service center. In 2005, a government reform (PASM) promoted a shift of mental health care from hospital-centered mental health services toward community-based (proximity) services in order to strengthen delivery of care at the primary care level (Ministère de la Santé et des Services Sociaux, 2005). This reform involved a transfer of financial resources and child mental health professionals including social workers, psychologists and specialized educators from hospital psychiatric teams to community institutions. In addition, the reform envisioned the community clinics as the doorway of entry for youth to access all mental health care services, which would be linked in a network of institutions providing increasing levels of mental health care (from community

care to mental health care specialty and subspecialty outpatient care to hospitalization) accessed by the creation of service networks between the institutions. Community services were also supported by creating a new role of "responding psychiatrist" which consisted in supporting primary care professionals through on-site capacity-building activities ranging from case conferences, direct consultations with patients, training opportunities and ad hoc telephone discussions of clinical issues.

The collaborative care model has been the subject of much challenge, resistance and debate. On the one hand, primary care professionals, including family physicians who already are underrepresented in Montreal, noted that the addition of community-based mental health care to their existing community responsibilities was particularly challenging given their limited resources. Hospital-based services also resisted the reform, because the shift of services was not accompanied by new money or personnel, but instead involved a transfer of funds and care providers from existing hospital services to the community clinic. The challenge, therefore, has been to build partnerships that respect the realities on the ground and offer more benefit than burden for all of the partners as they work to provide appropriate mental health care to an underserved population. In the government plan, the community clinics were identified as the main place where this new challenge was to be met. A recent report by the Commissioner of Health and Well-being of the province reiterated the importance of primary care settings and community organizations in providing mental health care (Commissaire à la santé et au bien-être, 2012).

In the summer of 2007, three child psychiatrists specialized in transcultural mental health moved from the pediatric hospital to work in the community clinics of the CSSS. With them came a research group devoted to immigrant and refugee children and their families. At the same time, the community clinics started to build a youth mental health team, which included both professionals already working in the community clinic and professionals transferred from hospital-based child mental health teams. This Youth Mental Health Team aimed to provide mental health care directly to youth and their families and support the work of other teams in the community clinic. When the project began, the group was determined to work closely with community organizations. This determination stemmed from previous clinical experience, which highlighted the importance for refugee and immigrant families of the barriers to care and the power imbalances in health care delivery (Nadeau, 2004). Establishing bridges with community organizations provided a channel for the expression of individual and family concerns. Understanding a family's community links during the consultation process facilitated the appraisal of the child and family's difficulties within broader social and cultural perspectives.

The CSSS staff already worked closely with community organizations. These professionals' experiences and their sense of familiarity with the different ethnic communities enhanced the partnerships formed around youth mental health care. Social workers, educators, dieticians and nurses from the CSSS also worked closely with daycare facilities and schools. Primary care health and social service organizations, meant to be frontline services for the population, faced the challenge of establishing respectful partnerships with community organizations. Health institutions go through restructuring phases, changing their organizational models, their leaders or their programs' vocations which may interfere with the continuity of community partnerships, putting at risk the slowly developed personalized links which have been forged with community organizations. As well, child psychiatrists and the youth mental health collaborative care initiative, including all of the restructuring it entailed, were newer additions to the community-based model, and this could be destabilizing at times or even threatening because of the shadow of hospital-centered and hierarchical professional models.

Service Delivery by the Youth Mental Health Team

The child or adolescent mental health referrals to the Youth Mental Health Team are first reviewed by the "Guichet d'accès" (triage team) and then assigned to a specific community-based youth mental health team. Depending on the clinical situation, a youth mental health team member may become a key person in the care of this patient or alternatively may provide backup to a first-line professional from another team already involved in the care. The triage team also decides if a child psychiatric consultation is necessary (either directly with the child and family or indirectly through a case discussion among professionals).

Child psychiatry consultations are always done in the presence of the main primary care provider and often with other professionals involved in the care of the child or youth. The role of the main care provider is reinforced during the consultation and he or she remains responsible for implementing the treatment recommendations and insuring continuity of care. Consultations have three main aims: (1) providing the frontline professional with therapeutic tools by establishing or clarifying a diagnosis, exploring individual and family dynamics, elaborating a treatment plan and transmitting therapeutic know-how; (2) supporting the professional during complex therapeutic work through clinical supervision, allowing the expression of feelings of uncertainty, ambivalence and sharing the perceived burden of care; and (3) facilitating access to specialized services in mental health care. The consultation process is flexible and varies according to circumstances: it may consist of a punctual consultation or can involve repeated meetings with the patient and or the treatment team at the request of the primary treating professional.

The WHO and WONCA report (2008) underlined the efficacy of modalities using experiential ongoing training for primary care professionals built in their core work experience:

> The effects of training are nearly always short-lived if health workers do not practise newly-learnt skills and receive specialist supervision over time. Ongoing support and supervision from mental health specialists are essential. Collaborative or shared care models, in which joint consultations and interventions take place between primary care workers and mental health specialists, seem especially promising. (p. 67)

Addressing power issues within interprofessional care is a cornerstone of collaborative mental health care. Professionals often renegotiate their roles within the process of care, either at the time of the consultation or following it. The consultation creates an opportunity to identify roles and responsibilities, to express concerns and to review treatment strategies. Most often, all professionals working with the identified patient and family are invited to the consultation.

In the presence of the family, the consultation process is described as one of sharing views, thus allowing families to voice their concerns and interpretation of the situation. This hopes to be an empowering process, counteracting some of the voicelessness that migrants may experience in the host society. The establishment of a dialogue is an explicit recognition of the knowledge that migrants and minority ethnic groups have of their own predicament and of their agency in seeking solutions.

Mental health issues may complicate this process of dialogue when the stigma of mental illness adds to the exclusion associated with minority status. At times, the internalization by migrants of paternalistic and hierarchical representations of mental health professionals act as barriers to the empowerment process.

The consultation is often an occasion to have a joint meeting with other institutional and community partners involved in a child's care, if a family is open to their presence and it is clinically relevant. These networking meetings favor collegial discussion and co-construction of a plan among the family and the multiple professionals involved in the child's care. Although professionals may disagree about treatment directions, this form of consultation decreases misunderstandings and improves communication, facilitating mediation between potentially divergent views. The inclusion of community organization members in the consultation may also facilitate the alliance with the family, as illustrated in the following vignette.

Case Vignette 9-2

Carlos, a 10-year-old boy from Peru who had academic difficulties, mentioned to a school psycho-educator that on occasions he was hearing voices. The school asked for a psychiatric consultation because they were worried by these symptoms. Within the consultation, the parents were invited to share their views on the boys' symptom. They disclosed that according to the family Carlos was the bearer of a transgenerational gift: he had some shamanic powers, which were associated with the voices he heard. The parents then thanked the consultation group members for their openness and respect toward this interpretation of his "problems." While the parental explanatory model was acknowledged, the consultation also emphasized the boy's anxiety and his dissociative symptoms. This intervention helped to strengthen the alliance with the school and the health care system and facilitated follow-up intervention by simultaneously addressing the strengths and the vulnerabilities of the family and of the boy, without pathologizing them.

Case Vignette 9-3

Anika, a 7-year-old girl from Bangladesh was referred by her school social worker for consultation for symptoms of anxiety and depression. Her mother was reported to have been noncooperative at an earlier interpreter-assisted school meeting to discuss her daughter's difficulties. The description of the difficulties communicating with the mother was such that the Youth Mental Health Team, prior to the meeting, raised the possibility that she might be suffering from paranoid symptoms. With the mother's approval, a representative from a community organization, who was already known to her, was invited to the consultation with the objective of better understanding the mother's worries and of finding acceptable strategies to help her and her child.

In the community organization worker's presence, the mother was able to explain how she felt bewildered in the host

(continued)

society because she was suffering from intimate partner violence. She had been kept isolated and threatened by her partner and had no information about what services the host society could offer. The meeting shifted the perception of the consulting team, who now perceived the mother's avoidance as trauma-related rather than a sign of paranoia. Her linguistic communication problems and her sparse knowledge of the host society aggravated her fear and withdrawal. The support provided to her by community organization members who were familiar with her social and cultural circumstances enabled the team to establish a working alliance to respond to her child's needs.

Interpreters are also major players in building bridges toward communities. They are important members of the multidisciplinary team and play a key role in the consultation process, not limited to translation (Leanza, 2007; Rousseau, Measham, & Moro, 2011; see Chapter 5). Unfortunately, the inclusion of interpreters in health institutions across the province tends to remain limited to situations where communication is expected to be very restricted or impossible without their presence. At the CSSS, interpreters are asked to join consultations when the professional organizing the consultation deems this necessary. Because mental health consultations touch upon sensitive and complex emotional issues often requiring a rich vocabulary, and because family members may differ in their knowledge of the host country languages, liberal use of interpreters in consultations is essential in the work of the Youth Mental Health Team. Interpreters also often play the role of cultural brokers, alerting the group to possible misunderstandings and to cultural issues (Kaufert & Putsch, 1997). They can give advice about how to interpret the cultural elements of a narrative and can help to distinguish signs of pathology from culturally normative behavior. Their presence

may support the family disclosure of adverse experiences in the community of origin or in the host country community. At the same time, the presence of an interpreter adds a new figure to the consultation and collaborative care process. Exchanges through interpreters take more time and require an adjustment of assessment and treatment practices. This new presence can be integrated in order to bring collaboration and clarification rather than confusion in the clinical process. Finally, the very presence of an interpreter or cultural broker conveys a message that the family's cultural background is deemed important within the consultation. The need for the family to experience a sense of a culturally safe space gets explicitly named during the consultation interview.

Case Vignette 9-4

Kiara, a 12-year-old girl was referred to the clinic for symptoms of anxiety. The family, from the Philippines, had to deal with the challenge of the mother suffering from a disabling chronic illness. The parents needed help navigating the health and social services systems. The whole family experienced anxiety because of mother's illness, which had drastically changed their hopes around immigration. The family wished to have another family member, living in their country of origin, come to help them deal with the mother's illness but felt disempowered to take action toward such a request. The presence of a professional interpreter who was very knowledgeable about social services, health networks and immigration procedures was key to conveying health information in a culturally safe manner and to accompanying through the multiple steps needed to get help within the local health network and proceed with the request to have the family member to come for a few months to Canada. They were reassured and able to envision possible steps forward.

Addressing Culture and Immigration

For the vast majority of the child psychiatry consultations taking place within the CSSS project, the meeting with the family provides an opportunity to discuss the cultural roots and sense of belonging of families. Meeting with migrant families also acts as a reminder for clinicians' of their own values and representations, both individual and collective. Many care providers have become more aware of how their own identities are implicated in the clinical process and are learning to make intentional use of these identities within the clinical work (Nadeau et al., 2009).

In addition to training in cultural competence, collaborative care requires that frontline professionals acquire the knowledge, skills and attitudes essential to provide mental health care. This includes core information about the epidemiology, identification and treatment of major mental health disorders, the relationship between physical and mental health problems and communication skills to enhance the patient–clinician relationship (WHO & WONCA, 2008). Mastering the new roles associated with collaborative care and becoming aware of impact of one's own identity in the clinical process can be challenging (Murphy, 1987) and requires the ability to suspend judgment and learn from others (Lu, Lim, & Mezzich, 1995; Toniolo, 2007).

Training modalities need to adapt to this transformation of practices and to provide support to clinicians. Learning to tolerate uncertainty, while at the same time being supported in new experiences of clinical work can increase professional confidence. Joint clinical work and case discussion seminars over a period of time can help professionals expand their clinical knowledge, skills and attitudes in the encounter with "otherness."

Case Vignette 9-5

Nader, a 10-year-old boy presented with conflictual peer relationships and intrafamilial verbal aggressivity with the use of threatening and disrespectful language.

He also had academic difficulties. His family was from Lebanon and the parents were separated. There were some attachment difficulties with the mother who was suffering from lupus and obsessive-compulsive disorder. After the initial consultation, a follow-up was organized for the parents to review parenting issues. Individual therapy was offered to Nader, in order to support him while his parents' conflictual relationship was addressed. During the treatment, the primary care professionals were faced many family crises. The boy's verbal threats were reassessed in relation to the family's cultural background. For example, when the boy said to his parents "I will kill you," this was viewed as a homicidal threat by the service providers who were worried by the level of conflict in the family and were afraid of the risk of a violent acting out. A culture broker emphasized that in Lebanon these utterances would mainly be understood as an expression of anger with no real intention to inflict physical violence. This reframing and repeated contacts and discussions between care providers allowed them to better understand the family dynamics and to interpret the boy's aggressive verbalizations in cultural context, avoiding a more intrusive intervention through youth protection. The collaborative care model facilitated the discussion of specific cultural manifestations of family turmoil and supported their resolution.

Adapting services also means taking into account the sociopolitical context of the patient's history, acknowledging pre-migratory experiences (such as organized violence) as well as post-migratory experiences such as discrimination and poverty. These experiences modulate the illness experience, difficulties encountered and the response given to proposed treatments (Kleinman, Das, & Lock, 1997; Porter & Haslam, 2005).

The consultations with the child psychiatrist often provide an occasion to ask the family to narrate their migration process including some of their pre- and post-migratory challenges, stresses and successes. Frontline professionals who familiarise themselves with these experiences deepen their understanding of the family's unique history. At the same time, the consultation process is not only about obtaining specific information from families; it is also about deciding what information needs to be gathered and when and how this can be done. When sensitive information, such as traumatic events, is involved, the timing of disclosure of this information with the family is a delicate issue (Measham & Rousseau, 2010).

The stigma associated with mental illness may also need to be addressed because it is a major barrier to access services for many people. Stigma may be particularly severe for some cultural groups, for example, if mental illness was highly stigmatized in their country of origin or they already have experiences of discrimination or exclusion due to their minority status in the host country. Primary care settings may be viewed as less stigmatizing than mental health services making it easier to deliver mental health care (Kates, 2008).

The consultations are also an occasion to learn know-how regarding fostering attention to diversity and culture. Primary care professionals themselves represent the growing diversity of society. In the consultation process, the diversity of cultural identities within the group of professionals can implicitly represent the multiplicity of interpretations available to give meaning to a clinical situation. This can encourage families to share their own understandings of the clinical situation. At times, the consultation may acknowledge this diversity explicitly by inviting both service users and professionals to share their own interpretations with the group.

Case Vignette 9-6
At the onset of a consultation for David, a 6-year-old first-born son of two university parents from Togo, the child psychiatrist evoked the diversity of professions and cultural origins of the team present at the assessment and explained their presence as an opportunity to think through the issues together using different lenses or ways of interpreting the difficulties to identify strategies to improve the situation. Meeting a child psychiatrist alone might have led the parents to refer mostly to the Western biomedical models they were familiar with through their studies. The invitation to discuss different interpretations, together with the initiative of one of the team members professional to comment on traditional views on first-born sons, allowed them to share the extended family discourse on the privileged place of this son as the first-born grandchild. His oppositional behavior could then be reinterpreted in the light of the specific dynamics around this cherished child.

Allowing for the expression of the multiple points of views of patients, their family members and the different primary care providers needs to be considered in the context of the imagined legitimate public expression of thoughts and emotions within the framework of both the cultural manners one feel bound to and the host society current discourses on migrants. It talks about providing a safe space to discuss alternative ways to Western models of healing. It stimulates clinicians' awareness of their expectation regarding the style of emotional expression and communication strategies within the clinical encounter. It also solicits in a modulated manner a discourse on the country of origin.

Furthermore, the institutional culture in the Western world often frames the patient-service provider clinical encounter in a dyadic way. Some patients used to a more collective way to envisage solutions when facing adversity, may feel estranged by a purely dyadic process. The primary care professionals differ in their training on this aspect: some will have been used to almost exclusively to a dyadic process, whereas others have been more exposed to systemic approaches.

Training Methods to Support Collaborative Care for Culturally Diverse Populations

The implementation of the collaborative youth mental health project in an urban setting was supported by a continuing education program based on the synergy between seminars, supervisions and didactic teaching. Inter-institutional case discussion seminars promote a shared place of dialogue between partners who work in different organizational cultures. They can work to decrease service fragmentation, offer support to primary workers and transmit clinical know-how (De Plaen et al., 2005; Rousseau et al., 2005). By regularly bringing together workers from different neighborhood institutions to discuss the same case, these seminars allow clinicians to develop trusting working relationships and to co-construct their clinical practices within a theoretical framework that facilitates the transformation of these practices to better address the specificities of the clinical situation at stake. Training in the form of group and individual clinical supervision provides complementary modalities together with didactic clinical and theoretical teaching. This training takes into account the time and clinical load constraints of primary care workers. The training content focuses on issues pertinent to primary care including adaptations of clinical detection and intervention tools for youth with mental health difficulties to fit the reality of primary care in multiethnic urban neighborhoods. There is also a focus on promoting awareness of the historical and sociocultural specificities of the communities served.

These hands-on training activities seem to benefit the collaborative partnership. Shared discussions and teaching strengthen the network and increase understanding of each other's responsibilities, limits, mandates and traditions (Nadeau & Measham, 2006). Shared clinical discussions also offer a forum to merge different clinical points of view, which is an essential part of developing collaborative care. Rather than aiming at a consensus of points of view, these discussions provide a space for different interpretations to be heard, considered and integrated within a coherent treatment plan. In initiatives combining collaborative mental health care and services to a culturally diverse population, the mix of different modalities including case discussions within seminars and supervision as well as didactic teaching facilitates the reflection on one's own work that is needed to enable the patient's voice to be heard (Katz & Shotter, 1996). As such, it helps to avoid two pitfalls: stereotyping the culture of the patient and being color blind and attributing no importance to cultural aspects.

In describing our approach to collaborative care, we have used case vignettes involving children and youth, reflecting our practice as child psychiatrists. While the general principles discussed in this chapter also apply to adult populations, adults face specific challenges in a culturally diverse population (e.g., work, lodging) that must be addressed accordingly. As well, collaborative care in adult mental health requires specific partnerships and resources (e.g., crisis centers) that differ from those most relevant in child and youth mental health.

Conclusion: Collaborative Mental Health Care in Transcultural Contexts

Collaboration between primary, secondary and tertiary care professionals can provide better continuity of care and efficient use of limited resources. Of course, collaboration across different professions demands its own share of adjustments, and much work must be done with partners and stakeholders at the onset to clarify roles and build effective teams. Multidisciplinary teams can facilitate understanding of cultural contexts and promote negotiation of differences and the provision of culturally appropriate care. Indeed, the focus on cultural formulation can itself facilitate the interdisciplinary exchange by giving explicit place for the insights of professions like social work, nursing and social sciences focussed on the lifeworld of patient and family (Dinh, Groleau, Kirmayer, Rodriguez, & Bibeau, 2012).

At its roots the model of collaborative mental health care encourages all actors to be partners in care and promotes a partnership role for families as well. At the same time, true collaboration remains a major challenge as both illness and migration may strain the voice and agency of families as they struggle with new predicaments. Families come to a new country with an expected model of care in mind, unconsciously if not consciously. Migrants become expert at adapting to new realities, but in so far as mental health problems mobilize defence mechanisms, they can provoke fears about an unfamiliar system of care which is perceived as stigmatizing and unresponsive. Introducing a multiplicity of voices within collaborative care symbolically conveys that all perspectives are important and this process can be empowering for families.

Multidisciplinary collaboration and inviting a multiplicity of voices, however, runs the risk of disorganization if no one acts as leader. The consultation process needs to avoid a cacophony of voices while promoting a stimulating diversity of actors. To insure coordination and coherence, the process needs to be led by a designated care provider, usually the main primary care provider who will remain in charge of the follow-up. Having the primary care provider take this lead role reorganizes the traditional hierarchy between psychiatrists and other health care providers and may at times be destabilizing. It also confronts primary care providers with all the complexities and uncertainties of mental health issues. It is thus essential that opportunities are provided within both training and practice settings to regularly discuss the transformation of roles and to support workers who face difficulties with the new modes of practice. This underscores the need to introduce opportunities for debate about the impact of collaborative care ventures during the implementation of new models. Introducing spaces to express doubt and uncertainty is especially important at the outset of the implementation of collaborative care projects when everyone is struggling to understand what exactly the project will entail in terms of new roles.

In summary, models of consultation in collaborative care base their efficacy on partnerships.

The mental health consultation model described in this chapter promotes close partnerships among professionals but also with families and communities through which traditional power imbalances within the medical system can be challenged and transformed. The model also can be used to promote greater awareness of the diverse cultures that permeate the collaborative care in multiethnic populations, and tries to avoid cultural stereotyping by giving voice to the diversity of perspectives within communities, including those of women and youth. Because this model presents a double challenge to primary care professionals' in terms of role and cultural identity, training modalities must directly address the feelings of adequacy or competence of primary care workers as well as the notion of cultural safety for both families and professionals.

References

Ang, S., & Van Dyne, L. (2008). *Handbook of cultural intelligence: Theory, measurement, and applications.* Armonk, NY: ME Sharpe.

Benigeri, M., Bluteau, J.-P., Roberge, M., Provencher, P., & Nadeau, L. (2007). *L'utilisation des services de santé mentale par les Montréalais en 2004–2005.* Montreal, Quebec, Canada: Carrefour montréalais d'information sociosanitaire, Agence de la santé et des services sociaux de Montréal 2007.

Berry, J. W. (1998). Acculturation in health. In S. Kazrin & D. R. Evans (Eds.), *Cultural clinical psychology.* New York, NY: Oxford.

Bibeau, G. (1998). Tropismes Québecois. Je me souviens dans l'oubli. *Anthropologie et Sociétés, 19*(3), 151–198.

Bibeau, G., Chan-Yip, A., Lock, M., & Rousseau, C. (1992). *La santé mentale et ses visage: Vers un québec plus rythmique au quotidien.* Montréal, Quebec, Canada: Gaeten Morin.

Bilodeau, A., Lapierre, S., & Marchand, Y. (2003). *Le partenariat: Comment ça marche.* Montreal, Quebec, Canada: Régie régionale de la santé et des services sociaux de Montréal- centre, Direction de la santé publique.

Bowen, S. (2001). *Language barriers in access to health care "certain circumstances": Equity in and responsiveness of the health care system to the needs of minority and marginalized populations* (pp. 145–160). Ottawa, Ontario, Canada: Health Canada.

Brascoupé, S., & Waters, C. (2009). Cultural safety: Exploring the applicabiity of the concept of cultural safety to Aboriginal health and community wellness. *Journal of Aboriginal Health, 7*(1), 6–40.

Brauner, C. B., & Stephen, C. B. (2006). Estimating the prevalence of early childhood serious emotional/behavioral disorders: Challenges and recommendations. *Public Health Reports, 121*(3), 303–310.

Burns, B. J., Costello, E. J., Angold, A., Tweed, D., Stangl, D., Farmer, E. M., et al. (1995). Children's mental health service across service sectors. *Health Affairs, 14*(3), 147–159.

Canadian Collaborative Mental Health Initiative. (2006). *Establishing collaborative initiatives between mental health and primary care services for ethnocultural populations. A companion to the CCMHI planning and implementation toolkit for health care providers and planners.* Mississauga, Ontario, Canada: Canadian Collaborative Mental Health Initiative. Retrieved from http://www.ccmhi.ca

Canadian Mental Health Association. (2003). *Access to mental health services: Issues, barriers and recommendations for federal action: A brief to the standing senate committee on social affairs.* Ottawa, Ontario, Canada: Science and Technology.

Chen, A. W., Kazanjian, A., Wong, H., & Goldner, E. M. (2010). Mental health service use by Chinese immigrants with severe and persistent mental illness. *Canadian Journal of Psychiatry, 55*(1), 35–42.

Chenven, M. (2010). Community systems of care for children's mental health. *Child and Adolescent Psychiatric Clinic of North America, 19*, 163–174.

Commissaire à la santé et au bien-être (2012). *Rapport d'appréciation de la performance du système de santé et de services sociaux 2012 – Pour plus d'équité et de résultats en santé mentale au Québec*, Québec, Gouvernement du Québec, 179 p.

Corin, E., Uchoa, E., Bibeau, G., & Koumare, B. (1992). Articulation et variations des systèmes de signes, de sens et d'action. *Psychopathologie Africaine, 24*(2), 183–204.

Costello, D. M., Swendsen, J., Rose, J. S., & Dierker, L. C. (2008). Risk and protective factors associated with trajectories of depressed mood from adolescence to early adulthood. *Journal of Consulting and Clinical Psychology, 76*(2), 173.

D'Amours, D. (2005). De l'individuel au collectif. *Le point en administration de la santé et des services sociaux, 1*(3), 12–13.

DePlaen, S., Alain, N., Rousseau, C., Chiasson, M., Lynch, A., Elejalde, A., et al. (2005). Mieux travailler en situations cliniques complexes: L'expérience des séminaires transculturels institutionels. *Santé Mentale au Québec, 30*(2), 281–299.

Dewar, S. (2000). Collaborating for quality: The need to strengthen accountability. *Journal of Interprofessional Care, 14*(1), 31–38.

Dinh, M. H., Groleau, D., Kirmayer, L. J., Rodriguez, C., & Bibeau, G. (2012). Influence of the DSM-IV outline for cultural formulation on multidisciplinary case conferences in mental health. *Anthropology & Medicine, 19*(2), 261–276.

Ewing, K. P. (1990). The illusion of wholeness: Culture, self, and the experience of inconsistency. *Ethos, 18*(3), 251–278.

Fenta, H., Hyman, I., & Noh, S. (2006). Mental health service utilization by Ethiopian immigrants and refugees in Toronto. *The Journal of Nervous and Mental Disease, 194*(12), 925–934.

Gorman, W. (2001). Refugee survivors of torture: Trauma and treatment. *Professional Psychology: Research and Practice, 32*(5), 443.

Hickie, I. B., Fogarty, A. S., Davenport, T. A., Luscombe, G. M., & Burns, J. (2007). Responding to experiences of young people with common mental health problems attending Australian general practice. *Medical Journal of Australia, 187*(7 Suppl), S47–S52.

Hyman, I. (2004). Setting the stage: Reviewing current knowledge on the health of Canadian immigrants. *Canadian Journal of Public Health, 95*(3), 1–4.

Kates, N. (2008). Promoting collaborative care in Canada: The Canadian collaborative mental health initiative. *Families, Systems & Health, 26*(4), 466–473.

Kates, N., Mazowita, G., Lemire, F., Jayabarathan, A., Bland, R., Selby, P., et al. (2011). The evolution of collaborative mental health care in Canada: A shared vision for the future. *Canadian Journal of Psychiatry, 56*(5), 1–10.

Katon, W. J., & Seelig, M. (2008). Population-based care of depression: Team care approaches to improving outcomes. *Journal of Occupational and Environmental Medicine, 50*(4), 459–467.

Katz, A. M., & Shotter, J. (1996). Hearing the patient's "voice": Toward a social poetics in diagnostic interviews. *Social Science & Medicine, 43*(6), 919–931.

Kaufert, J. M., & Putsch, R. W. (1997). Communication through interpreters in healthcare: ethical dilemmas arising from differences in class, culture, language, and power. *The Journal of Clinical Ethics, 8*(1), 71–87.

Kirmayer, L., Narasiah, L., Muñoz, M., Rashid, M., Ryder, A., Guzder, J., Rousseau, C. (2011). Common mental health problems in immigrants and refugees: General approach to the patient in primary care. Canadian Medical Association Journal, 183(12), E959-967. doi: 10.1503/cmaj.090292.

Kleinman, A., Das, V., & Lock, M. (Eds.). (1997). *Social suffering.* Berkeley, CA: University of California Press.

Koptie, S. (2009). Irihapeti Ramsden: The public narrative on cultural safety. *First Peoples Child & Family Review, 4*(2), 30–43.

LaFromboise, T., Coleman, H. L., & Gerton, J. (1993). Psychological impact of biculturalism: Evidence and theory. *Psychological Bulletin, 114*(3), 395–412.

Leaf, P. J., Alegria, A., Cohen, P., Goodman, S. H., Horwitz, S. M., Hoven, C. W., et al. (1996). Mental health service use in the community and school: Results from the four-community MECA study. *Journal of the American Academy of Child and Adolescent Psychiatry, 35*(7), 889–897.

Leanza, Y. (2007). Roles of community interpreters in pediatrics as seen by interpreters, physicians and researchers. In F. Pöchhacker & M. Shlesinger (Eds.), *Healthcare interpreting: Discourse and interaction.* Philadelphia, PA: John Benjamins Publishing Compay.

Leckman, J. F., & Leventhal, B. L. (2008). Edtorial: A global perspective on child and adolescent mental health. *Journal of Child Psychology and Psychiatry, 49*(3), 221–225.

Lesage, A., Vasiliadis, H. M., Gagne, M.-A., Dudgeon, S., Kasman, N., & Hay, C. (2006). *Prévalence de la maladie mentale et utilisation des services connexes au Canada: Une analyse des donneés de l'Enquête sur la santé dans les collectivités canadiennes.* Mississauga, ON: Canadian Collaborative Mental Health Initiative.

Lu, F. G., Lim, R. F., & Mezzich, J. E. (1995). Issues of assessment and diagnosis of culturally diverse individuals. In J. M. Oldham & M. B. Riba (Eds.), *Review of psychiatry* (Vol. 14). Washington, DC: American Psychiatric Press.

Measham, T., & Rousseau, C. (2010). Family disclosure of war trauma to children. *Traumatology, 16*(4), 85–96.

Mental Health Commission of Canada. (2012). *Changing directions, changing lives: The mental health strategy for Canada.* Ottawa, Ontario, Canada: Mental Health Commission of Canada.

Ministère de la santé et des Services sociaux. (2005). *Plan d'action en santé mentale 2005–2010: La force des liens.* Québec, Canada: Gouvernement du Québec.

Murphy, H. B. M. (1987). Migration, culture and our perception of the stranger. In E. Corin, S. Lamarre, P. Migneault, & M. Tousignant (Eds.), *Regards anthropologiques en psychiatrie* (pp. 77–86). Outremont, Quebec, Canada: Production Immédia.

Nadeau, L. (2004). *Altérité et relations de pouvoir dans le processus thérapeutique d'une clinique de pédopsychiatrie transculturelle.* Master's thesis, Department of Psychiatry, McGill University, Montreal, Quebec, Canada.

Nadeau, L. (2007). L'altérité dans la rencontre de pédopsychiatrie transculturelle. In M. Cognet & C. Montgomery (Eds.), *Éthique de l'altérité. La question de la culture dans le champ de la santé et des services sociaux* (pp. 177–190). Montréal, Quebec, Canada: Les Presses de l'Université Laval.

Nadeau, L., & Measham, T. (2006). Caring for migrant and refugee children: Challenges associated with mental health care in pediatrics. *Journal of Development and Behavioral Pediatriacs, 27*(2), 145–154.

Nadeau, L., Rousseau, C., Séguin, Y., Moreau, N. (2009). Évaluation préliminaire d'un projet de soins concertés en santé mentale jeunesse à Montréal : faire face à l'incertitude institutionnelle et culturelle. *Santé mentale au Québec, 34*(1), 127–142.

Papps, E., & Ramsden, I. (1996). Cultural safety in nursing: The New Zealand experience. *International Journal for Quality in Health Care, 8*(5), 491–497.

Paquin, C. (2008). *Profil statistique de la population du territoire du CSSS de la Montagne 2006.* Montreal, Quebec, Canada: Centre de santé et des services sociaux de la Montagne.

Patel, V., Flisher, A., Hetrick, S., & McGory, P. (2007). Mental health of young people: A global public health challenge. *The Lancet, 369*(9569), 1302–1313.

Pautler, K., & Gagné, M.-A. (2005). *Bibliographie annotée des soins de santé mentale axés sur la collaboration.* Mississaugua, Ontario, Canada: Initiative canadienne de collaboration en santé mentale. Available from Disponible au, www.iccsm.ca

Pauzé, E., Gagné, M.-A., & Pautler, K. (2005). *Collaborative mental health care in primary health care: A review of Canadian initiatives. Vol. 1: Analysis of initiatives.* Mississauga, ON: Canadian Collaborative Mental Health Initiative (CCMHI).

Porter, M., & Haslam, N. (2005). Predisplacement and postdisplacement factors associated with mental health of refugees and internally displaced persons: A meta-analysis. *Journal of the American Medical Association, 294*(5), 602–612.

Pottie, K., Greenaway, C., Feightner, J., Welch, V., Greenaway, C., Swinkels, H., et al. (2011). Review: Evidence-based clinical guidelines for immigrants and refugees. *Canadian Medical Association Journal, 183*, E824–E925. doi:10.1503/cmaj.090313.

Pottie, K., Tugwell, P., Feightner, J., Welch, V., Greenaway, C., Swinkels, H., et al. (2010). Summary of clinical preventive care recommendations for newly arriving immigrants and refugees to Canada. *Canadian Medical Association Journal.* doi: cmaj.090313 [pii] 10.1503/cmaj.090313

Regier, Darrel A.; Narrow, William E.; Rae, Donald S.; Manderscheid, Ronald W.; Locke, Ben Z.; Goodwin, Frederick K. (1993). The de facto US mental and addictive disorders service system: Epidemiologic Catchment Area prospective 1-year prevalence rates of disorders and services. *Archives of General Psychiatry, 50*(2), 85–94.

Rousseau, C., Alain, N., De Plaen, S., Chiasson-Lavoie, M., Elejalde, A., Lynch, A., et al. (2005). Repenser la formation continue dans le réseau de la santé et des services sociaux: L'expérience des séminaires interinstitutionnels en intervention transculturelle. *Nouvelles Pratiques Sociales, 17*(2), 109–125.

Rousseau, C., Ammara, G., Baillargeon, L., Lenoir, A., & Roy, D. (2007). *Repenser les services en santé mentale des jeunes. La créativité nécessaire.* Montréal, Quebec, Canada: Les Publications du Québec.

Rousseau, C., de la Aldea, E., Viger Rojas, M., & Foxen, P. (2005). After the NGO's departure: Changing memory strategies of young Mayan refugees who returned to Guatemala as a community. *Anthropology & Medicine, 12*(1), 3–21.

Rousseau, C., Measham, T., & Moro, M. R. (2011). Working with interpreters in child mental health. *Child and Adolescent Mental Health, 16*(1), 55–59.

Rousseau, C., Measham, T., & Nadeau, L. (2012). Addressing trauma in collaborative mental health care for refugee children. *Clinical Child Psychology and Psychiatry, 18*(1), 121–136.

Rushton, J., Bruckman, D., & Kelleher, K. (2002). Primary care referral of children with psychosocial problems. *Archives of Pediatrics & Adolescent Medicine, 156*(6), 592–598.

Sadavoy, J., Meier, R., & Ong, A. Y. (2004). Barriers to access to mental health services for ethnic seniors: The Toronto study. *Canadian Journal of Psychiatry, 49*(3), 192–199.

Schwartz, S. J., Unger, J. B., Zamboanga, B. L., & Szapocznik, J. (2010). Rethinking the concept of acculturation: Implications for theory and research. *American Psychologist, 65*(4), 237–251.

Sévigny, D., Viau, A., & Rabhi, K. (2002). *Portrait socio-culturelle des élèves inscrits dans les écoles publiques de l'Île de Montréal: Inscriptions au 31 Septembre 2001.* Montréal, Quebec, Canada: Conseil scolaire de l'Île de Montréal.

Smye, V., Josewski, V., & Kendall, E. (2010). *Cultural safety: An overview.* Ottawa, Ontario, Canada: First Nations, Inuit and Métis Advisory Committee, Mental Health Commission of Canada.

Spenser, H. R., Gilles, A., & Maysenhoelder, H. (2009). The CHAT project: Paediatricians and mental health clinicians: Working together for the sake of the children. *Journal of Canadian Academy of Child and Adolescent Psychiatry, 18*(2), 110–116.

Sue, D. W. (2001). Multidimensional facets of cultural competence. *The Counseling Psychologist, 29*(6), 790-821.

Swinkels, H., Pottie, K., Tugwell, P., Rashid, M., & Narasiah, L. (2011). Development of guidelines for recently arrived immigrants and refugees to Canada: Delphi consensus on selecting preventable and treatable conditions. *Canadian Medical Association Journal.* doi: cmaj.090290 [pii] 10.1503/cmaj.090290

Toniolo, I. (2007). Psychiatric dosorders in a transcultural setting. *Clinical Neuropsychiatry, 4*(4), 160–178.

Trickett, E. J. (2009). Multilevel community-based culturally situated interventions and community impact: An ecological perspective. *American Journal of Community Psychology, 43*(3), 257–266.

Verhulst, F. C., VanderEnde, J., Ferdinand, R. F., & Kasius, M. C. (1997). The prevalence of DSM-III-R diagnosis in a national sample of Dutch adolescents. *Archives of General Psychiatry, 54*(4), 329–336.

Waddell, C., McEwan, K., Shepherd, C. A., Offord, D. R., Huam J. M. (2005). A public health strategy to improve the mental health of Canadian children. *Canadian Journal of Psychiatry, 50*(4), 226–233.

WHO & WONCA (2008). *Integrating mental health into primary care: A global perspective. Geneva*: World Health Organization.

Yeung, A., Kung, W. W., Chung, H., Rubenstein, G., Roffi, P., Mischoulon, D., et al. (2004). Integrating psychiatry and primary care improves acceptability to mental health services among Chinese Americans. *General Hospital Psychiatry, 26*(4), 256–260.

Consultation to Remote and Indigenous Communities

11

Marie-Eve Cotton, Lucie Nadeau,
and Laurence J. Kirmayer

Introduction

Most models of mental health services have been developed in urban settings, with large populations and many specialized resources. Rural and remote communities pose challenges to these models for reasons of geography, social structure and culture. In Canada and other countries, rural and remote communities include a high proportion of Indigenous peoples, with important cultural differences from the urban population. In this chapter, we discuss the role of cultural consultation in providing mental health services for remote and rural communities, with an emphasis on the mental health of Indigenous peoples in Canada. The authors have worked as psychiatric consultants to First Nations and Inuit communities in Northern Quebec and draw from this experience and the work of the CCS to outline key issues for cultural consultation in this setting.

The Context of Rural and Remote Communities

Rural and remote communities can be defined in various ways reflecting relative size and density of population, level of infrastructure and distance from urban centers (Hart, Larson, & Lishner, 2005). A rural community is located outside an urban area has smaller size, lower population density and less infrastructure. A remote community is situated at a great distance from a metropolitan region and is difficult to reach by regular transportation. Such communities typically have a small population and low population density and usually have very limited infrastructure. The costs of providing mental health services in such settings are high.

In Canada, the population of most remote communities is predominately Aboriginal peoples (First Nations, Inuit or Métis).[1] Although more than 50% of the Indigenous population live

M.-E. Cotton, M.D. (✉)
Hôpital Louis-H. Lafontaine, 7401, rue Hochelaga,
Montréal, QC, Canada H1T 3M5
e-mail: marieevecotton@hotmail.com

L. Nadeau, M.D., M.Sc., F.R.C.P.(C)
CSSS de la Montagne (CLSC Parc Extension),
7085 Hutchison, #204.10, Montreal,
QC, Canada H3N 1Y9
e-mail: lucie.nadeau@mcgill.ca

L.J. Kirmayer, M.D.
Culture & Mental Health Research Unit,
Institute of Community & Family Psychiatry,
Jewish General Hospital, 4333 Cote Ste Catherine Road,
Montreal, QC, Canada H3T 1E4
e-mail: laurence.kirmayer@mcgill.ca

[1] Although "Aboriginal" is the official term used by government to designate the Indigenous peoples of Canada (including First Nations, Inuit and Métis), in this chapter we will use the term "Indigenous" which is increasingly preferred by groups internationally.

L.J. Kirmayer et al. (eds.), *Cultural Consultation: Encountering the Other in Mental Health Care*, International and Cultural Psychology, DOI 10.1007/978-1-4614-7615-3_11, © Springer Science+Business Media New York 2014

in cities, and many live in reserves located near cities, according to Statistics Canada (2008), approximately 20% of Indigenous people in Canada live in rural or remote non-reserve communities. In this context, rural and remote includes wilderness areas and agricultural lands, as well as small towns, villages and other populated places with a population of less than 1,000 and a density of less than 400 persons per square kilometer. Many of these communities are located in Canada's northern regions. The social, cultural and political issues of Indigenous peoples combined with logistical issues of geographical location and scale pose distinct challenges for mental health services.

Fully 90% of Indigenous communities across Canada consist of less than 1,000 people. These communities are often located in regions with very low population density. Some of these communities, especially arctic and northern communities, are more than 2,000 km from a major city. Access to many of these centers from rural and remote areas is often difficult. Few roads connect some of the smaller communities, which may be hundreds of kilometers from neighboring communities.

Small communities have some advantages with regard to mental health. There can be greater social cohesion, easy access to social and family support systems, a strong informal network of helpers and widely shared knowledge of the community and available resources. In small communities, personal networks and professional relationships are likely to overlap. This can be an advantage when an immediate response is needed to avert a crisis but can be a disadvantage to both clinicians and clients when privacy and professional distance is desired. Community workers may be closely connected to the people they are supposed to help, implicated in their conflicts, and may never have any respite from their role as caregivers.

A variety of forms of mental health service have been provided to rural and remote Indigenous communities, including primary care, crisis intervention, prevention and health promotion programs. However, many people living in rural or remote areas do not have ready access to professional mental health care. Larger communities may have a primary health clinic staffed by a physician and other health or social service professionals. Smaller communities may have a nursing station, with nurse practitioners, assisted by visits from other health professionals on a rotating basis. Specialist, secondary and tertiary services are generally not readily available in smaller rural and remote communities. Patients with serious health problems may therefore need to travel long distances at considerable expense to receive the appropriate medical care.

This situation is compounded by common difficulties faced in the provision of mental health services in rural and remote settings. These include (1) shortage of trained professionals or other helpers, (2) the pressure on the mental health workers living in a small community who work alone with limited access to ongoing clinical supervision and continuing education, (3) the difficulty of ensuring confidentiality when people live in close proximity, (4) stigma associated with mental illness that is difficult to conceal in small communities and (5) the costs and logistical challenges associated with transportation of providers or patients (McDonel et al., 1997; Nagarajan, 2004).

In addition to the challenges associated with geographical remoteness, rural and remote communities face similar challenges to those faced by Indigenous people across Canada. Many remote Indigenous communities have social problems including housing shortages, overcrowding, poverty, unemployment as well as issues of substance abuse and domestic violence that may reduce wellbeing and increase the prevalence of mental health problems (King, Smith, & Gracey, 2009; Kirmayer, Tait, & Simpson, 2008). Social and mental health services may be underfunded, while rates of substance abuse, violence and suicide often are high (Kirmayer, Whitley, & Fauras, 2010).

Beyond the geographical and environmental challenges associated with remoteness, there are dilemmas for health service delivery in remote and rural communities reflecting jurisdictional issues in the ways that services have developed (Macdonald, 2008; McCormick & Quantz, 2009):

• Services tend to be provided in reaction to crises, with fewer resources invested in primary and secondary prevention or mental health promotion activities.

- Services are often fragmented with lack of continuity of care over time and across sectors. The lack of temporal continuity results from staff shortages, high levels of staff turnover, and shortages of resources. Remote and rural communities often rely on locum or itinerant physicians and nurses on rotation (Armstrong, 1978; Group for the Advancement of Psychiatry, 1995). Discontinuity across sectors occurs because services are segmented in silos, i.e. substance use disorder services, mental health services, social services and education are not integrated and may provide contradictory advice or interventions.
- Often services are provided through specific time-limited projects or initiatives. Funding tends to be available for pilot projects on a short-term basis, with promising and innovative projects terminated just as communities are becoming more comfortable with the intervention.
- Program evaluation is less common in rural mental health than in urban settings, due to the shortage of resources, costs of hiring outside researchers to evaluate projects and the lack of trained personnel on the ground to conduct evaluation. There may also be a heightened sensitivity on the part of providers about the potential perception of urban-based outsiders that their services are of an inferior quality. The result of all this is that there is a lack of rigorously evaluated, evidence-based interventions relevant to promoting mental health and well-being in rural and remote regions.

In the absence of a comprehensive service, it has been suggested that a community mental health liaison service or related models of collaborative care can provide support for primary care practitioners, while also assisting family carers, though again this model has not been rigorously tested (Hazelton, Habibis, Schneider, Davidson, & Bowling, 2004).

In additional to these pragmatic and logistical considerations, there is increasing recognition that conventional services may create situations that are unsafe for Indigenous peoples and other groups that have experienced oppression. Building on work by Maori nurses in New Zealand (Papps & Ramsden, 1996), Indigenous scholars and organizations have endorsed the notion of cultural safety as a way to highlight and address issues of power, institutionalized racism, and discrimination in the health care system (Brascoupé & Waters, 2009; Koptie, 2009; Smye, Josewski, & Kendall, 2010). The Indigenous Physicians Association of Canada (2009) has produced a curriculum for training health professionals to give them some of the basic historical and contemporary background knowledge needed to understand the experience of Indigenous patients and to begin to address their own attitudes and stereotypes. Any approach to services for Indigenous peoples must engage these principles of cultural safety to insure that the context of health care delivery and the modes of interaction acknowledge and redress the legacy of colonialism and ongoing power disparities that continue to affect the health and well-being of Indigenous individuals and communities.

Social Determinants of Mental Health in Rural and Remote Settings

As a result of the social, economic and technological changes in developed countries in the last 200 years, there has been an enormous migration from rural to urban regions. One result of this migration is the preferential move of young people to urban centers, with a corresponding aging of rural populations (Judd et al., 2002). A more recent phenomenon is counter-urbanization, with the movement of low-income families from urban zones towards rural areas, often searching for housing at lower costs (Fitchen, 1995). Increased mobility has also resulted in greater circulation of people back and forth between urban rural and remote communities.

Generally speaking, health indicators in urban and rural regions are similar, and both present a profile that is less favorable than the profile found in suburban regions that are comprised of a large proportion of high-income families. In the United States, many rural regions have higher rates of premature mortality (before 75 years of age), child mortality, suicide, accidents, tobacco consumption and chronic obstructive pulmonary disease (Eberhardt & Pamuk, 2004).

Few studies have considered area of residence (rural, urban or suburban) as a risk factor for psychiatric illness. The prevalence of illness seems to be influenced more by socioeconomic factors (such as unemployment, poverty, social support networks) that vary within rural and urban zones as well as between them (Judd et al., 2002). The socioeconomic profile of rural areas in North America has evolved in the last decades, but the populations remain disadvantaged in many ways in comparison to urban centers, with lower employment rates and average salaries, higher poverty rates and a larger proportion of individuals depending on social security, as well as a globally lower level of education (Gamm, 2004; Judd et al., 2002; Nelson, Pomerantz, & Schwartz, 2007).

Further, the lifestyle in rural communities differs in many ways from the lifestyle in cities. Many authors use the concept of subculture to describe the particularities of values, traditions, religious practices and attitudes towards illnesses that are common in rural populations. As an example, some authors cite the prevalence in rural areas of the values of independence, self-management and a strong work ethic (Fuller, Edwards, Procter, & Moss, 2000; Hoyt, Conger, Valde, & Weihs, 1997; Nelson et al., 2007; Strasser, 1995). The church holds a place of prominence in many communities (Judd & Humphreys, 2001), and there is evidence that, when dealing with issues of mental illness, rural residents have a tendency not to use health services and are more inclined to rely on informal support including neighbours, the church, police, teachers and community groups (Bushy, 1994; Fuller et al., 2004; Judd et al., 2002).

The standard models of mental health services and interventions, which have been developed mainly for urban contexts, must be adapted to fit rural situations (Gamm, 2004). This may involve considering issues of lifestyle, values, community dynamics and the overall organization of place and time. The values and perspectives of rural communities may be unfamiliar to health professionals who have been born, raised and trained exclusively in urban centers. For example, in some rural regions where hunting is an important activity, patterns of health utilization reflect the impact of the migration of animals. Adapting the hours of service availability to respect this community activity is a simple expression of respect for local values and priorities. Providing mental health services in remote regions also poses many logistical challenges. Rural populations may be dispersed across large areas, with a low population density, long distances for patients to travel to see clinicians and difficult climatic conditions that cause transportation problems and make it more difficult to organize services efficiently (Gamm, 2004; Nelson et al., 2007).

One of the most common problems in providing mental health services in remote regions is the lack of professionals and other appropriately trained staff. This problem affects mental health providers, general practitioners and psychiatrists. In industrialized countries such as Australia, Canada and the United States, approximately 20% of the total population lives in rural areas, whereas only 10% of physicians practise in these areas (Gamm, 2004; Judd & Humphreys, 2001). These regions typically have limited access to specialized services. Various strategies have been used to improve access to services in remote areas, including the use of itinerant specialists, training community workers to address basic needs and transferring patients to urban regions where they can receive specialized care. Increasingly, telemedicine and telepsychiatry have been used as ways to provide assessment and treatment for patients as well as consultation and support for providers (Calloway, Fried, Johnsen, & Morrissey, 1999; Judd et al., 2002).

Although technology has influenced the organization of mental health services in rural areas, there are continuing problems of engagement and retention of professionals to support local workers. Furthermore, local resources including community organizations may also be limited in rural areas. Small communities may have a few community workers who may be integrated within the health and social services system but rarely have an organization of their own. The Internet has allowed a growing number of support networks for people with mental health problems and concerns. Yet access to the Internet may be less available and reliable in remote areas where such networking is most needed. Overall, therefore, access to mental health services remains limited in rural regions, and as a result, patients, their families and relatives all face greater challenges than their urban counterparts (Judd & Humphreys, 2001).

Mental health services in rural areas face specific challenges in relation to stigmatization and the protection of patient confidentiality. In small communities where everyone knows each other and a clinic visit will not go unnoticed, the fear of being identified and stigmatized as mentally ill can be a major barrier to help-seeking. This reality of the proximity of caregivers to patients can lead to delays or avoidance in seeking professional help.

Rural populations have been described as holding negative attitudes towards mental illness and as being prone to stigmatizing individuals struggling with mental illness. Stigmatization, shame, social exclusion and isolation can occur because individuals are identified as "carriers" of mental illness or because they have displayed inappropriate behavior in public situations (Crawford & Brown, 2002; Fuller et al., 2004; Judd et al., 2002; Lambert & Hartley, 1998; Nelson et al., 2007). However, some studies also demonstrate greater acceptance and better social integration in rural areas of individuals with mental health problems. Thus, rural communities, particularly those in remote regions, may display a greater tolerance of individual idiosyncrasies or social deviance because the community may view each person in terms of their network of social relations.

Case Vignette 11-1
Markoosie was a 32-year-old Inuit man living in a remote village in northern Quebec. He had auditory and somatic hallucinations and a persistent delusion that three men from the south, who he had never met, were planning to come north to kill him. One day he mistook three co-workers driving the water truck for his southern assassins and shot at them with his rifle. He fled home in fear and was brought to the nursing station by police who asked that he be taken south to be hospitalized. On assessment at a hospital in Montreal, he received a diagnosis of paranoid schizophrenia and was put on neuroleptic medication. When he returned to his community, he was soon put back to work as the village dog catcher, shooting stray dogs with his rifle. Although he continued to have auditory hallucinations and delusions, even on neuroleptic medication, he kept these experiences to himself and was viewed by many community members as recovered.

The community's acceptance of Markoosie as recovered, partially reflected Inuit notions of the nature of mental illness as a potentially transient or reversible state of mind (Kirmayer, Fletcher, & Boothroyd, 1997b). However, it also seemed to result from the familiarity people had with him as an individual, with a long history in the community and many connections to cousins and other members of his extended family. The sense of interconnectedness and familiarity with individuals can contribute to a sense of community cohesion, responsibility and solidarity that encourages support and integration of individuals suffering from severe mental illnesses (Fuller et al., 2000; Hoyt et al., 1997; Judd et al., 2002; Lambert & Hartley, 1998; Sommers, 1989). Of course, not all communities function this way for all afflicted members, and this portrait of the cohesive rural community caring for its mentally ill members has been criticized as a romantic ideal by some authors (Murray & Kelleher, 1991). Supporting patients in the face of potential stigmatization is a major challenge for community mental health.

From the point of view of clinicians working in small rural communities, the challenge of maintaining confidentiality in health clinic depends on the discretion with which the services can be delivered. Unfortunately, maintaining the most rigorous confidentiality may require holding oneself apart from the community in ways that are neither practical nor positively viewed in the community. While communication that occurs in the clinical consultation must remain private, the consultant's everyday presence in the community and interactions with others afford a more ecologically meaningful, contextualized understanding of patients' problems that can point to creative solutions. Modifications of conventional mental health professional strategies around boundaries should be made when needed, after weighing the potential risks and benefits (Savin & Martinez, 2006).

Indigenous Communities

In certain industrialized countries such as Australia, Canada, New Zealand and the United States, Indigenous peoples constitute a larger proportion of rural and remote populations. Indigenous populations suffer from the legacy of colonization and subsequent policies of forced assimilation that have resulted in loss of cultural traditions and rapid changes in way of life. These communities continue to face serious political, economic and social challenges that are reflected in poor health (King et al., 2009; Reading, 2009; Reading & Wien, 2009).

Many Indigenous communities have high rates of mental health and social problems including suicide, depression, substance abuse, violence, sexual abuse, conjugal violence, incarceration, accidents, child mortality, type II diabetes, tuberculosis, hepatitis, and chlamydia (Adelson, 2005; Canadian Medical Association, 2003; Gamm, 2004). Life expectancy in Australia, Canada, New Zealand and in the United States for Indigenous peoples is less than in the general population (Cass, 2004; Durie, Milroy, & Hunter, 2008). In Canada, this difference is of 7.4 years in men and 5.2 years in women. The discrepancy in health indicators for Indigenous populations is largely determined by socioeconomic factors including income, employment, education, housing, infrastructure and environment (Adelson, 2005; Cass, 2004; King et al., 2009). In Canada, a high proportion of Indigenous peoples live in overcrowded housing and lack basic services. Although academic enrolment is improving, the level of education attained by students is still significantly below the national average. The employment rate is one-third that of the rest of the population (Tang & Browne, 2008). The average income is also greatly inferior to the national average (Adelson, 2005). Given these disparities, improvement in the health of Indigenous communities depends not only on providing services but on the correction of social and economic inequalities, which requires political will (Canadian Medical Association, 2003).

Health services in Indigenous communities face several challenges. Despite the high prevalence of psychosocial distress and substance abuse in these communities, there is a lack of specific services to address these problems (Gamm, 2004). The provision of health care services faces challenges in language and communication, the cross-cultural validity of diagnosis and the fit with indigenous concepts of health and illness (Judd et al., 2002). Indigenous concepts of well-being include notions of physical, emotional, mental and spiritual wellness of the person at hand. The individual is understood as an element in a larger ecosocial system, involving the family, community and environment (Adelson, 2005; Kirmayer, Fletcher, & Watt, 2008). Various forms of indigenous healing and helping may be preferred ways to address common mental health problems (Gamm, 2004).

Biomedical health care was established in Indigenous communities as part of the process of internal colonization. Today, there is increasing awareness of the need to provide culturally responsive services and to insure that non-Indigenous health workers have knowledge of cultural values and perspectives and the ability to work across cultures (Canadian Medical Association, 2003). Contemporary health services in Indigenous communities often repeat and perpetuate the hierarchical, paternalistic and even racist attitudes of the colonial process. Clinicians have a tendency to assume they understand the nature of the problem and the best intervention, to the exclusion of indigenous ways of knowing and healing. These issues lead to a failure to engage and support the capacity of local resources (McCallum, 2005).

Indigenous people making use of mainstream health services may face institutional racism and discrimination (Currie, Wild, Schopflocher, Laing, & Veugelers, 2012). One of the more prevalent discriminatory beliefs in the non-Indigenous health community involves assumptions that the disparity of health issues in Indigenous communities results from their own poor choices. This reflects general ignorance of the historical impact of colonization, sedentarization and the systematic destruction of Indigenous culture and identity through the Indian Residential Schools and other methods of forced assimilation (Tang & Browne, 2008). Other expressions of bias and discrimination may take subtler forms. The remote regions inhabited by Indigenous peoples may be described as harsh and unyielding and the Indigenous peoples perceived in romanticized and exoticized ways, while the non-Indigenous health professionals may describe themselves in paternalistic language reminiscent of the era of colonization as heroic workers "saving" the community (McCallum, 2005).

In recent years, Indigenous peoples in Canada have gained an increasing measure of control over health services in their own communities. This has been driven in part by top-down policies of "devolution" that seek to transfer responsibility for health care from centralized government institutions to regional and local authorities. It also reflects ongoing efforts to reassert community autonomy and local control. While the devolution process has tended to lead to the replication of bureaucratic models of health care regulation at different levels, the assertion of local autonomy suggests that services and intervention models must be revised to fit local aspirations as part of a process of decolonization and reconstruction (Kirmayer, Brass, & Valaskakis, 2008; MacKinnon, 2005).

There is evidence that local control of health services along with other key services and institutions is associated with better community health, including lower suicide rates (Chandler & Lalonde, 1998, 2008). The maintenance, strengthening or reintroduction of traditional healing

practices is also an important part of cultural revitalization, spirituality and identity for many Indigenous people (McCormick, 2008). Many questions remain about how best to integrate or achieve the effective coexistence of mainstream mental health services and traditional or indigenous healing systems. For example, some Aboriginal clinicians argue for integration of indigenous healing with professional mental health services (Wieman, 2008), while others suggest they should remain separate to insure that the conventional health care system does not simply appropriate community-based indigenous approaches and apply them in ways that undermine or betray their fundamental values and principles (McCormick, 2008; Mussell, 2005).

Increasing representation of professionals with Indigenous background in the milieu of health professionals is an important dimension of this self-determination. At present, health services in most Indigenous communities are still provided by a majority of non-Indigenous practitioners, including nurse practitioners or family physicians living in communities and other itinerant, periodic visitors. Although the number of Indigenous professionals in health services is growing, and measures have been taken to promote their training, they remain under represented in the health professions, particularly medicine and nursing (Lecompte & Baril, 2008). There has been greater progress in Indigenous representation in alternative professions such as midwives and natural medicine practitioners.

Service Models

Service models in rural and remote regions must adapt to a multitude of factors that vary considerably from one region to another. These factors include the size of a community, the demography and population density, the distance of the region from urban centers, the health profiles of the communities, the acceptance of health services within the community subcultures, socioeconomic conditions as well as the infrastructure and the available professional staff on location (Judd et al., 2002; Kirmayer et al., 2010).

The organization of health services in a specific geographical area must take into account the economic factors that define the service threshold, i.e., the minimum population required to justify the development and sustain the provision of a particular service over time. Some services with a very high threshold, such as a unit specialized in nutrition problems, can be justified only as regional programs for an entire province or region. Small rural populations with a low population density, however, cannot sustain even low threshold services, despite the fact that these communities might need certain specialized services, particularly in mental health (Judd et al., 2002). Clearly, the service threshold is not only an economic issue but depends on political choices that reflect cultural, social and moral values.

In urban centers in Canada, mental health service models have been built around hospital services with medical specialists as key providers. This organization persists despite the fact that there is evidence that many patients with mental health problems are treated exclusively in primary care. Recent efforts in Quebec to redefine the role of psychiatrists as consultants to primary care providers have been slow to take hold not only because the primary care system is overburdened but also because patients with mental health problems pose particular challenges in terms of time, resources and skills that may be difficult to provide in overburdened family medicine settings. Successful collaborative care demands adequate support for primary care practitioners and a reorientation towards community-based care among tertiary care mental health practitioners (see Chapter 10).

The rural model is structured differently, as it is built around frontline professionals. The family physician or general practitioner is the key medical resource. Interdisciplinary teams specialized in mental health are developed within the community making use of other professionals or local social workers, educators and others. In remote or dispersed communities, the key resource person is more often a nurse practitioner who must work with community workers or others with less professional training and support.

Ironically, then, those with less training and resources must provide the broadest range of services (Judd et al., 2002; Tobin, 1996).

Local teams of frontline workers in mental health must be supported and complemented by specialized services made available in rural areas through outreach strategies. There are three common strategies to provide this support: (1) mobile and itinerant services involving specialized workers in mental health, such as psychiatrists that make periodic visits to isolated communities; (2) telepsychiatry, which refers to the use of audio–visual communication technologies to provide psychiatric services and support for frontline professionals on either a regular schedule or an urgent basis; and (3) the use of satellite services established through agreements between rural mental health teams and large psychiatric centers in urban settings that provide isolated communities with resources that they lack, including psychiatric hospitalization, medico-legal evaluation and residential substance abuse treatment (Henderson, Vanier, & Noel, 1991; Judd et al., 2002; Owen, Tennant, Jessie, Jones, & Rutherford, 1999; Samuels & Owen, 1998; Yellowlees, 1992). In primary care models for rural services, the main role of the psychiatrist or mental health practitioner is no longer the direct provision of care. Instead, the specialist's tasks are those of consulting, training, education and support of general practitioners and other health professionals in frontline positions.

Onsite Service Delivery

The challenges of providing mental health services in remote or isolated communities include developing a practical and efficient organization, training and sustaining an adequate team of providers and addressing the unique personal and professional dilemmas of working in a small community.

Small rural and remote communities generally have access only to general health services. Specialized services usually are available to the population only via outreach strategies. Furthermore, because there is a shortage of health professionals in rural regions, frontline professionals face additional challenges. Professionals with limited training in psychiatry must address a wide range of clinical problems, broadening the scope of their professional functions and playing a more polyvalent role compared to practice in urban settings (Humphreys, Hegney, Lipscombe, Gregory, & Chater, 2002).

This type of work requires flexible organization among professionals who must collaborate to meet the needs of a rural community. To work well in this setting, professionals must be flexible, eclectic and creative (Fuller et al., 2004). For example, in isolated regions, social workers are often called upon to play multiple roles simultaneously, including the psychosocial follow-up of children, adults and the elderly, social interventions for medical or psychiatric conditions, ensuring the application of child protection laws, evaluating potential danger for self-injury or violence, crisis intervention and psychotherapeutic interventions. This work cannot all be carried out in the confines of a clinic office and may require extensive travel for home visits in rural populations that are widely dispersed.

Developing human resources for mental health services constitutes a significant problem in isolated regions. Recruiting well-trained professionals is difficult and there is often a high rate of turnover of professionals who stay for only brief periods in communities. The difficulty of recruiting and of retaining professionals can be attributed to several factors, including professional isolation, poor collegial support (due to limited resources), the scarcity of professional development opportunities, heavy workload and responsibilities and the demand for an unusually wide range of skills. As well, there is often some stigma associated with being a mental health worker who is known and identified as such by the entire community (Judd et al., 2002; Nelson et al., 2007). Academic issues are also part of the problem in recruiting as mental health professionals are often poorly prepared to practise in isolated regions during their training. Most professionals are trained exclusively in urban centers, and their training does not include the needs and realities of practice in rural contexts (Gamm,

2004; Merwin, Goldsmith, & Manderscheid, 1995).

Given the lack of local professionals, isolated regions frequently rely on outside aid workers who rotate through communities every few weeks or months. Although these teams insure basic services, they have many limitations. They cannot provide continuity of care at the level of clinical follow-up of patients, communication and transfer of information or provision of supervision of medication and treatment. The lack of continuity can increase the risk of deterioration in patients with unstable chronic conditions. The responsibility for maintaining follow-up then falls more often on patients and their families, despite the fact that they may lack the necessary skills and resources to deal with the problems or may be acting in ways that contribute to stressors. Because of limited human resources, these regional organizations tend to privilege short-term services, such as emergency care, to the detriment of long-term services focussed on prevention and health promotion, screening, counselling and adequate supportive care for the chronically ill (Fuller et al., 2004; Minore et al., 2005).

Additional problems arise from the rotation system of itinerant professionals. These workers have little opportunity for immersion in the community in which they work and therefore have limited knowledge of the social and cultural context. Consequently, they are ill-prepared to culturally adapt their services and interventions. In such a system, it is the patients who must continually adapt to new professionals with whom they must communicate intimate problems as they tell the same story over and over again. Patients also face the repeated threat of losing the aid worker, which places them in the precarious and uncertain position of anticipated loss. As a result, they may eventually become reticent or resistant to invest in a therapeutic relationship and may maintain a dubious or disengaged attitude towards health services. For professionals working in remote communities, it is a common observation that the local population takes a certain period of time to accept and "adopt" professionals; this period of reticence gives locals a chance to assess the durability of the helper's presence in the community. Local community and health care workers also experience the discontinuities in this model of care, since they must train new visiting professionals regularly and adapt to their differing styles of working (Fuller et al., 2004; Gamm, 2004; Minore et al., 2005).

Several measures have been proposed to minimize the negative impact of rotating professionals. Encouraging and supporting the recruitment of aid workers from within the communities where services are dispensed will provide a stronger base for the outside worker. Itinerant professionals need training in the organizational and interpersonal dynamics of episodic work and more specifically in the sociocultural realities of the communities in which they are to work, as well as in how local services function. This formal training should be a prerequisite for working in rural and remote communities. In situations where the use of rotating teams and outside professionals is necessary, it is important to assign the same professionals to the same communities during their rotations in order to minimize the discontinuity of care (Minore et al., 2005).

The work of local aid workers in mental health in small rural communities raises distinctive issues of professional limits. In contrast to the usual anonymity of practice in urban settings, the social and geographical isolation and scale of small communities put professionals in direct interaction with patients in public areas and social events. Professionals living and working in small communities then must provide services to individuals with whom they have frequent informal contacts and ongoing personal relationships. For example, a psychiatrist may meet patients while grocery shopping, be obliged to intervene medically with a neighbor or a colleague or find that his child's teacher is a patient (Crawford & Brown, 2002; Judd et al., 2002; Nelson et al., 2007). This phenomenon of multiple or overlapping relationships requires rethinking professional roles, boundaries and rules designed to maintain ethical standards.

Mental health workers in small rural communities are known by the entire population. They must build trust and earn the respect of community members, as well as accepting that their private life will be the object of scrutiny. This demands high standards of comportment to maintain one's good standing and leaves the worker with little privacy (Minore et al., 2005). Of course, this proximity also has benefits and other authors have emphasized the advantages for assessment and intervention where the practitioner is able to observe patients in their alternative environments (Jennings, 1992).

For example, when working in small remote communities with a population, the consultant will regularly meet patients at the grocery store, airport or on the street. These meetings provide important information about patients' social functioning, support networks, resources as well as the ways in which their community view them. Seen in community context, many patients appear more functional than when assessed only within the narrow confines of the clinical setting.

Certain rules of conduct in mental health are not applicable in isolated regions. For example, psychiatrists are usually dissuaded from providing care for several members of the same family, in order to better preserve boundaries, confidentiality or a position of neutrality. In small communities, where there is a single consultant, this rule cannot be observed, as the inhabitants would then be deprived of medical services. The same clinician may have to deal with simultaneously treating a spouse, a parent and a child, siblings and others within an extended social network. This state of affairs can lead to challenging clinical issues, as illustrated by the following case.

Case Vignette 11-2

In the context of ongoing consultation work in an isolated First Nations community of 600 inhabitants, a psychiatric consultant provided care for Mary, a 40-year-old woman suffering from schizoaffective disorder, and her 23-year-old son, with schizophrenia. When the son presented with a psychotic decompensation with aggressive behavior, the psychiatrist had to arrange for

(continued)

his hospitalization against his will. This event strongly impacted on the clinician's therapeutic relationship with the mother, who was staunchly opposed to the hospitalization of her son. The mother's position was influenced by several factors. She had maintained denial of her own condition in parallel with the denial of her son's symptoms. In this way, she demonstrated solidarity with him against the threat of psychiatric services, which she viewed as persecutory. The procedure of hospitalizing her son awakened memories of her own compulsory hospitalizations earlier in her life during acute relapses, which were traumatic and difficult for her to integrate. To help her come to terms with her son's need for hospitalization, the psychiatrist had to address and work through some of these past traumatic experiences with psychiatric services.

Although we have touched upon some of the difficulties that occur when dealing with local mental health services in isolated regions, there are advantages as well. In particular, the smaller community may provide a strong support network for patients, information about patients may be easier to obtain, and there may be fewer communication problems than in urban settings (Calloway et al., 1999; Judd et al., 2002).

Itinerant Consultants

Some mental health professionals work as itinerant consultants, making periodic short visits to isolated regions. In mental health, psychiatrists are the practitioners who use this approach most frequently, providing consultation to general practitioners and frontline workers, as well as training and continuing education to support mental health teams in the communities. Itinerant psychiatrists may also offer certain specialized services directly to patients. Because the services provided by itinerant workers are intermittent,

they cannot provide reliable emergency care. For local teams, effective use of itinerant consultants depends on close coordination of services and logistical arrangements for transportation and housing. Compared with the services provided by local teams, the work of itinerant professionals has its own particularities, advantages and limitations.

First, an itinerant consultant is less subject to the multiple or overlapping relationships which constitute a major issue for local professionals and the population. Thus, the itinerant consultant, who is usually a stranger to the intricate social structure of small communities, can avoid some of the difficulties that can arise from encountering patients in social settings. From the patient's perspective, the caregiver may be the only person they have never had personal interactions with, and therefore they can offer a fresh account and reflection on their problems to someone with a "neutral" or outsider perspective. As an outsider and temporary visitor, the itinerant clinician can offer greater confidentiality and less potential for stigmatization compared to relationships with local caregivers (Fuller et al., 2004). This outsider position may provide a comfortable distance between patient-therapist that allows some patients a safe space to discuss sensitive topics. This distance may be particularly useful in dealing with the impact of traumatic events within the community or within their families of origin.

Case Vignette 11-3

Paulusie, a 45-year-old Inuit man, asked the community nurse for a meeting with the visiting psychiatrist to discuss some private matters. Alone with the consultant, he divulged his concerns about his wife's mental health. She had become intensively involved in a local Pentecostal church and was urging him to join as well. He felt uncomfortable about this and found her overzealous. The discussion centered on

(continued)

strategies for him to improve his communication with his wife. Several weeks after the consultant has returned to the south, he received a long letter from Paulusie describing his own traumatic experiences that, he said, had made him especially insecure and apprehensive about his wife's religious involvement. He had never disclosed these events, and apologized for using the letter this way, but said it made him feel better to write this down to someone he trusted.

The visiting consultant is outside local systems, better able to provide confidentiality, and potentially can provide a safe place to confide painful or shameful secrets. The consultant can symbolically hold or contain the traumatic secret. The departure of the consultant from the community may then provide symbolic distance from the painful memories and can diminish the threat posed by ongoing therapeutic work.

For local aid workers, the itinerant consultant can be a precious source of professional support, in addition to performing their standard tasks. The position of outsider to the local social and professional systems has certain advantages. The outsider can provide alternative viewpoints and fresh thinking about clinical issues and organizational challenges in work relationships.

Of course, the position of itinerant consultant also has limitations. As a stranger to the community, the itinerant consultant has but brief exposure to local issues and may have very limited knowledge of the sociocultural milieu. The periodic nature of visits does not promote continuity of care, with stable and reliable access to the consultant's services, nor does it allow for the timely management of emergency and crisis situations that emerge between visits. The itinerant consultant may lose therapeutic momentum due to the episodic nature of interactions with the community and have to rebuild trust and renew working relationships to some degree on each visit (Fuller et al., 2004). The problems associated with lack of continuity can be reduced when the consultant is able to provide telephone or video services between visits. Using telecommunication to maintain a link can be extremely useful for local professionals working in isolated situations.

Telepsychiatry

Telepsychiatry refers to the use of telephone, interactive video, electronic medical records and the Internet to allow communication between doctors, patients and other health care personnel for the assessment, treatment or prevention of mental health problems. Many different types of service can be dispensed through telepsychiatry, including clinical evaluations, medico-legal evaluations, legal audiences, neuropsychological assessment, consulting with frontline teams and clinical supervision, individual, family or group psychotherapy and continuing professional education both in didactic presentations and clinical case conferences.

Telepsychiatry is a particularly important strategy for providing specific mental health services and reducing health disparities for people in remote areas where specialist providers are not available (Hilty, Yellowlees, Sonik, Derlet, & Hendren, 2009). Telepsychiatry can reduce the need for lengthy, expensive and arduous trips for patients or health care personnel to and from urban centers. It can increase access to psychiatric services and reduce professional and frontline worker isolation in under-serviced regions (Hilty, Marks, Urness, Yellowlees, & Nesbitt, 2004; Hilty, Servis, Nesbitt, & Hales, 1999). Telepsychiatry is also consistent with efforts to provide community-based care and promote community involvement in and control of service delivery.

There is increasing evidence that telepsychiatry can be an effective method to deliver mental health services for both children and adults. It can be used for training, supervision, team building, assessment and intervention. It may allow teams to feel supported and sustain their work in challenging clinical situations. Telepsychiatry can be a reliable method of assessing psychiatric disorders (Shore, Savin, Orton, Beals, & Manson, 2007) and a cost-effective method of assessing suicidal patients (Jong, 2004). Studies have demonstrated the reliability of diagnostic evaluations using telepsychiatry compared to live evaluations (Baigent et al., 1997; Bear, Jacobson, Aaronson, & Hanson, 1997; Elford et al., 2000; Hilty, Luo, Morache, Marcelo, & Nesbitt, 2002; Hilty et al., 2004; Ruskin et al., 1998; Singh, Arya, & Peters, 2007). Several studies have found that videoconferencing and face-to-face meetings have comparable effectiveness for diagnostic and therapeutic intervention (Elford et al., 2000; O'Reilly et al., 2007). Telepsychiatry also can work well for providing specialized services in child and adolescent mental health, including cognitive behavioral interventions (Lingley-Pottie & McGrath, 2008; McGrath et al., 2011; Myers, Valentine, & Meltzer, 2007; Nelson, Barnard, & Cain, 2003; Paing et al., 2009).

Patients and clinicians, both in the general population and in Indigenous communities, generally report high levels of satisfaction with telepsychiatry services (Alexander & Latanzio, 2009; Greenberg, Boydell, & Volpe, 2006; Hilty et al., 2009). Both mental health providers and patients tend to be comfortable with this method, in part because it allows them to avoid lengthy and costly travel and stay in their work setting or community while giving (or receiving) consultation (Hilty, Yellowlees, & Nesbitt, 2006; Kennedy & Yellowlees, 2000).

Although some patients and clinicians express scepticism or apprehension when first presented with the idea of telepsychiatry, most quickly adapt to the situation. In a study with rural American Indian youth, patients expressed some concern at the beginning of videoconferencing about "talking to a box" (Savin, Garry, Zuccaro, & Novins, 2006). However, knowing that the session was conducted by an expert, and having their own local clinician present in the room, helped them become comfortable with the process. Clinicians sitting-in with the patient at the teleconference reported that the sessions acted as training experiences, increasing their knowledge and skills as clinicians. They also reported feeling less professionally isolated and appreciated

the regular contact that the teleconferences allowed as a better format for learning than irregular and infrequent visits to the city. Consultants did express apprehension about the potential for decreased rapport with the patients seen only by teleconference and the challenge of collecting all the needed information for clinical assessment through teleconference. However, these concerns subsided with increased familiarity with telepsychiatry.

There are several different models of telepsychiatry based on the available resources at each end of the link (Janca, 2000). The community primary care clinic may have general practitioners, nurse practitioners, social workers or Indigenous community mental health workers with varying level of training. The outside consultant may be a psychiatrist, psychologist, psychiatric nurse or social worker or a multidisciplinary team consisting of some or all of these types of practitioners.

Telepsychiatry can facilitate communication between a centrally located mental health care team (generally consultant psychiatrists in urban centers) and scattered primary care providers practicing in geographically remote locations (Hilty et al., 2006). A collaborative care model can be implemented for remote rural areas through telepsychiatry (Fortney et al., 2007). Telepsychiatry can be used to build a mental health team (Cornish et al., 2003) and can be used to network clinicians located in remote communities. Community mental health workers or teams operating in rural and remote areas can use telepsychiatry for training, supervision and support, to the specific needs of clients with persistent difficulties, or simply for routine follow-up appointments.

To work effectively, mental health professionals and mental health workers on both ends of the line must be trained in the use of telepsychiatry (Szeftel et al., 2008). Outside professional consultants should have expertise in working with multidisciplinary teams and knowledge of the Indigenous communities where the patients involved live. In some circumstances, the outside consultant may be chosen for their specific expertise in Indigenous mental health. This might include Indigenous mental health workers from one community or organization consulting with another community where such expertise is not available.

Telepsychiatry may be safest and most effective when used in conjunction with local community mental health workers. Community workers can provide support on the ground for people with mental health problems under the supervision of psychiatrists based elsewhere. Telepsychiatry can be used to deliver training programs, case supervision and case conferences as part of the development and continuing education of a cadre of community-based mental health works. Telepsychiatry also can provide essential backup for the assessment and management of challenging cases. Without adequate training and supervision, however, telepsychiatry may be ineffective (Bartik, Dixon, & Dart, 2007; Crowe, Deane, Oades, Caputi, & Morland, 2006; McBride & Gregory, 2005).

Given the increasing use of Internet communications, familiarity with and acceptance of the use of telepsychiatry is likely to grow over time. Nevertheless, many patients do prefer face-to-face mental health assessment. In addition to patient preferences, being present in a community allows a consultant to gain a much greater appreciation of social context and environment and may allow various forms of networking, mobilizing and negotiating with others that can lead to new clinical strategies.

The Internet and electronic media can be used in other ways to deliver educational health promotion and training materials. There is evidence that Internet-based programs are well received and may be especially appealing to youth who make use of such technologies for social networking (Di Noia, Schwinn, Dastur, & Schinke, 2003). Such communications technology can provide a way to disseminate and share resources to be used by individuals on their own in self-management of mental health problems or as an adjunct to other forms of mental health promotion (Griffiths & Christensen, 2007).

There is evidence that with proper attention to local protocols, telepsychiatry and tele-mental health can be used effectively in Indigenous communities (Muttitt, Vigneault, & Loewen, 2004; Shore, Savin, Novins, & Manson, 2006). A recent study that examined the acceptability of telepsychiatry in American Indian communities found that, in comparison to interviews in person, the use of this technology did not present patients with any significant difference in level of comfort, satisfaction and cultural acceptance (Shore et al., 2008). To be most effective, however, teleconferencing should be a complement to, not a replacement for face-to-face services.

Studies that have examined the effects of telepsychiatry on the therapeutic relationship show that a good therapeutic alliance is possible despite some difficulties in reading nonverbal or body language cues (Hilty et al., 2004; McLaren, Ball, Summerfield, Watson, & Lipsedge, 1995; Nelson & Palsbo, 2006; O'Reilly et al., 2007). Research on the nature of online communication offers support for the position that with sufficient bandwidth, electronic communication can provide a satisfying level of emotional rapport. A sense of contact can certainly be created through language alone (Havens, 1986). Nevertheless, the lack of physical presence experienced by clinician and patient when sitting together in the same room must have some effect on the nature of clinical communication and the therapeutic process, changing its rhythm and increasing the possibility of miscommunication or ruptures when the quality of transmission is poor or timing lags (Kappas & Krämer, 2011).

Another important challenge for telepsychiatry is the limited access that the long-distance consultant has to the everyday social contexts of the patient's life. A distinctive feature of work in small communities is the likelihood of seeing patients outside non-clinical settings—at the grocery store, at recreational facilities or other community activities or just walking about. This allows the clinician a view of patients in everyday contexts in ways that can inform diagnostic assessment, treatment and outcome. With telepsychiatry, there are few opportunities for this type of encounter. As well, the patient has little sense of how to locate the consultant in an institutional setting. The use of telecommunication technology may exacerbate the tendency in psychiatric assessment to focus only on symptoms and signs instead of the patient's experience and social context.

The consultant who will work repeatedly with patients from a particular region or community can gain some sense of the social and cultural context of a community through periodic visits. During these visits, in addition to doing consultations on site, the clinician spend time with community workers and others to learn something of local realities, including the physical environment, socioeconomic issues and the dynamics between community members and outside workers.

Satellite Services

Satellite services involve transferring patients from isolated regions to urban centers to provide care that is not available either from visiting services or through telecommunication technology. These services rely on agreements between rural service teams and urban medical centers. The most common satellite services are psychiatric hospitalization, inpatient on a specialized unit (medico-legal maternal-infant, eating disorder, etc.) and residential substance abuse programs. Satellite service provision demands careful attention to organization, communication and coordination between services for continuity of care. The logistical details extend to transport and housing supports for patients and their carers who are far from their homes (Judd et al., 2002). Clinicians working in satellite services must have a clear sense of the context that patients come from and to which they will return for effective assessment, treatment and discharge planning.

From the patient's perspective, a key issue is the separation from the familiar home and community environment at a time of crisis and sickness. This separation may be helpful because it reduces stressors that contribute to distress but it may also exacerbate illness or impede recovery because it constitutes a rupture in bonds of attachment and social support, as well as disrupting the cognitive, emotional and environmental landmarks that serve to anchor or orientate the self. Being ill in an alien environment and unable to access personal networks of family, friends and community may pose significant risks for patients. This disconnection from family and community supports and environment can be partially mitigated by maintaining telephone or Internet connections as well as by creating some forms of familiarity within the hospital environment such as visits by interpreters and providing traditional food.

Satellite services for children usually include the presence of at least one legal guardian; however, the options are often limited due to financial constraints and housing problems. Separations caused by hospital admissions are difficult for families in the best of circumstances. When such separations involve great distances and lack of contact for long periods, they provoke significant anxiety for patients and their families. If a parent accompanies a child to hospital, the stress of separation may still be high if this requires leaving younger children in the community. While for some adolescent or adult patients, being away from the family can foster new levels of autonomy and independence, this developmental benefit may occur only if the process of leave-taking and returning is predictable and controlled by the patient. The sense of disorientation, loss and disconnection found in foreign hospital settings may far outweigh any sense of discovery or stimulation provided by exploring a new place. These separations for hospitalization may also be experienced as resonant with stories of past forced separations experienced by others in the family or community. Many Indigenous people in Canada experienced long periods of forced separation and institutionalization in association with the residential school system or prolonged confinement in sanatoria for tuberculosis (Adelson, 2005; McCallum, 2005). For some Indigenous people, hospitalization outside their community may elicit memories or images of these oppressive experiences. When Indigenous patients from remote communities are sent to urban centers, they may also experience new forms of racism, discrimination and social exclusion.

From the point of view of the caregiving team, satellite services are equally challenging. Since the team cannot meet and consult with family members, it becomes imperative to find alternate ways to collect information, communicate intervention plans and provide a holding environment and ongoing support for the community-based care providers after the patient is discharged. In addition to the usual issues of cultural countertransference, health professionals may have their own biases or reactions to a patient who has been flown in from a remote community.

A Consulting Service to Inuit Children and Youth Communities in Nunavik, Quebec

The arctic region of northern Quebec, called Nunavik, is populated mainly by Inuit, who live in 14 communities scattered along the coast of Hudson's Bay and Ungava Bay, ranging from few hundred people to about 1,500. Demographically, the population is very young, with 40% of the population under the age of 15 (Auclair & Sappa, 2012). Like other Indigenous peoples in Canada, Inuit have struggled with many challenges that have followed from the history of colonization, sedentarization and bureaucratic control, including forced displacements, relocation and prolonged childhood separation and traumas suffered in residential schools or during hospitalization for tuberculosis (Kirmayer et al., 2008). The high levels of exposure to traumatic events, losses and abuse have influenced the mental health of the communities. In recent decades, there have been very high rates of youth suicide (Boothroyd et al., 2001; Kirmayer, Boothroyd, & Hodgins, 1998; Kirmayer, Fletcher, & Boothroyd, 1997a). Inuit are under represented in health and social service professions. Community members may be reluctant to invest in relationships with non-Inuit professionals coming from "the South." In this context, a culturally informed collaborative care consultation program has provided a useful supplement to local primary care services (see Chapter 9 for a general discussion of cultural consultation in collaborative care).

The Nunavik collaborative mental health care initiative consists of regular visits by a child psychiatric consultant to Inuit communities of the Hudson coast, supplemented by a weekly half-day of indirect consultation by telephone. During visits, the local health care service (nursing station or, in one of the larger communities, a hospital) provides the consultant with an interpreter, as Inuktitut is the main language used, with more than 90% of Inuit speaking Inuktitut at home. Work with interpreters is well organized in Nunavik, and visiting medical specialists are always paired with an interpreter. Interpreters are available throughout the visit and often function as culture brokers as well, providing information about the community dynamics at the time of the visit. Interpreters are often able to give a general sense of how the patient seems to be doing in the community, and this complements information available from family, caregivers or others. The interpreter thus becomes an essential member of the collaborative care team. Telehealth conferences were organized to provide the interpreters with an arena to discuss challenging aspects of mental health interpreting in a small community. These meetings also allowed the interpreters to provide the consultant with practical advice concerning clinical meetings with parents and families.

At the start of the project, while planning the visits to the communities, the consultant invited primary care workers, including social workers, community workers, primary care physicians and school professionals, to take part in the consultation in order to strengthen collaboration and to reinforce their role in the continuity of care. This proved difficult due to the workload of most primary care workers, who are often dealing with emergencies. The consultation process therefore has been approached as a two-step process including a meeting with the family providing the core of the consultation, supplemented by a number of discussions with other treating providers.

Finally, the consultation process relies on the supportive presence of another consulting pediatrician who has been regularly visiting this area and who represents an important asset in terms of continuity of care.

For the non-Inuit consultant, there are many challenges in building bridges with the communities. First, being white brings the shadow of colonization, with wariness about the potential for racism, discrimination and exploitation. Second, as a visiting professional with limited time to spend in the communities, the consultant's commitment may be questioned. As people in these isolated communities are accustomed to frequent brief visits by itinerant professionals, they may expect little from these relationships and remain guarded or hesitant to build new partnerships unless there is evidence that the relationship will be sustained. Third, cultural styles of communication raise complex issues. Inuit, traditionally, strive to avoid overt conflict or anger in interpersonal relations (Briggs, 1970). While avoiding discussion of conflictual issues and valuing non-interference with other's autonomy may contribute to family or community harmony, it may also reflect social pressures that silence individuals and the legacy of a history of individual and collective trauma.

For Inuit professionals participating in this collaborative care model, key challenges exist around the burden of expectations and community members' trust in confidentiality. Inuit mental health workers experience the double burden of professional and community expectations in their roles. Their working conditions are challenging, as few first-line professionals are employed in these communities. The limited availability of trained professionals restricts the multidisciplinary work that can be done in mental health promotion. Access and continuity of care remain major challenges. To be successful, interprofessional collaborative care must be sustained by an adequate structure and a diversity of collaborators (Pauzé, Gagné, & Pautler, 2005). The limited resources in the north present a major challenge to sustained collaboration.

Strategies to address these limitations have included providing support to primary care workers, sharing with them know-how to improve continuity of care in the community and creating opportunities to share their ideas around the care needed. Continued advocacy for sufficient community resources remains imperative. Supporting collective efforts may assist the community in voicing their concerns and proposing possible solutions (Kirmayer, Sedhev, Whitley, Dandeneau, & Isaac, 2009; Law & Hutton, 2007). Given the close ties and similarities in experience across families in many Indigenous communities, interventions focussed on one individual may have immediate relevance to others or to broader concerns in the community.

Building partnerships with Indigenous communities is a long process which must take into account the historical background and appreciate the constraints of everyday life in these communities. Partnerships may require constant adjustment and renegotiation in view of ongoing relationships with other individuals and institutions in the south. Each new interaction is measured against previous experiences, as well as on the actual results of the current collaboration and on the potential future of consequences of engaging with a new visiting health professional. This renegotiation demands understanding, respect and collaboration between health workers and community members.

Case Vignette 11-4

Adamie was a 27-year-old Inuit man with schizophrenia and substance abuse problem, living in a remote community in Nunavik. After an episode of psychotic decompensation, he drank heavily and became violent with several members of the community. Everyone in the community knew of these events and community members approached their general practitioner, a non-Indigenous professional from outside of Nunavik, for help. They

(continued)

requested intervention and hospitalization for the young man and safety for their community.

The general practitioner organized a medical evacuation and transfer of the patient to an urban general hospital affiliated with the region. At the hospital, Adamie was admitted to psychiatry and stabilized with neuroleptic medication. Hospitalization and medication reduced his psychotic symptoms and violent behavior. His time in the hospital also gave him an opportunity to reflect on his actions and his responsibility in seeking the community's forgiveness. Reclaiming the respect of the community was a critical reparation task for his reintegration.

Adamie recognized that his use of cannabis had contributed to a psychotic decompensation and that his alcohol abuse had caused disinhibition with aggressive outbursts against members of the community. He thus prioritized treatment for his substance abuse problems. Because there were no resources available for substance abuse within his community, he developed a creative plan to reach out to the community to help him with his addiction issue.

Back in his village, after his return, he requested permission from the mayor to speak on the community radio. He asked the community for forgiveness for his violence. He also asked the community, with support from the mayor, to no longer sell or give him drugs or alcohol. He explained that he was incapable of controlling his intake once he started drinking and the drinking led to uncontrolled aggression. His public plea served several functions: It displayed his honesty and integrity; it showed him to be someone who was reaching out to the community seeking their support and help to recover; it allowed him to seek pardon from the community and allowed the community, in turn, to include

him rather than exclude him. Importantly, it gave the community a central role in his recovery and reinforced a sense of collective agency to address local problems including substance abuse and violence. The intervention combined medical, social and community approaches in a creative cultural way, ultimately empowering the patient, his community and the care team.

As this case illustrates, community-based interventions for individual cases may have a broader impact. The approach taken in this case, emphasizing public apology, efforts at restitution and taking responsibility for obtaining care, fits well with Inuit values of maintaining connections and reincorporating the person who has transgressed (Drummond, 1997). In the criminal justice system, these values have led to methods of reparative and restorative justice. In the mental health field, they have been expressed through family group conferencing, decision making, network therapy and other methods that emphasize reintegrating the individual into family and community (Speck & Attneave, 1973). The cohesion of small, remote communities may allow interventions based on forms of solidarity and mobilization that are difficult to achieve in urban settings.

Conclusion

In Canada, as in many other countries, mental health services are limited in many remote and rural areas. Even where there are adequate primary health care services, community mental health workers or teams in rural and remote areas may lack access to experts who can assist them in case management. Innovative strategies for service delivery need to be developed to allow appropriate management of patients, support community workers and contribute to mental health promotion. Such methods may include telepsychiatry and mobile consultation teams as well as regional and national networking strategies. All of these programs require training and support of Indigenous and non-Indigenous community mental health workers who can deliver improved primary mental health care with the collaboration of outside consultants.

Mental health services for Indigenous communities need to be provided in culturally appropriate ways, both through supporting the use of traditional healing approaches and ensuring that mainstream mental health services are culturally safe and competent. Specific issues reflecting each community's social, cultural and historical context must be addressed. Because of the diversity of cultures, communities, populations, settings and individual needs, one model or approach will not suffice.

References

Adelson, N. (2005). The embodiment of inequity: Health disparities in Aboriginal Canada. *Canadian Journal of Public Health, 96*(Suppl 2), S45–S61.

Alexander, J., & Lattanzio, A. (2009). Utility of telepsychiatry for Aboriginal Australians. *Australia and New Zealand Journal of Psychiatry, 43*(12), 1185.

Armstrong, H. (1978). Providing psychiatric care and consultation in remote Indian villages. *Hospital & Community Psychiatry, 29*(10), 678–680.

Auclair, G., & Sappa, M. (2012). Mental health in inuit youth from Nunavik: Clinical considerations on a transcultural, interdisciplinary, community-oriented approach. *Journal of the Canadian Academy of Child and Adolescent Psychiatry, 21*(2), 124–126.

Baigent, M. F., Lloyd, C. J., Kavanagh, S. J., Ben-Tovim, D. I., Yellowlees, P. M., Kalucy, R. S., et al. (1997). Telepsychiatry: "Tele" yes, but what about the "psychiatry"? *Journal of Telemedicine and Telecare, 3*(Suppl 1), 3–5.

Bartik, W., Dixon, A., & Dart, K. (2007). Aboriginal child and adolescent mental health: A rural worker training model. *Australasian Psychiatry, 15*(2), 135–139.

Bear, D., Jacobson, G., Aaronson, S., & Hanson, A. (1997). Telemedicine in psychiatry: Making the dream reality. *The American Journal of Psychiatry, 154*(6), 884–885.

Boothroyd, L. J., Kirmayer, L. J., Spreng, S., Malus, M., & Hodgins, S. (2001). Completed suicides among the Inuit of northern Quebec: A case control study. *Canadian Medical Association Journal, 165*(6), 749–755.

Brascoupé, S., & Waters, C. (2009). Cultural safety: Exploring the applicabiity of the concept of cultural safety to Aboriginal health and community wellness. *Journal of Aboriginal Health, 7*(1), 6–40.

Briggs, J. L. (1970). *Never in anger: Portrait of an Eskimo family*. Cambridge, England: Harvard University Press.

Bushy, A. (1994). When your client lives in a rural area. Part I: Rural health care delivery issues. *Isues of Mental Health Nursing, 15*, 253–266.

Calloway, M., Fried, B., Johnsen, M., & Morrissey, J. (1999). Characterization of rural mental health service systems. *The Journal of Rural Health, 15*(3), 296–307.

Canadian Medical Association. (2003). The health of Aboriginal peoples 2002. *Canadian Medical Association Journal, 168*(10), 1315–1318.

Cass, A. (2004). Health outcomes in Aboriginal populations. *Canadian Medical Association Journal, 171*(6), 597–598.

Chandler, M. J., & Lalonde, C. E. (1998). Cultural continuity as a hedge against suicide in Canada's First Nations. *Transcultural Psychiatry, 35*(2), 193–211.

Chandler, M. J., & Lalonde, C. E. (2008). Cultural continuity as a moderator of suicide risk among Canada's First Nations. In L. J. Kirmayer & G. Valaskakis (Eds.), *Healing traditions: The mental health of Aboriginal peoples in Canada* (pp. 221–248). Vancouver, British Columbia, Canada: University of British Columbia Press.

Cornish, P. A., Church, E., Callahan, T., Bethune, C., Robbins, C., & Miller, R. (2003). Rural interdisciplinary mental health team building via satellite: A demonstration project. *Telemedicine Journal and e-Health, 9*(1), 63–71.

Crawford, P., & Brown, B. (2002). "Like a friend going round": Reducing the stigma attached to mental healthcare in rural communities. *Health & Social Care in the Community, 10*(4), 229–238.

Crowe, T. P., Deane, F. P., Oades, L. G., Caputi, P., & Morland, K. G. (2006). Effectiveness of a collaborative recovery training program in Australia in promoting positive views about recovery. *Psychiatric Services, 57*(10), 1497–1500.

Currie, C. L., Wild, T. C., Schopflocher, D. P., Laing, L., & Veugelers, P. (2012). Racial discrimination experienced by aboriginal university students in Canada. *Canadian Journal of Psychiatry, 57*(10), 617–625.

Di Noia, J., Schwinn, T. M., Dastur, Z. A., & Schinke, S. P. (2003). The relative efficacy of pamphlets, CD-ROM, and the Internet for disseminating adolescent drug abuse prevention programs: An exploratory study. *Preventive Medicine, 37*(6 Pt 1), 646–653.

Drummond, S. G. (1997). *Incorporating the familiar: An investigation into legal sensibilities in Nunavik*. Montreal, Quebec, Canada: McGill-Queen's University Press.

Durie, M., Milroy, H., & Hunter, E. (2008). Mental health and the indigenous peoples of Australia and New Zealand. In L. J. Kirmayer & G. Valaskakis (Eds.), *Healing traditions: The mental health of Aboriginal peoples in Canada* (pp. 36–55). Vancouver, British Columbia, Canada: University of British Columbia Press.

Eberhardt, M. S., & Pamuk, E. R. (2004). The importance of place of residence: Examining health in rural and nonrural areas. *American Journal of Public Health, 94*(10), 1682–1686.

Elford, R., White, H., Bowering, R., Ghandi, A., Maddiggan, B., St. John, K., et al. (2000). A randomised controlled trial of child psychiatric assessments conducted using videoconferencing. *Journal of Telemedicine and Telecare, 6*(2), 73–82.

Fitchen, J. M. (1995). Spatial redistribution of poverty through migration of poor people to depressed rural communities. *Rural Sociology, 60*(2), 181–202.

Fortney, J. C., Pyne, J. M., Edlund, M. J., Williams, D. K., Robinson, D. E., Mittal, D., et al. (2007). A randomized trial of telemedicine-based collaborative care for depression. *Journal of General Internal Medicine, 22*(8), 1086–1093.

Fuller, J., Edwards, J., Martinez, L., Edwards, B., & Reid, K. (2004). Collaboration and local networks for rural and remote primary mental healthcare in South Australia. *Health & Social Care in the Community, 12*(1), 75–84.

Fuller, J., Edwards, J., Procter, N., & Moss, J. (2000). How definition of mental health problems can influence help seeking in rural and remote communities. *Australian Journal of Rural Health, 8*(3), 148–153.

Gamm, L. D. (2004). Mental health care and substance abuse services among rural minorities. *The Journal of Rural Health, 20*(3), 206–209.

Greenberg, N., Boydell, K. M., & Volpe, T. (2006). Pediatric telepsychiatry in Ontario: Caregiver and service provider perspectives. *Journal of Behavioral Health Services and Research, 33*(1), 105–111.

Griffiths, K. M., & Christensen, H. (2007). Internet-based mental health programs: A powerful tool in the rural medical kit. *Australian Journal of Rural Health, 15*(2), 81–87.

Group for the Advancement of Psychiatry. (1995). *Mental health in remote rural areas: Concepts and cases*. Washington, DC: American Psychiatric Press.

Hart, L. G., Larson, E. H., & Lishner, D. M. (2005). Rural definitions for health policy and research. *American Journal of Public Health, 95*(7), 1149–1155.

Havens, L. L. (1986). *Making contact: Uses of language in psychotherapy*. Cambridge, MA: Harvard University Press.

Hazelton, M., Habibis, D., Schneider, R., Davidson, J., & Bowling, A. (2004). Effect of an extended-hours community mental health team on family caregiving in a semi-rural region of Australia. *Australian Journal of Rural Health, 12*(5), 220–222.

Henderson, C., Vanier, C., & Noel, P. (1991). A Canadian model for developing mental health services in rural communities through linkages with urban centers. *Journal of Mental Health Administration, 18*(2), 135–142.

Hilty, D., Luo, J. S., Morache, C., Marcelo, D. A., & Nesbitt, T. S. (2002). Telepsychiatry: What is it and what are its advantages and disadvantages? *CNS Drugs, 16*, 527–548.

Hilty, D. M., Marks, S. L., Urness, D., Yellowlees, P. M., & Nesbitt, T. S. (2004). Clinical and educational telepsychiatry applications: A review. *Canadian Journal of Psychiatry, 49*(1), 12–23.

Hilty, D. M., Servis, M. E., Nesbitt, T. S., & Hales, R. (1999). The use of telemedicine to provide consultation liaison service to the primary care setting. *Psychiatric Annals, 29*, 421–427.

Hilty, D. M., Yellowlees, P. M., & Nesbitt, T. S. (2006). Evolution of telepsychiatry to rural sites: Changes over time in types of referral and in primary care providers' knowledge, skills and satisfaction. *General Hospital Psychiatry, 28*(5), 367–373.

Hilty, D. M., Yellowlees, P. M., Sonik, P., Derlet, M., & Hendren, R. L. (2009). Rural child and adolescent telepsychiatry: Successes and struggles. *Pediatric Annals, 38*(4), 228–232.

Hoyt, D. R., Conger, R. D., Valde, J. G., & Weihs, K. (1997). Psychological distress and help seeking in rural America. *American Journal of Community Psychology, 25*(4), 449–470.

Humphreys, J., Hegney, D., Lipscombe, J., Gregory, G., & Chater, B. (2002). Whither rural health? Reviewing a decade of progress in rural health. *Australian Journal of Rural Health, 10*, 2–14.

Indigenous Physicians Association of Canada, & The Royal College of Physicians & Surgeons of Canada. (2009). *Cultural safety in practice: A curriculum for family medicine residents and physicians*. Ottawa, Ontario, Canada: IPAC-RCPSC Family Medicine Curriculum Development Working Group.

Janca, A. (2000). Telepsychiatry: An update on technology and its applications. *Current Opinion in Psychiatry, 13*, 591–597.

Jennings, F. L. (1992). Ethics in rural practice. *Psychotherapy in Private Practice, 10*(3), 85–104.

Jong, M. (2004). Managing suicides via videoconferencing in a remote northern community in Canada. *International Journal of Circumpolar Health, 63*(4), 422–428.

Judd, F., Fraser, C., Grigg, M., Scopelliti, J., Hodgins, G., Gonoghue, A., et al. (2002). Rural psychiatry: Special issues and models of service delivery. *Disease Management and Health Outcomes, 10*(12), 771–781.

Judd, F. K., & Humphreys, J. S. (2001). Mental health issues for rural and remote Australia. *Australian Journal of Rural Health, 9*, 254–258.

Kappas, A., & Krämer, N. C. (Eds.). (2011). *Face-to-face communication over the Internet: emotions in a web of culture, language, and technology*. Cambridge, UK: Cambridge University Press.

Kennedy, C., & Yellowlees, P. (2000). A community-based approach to evaluation of health outcomes and costs for telepsychiatry in a rural population: Preliminary results. *Journal of Telemedicine and Telecare, 6*(Suppl 1), S155–S157.

King, M., Smith, A., & Gracey, M. (2009). Indigenous health part 2: The underlying causes of the health gap. *The Lancet, 374*(9683), 76–85.

Kirmayer, L. J., Boothroyd, L. J., & Hodgins, S. (1998). Attempted suicide among Inuit youth: Psychosocial correlates and implications for prevention. *Canadian Journal of Psychiatry, 43*(8), 816–822.

Kirmayer, L. J., Brass, G. M., & Valaskakis, G. G. (2008). Conclusion: Healing/invention/tradition. In L. J. Kirmayer & G. Valaskakis (Eds.), *Healing traditions: The mental health of aboriginal peoples in Canada* (pp. 440–472). Vancouver, British Columbia, Canada: University of British Columbia Press.

Kirmayer, L. J., Fletcher, C., & Boothroyd, L. J. (1997a). Suicide among the Inuit of Canada. In A. Leenaars, S. Wenckstern, I. Sakinofsky, R. J. Dyck, M. J. Kral, & R. C. Bland (Eds.), *Suicide in Canada* (pp. 189–211). Toronto, Ontario, Canada: University of Toronto Press.

Kirmayer, L. J., Fletcher, C. M., & Boothroyd, L. J. (1997b). Inuit attitudes toward deviant behavior: A vignette study. *The Journal of Nervous and Mental Disease, 185*(2), 78–86.

Kirmayer, L. J., Fletcher, C., & Watt, R. (2008). Locating the ecocentric self: Inuit concepts of mental health and illness. In L. J. Kirmayer & G. Valaskakis (Eds.), *Healing traditions: The mental health of Aboriginal peoples in Canada* (pp. 289–314). Vancouver, British Columbia, Canada: University of British Columbia Press.

Kirmayer, L. J., Malus, M., & Boothroyd, L. J. (1996). Suicide attempts among Inuit youth: A community survey of prevalence and risk factors. *Acta Psychiatrica Scandinavica, 94*(1), 8–17.

Kirmayer, L. J., Sedhev, M., Whitley, R., Dandeneau, S., & Isaac, C. (2009). Community resilience: Models, metaphors and measures. *Journal of Aboriginal Health, 7*(1), 62–117.

Kirmayer, L. J., Tait, C. L., & Simpson, C. (2008). The mental health of Aboriginal peoples in Canada: Transformations of identity and community. In L. J. Kirmayer & G. Valaskakis (Eds.), *Healing traditions: The mental health of Aboriginal peoples in Canada* (pp. 3–35). Vancouver, British Columbia, Canada: University of British Columbia Press.

Kirmayer, L. J., Whitley, R., & Fauras, V. (2010). *Community team approaches to mental health services and wellness promotion.* Ottawa, Ontario, Canada: Health Canada, First Nations and Inuit Health Branch.

Koptie, S. (2009). Irihapeti Ramsden: The public narrative on cultural safety. *First Peoples Child & Family Review, 4*(2), 30–43.

Lambert, D., & Hartley, D. (1998). Linking primary care and rural psychiatry: Where have we been and where are we going? *Psychiatric Services, 49*(7), 965–967.

Law, S. F., & Hutton, E. M. (2007). Community psychiatry in the Canadian Arctic—Reflections from a 1-year continuous consultation series in Iqaluit, Nunavut. *Canadian Journal of Community Mental Health, 26*(2), 123–140.

Lecompte, E., & Baril, M. (2008). Comparison of the 1996 and 2001 census data for Aboriginal and non-Aboriginal workers in health care occupations. *Cahiers de Sociologie et de Démographie Médicales, 48*(1), 123–138.

Lingley-Pottie, P., & McGrath, P. J. (2008). Telehealth: A child and family-friendly approach to mental health-care reform. *Journal of Telemedicine and Telecare, 14*(5), 225–226.

Macdonald, M. E. (2008). A jurisdictional tapestry and a patchwork quilt of care: Aboriginal health and social services in Montreal. In L. J. Kirmayer & G. Valaskakis (Eds.), *Healing traditions: The mental health of Aboriginal peoples in Canada* (pp. 381–400). Vancouver, British Columbia, Canada: University of British Columbia Press.

MacKinnon, M. (2005). A First Nations voice in the present creates healing in the future. *Canadian Journal of Public Health, 96*(Suppl 1), S13–S16.

McBride, W., & Gregory, D. (2005). Aboriginal health human resources initiatives: Towards the development of a strategic framework. *Canadian Journal of Nursing Research, 37*(4), 89–94.

McCallum, M. J. (2005). This last frontier: Isolation and Aboriginal health. *Canadian Bulletin of Medical History, 22*(1), 103–120.

McCormick, R. (2008). Aboriginal approaches to counselling. In L. J. Kirmayer & G. Valaskakis (Eds.), *Healing traditions: The mental health of Aboriginal peoples in Canada* (pp. 337–355). Vancouver, British Columbia, Canada: University of British Columbia Press.

McCormick, R., & Quantz, D. (2009). *Improving mental health services and supports in the National Native Alcohol and Drug Abuse Program.* NNADAP Gap Paper. Ottawa, Ontario, Canada: NNADAP.

McDonel, E. C., Bond, G. R., Salyers, M., Fekete, D., Chen, A., McGrew, J. H., et al. (1997). Implementing assertive community treatment programs in rural settings. *Administrative Policy in Mental Health, 25*(2), 153–173.

McGrath, P. J., Lingley-Pottie, P., Thurston, C., MacLean, C., Cunningham, C., Waschbusch, D. A., et al. (2011). Telephone-based mental health interventions for child disruptive behavior or anxiety disorders: Randomized trials and overall analysis. *Journal of the American Academy of Child and Adolescent Psychiatry, 50*(11), 1162–1172.

McLaren, P., Ball, C. J., Summerfield, A. B., Watson, J. P., & Lipsedge, M. (1995). An evaluation of the use of interactive television in an acute psychiatric service. *Journal of Telemedicine and Telecare, 1*, 79–85.

Merwin, E. I., Goldsmith, H. F., & Manderscheid, R. W. (1995). Human resource issues in rural mental health services. *Community Mental Health Journal, 31*(6), 525–537.

Minore, B., Boone, M., Katt, M., Kinch, P., Birch, S., & Mushquash, C. (2005). The effects of nursing turnover on continuity of care in isolated First Nations communities. *Canadian Journal of Nursing Research, 37*(1), 86–100.

Murray, J. D., & Kelleher, K. (1991). Psychology and rural America: Current status and future directions. *American Psychology, 46*(3), 220–231.

Mussell, W. J. (2005). *Warrior-caregivers: Understanding the challenges and healing of First Nations men.* Ottawa, Ontario, Canada: Aboriginal Healing Foundation.

Muttitt, S., Vigneault, R., & Loewen, L. (2004). Integrating telehealth into Aboriginal healthcare: The Canadian experience. *International Journal of Circumpolar Health, 63*(4), 401–414.

Myers, K. M., Valentine, J. M., & Melzer, S. M. (2007). Feasibility, acceptability, and sustainability of telepsychiatry for children and adolescents. *Psychiatric Services, 58*(11), 1493–1496.

Nagarajan, K. V. (2004). Rural and remote community health care in Canada: Beyond the Kirby panel report, the Romanow report and the federal budget of 2003. *Canadian Journal of Rural Medicine, 9*(4), 245–251.

Nelson, E. L., Barnard, M., & Cain, S. (2003). Treating childhood depression over videoconferencing. *Telemedicine and e-Health, 9*, 49–55.

Nelson, E., & Palsbo, S. (2006). Challenges in telemedicine equivalence studies. *Evaluation and Program Planning, 29*, 419–425.

Nelson, W. A., Pomerantz, A., & Schwartz, J. (2007). Putting "rural" into psychiatry residency training programs. *Academic Psychiatry, 31*(6), 423–429.

O'Reilly, R., Bishop, J., Maddox, K., Hutchison, L., Fisman, M., & Takhar, J. (2007). Is telepsychiatry equivalent to face-to-face psychiatry? Results from a randomized controlled equivalence trial. *Psychiatric Services, 58*, 836–843.

Owen, C., Tennant, C., Jessie, D., Jones, M., & Rutherford, V. (1999). A model for clinical and educational psychiatric service delivery in remote communities. *The Australian and New Zealand Journal of Psychiatry, 33*(3), 372–378.

Paing, W. W., Weller, R. A., Weslh, B., Foster, T., Birnkrant, J. M., & Weller, E. B. (2009). Telemedicine in children and adolescents. *Current Psychiatry Reports, 11*, 114–119.

Papps, E., & Ramsden, I. (1996). Cultural safety in nursing: The New Zealand experience. *International Journal for Quality in Health Care, 8*(5), 491–497.

Pauzé, E., Gagné, M.-A., & Pautler, K. (2005). *Collaborative mental health care in primary health care: A review of Canadian initiatives. Vol. 1: Analysis of initiatives.* Mississauga, ON: Canadian Collaborative Mental Health Initiative (CCMHI).

Reading, J. (2009). *The crisis of chronic disease among Aboriginal peoples: A challenge for public health, population health and social policy.* Victoria, British Columbia, Canada: Centre for Aboriginal Health Research.

Reading, C. L., & Wien, F. (2009). *Health inequalities and social determinants of Aboriginal peoples' health.* Victoria, British Columbia, Canada: National Collaborating Centre for Aboriginal Health.

Ruskin, P. E., Reed, S., Kumar, R., King, M. A., Siegel, E., Rosen, M., et al. (1998). Reliability and acceptability of psychiatric diagnosis via telecommunication and audiovisual technology. *Psychiatric Services, 49*(8), 1086–1088.

Samuels, A. H., & Owen, C. (1998). A day in the country: A perspective on rural psychiatry. *Australasian Psychiatry, 6*, 283–286.

Savin, D., Garry, M. T., Zuccaro, P., & Novins, D. (2006). Telepsychiatry for treating rural American Indian youth. *Journal of the American Academy of Child and Adolescent Psychiatry, 45*(4), 484–488.

Savin, D., & Martinez, R. (2006). Cross-cultural boundary dilemmas: A graded-risk assessment approach. *Transcultural Psychiatry, 43*(2), 243–258.

Shore, J. H., Brooks, E., Savin, D., Orton, H., Grigsby, J., & Manson, S. M. (2008). Acceptability of telepsychiatry in American Indians. *Telemedicine and e-Health, 14*(5), 461–466.

Shore, J. H., Savin, D. M., Novins, D., & Manson, S. M. (2006). Cultural aspects of telepsychiatry. *Journal of Telemedicine and Telecare, 12*(3), 116–121.

Shore, J. H., Savin, D., Orton, H., Beals, J., & Manson, S. M. (2007). Diagnostic reliability of telepsychiatry in American Indian veterans. *The American Journal of Psychiatry, 164*(1), 115–118.

Singh, S. P., Arya, D., & Peters, T. (2007). Accuracy of telepsychiatric assessment of new routine outpatient referrals. *BMC Psychiatry, 7*(55), 1–13.

Smye, V., Josewski, V., & Kendall, E. (2010). *Cultural safety: An overview.* Ottawa, Ontario, Canada: First Nations, Inuit and Métis Advisory Committee, Mental Health Commission of Canada.

Sommers, I. (1989). Geographic isolation and mental health services utilisation among the chronically mentally ill. *Community Mental Health Journal, 25*(2), 132–144.

Speck, R. V., & Attneave, C. L. (1973). *Family networks: Retribalization and healing.* New York, NY: Pantheon.

Statistics Canada. (2008). *Aboriginal peoples in Canada in 2006: Inuit, Métis and First Nations, 2006 census.* Ottawa, Ontario, Canada: Ministry of Industry.

Strasser, R. (1995). Rural general practice: Is it a distinct discipline? *Australian Family Physician, 24*, 870–876.

Szeftel, R., Hakak, R., Meyer, S., Naqvi, S., Sulman-Smith, H., Delrahim, K., et al. (2008). Training psychiatric residents and fellows in a telepsychiatry clinic: A supervision model. *Academic Psychiatry, 32*(5), 393–399.

Tang, S. Y., & Browne, A. J. (2008). "Race" matters: Racialization and egalitarian discourses involving Aboriginal people in the Canadian health care context. *Ethnicity and Health, 13*(2), 109–127.

Tobin, M. J. (1996). Rural psychiatric services. *The Australian and New Zealand Journal of Psychiatry, 31*(1), 114–123.

Wieman, C. (2008). Six nations mental health services: A model of care for Aboriginal communities. In L. J. Kirmayer & G. Valaskakis (Eds.), *Healing traditions: The mental health of Aboriginal peoples in Canada* (pp. 401–418). Vancouver, British Columbia, Canada: University of British Columbia Press.

Yellowlees, P. (1992). Bush psychiatric services. *The Australian and New Zealand Journal of Psychiatry, 26*(2), 191–196.

Cultural Consultation for Refugees

12

Janet Cleveland, Cécile Rousseau,
and Jaswant Guzder

Around the world, some 36 million people have been forcibly displaced from their homes by mass conflict or individual violence (United Nations High Commissioner for Refugees, 2013). This includes over 19 million people who are internally displaced and over 14 million others who are either stateless or have fled to neighboring countries of the global South where they are often housed in refugee camps. A minority (less than a million people a year) seeks asylum in the higher-income countries of the global North.

The United Nations 1951 Convention and 1967 Protocol Relating to the Status of Refugees (UNHCR, 2010), ratified by 145 nations, defines refugees as people who have fled their country because of a well-founded fear of persecution linked to their political beliefs, ethnicity, religion,

J. Cleveland, Ph.D. (✉)
CSSS de la Montagne Research Centre,
7085 Hutchison Street, Montreal,
QC, Canada H3N 1Y9
e-mail: janet.cleveland@mail.mcgill.ca

C. Rousseau, M.D., M.Sc.
Centre de recherche et de formation,
CSSS de la Montagne, 7085 rue Hutchison, Montréal,
QC, Canada H3N 1Y9
e-mail: cecile.rousseau@mcgill.ca

J. Guzder, M.D.
Center for Child Development and Mental Health,
Institute of Community and Family Psychiatry,
4335 Cote St. Catherine Road, Montreal, QC,
Canada H3T 1E4
e-mail: jaswant@videotron.ca

gender, sexual orientation, or similar reasons (Hathaway, 2005; United Nations High Commissioner for Refugees, 2010). Destination countries are prohibited from sending refugees back to their home country if they would be exposed to such persecution, and may not penalize refugees for entering the destination country irregularly or without official documents (Edwards, 2011; Hathaway, 2005; United Nations High Commissioner for Refugees, 2010). Some countries, including Canada, also recognize refugees as people who, if returned to their home country, would face a danger of torture, a risk of cruel and unusual treatment, or a risk to their life that does not stem from inadequate health care or conditions such as natural catastrophes that affect the population in general (Immigration and Refugee Protection Act, 2001).

In Canada, as in many other countries, refugees fall into two groups. The first group is *resettled refugees* sponsored either by the government (Government Assisted Refugees) or by private groups such as churches (Privately Sponsored Refugees). Resettled refugees, often coming from refugee camps, have already been recognized as refugees and granted permanent resident status before arriving in Canada. The second group of refugees are individuals who come to Canada on their own without prior government authorization and make a well-founded claim for refugee status. During the claims process, they are known as *refugee claimants* or *asylum seekers*. Refugee claimants have the right to remain in

L.J. Kirmayer et al. (eds.), *Cultural Consultation: Encountering the Other in Mental Health Care*,
International and Cultural Psychology, DOI 10.1007/978-1-4614-7615-3_12,
© Springer Science+Business Media New York 2014

Canada until final adjudication of the merit of their claim by an independent administrative tribunal, the Immigration and Refugee Board (IRB), including any appeal or judicial review proceedings. If the initial claim is rejected, during subsequent appeals, the person retains legal status and is known as a *rejected* or *failed claimant*. Acceptance of the claim confers secure refugee status and is the first step on the path to citizenship. If the claim is definitively rejected, the person will be ordered to leave the country (Immigration and Refugee Protection Act, 2001). If he or she does not comply with the deportation order, she loses her legal status and is known as an undocumented or nonstatus migrant.

In many countries, including Canada, it is also possible to apply for permission to remain in the country on humanitarian and compassionate (H&C) grounds. In Canada, as a result of recently adopted legislation (PCISA, 2012), most rejected claimants must now wait 1 year after definitive rejection of their claim before submitting an H&C application, during which time they will almost certainly be deported (unless they go underground). However, it remains possible to submit an H&C application immediately after final rejection of the refugee claim if it is based primarily either on a medical condition or the best interests of a child. Unlike appeal procedures, submitting an H&C application does not automatically prevent deportation but it may be possible to apply to the Federal Court for a stay of deportation while the H&C application is being examined. Humanitarian applications will not be further discussed in this chapter, because the criteria vary considerably from country to country.

Most resettled refugees have suffered years of privation and marginalization in transit countries, often in refugee camps, in addition to the traumatic events that initially led them to leave their country. Many have major physical or mental health problems due to trauma and hardship in both the home and transit countries, as well as the challenges of integrating into a new society (Fazel, Reed, Panter-Brick, & Stein, 2012; Fazel, Wheeler, & Danesh, 2005; Lie, 2002; Marshall, Schell, Elliott, Berthold, & Chun, 2005; Steel et al., 2009; Steel, Silove, Phan, & Bauman, 2002; Turner, Bowie, Dunn, Shapo, & Yule, 2003; Vaage et al., 2010). Upon arrival in Canada, however, they have secure, permanent status and are on the road to citizenship, factors that are associated with long-term improvement of mental health (Beiser, 1999, 2009; Nickerson, Steel, Bryant, Brooks, & Silove, 2011; Porter & Haslam, 2005; Schweitzer, Melville, Steel, & Lacharez, 2006; Steel et al., 2011).

Refugee claimants, on the other hand, face the challenge of trying to prove the well-foundedness of their refugee claim before the IRB, failing which they will be forcibly sent back to their country of origin (repatriation or deportation). Thus, in addition to the trauma experienced in the country of origin, refugee claimants face insecurity and precarious status in the receiving country. In this chapter, we will focus primarily on the situation of refugee claimants. After presenting the legal definition of a refugee, there is a brief overview of pre-migratory, transit, and postmigratory factors that may affect refugee claimants' psychosocial status, including a more detailed discussion of two common postmigratory problems: detention and family separation. The next section examines clinical intervention with refugee claimants, particularly the assessment and treatment of posttraumatic symptoms. Finally, there is a discussion of the ways in which clinicians may act upon the social determinants of refugee claimants' health, including a detailed explanation of how to write a report in the context of refugee status proceedings.

Refugees and Refugee Claimants: Legal Principles

Clinicians generally adhere to an ethos of care which prescribes that people who are ill should receive treatment, irrespective of their migration status. Many clinicians feel that the laws and policies defining migrants' rights are not relevant to their clinical practice with this population. Yet, migratory status has a huge impact on migrants' physical and mental health because it determines access to jobs, health care, social assistance, schooling, ability to reunite with family, and, most fundamentally, secure status in the destination country.

Sovereign states generally have the power to decide who may enter and remain in their country and on what terms and to expel those who do not comply. United Nations 1951 Convention and 1967 Protocol Relating to the Status of Refugees (UNHCR, 2010) is an exception to this rule. A person may enter and remain in a country other than her own if she would be in danger because of her ethnicity, religion, gender, sexual orientation, political opinions, or similar reasons if returned to her home country (Hathaway, 2005; Immigration and Refugee Protection Act, 2001; United Nations High Commissioner for Refugees, 2010). In Canada, a person may also be accepted as a refugee if she would be exposed to a risk of torture, cruel and unusual treatment, or an individualized threat to her life if returned to her country of origin. An individualized threat to life must go beyond the risks affecting the general population (e.g., epidemics, environmental disasters, earthquakes, famine) and excludes risks linked to lack of adequate health care (Immigration and Refugee Protection Act, 2001).

In Canada, refugee claimants present their case at a hearing before the IRB, which decides if their claim is well founded. The refugee claimant has the burden of proving three main elements. First, that she would be in danger of persecution if sent back to her country of origin and that this danger is linked to one of the grounds mentioned in the refugee definition (ethnicity, religion, gender, sexual orientation, political opinions, risk of torture, etc.). To prove this, the person must usually establish that they suffered severe mistreatment for one of these reasons in their home country, or were in imminent danger of suffering such mistreatment. Second, that the government of her country is unwilling or unable to protect her against this persecution. In some cases, this is obvious because government agents such as the military were directly responsible for the persecution. In others, the refugee claimant must prove that the police and judicial system did not offer adequate protection against her persecutors. Finally, the refugee claimant must demonstrate that she would not have been safe anywhere in her country, even if she had moved to a different region. The refugee claimant must prove all of these elements; otherwise, her claim will be rejected (Hathaway, 2005; Immigration and Refugee Protection Act, 2001). Between 2006

and 2011, on average, 41% of refugee claims were accepted annually in Canada (The Refugee Forum, 2012).

Many refugee claimants travel with false documents, for a number of reasons. In many cases it would be dangerous to apply to their government for a passport or other travel document because the government is involved or complicit in their persecution. At times, staying in the country long enough to obtain official documents would place the person in danger. Finally, many refugee claimants would be unable to obtain a visa even if they asked for one, for there is no such thing as a visa to flee persecution (Hathaway, 2005; Phillips, 2011).

Under international law, states are not allowed to penalize refugees for entering the country with false documents (Edwards, 2011; Hathaway, 2005; Phillips, 2011; United Nations High Commissioner for Refugees, 2010). Since the 1990s, however, governments in destination countries in the global North have increasingly adopted policies such as detention and visas designed to limit the flow of refugee claimants, as well as a discourse portraying them as "illegal" and potentially dangerous intruders, "bogus" refugees bent on taking advantage of the local population (Crépeau, Nakache, & Atak, 2007; Hathaway, 2005; Hyndman & Mountz, 2008). This discourse tends to reinforce implicit xenophobic stereotypes and may contribute to hostility toward refugee claimants in destination countries (Rousseau, Hassan, Moreau, & Thombs, 2011).

The Refugee Experience: Premigration, Transit, and Postmigration Stressors

Every year, thousands of people seek asylum in Canada (The Refugee Forum, 2012). Many have experienced traumatic events such as torture, sexual or physical assault, spousal violence, armed conflict, arbitrary imprisonment, murder of loved ones, or other forms of violence, often in the context of mass conflict or state failure. During their journey in search of a safe country, they often experience considerable hardship. When they finally arrive in the destination country, refugee claimants face not only the integration challenges common to all new immigrants, but also specific challenges such as living in constant fear of deportation should they fail to convince immigration authorities that they are entitled to protection as refugees. Postmigration stresses experienced during the asylum-seeking process, such as fear of deportation, may exacerbate consequences of premigratory traumas. To fully understand refugee claimants' experience, therefore, it is crucial to examine the potentially traumatic events and stressors that they have faced in their country of origin, in transit, and since their arrival in the destination country.

In many cases, multiple traumatic events may have disrupted the person's daily life over an extended period. A recent meta-analysis of 181 surveys involving over 80,000 adult refugees and other persons affected by mass conflict showed that cumulative exposure to trauma was a strong predictor of PTSD and depression, particularly the latter outcome (Steel et al., 2009). Populations granted secure, permanent status in another country had lower PTSD rates than persons who were internally displaced or living in camps, suggesting that a positive post trauma environment can help mitigate the impact of trauma and foster recovery. This is consistent with another meta-analysis on refugee mental health showing that favorable post-displacement conditions such as access to employment and adequate housing significantly reduced the negative impact of trauma exposure (Porter & Haslam, 2005). Longitudinal Canadian studies have shown that most adults and children with secure refugee status adapt well despite high levels of premigratory trauma exposure (Beiser, 1999; Rousseau & Drapeau, 2003). However, negative postmigration conditions may adversely affect refugee claimants' mental health. Some postmigratory stressors, such as language difficulties (Pottie, Ng, Spitzer, Mohammed, & Glazier, 2008), cultural differences (McKeary & Newbold, 2010), lack of recognition of qualifications, loss of social support (Schweitzer et al., 2006), discrimination (Rousseau, Hassan, et al., 2011), or a combination of such factors (Kirmayer, Narasiah, et al., 2011), also affect many other newly arrived migrants. However, refugee claimants often face additional difficulties that may aggravate the negative impact of past trauma,

including detention (Cleveland, Dionne-Boivin, & Rousseau, 2013; Cleveland & Rousseau, in press; Ichikawa, Nakahara, & Wakai, 2006; Keller et al., 2003; Kronick, Rousseau, & Cleveland, 2011; Lorek et al., 2009; Mares, Newman, Dudley, & Gale, 2002; Momartin et al., 2006; Newman, Dudley, & Steel, 2008; Robjant, Hassan, & Katona, 2009; Robjant, Robbins, & Senior, 2009; Silove, Austin, & Steel, 2007; Steel et al., 2006; Steel, Momartin, et al., 2004); lengthy refugee claim proceedings and protracted precarious status (Laban, Gernaat, Komproe, Schreuders, & De Jong, 2004; Momartin et al., 2006; Steel et al., 2006, 2011); limited access to health and social services (Arya, McMurray, & Rashid, 2012; Taylor, 2009); limited job access due to the temporary nature of refugee claimant work permits; or a combination of these factors (Laban et al, 2005; Nickerson, Bryant, Steel, Brooks, & Silove, 2010; Nickerson, Steel, et al., 2011; Porter & Haslam, 2005; Ryan, Benson, & Dooley, 2008; Ryan, Kelly, & Kelly, 2009; Silove, Sinnerbrink, Field, Manicavasagar, & Steel, 1997; Steel et al., 2009; Steel, Silove, Bird, McGorry, & Mohan, 1999).

When refugee claimants flee their country, they generally leave behind close family members, including spouse and children, and must often wait for years before being reunited, given the lengthy delays involved in the refugee status and family reunification proceedings (Nickerson et al., 2010; Rousseau, Mekki-Berrada, & Moreau, 2001; Rousseau, Rufagari, Bagilishya, & Measham, 2004). In addition to the pain of separation, refugee claimants may fear for the safety of family members left behind. This fear of future harm to family may aggravate posttraumatic stress and depression symptoms, as may fear of future harm to self such as deportation (Nickerson et al., 2010).

In short, refugee claimants are simultaneously faced with the task of rebuilding their lives in an unfamiliar environment, while having to deal with past trauma and multiple ongoing stressors, including separation from family; anxiety about family back home; limited access to employment, social assistance, and health care; and fear of deportation should their claim be rejected.

Table 12.1 provides an overview of the factors affecting refugee claimants' health and

Table 12.1 Factors affecting refugee mental health and well-being

Premigration factors	Potentially traumatic events (PTEs) in home country
	• Single or multiple
	• Discrete event or continuing situation
	Living conditions
	• Socioeconomic circumstances
	• Family situation
	• Situation of membership group (ethnic, religious, etc.)
	Personal history
	• Vulnerability factors
	• Protective (resiliency) factors
Transit factors	Direct trip to destination country vs. stays in transit locations
	If transit through other locations
	• Refugee camps (internal or in transit country)
	• Stays in transit countries
	– Clandestine (nonstatus) or with status
	– Economic situation, access to care, etc.
	– Detention linked to migratory status
	Travel with official documents or false documents
	If obtained from a smuggler
	• Cost and impact on the person's finances
	Exposure to PTEs during transit
	• Exploitation by smugglers
	• Poverty
	• Protracted experience of marginalization, helplessness, being stuck (e.g., refugee camp)
	• Physical injuries or mental stress linked to clandestine entry (e.g., exposure to the elements, hunger, confinement)
	Strengths acquired during transit
Postmigration factors	Obstacles upon arriving in destination country
	• Interviews by immigration officers
	• Detention
	• Challenges to admissibility
	Ongoing threat: fears for the future, feeling of not being safe
	• Protracted uncertainty about legal status
	• Anxiety about testifying at refugee status hearing
	• Fear of being sent back to country of origin
	• Fears about safety of family members back home
	• Fear that their membership group (ethnic, religious, political, or other) is under threat in country of origin
	Current living conditions
	• Loss of social identity (role as provider, community member, member of extended family, social recognition of competence, etc.)
	• Limited access to employment, health care, social services, education, etc.
	• Separation from family
	• Poverty
	• Limited social support
	• Marginalization or discrimination linked to migratory status, ethnicity, language, etc.
	• Settlement challenges: finding a place to live, a job, adapting to a different culture, learning a language, etc.

well-being during the different phases of migration. Many of these factors apply to any migration situation but have specific features for refugee claimants. We will discuss two postmigration stressors mentioned in Table 12.1 in greater detail—detention and family separation—because these are especially challenging aspects of the refugee's predicament.

Detention

In Canada, about 5–10% of refugee claimants are detained upon arrival, most often pending identity checks (Nakache, 2011). Detention is generally unrelated to any criminal wrongdoing, and detained claimants are very rarely even suspected of being a security risk (Nakache, 2011). Yet nearly a third of detained refugee claimants are held in high-security provincial jails with the criminal population, while the others are placed in Immigration Holding Centres that are operated as prisons, with razor-wire fences, centrally controlled locked doors, and constant surveillance by cameras and uniformed guards, as documented by recent studies (Cleveland et al., 2013; Cleveland & Rousseau, in press). Men and women are held in separate wings, with a special section for children detained with their mothers. All aspects of daily life are controlled by rigid rules, and failure to respect rules may be punished by solitary confinement. There are virtually no activities except watching television. Basic medical care is provided, but no counselling or mental health support. Suicidal detainees are either placed under 24/7 individual surveillance, usually in solitary confinement, or transferred to a provincial jail. All detained refugee claimants except pregnant women and minors are handcuffed, and sometimes shackled, during transportation, notably when in need of specialized medical care at a hospital. Detained claimants may be chained during medical procedures. For example, a claimant recounted being handcuffed to the dentist's chair during surgery for an abscessed tooth (Cleveland et al., 2013). If hospitalized, detainees, including women who have

just given birth, are almost always chained to their beds as well as being under guard. Some claimants forego medical treatment rather than enduring the shame of being seen in public handcuffed like a criminal (Cleveland et al., 2013).

Studies from around the world have consistently shown high levels of psychiatric symptoms among detained refugee claimants, even after short periods (Cleveland et al., 2013; Cleveland & Rousseau, in press; Ichikawa et al., 2006; Keller et al., 2003; Kronick et al., 2011; Lorek et al., 2009; Mares et al., 2002; Momartin et al., 2006; Newman et al., 2008; Robjant, Hassan, et al., 2009; Robjant, Robbins, et al., 2009; Silove et al., 2007; Steel et al., 2006; Steel, Momartin, et al., 2004). Symptoms tend to worsen over time (Keller et al., 2003; Steel et al., 2006). Depression and posttraumatic stress are the most common psychiatric problems among detained refugee claimants. In the United Kingdom, after about 30 days in detention, 76% of detained refugee claimants were clinically depressed compared to 26% of a nondetained comparison sample (Robjant, Robbins, et al., 2009). In the United States, after about 5 months in detention, 86% of refugee claimants showed clinical levels of depression, 77% clinical anxiety, and 50% clinical posttraumatic stress disorder (Keller et al., 2003). At follow-up a few months later, the mental health of those who were still detained had continued to deteriorate, whereas it had substantially improved among those who had been released and granted permanent status. In Australia, in 2010–2011, there were over 1,100 incidents of self-harm in immigration detention centers, including 6 suicides (Suicide Prevention Australia, 2011), for a population of about 6,000 people detained for a median of 10 months (Australian Department of Immigration and Citizenship, 2011).

In Canada, researchers conducted a study involving 122 adult refugee claimants detained in immigration holding centers and a comparison group of 66 never-detained refugee claimants (Cleveland et al., 2013; Cleveland & Rousseau, in press). Claimants in both groups had experienced an average of 9 serious traumatic events such as being physically assaulted, having family or friends who were assaulted and/or murdered, and being at risk of death. After an average detention of only 31 days, over three-quarters of the detained participants scored above clinical levels for depression, about two-thirds for anxiety, and about a third for posttraumatic stress symptoms. Detained refugee claimants were almost twice as likely as their nondetained peers to report clinically significant levels of posttraumatic stress symptoms (32% for detained participants, 18% for nondetained), while clinically significant depression rates were 50% higher among detained claimants than among their nondetained peers (78% for detained participants, 52% for nondetained). This reflects a response to factors such as disempowerment, loss of agency, inability to modify or escape from a painful situation, isolation, and stigmatization.

Detention is also harmful for asylum-seeking children (Kronick et al., 2011). In the UK, after an average 43-day detention, asylum-seeking children showed symptoms such as posttraumatic stress, depression, suicidal ideation, behavioral difficulties, and developmental delay as well as weight loss, difficulty breast-feeding in infants, food refusal, and regressive behaviors (Lorek et al., 2009). An Australian study of ten asylum-seeking families (14 adults and 20 children) detained for a prolonged period found that all but one child suffered from major depressive disorder and half from PTSD (Steel, Momartin, et al., 2004). A majority of children frequently contemplated suicide, and five had self-harmed. Most of the younger children showed developmental delays as well as attachment and behavioral problems. A third of the parents had attempted suicide. In 2004, an Australian government inquiry found that a high proportion of detained asylum-seeking children had psychological problems such as developmental delays, bed-wetting, nightmares, separation anxiety, sleep disturbance, depression, and suicidal behaviors (Newman et al., 2008; Silove et al., 2007). Previously competent parents, notably women

giving birth during detention, were often too depressed to adequately care for their children.

In January 2012, four asylum-seeking children won a six-figure settlement from the UK government in compensation for the negative impact of their 13-month detention (Taylor & Hattenstone, 2012). During detention, the children had developed multiple problems including hand tremors, refusal to eat, hair loss, recurrent nightmares, and severe anxiety. Eight years after release, the four children still had numerous symptoms, including insomnia, intrusive frightening memories of detention, phobic reactions, and reduced ability to concentrate and study. Their academic performance, which had been excellent before their detention, remained impaired.

Case Vignette 12-1

A family with two Canadian-born children aged 5 and 7 was detained for 5 days following rejection of their refugee claim. During the arrest, the parents were handcuffed in front of the children. The 5-year-old boy tried to escape and was physically forced into the van.

After release from detention the 7-year-old girl, who was previously healthy and doing well at school, became severely withdrawn and had difficulty speaking with adults and peers. Her academic performance declined. She also had regular nightmares and difficulty falling asleep. The 5-year-old boy developed phobias of police, dark-colored vans, and dogs and refused to go to preschool for the first 6 months after detention because he was too frightened to leave the house. He had regular temper tantrums, was unable to fall asleep without his parents present, and would not tolerate being in a room with the door closed. A year after detention, the two children were still struggling with anxiety, sleep problems and irritability, and met diagnostic criteria for PTSD.

In some cases, children may be separated from detained asylum-seeking parents, particularly when parents are held in regular jails, which do not accept young children. Forced separation is particularly likely to be harmful to children who have been exposed to violence in their home country; who leave behind relatives, friends, school, and everything with which they are familiar; and who arrive in a strange country where they may not even speak the language. Most are unlikely to have close relatives in Canada and would be placed in institutional care or in foster care with strangers, which is generally more harmful than fostering by relatives (Holtan, Rønning, Handegård, & Sourander, 2005).

Asylum-seeking Sudanese youth in the USA who were separated from their immediate family were at increased risk of PTSD, especially those placed in foster homes with strangers rather than with other Sudanese families (Geltman et al., 2005). Children separated for over a month from parents detained in US immigration prisons had high rates of sleep disturbance, aggressiveness, and withdrawal (Chaudry et al., 2010). On the other hand, when children fleeing organized violence are able to maintain secure attachments to family members, they are protected from some of the psychological consequences of trauma (Rousseau, Said, Gagne, & Bibeau, 1998).

Family Separation and Reunification

Separation of family members is a central stressor for refugees. Barudy (1989) distinguished three main stages in the family separation and reunification process: before the separation, during the separation, and the reunion itself. Each of these stages defines a new balance or imbalance in the family and determines, in part, what will become of the family. As in the case of other migrants, separations and cultural uprooting change family relationships, roles, and strategies (Williams, 1990), but for refugee families, these reorganizations take on distinctive characteristics.

Refugees repeatedly must face the question of what an extended separation means to the various members of their family. Family members who have fled abroad may be in a very difficult situation; the refugee who has found safe haven may feel guilty, powerless, and depressed about a separation over which they have little or no control (Fox, Cowell, & Johnson, 1995; Nickerson et al., 2010; Tseng, Cheng, Chen, Hwang, & Hsu, 1993). Those who remain behind may feel abandoned or even betrayed or deceived (Moreau, Rousseau, Meikki-Berrada, TCMR, & ERASME, 1999; Suarez-Orozco, Bang, & Kim, 2011). The long absence of one or more members first leads to a reconfiguration of roles within the family. Sometimes one of the parents must play the role of both mother and father; sometimes the older children must assume adult responsibilities or symbolically take the place of one of the parents (Barudy, 1989). This reorganization may also involve the use of surrogates, including members of the extended family, outsiders, and sometimes even divine figures. The temporary nature of this initial reconfiguration of roles may make the family all the more vulnerable (Williams, 1990).

When adolescents were reunited with their parents after having been left with close relatives for a few years while their parents settled in the USA, those who had been separated from one or both parents for over 2 years had significantly higher levels of depression and anxiety than those who had not been separated (Suarez-Orozco et al., 2011). Symptom severity increased with length of separation. Family reunification was often fraught with conflict. Especially in cases of lengthy separation, many children felt estranged from their parents and were deeply distressed at the separation from their alternate caregivers. Some children showed withdrawal, lack of trust, and depressive symptoms, while others showed increased anger and aggression. The emotional scars of long-term separation typically took years to heal.

Refugees often see family reunification as an event that will bring a happy ending to a long series of losses. Although refugees may eventually mention problems ensuing from reunification, it is initially presented as a time for celebration. While the family reunion is a turning point that can lend meaning to the many losses refugees have endured in their long journey, it also disrupts the fragile balance that has been established during the waiting period. The family reunion thus represents both renewal of highly significant family bonds and at the same time another loss of the new equilibrium, which may be difficult to cope with because it often cannot be mentioned. Once the family has been reunited, it has another crisis to face in trying to unite members who may have had very different experiences. The longer members of the family have been apart, the more difficult it may be for the family unit to regain its balance (Barudy, 1989). Roles must be redefined, taking into account the past (family history and ideas of the home culture) and the present (the realities of the host country, the cultural gaps between family members across generations). For those who have experienced trauma, this process may be particularly difficult if they need to hold on to well-defined roles in order to rebuild their identity (Rousseau et al., 2004). For further discussion of issues of reunification see Chapter 13.

Responding to Refugee Trauma and Loss: When and How?

Primary care practitioners have a key role in the recognition and management of mental health problems in immigrant and refugee patients for three main reasons (Kirmayer, Narasiah, et al., 2011). First, general practitioners are the gateway to health care for immigrants and refugees, who, as a group, underutilize mental health services in Canada. Second, immigrants and refugees report elevated rates of extreme trauma, such as torture and rape, that can have severe and long-lasting consequences for both physical and mental health and require integrated treatment approaches. Third, although a particular family member may present as the identified patient, a family perspective is essential because trauma stemming from organized violence tends to affect the whole family, especially, children, who may not display dramatic or easily recognizable symptoms. Because of the complexity of these situations and the emotional burden that they represent, the primary care practitioners can benefit from cultural consultation to help them address the entanglements of past and present contextual factors with cultural issues.

In many places, health care services for refugees are limited. In Canada, the federal government has recently made major cuts to health care for refugee claimants (Arya et al., 2012). The new Interim Federal Health Plan covers only medical acts by physicians or nurses and explicitly excludes coverage of psychotherapy or any services provided by psychologists or other non-medical health professionals. Medication coverage by the federal government is also very limited, although this may be mitigated by provincial plans. As a result, primary care practitioners will face the challenge of managing refugee claimants' mental health problems with very limited resources.

Primary care practitioners need to be aware that immigrants and refugees may have undergone premigratory trauma. A warm and empathic stance is essential to create a safe environment for disclosure (Rousseau, Measham, & Nadeau, 2012). It is important to include an interpreter when language may impede accurate and empathetic communication (see Chapter 5). The choice of interpreter (gender, ethnicity, religion) should be discussed with the patient. Interpretation over the telephone is not recommended because of the mistrust and shame often associated with a traumatic experience.

Assessment of traumatic symptoms cannot be separated from potential interventions. If a patient discloses a traumatic experience, acknowledging the pain and suffering associated with the event may be helpful. Practitioners may explain that the reaction is common in persons who have undergone trauma (normalization) and provide information. When patients face misunderstanding or incredulity elsewhere in health care, social service, or legal systems, practitioners may need to move away from offering a neutral stance and adopt a clear position of advocacy (Kirmayer, 2001; Rousseau et al., 2012). Offering empathetic reassurance that help will be provided and that the situation is likely to get better is an important first step. For refugee patients, practical family and social support is most often provided in Canada by community organizations. Family physicians may find it helpful to establish partnerships with these organizations in order to reduce the isolation of families and to help them obtain support in the initial phases of resettlement.

Although not supported by clinical trials, National Institute of Clinical Excellence (NICE) (National Collaborating Centre for Mental Health, & Royal College of Psychiatrists' Research Unit, 2005) recommends a phased model, reflecting a pragmatic clinical approach for refugee and refugee claimants who face the possibility of being returned to a traumatic environment. Phase I is defined as the period in which safety has not yet been established, during which intervention should focus on practical family and social support. Advocacy by health professionals may be essential at this stage to help establish a sense of safety. Phase II and III should focus on patient priorities, which may include social integration and/or treatment of symptoms. Trauma-focused psychological treatment should be offered because it has been shown to be effective even years after trauma occurred (Rousseau et al., 2001).

There is some evidence that even for accepted refugees the effect of social factors like unemployment, isolation, and discrimination may overshadow the efficacy of mental health treatment in many patients (Gorst-Unworth & Goldenberg, 1998). This adds support to the idea that a multilevel response to traumatic stress is needed for refugee and immigrant populations, with interventions that include primary care, community organizations, and other social institutions (Nickerson, Bryant, Silove, & Steel, 2011; Silove, 1999).

Clinical Assessment of Trauma and Its Consequences

Exploration of trauma and its consequences is not typically recommended in the first meeting with a patient unless it is the patient's primary complaint. Otherwise, exploration of mental health issues can be delayed to subsequent interviews when a trusting relationship has been established (Weinstein, Dansky, & Iacopino, 1996). However, certain symptom presentations should alert clinicians to assess for PTSD, including unexplained physical complaints that may not be presented as PTSD (Burnett & Peel, 2001; Lustig et al., 2004), but suggest the possibility of psychological distress and PTSD as differential diagnoses (New Hampshire State, 2005). Similarly, trauma and torture can lead to a wide range of psychological pathologies that have significant comorbidity with PTSD. The most common are depression, panic disorder, and somatoform disorder (Fazel et al., 2005; Hinton et al., 2005). Other presentations, such as severe dissociation mimicking brief reactive psychosis, dissociative disorders involving amnesia and conversion symptoms (Van Ommeren et al., 2001), and psychotic depression, although less frequent, may also be related to PTSD. Key elements of the assessment include the level of psychological distress, impairment associated with the symptoms in the patient and his or her family, substance abuse, and suicidality. In children, particularly under age 8, the presence of sleep disturbance, emotional or behavioral problems should alert clinicians to the possibility of PTSD (National Collaborating Centre for Mental Health, & Royal College of Psychiatrists' Research Unit, 2005).

Interviews should be carried out in the presence of professional interpreters if the language ability of the patient is not adequate to express psychological distress and narrate their experience (Moreno & Grodin, 2002; National Collaborating Centre for Mental Health, & Royal College of Psychiatrists' Research Unit, 2005). Disclosing traumatic experience through relatives, family members or, particularly, through children can be traumatic and can discourage the patient from doing so. Efforts should be made to ensure the patient feels safe and understands that the assessment will be kept confidential. Assessment of children should be done directly in a culturally sensitive manner rather than relying solely on information from parents or guardians who may tend to minimize or ignore symptoms.

Treatment Interventions, Recovery, and Resilience

For refugees and others recovering from the impact of trauma and forced migration, intervention involves personal, family, and sociocultural collective dynamics with the aim of restoring a sense of normality by allowing life to go on (social integration) and overcoming the paralysis that terror and grief can cause (symptom reduction) (Nickerson, Bryant, Brooks, et al., 2011; Nickerson, Bryant, Silove, et al., 2011). Although they are affected by many of the same processes, social integration and symptom reduction are not given the same weight in the specific treatment interventions. The chief target of psychotherapy and medication is symptom reduction, and their effectiveness is usually measured in these terms; gains in terms of reduction of impairment and improvement in functioning are often not considered, although their relation to symptoms is not linear (Pynoos et al., 2009). Consideration of patients' own concerns and their social context, however, makes it clear that restoring the continuity of life by facilitating a person and family's social integration into the host country is just as important as symptom reduction.

Trauma-related anxiety disorders (which have been mainly studied in relation to PTSD), depression stemming from multiple losses in an exile setting, and the interaction of the two can be treated through various forms of psychotherapy, psychopharmacology, or alternative therapies including traditional treatments (Hinton, Hoffmann, Pollack, & Otto, 2009). In primary care settings, the recommendation of one type of treatment over another must be based on considerations that include the resources available and the cultural and clinical appropriateness of these resources. Acknowledging at the start that access to specialized therapeutic resources in the host country is limited can safeguard the referring clinician and the patient against unrealistic expectations. Drawing up an inventory of available resources prior to consultation is essential for a realistic treatment plan. In many settings, specialized psychotherapy for refugee trauma or torture-related issues may not be widely available, but committed community workers and primary care professionals can provide excellent therapeutic support and a forum for empathic listening that can provide relief for patients.

Trauma-focused psychotherapy helps reduce the fragmentation of memory caused by trauma by providing the patient with a coherent account. Diverse methods of psychotherapy that elicit a trauma narrative—some emphasizing structure, others the value of openness to what emerges—may be successful and can be chosen to fit the patient's expectations and the clinician's skills. In clinical practice, some patients seem to need to borrow an external structure in order to reconstruct coherence. They may prefer a culturally distant frame of reference, like cognitive behavior therapy (CBT) (Bolton et al., 2007) or narrative exposure therapy (NET) (Neuner et al., 2008), for example, or opt for a more traditional framework that emphasizes the coherence of their experience within the range of representations of their culture of origin (Peltzer, 1997). Other patients will resist such structures because they see them as representing a repetition of the constraints to which they were subjected. They need to talk at length and to be the architects of their life stories. The therapist, provided he or she does not enter into a struggle for control, can help them to avoid the vicious circle of traumatic repetition and to reintroduce key fragments of their past to help them with their posttraumatic reconstruction (Rousseau & Measham, 2007).

Unilateral imposition of either Western expertise (no matter how "cutting edge") or culturally sensitive modalities (no matter how rooted in tradition) may be experienced as coercive if the choice of the individual or family is not taken into account. Creative arts based therapies, such as art therapy, are sometimes preferred by refugee families, in part because these therapies often emphasize nonverbal therapeutic methods, thus helping people who are reluctant to engage in verbal therapy (Rousseau & Guzder, 2008). This reluctance may reflect either cultural attitudes or the fact that verbal approaches may be seen as being disrespectful of cultural values of emotional containment or restraint. Some clinicians may regard nonverbal therapies as potentially colluding with the avoidance that is part of the psychopathology of PTSD. But avoidance is not uniformly harmful, nor is it always a sign of psychopathology. While psychotherapists in the West (and popular culture) may favor more direct working-through of trauma, focusing therapeutic work explicitly on trauma, other cultural traditions prefer to work "around" trauma, institutionalizing avoidance as a collective strategy. At one end of the spectrum stands the culture of Jewish Holocaust survivors, in which collective pressure to remember has resulted in a "duty of memory", and at the other end are cultural strategies like those adopted by Cambodian survivors of Pol Pot, who seek to set aside the past in order to move on (Kidron, 2012). The duty of memory serves collective goals of communal solidarity, moral pedagogy, and even nation building, but it is not always associated with individual healing (Semprun, 1994). The preferred strategy in some cultures is to avoid direct individual or collective references to specific trauma and instead emphasize survival and continuity through a peoples' ability to overcome adversity (Rousseau, de la Aldea, Viger Rojas, & Foxen, 2005).

In addition to emotional problems, refugees who have experienced trauma may display other stress-related symptoms, which may be very impairing (Ehntholt & Yule, 2006; Kinzie, 2007). Sleep is often a major problem for PTSD patients; nightmares being one of the most frequent and disabling symptoms. NICE recommends the short-term use of hypnotic medication for adults or, if longer-term treatment is required, the use of suitable antidepressants to reduce the risk of dependence. Trials of cognitive behavioral treatments of nightmares have very promising results, and although they have not been tested in refugee and immigrant patients, their mode of action (cognitive restructuring and replacing negative by positive appraisals) may fit well with the ways in which certain cultures normalize nightmares rather than considering them symptoms

per se. Medically unexplained symptoms and various forms of chronic pain also warrant attention. The Rehabilitation and Research Centre for Torture Victims in Copenhagen (Sjölund, 2007) has produced a very useful manual to help practitioners address these symptoms which need to be taken seriously even if they are not related to clear organic pathology.

Case Vignette 12-2

Begum was a 30-year-old Bangladeshi Muslim mother who had fled her country after repeated domestic violence. After she had attempted to leave her husband, he abducted her from her family, vandalized her parent's home, and assaulted them. With the help of her parents, she left Bangladesh with her 4-year-old son. En route to Canada, she was detained in New York by the agents who had arranged her passage with her parents. She was taken to an apartment with other refugees and raped before being returned to the airport.

She applied for refugee status in Canada, but was too ashamed to recount her rape en route and the history of rape within her marriage. The refugee board rejected her claim because her testimony differed from her initial written claim, and she had dissociated during the hearing when attempting to recount her traumatic journey. Her appeal process continued for 6 years. During much of this time, she was suicidal and depressed, at times threatening to kill both her children as she felt unsafe to return to Bangladesh where her husband continued to be involved in antisocial gang activities. She was particularly terrified that she might be returned to New York, which triggered re-experiencing of her rape and helplessness. Both of her parents died in Bangladesh during this period and this further complicated her adaptation. Her depression undermined her parenting capacity and her children also suffered from depression.

(continued)

The role of the CCS consultant was to advise her primary care clinicians on the management of Begum's complicated grief, PTSD, her threats of suicide and infanticide, as well as the depression of her children during the protracted period of her unresolved status. Initially, she had been assessed by a male Euro-Canadian psychiatrist and refused to speak because cultural and gender differences precluded a sense of cultural safety. Her primary care team, comprised of a female general practitioner and social worker, worked with interpreters, her children's school, the Department of Youth Protection, and other resources to stabilize her functioning. Her functioning improved significantly after her refugee status was confirmed, but her children remained fragile and continued to have significant mental health problems.

Writing Reports for the Determination of Refugee Status

During the refugee status determination process, claimants must explain the events that have led them to seek refugee status. When they first claim refugee status at the port of entry, they will be questioned by immigration officials, primarily about identity and security issues. Under new Canadian legislation that came into force in December 2012 (PCISA, 2012), refugee claimants must complete and submit a detailed written Basis of Claim form explaining the reasons for their claim to the IRB within 15 days of arrival. Later, they will give an in-depth oral account of the events underlying their claim at a hearing before the IRB, which then determines whether the claimant meets the legal criteria for recognition as a refugee. The new law provides that most claimants will (for the first time in Canada) have access to a full appeal on the merits before the Refugee Appeal Division (RAD) of the IRB. The RAD appeal is generally based solely on the transcript and other documentary evidence already on file, so the claimant will not testify anew at this stage.

In general, the refugee claimant is the only witness; everything hinges on the believability of the claimant's testimony, as there are generally no witnesses to corroborate her account and little documentary evidence beyond general information on country conditions. Credibility assessment is largely based on the coherence, consistency, level of detail, and plausibility of the claimant's account (Herlihy, Scragg, & Turner, 2002; Steel, Frommer, et al., 2004). In addition, Board members are inevitably influenced by factors such as the claimant's demeanor, nonverbal signals, and expressed emotions as well as their own emotional response to the claimant's story (Macklin, 1998; Rousseau, Crépeau, Foxen, & Houle, 2002). Consistency is of paramount importance, and discrepancies between the claimant's testimony before the Board and previous oral or written accounts tend to be viewed with suspicion. Claimants are generally expected to give a reasonably coherent, linear account of their traumatic experiences, including precise dates and locations.

Consultants may be requested by the patient, a lawyer or other health care practitioners, to provide a written report on the refugee claimant's mental health and capacity to take part in the IRB hearing. When preparing this report, there are two essential questions to consider: (1) What are the precise issues of concern to the decision-maker who will read the report? and (2) What aspects of the refugee claimant's psychological state are relevant to these issues?

As already mentioned, refugee claimants must prove three main elements in order to be accepted as refugees. First, that if sent back to their country of origin, they would be in danger of severe mistreatment linked to one of the grounds mentioned in the refugee definition (ethnicity, religion, gender, sexual orientation, political opinions, risk of torture, etc.). Although in theory all that is necessary is to prove that the person would be at risk of persecution if returned to their country (future risk), in practice this almost always implies showing that they have already suffered persecution in their home country for one of these reasons and would still be in danger if sent back. Second, refugee claimants must show that they made reasonable efforts to obtain protection in their own country, but that their government was unwilling or unable to protect them. If the government is directly responsible for the persecution (e.g., ethnic minority civilians targeted by government troops during a civil war), state protection is clearly unavailable. In other cases, the refugee claimant will have to show that he made diligent but unsuccessful efforts to seek protection from local authorities, or that he had serious reasons not to seek protection (e.g. in his country, police officers consistently beat up or ignore gay men who try to make a complaint). Finally, the refugee claimant must prove that she would still have been at risk if she had moved to a different region within her country.

These criteria are specific to refugee claim proceedings. If the report is submitted in the context of a different type of procedure, the issues to be addressed will be different. For example, in Canada a failed refugee claimant can apply for permanent residence based on humanitarian and compassionate grounds (H&C application) if she can demonstrate that her deportation would be contrary the best interests of her children or severely detrimental to her own physical or mental health. She must also show that she is well integrated into Canadian society (e.g., employed, studying or involved in volunteer work, reasonably fluent in one of the official languages). All these issues are largely irrelevant in the context of a refugee claim. The content of the report therefore will differ depending on the nature of the proceeding and the specific factors to be considered by the decision-maker. As already mentioned, only reports in the context of refugee claim proceedings will be discussed because the grounds for humanitarian applications differ considerably from one country to another, whereas the criteria for successful refugee claims are relatively uniform throughout the 145 countries that have ratified the United Nations 1951 Convention and 1967 Protocol Relating to the Status of Refugees (UNHCR, 2010).

The following comments on writing expert reports apply in cases in which the consultant has no serious reasons to suspect that the claimant is malingering or fabricating her story. When the consultant feels uneasy about writing a report, the consultant would share with the refugee claimant that the report may not be helpful to his or her case.

In the context of refugee claim proceedings, there are four main issues that mental health professionals may potentially need to address: (1) whether the person's symptoms and clinical presentation are consistent with the alleged traumatic events on which the refugee claim is based; (2) whether certain apparently unreasonable or surprising behaviors might be linked to the person's psychological difficulties. For example, shame, disempowerment, and fear of authority figures might help explain why a woman in an abusive relationship failed to seek protection from local police and later failed to tell immigration officers about the abuse; (3) whether being sent back to her country might be a threat to her life or psychological integrity (e.g., risk of decompensation or suicide); and finally, (4) whether the person's ability to adequately present their case may be diminished due to cognitive, psychological, or emotional difficulties. Such difficulties may affect the person's ability to tell her story coherently, to describe certain particularly traumatic events, to attend a hearing on a particular date, or even to understand the proceedings (Herlihy et al., 2002; Prabhu & Baranoski, 2012; Rousseau et al., 2002; Steel, Frommer, et al., 2004).

In writing the report, it is important to try to make the person come alive as a unique individual for the reader. Board members see dozens of reports from mental health professionals, most of which state that the person suffers from PTSD. Of course, this is because refugee claims are usually based on traumatic events, so PTSD is not only frequent among refugee claimants, but is also the diagnosis that is most likely to be relevant to the issue at stake, namely, whether the refugee claimant's story of traumatic persecution is credible. Unfortunately, the ubiquity of PTSD in reports submitted in support of refugee claims tends to generate the impression that the diagnosis

Table 12.2 Outline of the mental health consultant report for refugee determination

The report should generally be about 2–4 pages long and include the following information:

- Professional qualifications
- Context of consultation and nature of relationship (assessment requested by a lawyer, progress report of an ongoing therapy)
- Method of assessment
- Clinically relevant elements of the refugee claimant's story
- Clinical signs and symptoms
- Diagnosis
- Potential limitations to the person's ability to adequately present their case
- Recommendations

is overused. This impression is strengthened if, as sometimes happens, the report is simply a generic list of symptoms such as insomnia, nightmares, and loss of appetite followed by a diagnosis of PTSD, based on a single assessment interview. In this context it is all the more essential to provide a clearly individualized report.

Table 12.2 outlines the key elements of the report. The overall tone of the report should be professional and objective while conveying the suffering experienced by the patient. To be credible, it is important to speak as a professional, not as an advocate (e.g., not to write "I urge you to accept Mr. X's refugee claim"). The report should focus on issues relevant to refugee status, particularly the symptoms consistent with acts of persecution that would entitle the person to protection as a refugee. It should be presented in terms that an educated layperson will readily understand. Technical jargon may be misunderstood by the decision-maker and should be avoided except when precise technical terms are essential, such as for the diagnosis, in which case the term should be briefly explained. For example, instead of "negative affect", it is preferable to use terms such as "negative emotions" or, better yet, more vivid and specific terms such as anger, sadness, or tears.

Professional Qualifications

In legal proceedings such as the refugee claim process, opinions are generally not admissible. The sole exception to this rule is opinions expressed by qualified experts, and only to the extent that the opinion is within their field of expertise (Paciocco & Stuesser, 2008; R. v. Lavallee, 1990). Consultants' opinion will not be taken into consideration unless they establish their expertise, primarily by listing their professional title (e.g., licensed psychologist) and relevant degrees. To further establish expertise, the consultant can mention relevant experience with certain populations or disorders (e.g., experience with refugees or trauma survivors), institutional affiliation (e.g., cultural consultation service, multidisciplinary treatment team), academic position, publications, and so on.

Context of Consultation and Nature of Relationship

Indicate whether the report is based on a one-off assessment requested by a lawyer or on an ongoing therapeutic relationship. If requested by a lawyer, the report may mention the specific questions that were posed. Otherwise, simply describe the person's reasons for consultation and whether she was referred by a colleague. If the consultation was requested because of physical or mental health problems, rather than simply because of an upcoming hearing, this is worth mentioning because it may contribute to making the patient's health problems credible.

Method of Assessment

Indicate the time frame, number, and length of assessment interviews or therapy sessions. Reports based on several assessment interviews or on a reasonably long-term therapy process are more credible than those based on a single brief interview, so it is important to emphasize that time was taken to do a full assessment if such is the case. If tests were used, briefly describe their purpose and validity, the results, and the interpretation.

Clinically Relevant Elements of the Refugee Claimant's Story

References to the refugee claimant's story should be limited to essentials, including only elements that are both relevant to the refugee claim and indispensable to explain the clinical assessment of the person's psychological state. In particular, keep details such as date, time, and place to the absolute minimum needed to make the account comprehensible. This is vitally important, for three main reasons. First, the more narrative details included, the higher the risk of contradictions between the report and the refugee claimant's testimony at the IRB hearing. At the hearing, claimants are under a tremendous amount of stress and may easily get confused about certain aspects of their story, particularly dates or names. Memories will be less reliable with the passage of time. The consultant may also have misunderstood certain details, such as the name of a town or a paramilitary group. During the interview, the claimant may describe a person as her brother and later call him a cousin during the IRB hearing. Including such details increases the risk of inconsistencies that may harm the claimant's credibility. Consulting the refugee claimant's Basis of Claim narrative before writing your report may be helpful to minimize inconsistencies, although this type of detail should in any case be limited to the strictly essential.

The second reason for keeping the summary of the claimant's story to a minimum is that the consultant usually has no personal knowledge of the facts that the claimant recounts and no means to check their veracity. In any case, this fact checking is not the consultant's job. Eliciting a detailed account of the facts on which the claim is based and assessing the refugee claimant's credibility is at the heart of the IRB's jurisdiction and will be the main focus of the hearing. For the

same reason, it is also crucial to always use expressions like "Mr. Y reported" or "Ms. Z said" rather than stating that an event actually occurred.

Finally, if the diagnosis appears to be based primarily on the claimant's story, and the Board does not believe the claimant, then the report is likely to be ignored. Board members frequently use this rationale to justify ignoring a clinical report: "The report was based on the refugee claimant's account, and I don't believe the refugee claimant, therefore I do not need to take the report into account." On the other hand, if the report is primarily based on specific clinical signs and symptoms, especially the consultant's own observations, it is much harder to set aside.

In the context of a therapeutic relationship, claimants may sometimes reveal important facts that they had not previously disclosed to immigration authorities or to their lawyer (e.g., sexual assault). When a claimant adds new details to her story at an advanced stage of the proceedings, there is a risk that the Board may suspect that the claimant is embellishing or making up facts to try to strengthen her claim. At the least, the claimant will need to explain the reasons for the late disclosure. Ideally, it is preferable to ask the lawyer whether the newly disclosed fact should be mentioned in the report. If the fact has little relevance to the claim, it may be as well not to include it. If, on the other hand, it is highly relevant, it is important to mention it and explain the reasons that the person did not disclose earlier (e.g., shame, fear) and did disclose to the consultant (e.g., having developed a relationship of trust). Simply stating that "rape victims often feel ashamed," for example, may not be sufficient. Board members will undoubtedly have heard such explanations before, as refugee claims are almost always based on acts of interpersonal violence.

Childhood trauma or other painful events unrelated to the refugee claim should usually be left out of the report. No matter how much a person may have suffered during their lives, this does not entitle them to refugee status unless the events fall within the scope of the legal refugee definition. On the other hand, for example, it could be relevant to mention that a woman had been a victim of incest as a child if this helps to explain why she stayed in an abusive relationship or was too ashamed to report spousal violence. More generally, psychological problems may have affected the person's ability to seek state protection or to relocate within the country of origin.

Clinical Signs and Symptoms

A description of the relevant clinical signs and symptoms is at the heart of the consultant's expertise. Reports based solely on self-reported symptoms may be seen as less persuasive because of the perception that claimants could be making them up. It is therefore important to explain the congruence between the symptoms reported by the claimant and the signs that you personally observed, and how the overall presentation is clinically plausible. Clinical signs are particularly important because they are directly observed by the clinician and cannot be entirely disregarded by the Board even if it does not believe the claimant. Potentially relevant clinical signs include: psychomotor slowing or similar physical signs consistent with depression; inability to stay focused or to tell the story coherently because of emotional distress or problems with memory or concentration; and nonverbal expressions of emotions such as tears, choked voice, shaking, tension, agitation, and tone of voice. Linking nonverbal emotional expression to trauma may make it more credible (e.g., "As he described seeing his father being killed, tears ran down his face").

Similarly, in describing the symptoms reported by the claimant, particular attention should be paid to symptoms consistent with the alleged traumatic antecedents. This may include intrusive thoughts or images, ruminations, recurrent themes in nightmares, situations that trigger strong emotions or avoidance, suicidal ideation, and so on. A brief quote from the claimant that illustrates her pain about past trauma, current suffering, or fear of future harm may be useful to include. In the context of a hearing, the claimant may not be able to express her feelings in a way that is as vivid or personal as in a clinical setting. In any case, refugee claim hearings tend to focus more on claimants' objective actions and cognitions than on

their inner world, so the consultant's report may be an occasion to highlight dimensions of the claimant's subjective experience that are relevant to the refugee claim but might not otherwise be mentioned. For example, recurrent nightmares of men hammering on the door would be highly relevant if the claim centers on an incident of arbitrary arrest and imprisonment, yet this is unlikely to come up at the hearing unless included in the report.

Faced with the difficult task of assessing a claimant's credibility, Board members often look for specific details that "ring true." For example, a young man from a persecuted religious minority recounted how, hidden in his parents' house, he had listened helplessly to his mother being insulted and threatened by police who were looking for him. In a choked voice, he reported being tormented by persistent feelings of shame at having exposed his mother to danger and having failed his duty as a man and a son to protect her. This type of snapshot of vivid, emotionally charged memories may contribute to the credibility of the claimant's account, especially when they involve feelings that most people can readily identify with.

Mentioning that the claimant is afraid of being repatriated is relevant, as this is one of the elements that must be established for the claim to be successful. However, it is rarely useful to expand on the hardships such a return may involve for the claimant and her family (e.g., disrupting children's schooling) because this has no bearing on the merit of the refugee claim, although the same information would be highly relevant to an application based on humanitarian and compassionate grounds. On the other hand, the heightened vulnerability of psychologically disturbed persons may be a relevant factor when assessing the risks they would face if returned to their country of origin. For example, a Roma woman who had suffered for years from severe depression, anxiety, and agoraphobia following an attack by skinheads was found to have compelling reasons not to return to Hungary, although the Board judged that the risks that she would face there would not amount to persecution for a less psychologically fragile person (ReX, 2008). Similarly, the claim of an Ethiopian refugee claimant with bipolar disorder and a history of suicide attempts was accepted on the grounds that the severe stigmatization and discrimination that she would experience in Ethiopia because of her mental illness amounted to persecution likely to lead to suicide (Re X, 2007). More generally, if there are serious reasons to believe that forced repatriation is likely to cause clinical decompensation, a suicide attempt or other consequences that could put the claimant's life at risk, this should be explained.

Generally, it is important to indicate whether the clinical presentation is consistent with the alleged trauma. However, never write that the claimant's symptoms are *caused* by the traumatic events, but rather that they are *consistent* with the alleged events. Causality is impossible to prove, and in any case the consultant has no personal knowledge whether the alleged events actually occurred.

Diagnosis

When posing the diagnosis (or clinical impressions), it may be useful to very briefly summarize the main factors on which the diagnosis is based that are set out in greater detail elsewhere in the report.

Potential Limitations to the Person's Ability to Adequately Present Their Case

Refugee status hearings are extremely stressful for claimants because the outcome will determine whether they will obtain secure, permanent status and the chance to build a new life in a safe country, or be forcibly sent back to a country where they may face grave danger. To establish that their claim is well founded, refugee claimants have to describe, sometimes in considerable detail, the traumatic experiences that form the basis of their claim. They may face close, sometimes confrontational, questioning, and their credibility may be challenged. Many claimants are particularly psychologically vulnerable because of the multiple hardships they have endured.

If the claimant may be unable to adequately present her case before the IRB because of cognitive, psychological, or emotional difficulties, this should be explained in the report. However, although the consultant may recommend that the Board be particularly sensitive when questioning the claimant about certain topics, the claimant generally will have no choice but to testify about the traumatic events on which her claim is based in order to prove that it is well founded.

The IRB has adopted the Guideline on Procedures with Respect to Vulnerable Persons Appearing Before the Immigration and Refugee Board of Canada (Guideline 8) to encourage decision-makers to make procedural accommodations if required to ensure that vulnerable refugee claimants are not disadvantaged in the presentation of their case (Cleveland, 2008; Immigration and Refugee Board of Canada, 2006). The focus is more on ensuring fairness than on minimizing distress, although decision-makers are also encouraged to "prevent vulnerable persons from becoming traumatized or re-traumatized" by IRB proceedings. Procedural accommodations include expediting or postponing a hearing, allowing the presence of a support person, keeping questions about certain particularly painful areas to a minimum, and so on.

Some claimants may have cognitive or psychological problems that impair their ability to understand the nature of the proceedings, such as an intellectual handicap, dementia, traumatic brain injury, or certain psychotic conditions. In such cases, the Board will appoint a designated representative who will find a lawyer and provide support to the claimant during the proceedings. Designated representatives are also automatically appointed to assist unaccompanied minors.

Other claimants may have difficulty telling their story coherently and convincingly due to psychological difficulties, sometimes compounded by sociocultural factors such as illiteracy, language difficulties, or traditional gender roles (Cleveland, 2008; Herlihy et al., 2002; Prabhu & Baranoski, 2012; Rousseau et al., 2002; Steel, Frommer, et al., 2004). The consequences can be extremely grave; if the Board member does not believe the claimant's story, the claim will be rejected. Board members often rely on narrative characteristics such as coherence, consistency, and emotional congruence to assess credibility, yet these same characteristics may be detrimentally affected by psychological or emotional problems. Therefore, if there are serious reasons to believe that a claimant may have difficulty presenting her case, it is important to mention this in the report and to explain the basis for these difficulties. Board members are generally aware that psychological problems may negatively impact claimants' ability to testify. The issue is to establish why this particular person is especially likely to have difficulties. This should be based on observations during the consultation (e.g., confusion, incoherence, numbing, intense emotions, dissociation), the clinical history, and psychological state. Behavior that the consultant has personally observed may be very persuasive; for example, claimants who are distressed to the point of incoherence when describing certain events systematically avoid certain topics, or display frequent or severe attention or concentration problems. However, the consultant should avoid making specific statements about how the patient will behave at the IRB hearing because it is difficult to predict how claimants will respond in this high-stress context. Some claimants may be very emotional, others may freeze, while still others may marshal all their inner resources and be very functional.

Board members' assessment of a claimant's credibility is likely to be influenced by the degree of congruence between the emotions expressed by the claimant and the content of her narrative. If the claimant displays flat affect, numbing, or excessive detachment, therefore, it is particularly important to explain that this may be a largely involuntary coping mechanism to ward off unbearable emotional pain. Lack of apparent emotion due to avoidance, dissociation, depression, or rigid self-control may easily be mistaken for untruthfulness.

Recommendations

If the claimant's ability to understand the IRB proceedings is impaired, recommend that a designated representative be appointed. If the claimant may have serious difficulty telling her story at the hearing, the consultant can recommend procedural accommodations such as expediting or postponing the hearing, minimizing questions about certain traumatic events, and so on. It is preferable to check with the claimant's lawyer before finalizing such recommendations to make certain that they are feasible and likely to be helpful.

To illustrate writing an effective report, Box 12.1 presents examples of incorrect and correct styles.

Box 12.1: Examples of Refugee Claimant Report Writing

Example A: INCORRECT
X was raped on September 3, 2010 in her home in YZ. The rape was perpetrated by M21 paramilitaries who were targeting her husband for his political opposition to the ruling regime. Five men, armed with rifles, broke into her house around 1:30 AM, while she and her husband were asleep. One man guarded the door, while two men dragged her husband to another room, tied him up, and hit him with the butt of a gun. The other two men forced X to undress and then one of them raped her.

X presents with primarily flat affect, although she briefly displays aversive negative arousal. She is currently suffering from insomnia, nightmares, anxiety, and feelings of hopelessness caused by her rape.

Example B: CORRECT
X initially appears tense and somewhat withdrawn. She reports having been raped in 2010 when several men broke into her home at night, apparently targeting her husband for his political opposition to the ruling regime. She first recounts the incident in a detached tone with little visible emotion. However, when she describes being rejected by her husband following the rape, she breaks down and weeps uncontrollably. She says "I have told my story so many times, I am tired of crying. I don't want to cry any more," but remains tearful for much of the rest of the interview.

(continued)

Box 12.1 (continued)

X reports that she sleeps very poorly. She often imagines men breaking into her room and becomes terrified, and cannot sleep at all without having a light on. She also reports frequent nightmares with themes of intrusion (e.g., men breaking down her door) and helplessness (e.g., being unable to flee). X says that at times when she is walking on the street and notices a man walking behind her, she panics and speeds up, fearing attack. She is particularly afraid of men who show signs of drunkenness because this reminds her of her rapist. According to X, all these symptoms (sleep problems, nightmares, fear of men) started after the rape. When asked how she sees her future, she replies in a despairing tone "The future is dark, it is like the past." Yet, she also expresses hope that she will find safety, saying that she has come to Canada because women are protected here.

There are several problems with Example A. There is far too much factual detail about the alleged rape, increasing the risk of inconsistencies between the report and the claimant's testimony at the hearing, which could seriously harm her credibility. Claimants may easily misremember details such as the date, time, sequence of events, precise identity, and even the number of attackers, either when recounting the story to you or to the Board. On the other hand, there is too little detail about clinical observations—the emotions, signs, and reported symptoms that are within the clinician's field of expertise and contribute to making this woman's story come alive. The clinical part of the report is generic and contains jargon terms such as "flat affect" and "aversive arousal" that may be meaningless to the Board member. Events are described as if the clinician could attest that they actually occurred, and the alleged rape is presented as the cause of the woman's symptoms. Example B avoids these errors, presenting a much more individualized picture that weaves together the claimant's symptoms, emotional presentation, and the core traumatic event.

Conclusion

Cultural consultation for refugees is challenging because clinicians must often go beyond their usual clinical role and take a position of advocacy that actively acknowledges and engages with the predicament of forced migration. Caring for refugees and their families involves medical and mental health interventions to mitigate the consequences of past violence and loss as well as current adversities. At the same time, consultants need to take on the role of advocate to contribute to illness prevention and mental health promotion by addressing the social determinants of health which include precarious migratory status, harsh practices of detention, prolonged uncertainty about the future, and obstacles to family reunification. Many of these issues are important for the long-term well-being and social integration of all refugees, including those who are not symptomatic or who do not request services.

Recent years have seen increasing ambivalence in most high-income countries toward refugees and refugee claimants, with considerable erosion of the international commitment to providing safe haven for the most vulnerable human beings. Clinicians who try to address these issues may be criticized by some individuals or institutions as taking an ideological position. Guidelines for medical training in Canada recognize that clinicians must be able to play the role of advocate both to provide care and work toward prevent and health promotion (Kirmayer, Fung, et al., 2012). In refugee health, there is simply no way to avoid the complex issues at the intersection of human rights, ethics, and politics.

In caring for refugee claimants, clinicians typically focus on helping the person to heal from past traumatic experiences and deal with the challenges of resettlement and adaptation to the host society. Helping to change the external circumstances that negatively impact the client has not traditionally been seen as an integral part of the mental health practitioner's role. Yet, the ongoing threat of possible deportation and a variety of other real-life stressors play a major role in maintaining and exacerbating psychological problems among refugee claimants and other migrants without secure status. Providing a report or letter concerning their mental or physical health in the context of the refugee claim process is only one of the ways in which clinicians can play a key role in improving the health of people who are seeking refugee status. In order to prevent further harm, health professionals also need to join forces in order to advocate for protection of refugees and their access to the same rights and services as Canadian citizens.

References

Arya, N., McMurray, J., & Rashid, M. (2012). Enter at your own risk: Government changes to comprehensive care for newly arrived Canadian refugees. *Canadian Medical Association Journal, 184*(17), 1875–1876.

Australian Department of Immigration and Citizenship. (2011). *Immigration detention statistics summary, November 2011*. Retrieved from www.immi.gov.au/managing-australias-borders/detention/_pdf/immigration-detention-statistics-20111130.pdf

Barudy, J. (1989). A programme of mental health for political refugees: Dealing with the invisible pain of political exile. *Social Science & Medicine, 28*(7), 715–727.

Beiser, M. (1999). *Strangers at the gate: The 'boat people's' first ten years in Canada*. Toronto, Ontario, Canada: University of Toronto Press.

Beiser, M. (2009). Resettling refugees and safeguarding their mental health: Lessons learned from the Canadian Refugee Resettlement Project. *Transcultural Psychiatry, 46*(4), 539–583.

Bolton, P., Bass, J., Betancourt, T. S., Speelman, L., Onyango, G., Clougher, K. F., et al. (2007). Interventions for depression symptoms among adolescent survivors of war and displacement in northern Uganda: A randomized controlled trial. *Journal of the American Medical Association, 298*(5), 519–527.

Burnett, A., & Peel, M. (2001). Asylum seekers and refugees in Britain: The health of survivors of torture and organised violence. *British Medical Journal, 322*, 606–609.

Chaudry, A., Capps, R., Pedroza, J. M., Castañeda, R. M., Santos, R., & Scott, M. M. (2010). *Facing our future. Children in the aftermath of immigration enforcement*. Washington, DC: The Urban Institute.

Cleveland, J. (2008). The guideline on procedures with respect to vulnerable persons appearing before the Immigration and Refugee Board of Canada: A critical overview. *Refuge, 25*(2), 119–131.

Cleveland, J., Dionne-Boivin, V., & Rousseau, C. (2013). Droit d'asile et incarcération: l'expérience des demandeurs d'asile détenus au Canada. *Criminologie*.

Cleveland, J., & Rousseau, C. (in press). Psychiatric symptoms associated with brief detention of adult asylum seekers in Canada. *Canadian Journal of Psychiatry*.

Crépeau, F., Nakache, D., & Atak, I. (2007). International migration: Security concerns and human rights standards. *Transcultural Psychiatry, 44*(3), 311–337.

Edwards, A. (2011). *Back to basics: The right to liberty and security of person and 'alternatives to detention' of refugees, asylum-seekers, stateless persons and other migrants*. Geneva, Switzerland: Office of the United Nations High Commissioner for Refugees.

Ehntholt, K. A., & Yule, W. (2006). Practitioner review: Assessment and treatment of refugee children and adolescents who have experienced war-related trauma. *Journal of Child Psychology and Psychiatry, 47*(12), 1197–1210.

Fazel, M., Reed, R. V., Panter-Brick, C., & Stein, A. (2012). Mental health of displaced and refugee children resettled in high-income countries: Risk and protective factors. *The Lancet, 379*, 266–282.

Fazel, M., Wheeler, J., & Danesh, J. (2005). Prevalence of serious mental disorder in 7000 refugees resettled in western countries: A systematic review. *The Lancet, 365*, 1309–1314.

Fox, P. G., Cowell, J. M., & Johnson, M. M. (1995). Effects of family disruption on Southeast Asian refugee women. *International Nursing Review, 42*(1), 27–30.

Geltman, P. L., Grant-Knight, W., Mehta, S. D., Lloyd-Travaglini, C., Lustig, S., Landgraf, M. A., et al. (2005). The "lost boys of Sudan": Functional and behavioral health of unaccompanied refugee minors resettled in the United States. *Archives of Pediatrics & Adolescent Medicine, 159*(6), 585–591.

Gorst-Unworth, C., & Goldenberg, E. (1998). Psychological sequelae of torture and organised violence suffered by refugees from Iraq: Trauma-related factors compared with social factors in exile. *British Medical Journal, 172*, 90–94.

Hathaway, J. C. (2005). *The rights of refugees under international law*. Cambridge, England: Cambridge University Press.

Herlihy, J., Scragg, P., & Turner, S. (2002). Discrepancies in autobiographical memories—Implications for the assessment of asylum seekers: Repeated interviews study. *British Medical Journal, 324*, 324–327.

Hinton, D. E., Chhean, D., Pich, V., Safren, S. A., Hofmann, S. G., & Pollack, M. H. (2005). A randomized controlled trial of cognitive-behavior therapy for Cambodian refugees with treatment-resistant PTSD and panic attacks: A cross-over design. *Journal of Traumatic Stress, 18*(6), 617–629.

Hinton, D. E., Hoffmann, S. G., Pollack, M. H., & Otto, M. W. (2009). Mechanisms of efficacy of CBT for Cambodian refugees with PTSD: Improvement in emotion regulation and orthostatic blood pressure response. *CNS Neuroscience and Therapeutics, 15*(3), 255–263.

Holtan, A., Rønning, J. A., Handegård, B. H., & Sourander, A. (2005). A comparison of mental health problems in kinship and nonkinship foster care.

European Child & Adolescent Psychiatry, 14(4), 200–207.

Hyndman, J., & Mountz, A. (2008). Another brick in the wall? Neo-refoulement and the externalization of asylum by Australia and Europe. *Government and Opposition, 43*, 249–269.

Ichikawa, M., Nakahara, S., & Wakai, S. (2006). Effect of post-migration detention on mental health among Afghan asylum seekers in Japan. *The Australian and New Zealand Journal of Psychiatry, 40*(4), 341–346.

Immigration and Refugee Protection Act, S.C. 2001, c.27.

Immigration and Refugee Board of Canada. (2006). *Guideline 8: Guideline on procedures with respect to vulnerable persons appearing before the Immigration and Refugee Board of Canada.* Retrieved from http://www.irb-cisr.gc.ca/Eng/brdcom/references/pol/guidir/Documents/GuideDir8_e.pdf

Keller, A. S., Rosenfeld, B., Trinh-Shevrin, C., Meserve, C., Sachs, E., Leviss, J. A., et al. (2003). Mental health of detained asylum seekers. *The Lancet, 362*, 1721–1723.

Kidron, C. A. (2012). Alterity and the particular limits of universalism: Comparing Jewish-Israeli and Canadian-Cambodian genocide legacies. *Current Anthropology, 53*(6), 723–754.

Kinzie, J. D. (2007). PTSD among traumatized refugees. In L. J. Kirmayer, R. Lemelson, & M. Barad (Eds.), *Understanding trauma: Biological, psychological and cultural perspectives* (pp. 194–206). New York, NY: Cambridge University Press.

Kirmayer, L. J. (2001). Failures of imagination: The refugee's narrative in psychiatry. *Anthropology & Medicine, 10*(2), 167–185.

Kirmayer, L. J., Fung, K., Rousseau, C., Lo, H. T., Menzies, P., Guzder, J., et al. (2012). Guidelines for training in cultural psychiatry. *Canadian Journal of Psychiatry, 57*(3), Insert 1–16.

Kirmayer, L., Narasiah, L., Muñoz, M., Rashid, M., Ryder, A., Guzder, J., et al. (2011). Common mental health problems in immigrants and refugees: General approach to the patient in primary care. *Canadian Medical Association Journal, 183*(12), E959–E967.

Kronick, R., Rousseau, C., & Cleveland, J. (2011). Mandatory detention of refugee children in Canada: A public health issue? *Paediatrics & Child Health, 16*(8), e65–e67.

Laban, C. J., Gernaat, H. B. P. E., Komproe, I. H., Schreuders, B. A., & De Jong, J. T. V. M. (2004). Impact of a long asylum procedure on the prevalence of psychiatric disorders in Iraqi asylum seekers in the Netherlands. *The Journal of Nervous and Mental Disease, 192*(12), 843–851.

Laban, C. J., Gernaat, H. B. P. E., Komproe, I. H., van der Tweel, I., & De Jong, J. T. V. M. (2005). Postmigration living problems and common psychiatric disorders in Iraqi asylum seekers in the Netherlands. *Journal of Nervous and Mental Disorders, 193*(12), 825–832.

Lie, B. (2002). A 3-year follow-up study of psychosocial functioning and general symptoms in settled refugees. *Acta Psychiatrica Scandinavica, 106*, 415–425.

Lorek, A., Ehntholt, K., Nesbitt, A., Wey, E., Githinji, C., Rossor, E., et al. (2009). The mental and physical health difficulties of children held within a British immigration detention center: A pilot study. *Child Abuse & Neglect, 33*(9), 573–585.

Lustig, S. L., Kia-Keating, M., Knight Grant, W., Geltman, P., Ellis, H., Kinzie, D. J., et al. (2004). Review of child and adolescent refugee mental health. *Journal of the American Academy of Child and Adolescent Psychiatry, 43*(1), 24–36.

Macklin, A. (1998). Truth and consequences: Credibility determination in the refugee context. In *Proceedings of the 1998 annual meeting of the International Association of Refugee Law Judges "Realities of Refugee Determination on the Eve of a New Millennium"*. Haarlem, The Netherlands: International Association of Refugee Law Judges.

Mares, S., Newman, L., Dudley, M., & Gale, F. (2002). Seeking refuge, losing hope: Parents and children in immigration detention. *Australasian Psychiatry, 10*(2), 91–96.

Marshall, G. N., Schell, T. L., Elliott, M. N., Berthold, S. M., & Chun, C. A. (2005). Mental health of Cambodian refugees 2 decades after resettlement in the United States. *Journal of the American Medical Association, 294*, 571–579.

McKeary, M., & Newbold, B. (2010). Barriers to care: The challenges for Canadian refugees and their health care providers. *Journal of Refugee Studies, 23*(4), 523–545.

Momartin, S., Steel, Z., Coello, M., Aroche, J., Silove, D. M., & Brooks, R. (2006). A comparison of the mental health of refugees with temporary versus permanent protection visas. *Medical Journal of Australia, 185*(7), 357–361.

Moreau, S., Rousseau, C., Meikki-Berrada, A., TCMR, & ERASME. (1999). Politiques d'immigration et santé mentale des réfugiés: Profil et impact des separations familiales. *Nouvelles Pratiques Sociales, 11*(2), 177–196.

Moreno, A., & Grodin, M. A. (2002). Torture and its neurological sequelae. *Spinal Cord, 40*, 213–223.

Nakache, D. (2011). *The human and financial cost of detention of asylum-seekers in Canada.* Available from Refworld, United Nations High Commissioner for Refugees Web site, http://www.unhcr.org/refworld/docid/4fafc44c2.html

National Collaborating Centre for Mental Health, & Royal College of Psychiatrists' Research Unit. (2005). *Post-traumatic stress disorder. The management of PTSD in adults and children in primary and secondary care* (Vol. National Clinical Practice Guideline Number 26). London, England: Gaskell and the British Psychological Society.

Neuner, F., Onyut, P. L., Ertl, V., Odenwald, M., Schauer, E., & Elbert, T. (2008). Treatment of posttraumatic stress disorder by trained lay counselors in an African refugee settlement: A randomized controlled trial. *Journal of Consulting and Clinical Psychology, 76*(4), 686–694.

New Hampshire State. (2005). *Guidelines for initial medical screening and care of refugees resettled in New Hampshire.* Concord, NH: New Hampshire Department of Health and Human Services Division of Public Health.

Newman, L. K., Dudley, M., & Steel, Z. (2008). Asylum, detention, and mental health in Australia. *Refugee Survey Quarterly, 27*(3), 110–127.

Nickerson, A., Bryant, R. A., Brooks, R., Steel, Z., Silove, D., & Chen, J. (2011). The familial influence of loss and trauma on refugee mental health: A multi-level path analysis. *Journal of Traumatic Stress, 24,* 25–33.

Nickerson, A., Bryant, R. A., Silove, D., & Steel, Z. (2011). A critical review of psychological treatments of posttraumatic stress disorder in refugees. *Clinical Psychology Review, 31,* 399–417.

Nickerson, A., Bryant, R. A., Steel, Z., Brooks, R., & Silove, D. (2010). The impact of fear for family on mental health in a resettled Iraqi refugee community. *Journal of Psychiatric Research, 44*(4), 229–235.

Nickerson, A., Steel, Z., Bryant, R., Brooks, R., & Silove, D. (2011). Change in visa status amongst Mandaean refugees: Relationship to psychological symptoms and living difficulties. *Psychiatry Research, 187*(1–2), 267–274.

Paciocco, D., & Stuesser, L. (2008). *The law of evidence. Essentials of Canadian law* (6th ed.). Toronto, Ontario, Canada: Irwin Law.

Peltzer, K. ((1997). Counselling and rehabilitation of victims of human rights violations in Africa. *Psychopathologie Africaine, XXVIII*(1), 55–87.

Phillips, J. (2011). *Asylum seekers and refugees: What are the facts?* Available from the Parliamentary Library of the Parliament of Australia Web site, http://www.aph.gov.au/binaries/library/pubs/bn/sp/asylumfacts.pdf

Porter, M., & Haslam, N. (2005). Predisplacement and postdisplacement factors associated with mental health of refugees and internally displaced persons: A meta-analysis. *Journal of the American Medical Association, 294*(5), 602–612.

Pottie, K., Ng, E., Spitzer, D., Mohammed, A., & Glazier, R. (2008). Language proficiency, gender and self-reported health: An analysis of the first two waves of the longitudinal survey of immigrants to Canada. *Canadian Journal of Public Health, 99*(6), 505–510.

Prabhu, M., & Baranoski, M. (2012). Forensic mental health professionals in the immigration process. *Psychiatric Clinics of North America, 35,* 929–946.

Protecting Canada's Immigration System Act, S.C. 2012, c.17.

Pynoos, R. S., Steinberg, A. M., Layne, C. M., Briggs, E. C., Ostrowski, S. A., & Fairbank, J. A. (2009). DSM V PTSD diagnostic criteria for children and adolescents: A developmental perspective and recommendations. *Journal of Traumatic Stress, 22*(5), 391–398.

R. v. Lavallee (1990) 1 S.C.R. 852.

Re X (2007) CanLII 49705 (IRB).

Re X (2008) CanLII 45239 (IRB).

Robjant, K., Hassan, R., & Katona, C. (2009). Mental health implications of detaining asylum seekers: Systematic review. *The British Journal of Psychiatry, 94*(4), 306–312.

Robjant, K., Robbins, I., & Senior, V. (2009). Psychological distress amongst immigration detainees: A cross-sectional questionnaire study. *British Journal of Clinical Psychology, 48*(3), 275–286.

Rousseau, C., Crépeau, F., Foxen, P., & Houle, F. (2002). The complexity of determining refugeehood: A multidisciplinary analysis of the decision-making process of the Canadian Immigration and Refugee Board. *Journal of Refugee Studies, 15*(1), 43–70.

Rousseau, C., de la Aldea, E., Viger Rojas, M., & Foxen, P. (2005). After the NGO's departure: Changing memory strategies of young Mayan refugees who returned to Guatemala as a community. *Anthropology & Medicine, 12*(1), 3–21.

Rousseau, C., & Drapeau, A. (2003). Are refugee children an at-risk group?: A longitudinal study of Cambodian adolescents. *Journal of Refugee Studies, 16*(1), 67–81.

Rousseau, C., & Guzder, J. (2008). School-based prevention programs for refugee children. *Child and Adolescent Psychiatric Clinics of North America, 17,* 533–549.

Rousseau, C., Hassan, G., Moreau, N., & Thombs, B. D. (2011). Perceived discrimination and its association with psychological distress among newly arrived immigrants before and after September 11, 2001. *American Journal of Public Health, 101*(5), 909–915.

Rousseau, C., & Measham, T. (2007). Posttraumatic suffering as a source of transformation: A clinical perspective. In L. J. Kirmayer, R. Lemelson, & M. Barad (Eds.), *Understanding trauma: Integrating biological, clinical and cultural perspectives* (pp. 275–293). Boston, MA: Cambridge University Press.

Rousseau, C., Measham, T., & Nadeau, L. (2012). Addressing trauma in collaborative mental health care for refugee children. *Clinical Child Psychology and Psychiatry, 18*(1), 121–136.

Rousseau, C., Mekki-Berrada, A., & Moreau, S. (2001). Trauma and extended separation from family among Latin American and African refugees in Montreal. *Psychiatry: Interpersonal and Biological Processes, 64*(1), 40–59.

Rousseau, C., Rufagari, M. C., Bagilishya, D., & Measham, T. (2004). Remaking family life: Strategies for re-establishing continuity among Congolese refugees during the family reunification process. *Social Science & Medicine, 59*(5), 1095–1108.

Rousseau, C., Said, T. M., Gagne, M. J., & Bibeau, G. (1998). Between myth and madness: The premigration dream of leaving among young Somali refugees. *Culture, Medicine and Psychiatry, 22,* 385–411.

Ryan, D. A., Benson, C. A., & Dooley, B. A. (2008). Psychological distress and the asylum process: A longitudinal study of forced migrants in Ireland. *The Journal of Nervous and Mental Disease, 196*(1), 37–45.

Ryan, D. A., Kelly, F. E., & Kelly, B. D. (2009). Mental health among persons awaiting an asylum outcome in western countries. A literature review. *International Journal of Mental Health, 38*(3), 88–111.

Schweitzer, R., Melville, F., Steel, Z., & Lacharez, P. (2006). Trauma, post-migration living difficulties and social support as predictors of psychosocial adjustment in resettled Sudanese refugees. *The Australian and New Zealand Journal of Psychiatry, 40*, 170–187.

Semprun, J. (1994). *L'écriture ou la vie*. Paris, France: Gallimard.

Silove, D. (1999). The psychosocial effects of torture, mass human rights violations, and refugee trauma: Toward an integrated conceptual framework. *The Journal of Nervous and Mental Disease, 187*(4), 200–207.

Silove, D., Austin, P., & Steel, Z. (2007). No refuge from terror: The impact of detention on the mental health of trauma-affected refugees seeking asylum in Australia. *Transcultural Psychiatry, 44*(3), 359–393.

Silove, D., Sinnerbrink, I., Field, A., Manicavasagar, V., & Steel, Z. (1997). Anxiety, depression and PTSD in asylum-seekers: Associations with pre-migration trauma and post-migration stressors. *The British Journal of Psychiatry, 170*(4), 351–357.

Sjölund, B. H. (Ed.). (2007). *RCT field manual on rehabilitation*. Copenhagen, Denmark: Rehabilitation and Research Centre for Torture Victims.

Steel, Z., Chey, T., Silove, D., Marnane, C., Bryant, R. A., & van Ommeren, M. (2009). Association of torture and other potentially traumatic events with mental health outcomes among populations exposed to mass conflict and displacement: A systematic review and meta-analysis. *Journal of the American Medical Association, 302*(5), 537–549.

Steel, Z., Frommer, N., & Silove, D. (2004). Part I—The mental health impacts of migration: The law and its effects: Failing to understand: Refugee determination and the traumatized applicant. *International Journal of Law and Psychiatry, 27*(6), 511–528.

Steel, Z., Momartin, S., Bateman, C., Hafshejani, A., Silove, D., Everson, N., et al. (2004). Psychiatric status of asylum seeker families held for a protracted period in a remote detention centre in Australia. *Australian and New Zealand Journal of Public Health, 28*(6), 527–536.

Steel, Z., Momartin, S., Silove, D., Coello, M., Aroche, J., & Tay, K. W. (2011). Two year psychosocial and mental health outcomes for refugees subjected to restrictive or supportive immigration policies. *Social Science & Medicine, 72*(7), 1149–1156.

Steel, Z., Silove, D., Bird, K., McGorry, P., & Mohan, P. (1999). Pathways from war trauma to posttraumatic stress symptoms among Tamil asylum seekers, refugees, and immigrants. *Journal of Traumatic Stress, 12*(3), 421–435.

Steel, Z., Silove, D., Brooks, R., Momartin, S., Alzuhairi, B., & Susljik, I. (2006). Impact of immigration detention and temporary protection on the mental health of refugees. *The British Journal of Psychiatry, 188*(1), 58–64.

Steel, Z., Silove, D., Phan, T., & Bauman, A. (2002). Long-term effect of psychological trauma on the mental health of Vietnamese refugees resettled in Australia: A population-based study. *The Lancet, 360*, 1056–1062.

Suarez-Orozco, C., Bang, H. J., & Kim, H. Y. (2011). I felt like my heart was staying behind: Psychological implications of family separations and reunifications for immigrant youth. *Journal of Adolescent Research, 26*(2), 222–257.

Suicide Prevention Australia. (2011). *Submission to the joint select committee on Australia's immigration detention network*. Retrieved from http://www.aph. gov.au/Senate/committee/immigration_detention_ ctte/immigration_detention/submissions.htm

Taylor, K. (2009). Asylum seekers, refugees, and the politics of access to health care: A UK perspective. *British Journal of General Practice, 59*, 765–772.

Taylor, D., & Hattenstone, S. (2012, January 6). Child asylum seekers win compensation for 13-month detention. *The guardian*. Retrieved from http://www. guardian.co.uk/uk/2012/jan/06/child-asylum-seekers-win-compensation

The Refugee Forum. (2012). *By the numbers: Refugee statistics 1989–2011*. Available from Human Rights Research and Education Centre of the University of Ottawa Web site, http://www.cdp-hrc.uottawa.ca/projects/refugee-forum/projects/documents/ REFUGEESTATSCOMPREHENSIVE1999-2011.pdf

Tseng, W.-S., Cheng, T.-A., Chen, Y.-S., Hwang, P.-L., & Hsu, J. (1993). Psychiatric complications of family reunion after four decades of separation. *The American Journal of Psychiatry, 150*, 614–619.

Turner, S. W., Bowie, C., Dunn, G., Shapo, L., & Yule, W. (2003). Mental health of Kosovan Albanian refugees in the UK. *The British Journal of Psychiatry, 182*, 444–448.

United Nations High Commissioner for Refugees. (2010). *Convention and protocol relating to the status of refugees*. Retrieved from http://www.unhcr.org/protect/ PROTECTION/3b66c2aa10.pdf

United Nations High Commissioner for Refugees. (2013). *UNHCR global appeal 2013 update—Populations of concern to UNHCR*. Retrieved from http://www. unhcr.org/50a9f81b27.html

Vaage, A. B., Thomsen, P. H., Silove, D., Wentzel-Larsen, T., Van Ta, T., & Hauff, E. (2010). Long-term mental health of Vietnamese refugees in the aftermath of trauma. *The British Journal of Psychiatry, 196*, 122–125.

Van Ommeren, M., de Jong, J. J. T., Sarma, B., Komproe, I., Thapa, S. B., & Cardena, E. (2001). Psychiatric disorders among tortured Bhutanese refugees in Nepal. *Archives of General Psychiatry, 58*(5), 475–482.

Weinstein, H., Dansky, L., & Iacopino, V. (1996). Torture and war trauma survivors in primary care practice. *The Western Journal of Medicine, 165*(3), 112–118.

Williams, A. (1990). Families in refugee camps. *Human Organization, 42*(2), 100–109.

Cultural Consultation to Child Protection Services and Legal Settings

Myrna Lashley, Ghayda Hassan, and Begum Maitra

Immigrant or refugee families often leave their country of origin looking for a better future for themselves and especially for their children (Vatz-Laaroussi & Bessong, 2008). Although most immigrant families eventually integrate well into the mainstream society, they face many challenges in meeting their needs. These challenges can include systemic barriers to integrating into the labor market, loss of occupational status and poverty, difficulties securing adequate housing and coping with discrimination in the community, as well as unequal access to health care and social services (Barn, 2006; Dufour, Hassan, & Lavergne, 2012; Mitchell, 2005).

An additional challenge for migrant families stems from the necessity for parents to renegotiate their roles and adapt their child-rearing practices to the social norms, values and expectations of the dominant culture and its institutions. This task is particularly stressful for many immigrant parents, who may not be fully aware of these norms or associated laws and may struggle with host society values and the modes of their transmission to children that significantly differ from those of their culture of origin (Saulnier, 2004). The social conditions of migration and resettlement may influence parenting in many ways, including the renegotiation of cultural, ethnic or religious identity; family separation and reunification issues; changes in gender roles; parent–child authority issues and the loss of support networks of extended family and community (Battaglini et al., 2002; Dufour et al., 2012; Vatz-Laaroussi & Bessong, 2008).

Services that are designed by, and for, the host society majority group may not be adequate or appropriate for ethnic minority or immigrant families because these services do not take into account specific cultural, migratory and resettlement issues (Alegria, Atkins, Farmer, Slaton, & Stelk, 2010). There is increased awareness of the importance of such issues in understanding the mental health problems of children and families and in planning appropriate interventions. These issues are relevant to cultural consultants who may be asked to provide advice to a variety of social service and institutional settings, including youth protection and family services, law enforcement agencies and the judicial system, as well as non-governmental organizations (NGOs).

M. Lashley, Ph.D. (✉)
Culture & Mental Health Research Unit,
Institute of Community & Family Psychiatry,
Jewish General Hospital, 4333 Cote Ste Catherine Road,
Montreal, QC, Canada H3T 1E4
e-mail: myrna.lashley2@mcgill.ca

G. Hassan, Ph.D.
Département de psychologie, Université du Québec
à Montréal (UQAM), C.P. 8888, Succursale
Centre-Ville, Montréal, QC, Canada H3C 3P8
e-mail: hassan.ghayda@uqam.ca

B. Maitra, M.R.C.Psych., M.D.
Honorary Consultant Child and Adolescent
Psychiatrist at the Tavistock and Portman NHS
Foundation Trust, 38 Nant Road, London NW2 2AT, UK
e-mail: begummaitra@hotmail.com

L.J. Kirmayer et al. (eds.), *Cultural Consultation: Encountering the Other in Mental Health Care*,
International and Cultural Psychology, DOI 10.1007/978-1-4614-7615-3_13,
© Springer Science+Business Media New York 2014

In this chapter, we will focus primarily on consultation with youth protection and family services, law enforcement agencies and the judicial system. Despite frequent involvement with migrants, these services and systems remain insufficiently adapted to the diverse social and cultural contexts of the families they serve (Dufour et al., 2012; Hines, Lemon, Wyatt, & Merdinger, 2004; Stoltzfus, 2005). We begin with a description of how the context of migration may fuel family conflicts around identity and belonging. This is followed by discussion of a key area of intercultural conflict for migrant families, the role of physical discipline in child-rearing. We then explore how some migratory trajectories may be associated with specific challenges for family relations. We examine, in particular, some of the mental health issues related to family separation and reunification which may lead to involvement with youth protection or legal institutions. Next, we consider issues of domestic violence or intimate partner violence, which are highly challenging for clinicians as well as the legal system. In all of these sections, we make use of composite case to highlight key issues, while protecting confidentiality. Finally, we discuss approaches to improve the cultural competence and safety of organizations and institutions through consultation and training.

Migration and Family Conflicts

Migration and settlement in a new society often leads to changes in the roles of parents and children, which may destabilize the family system. Transmission of cultural identity is one of the most significant challenges which immigrant parents and children face in their new homeland. Immigrant children are exposed on a daily basis to role models from the host society, including media personalities, teachers and parents of children from the host society as well as other minority or migrant cultures, which may present cultural values that differ from, or even contradict, those of their culture of origin (Hassan, Rousseau, Measham, & Lashley, 2008). Some of these role models or competing values may prove to be more appealing to youth than the norms and

values of their own parents (Phalet & Schonpflug, 2001a, 2001b; Phinney, Ong, & Maden, 2000). Second-generation adolescents, who are born in the host society, may experience different challenges in identity negotiation compared to immigrant youth who arrive with their parents (Hassan et al., 2008; Phinney et al., 2000).

The basic discrepancies in outlook and expectations between immigrant parents and their children have been termed the "paradox of the migration condition" (Hassan & Rousseau, 2009a; Phalet & Schonpflug, 2001a). The paradox stems from the fact that in a new social environment, the transmission of parents' cultural values may be viewed as both more important and more difficult due to their children's immersion in competing cultural systems from a very early age and the weaker influence of their own ethnocultural group (Hassan et al., 2008). Parents and adolescents of many immigrant families are able to meet halfway to negotiate or resolve this paradox. However, in situations where parental identities are especially vulnerable—due to colonial histories, exposure to trauma or difficult resettlement conditions, including discrimination, poverty, unemployment and social isolation or exclusion—the paradox may lead to increased family conflict and stricter forms of child control or child discipline (Hassan & Rousseau, 2009a, 2009b). Further, from the perspective of children, parents may become less attractive models of identification when they are devalued by the host society through personal or institutional acts of discrimination or exclusion. Many immigrant parents, particularly fathers from targeted groups (e.g., Blacks, Arabs), experience significant difficulty in accessing employment and find themselves working in poor conditions, with low-status jobs that do not correspond to their competencies and educational levels. To support the family, many immigrant mothers enter the labor market, but they too must struggle with discrimination, low wages and lack of recognition of their educational and professional qualifications. Even for the most resilient individuals, these adverse conditions may lead to feelings of failure, high levels of stress and a sense of being humiliated in the eyes of their children. Indeed, there is evidence that immigrants who have lower status employment than what they are qualified for based on their educational attainment are at elevated risk for mental health problems (Chen, Smith, & Mustard, 2010).

While the family faces the challenges of adaptation, immigrant children and youth also become aware of how the norms and ideals of parent–child relationships may differ across cultures. They come to understand how authorities beyond the family, including those of school, health care, the legal system and other institutions, define the limits of what is acceptable and what may be thought of as "abuse". This awareness of societal norms and authority has implications for the family's own hierarchy and authority. Youth may use their knowledge of the workings of the host society's institutions to mobilize external authority in ways that undermine the usual family hierarchy. Indeed, the timing of "disclosure" of physical discipline or abuse by children may sometimes suggest a strategic use of external authority (Hassan et al., 2011). In this context, it is important to consider the potential significance of underlying intergenerational conflict when professionals are involved in assessing claims of abuse (Hassan et al., 2011). Failure by professionals to consider the socioeconomic challenges, cultural transmission paradox and intergenerational conflicts faced by migrant families, as well as the conflicts of loyalty between host and heritage cultures may lead to an escalation of conflict between parents and children or to the disinvestment of parents in their youth's upbringing (Hassan & Rousseau, 2009a). Both of these outcomes can significantly jeopardize the integration of the family and youth into their new society.

Case Vignette 13-1

A consultation was requested by Child Protection Services (CPS)[1] for Farah, a 15-year-old girl from Palestine who had

recently immigrated with her parents and siblings. Farah's family had left their home because of political instability. Her father, who was a surgeon, was unable to pursue his profession because of nonrecognition of the equivalence of his medical training and diploma in Canada. Consequently, Farah's mother had to work to help support the family, and she also managed to find a low-wage job for her husband in the grocery store where she worked.

Farah quickly adapted to her new school and social environment and became increasingly demanding of autonomy and independence within the family. She often accused her parents of being too strict and still living in their home country in their hearts, in comparison to her friends' parents. The family atmosphere became very tense as the family experienced financial, social and psychological strain. On one occasion, Farah's father noticed that she had drunk alcohol, which was forbidden according to the family's religious and cultural values. This provoked a serious confrontation that ended with Farah being hit by her father. When Farah shared this event with her friends at school, they spoke with a school counsellor and the CPS was alerted. Her parents were shocked by the involvement of the CPS and felt both shamed and powerless. They reacted angrily by refusing any cooperation with the CPS professionals and accused Farah of dishonoring the family. Her mother, who stood by her husband, was described by the CPS professionals, as being submissive. They warned the father that they would not tolerate his aggressive and authoritarian manner.

Based on CPS recommendations as well as Farah's request, the court ordered her placement in a foster family for 24 months and gave authority over her activity to the foster family. Farah was allowed to call home once a week, but visits with her family,

---

[1]Workers from child protection services, who are generally social workers or psychoeducators, are legally mandated by the child and family court to offer help and assistance to any child who has been recognized by that court to be a victim of child abuse and/or neglect based on local provincial or state laws.

(continued)

including her siblings, were withheld until the parents cooperated more fully with the agency. Over the ensuing months, Farah's health significantly deteriorated. She became depressed, lost her appetite and had disturbed sleep as well as suicidal thoughts. At this point, CPS requested cultural consultation and psychological assessment.

Farah's case illustrates some of the common issues involved in cultural consultations to CPS. The cultural consultant has several roles and tasks in cases like Farah's. One of the central aims of the cultural consultation was to help bridge the gap between Farah and her parents. To do this, the consultant had to help the CPS workers acknowledge and explore the multiple impacts of social exclusion and powerlessness on family dynamics and the mental health of each of the family members. The cultural consultant assisted the CPS worker in recontextualizing both Farah's demands and her parents' expectations and reactions. Farah's father had experienced drastic changes in his social and economic status. He was no longer the main provider for the family and had to adapt to a radical shift in his role and authority within the family. He also had to participate in household chores during the day, such as preparing lunch for the younger children and helping to clean the house, but had difficulty adapting to these changes, in part because he worked nightshifts and often needed to sleep during the day. During the consultations, Farah's father expressed deep shame at not being able to provide for his family, which affected his self-esteem and contributed to the emergence of depressive symptoms. Their financial difficulties isolated the parents and increased the barriers to their integration into the host society. Both parents expressed feelings of helplessness, powerlessness and failure. Moreover, the parents' situation sharply contrasted with the rapid integration of their children. Farah, as the eldest child, was expected to assist in family chores. Her increasing demands to go out by herself, and for money, irritated her parents, who perceived

these behaviors as a threat to their cultural identity by breaching the important religious and cultural values, which had always guided their lives. The cultural consultation helped to show how, on a symbolic systemic level, the widening gap and conflict between Farah and her parents was similar, in many respects, to the widening gap between her parents in terms of their integration into host society. This, in turn, helped to explain why the family situation had become explosive, leading to episodes of physical abuse.

Although placement decisions by CPS are triggered by the legitimate duty to protect the child from further physical abuse, these decisions may nevertheless have unintended consequences, particularly given the emphasis on values of individualism, autonomy and choice in health and social service institutions. The cultural consultation revealed that Farah's dilemmas were closely related to her family's predicament, and that the CPS professionals' quick agreement with her wishes to leave the family may have reflected their own cultural biases rather than her own best interests or long-term needs. By establishing trust with the parents through openness to the family's concerns for their daughter, the consultant helped the CPS professionals become aware of how their own cultural values and prejudices might have interfered with their professional mandate. For example, CPS workers were outraged by the possibility that Farah's parents' restrictions on her behavior were motivated by culturally and religiously based gender norms congruent with their wish to raise her to be obedient and dependent on her family, rather than independent and assertive. The CPS workers believed that Farah's parents were too strict and her father is too authoritarian. Moreover, they felt that Farah was resisting pressure to be submissive and that, as professionals, they had a responsibility to assist her in her efforts at autonomy. Their apparent agreement with Farah's own view of her needs was problematic at several levels and produced many negative side effects.

The decision to place Farah and, most importantly, to give the authority over her activities to the foster family was a catalyst for her parents' disinvestment in their daughter. Farah's parents, like many immigrant parents in their situation, were too vulnerable to be able to challenge the authority of host society institutions. They saw themselves as harshly judged, helpless and abandoned, not only by the host society and its institutions but also by their own child. Feeling completely powerless, unable to "fight" the institution or make their voices heard, Farah's parents' self-protective reaction was to reject her. Farah had switched her loyalty to the host society, while in the eyes of the CPS, the parents remained committed to an oppressive cultural value system. Giving Farah over to the institutional representatives of the host society was an attempt by the parents to regain some sense of control over their family's future and block what they considered to be Farah's negative influence on her siblings. Their unwillingness to accept the opinion of CPS professionals became entrenched as a strategy of resistance while underlying issues of betrayal, powerlessness and lack of agency were not explored. Unfortunately, this desperate and angry gesture by the parents further reinforced the CPS view of the parents as rigid and rejecting. The cultural consultation recommended mediation services between Farah and her parents, restoring parental authority and reestablishing visits with her siblings in order to reconnect her with her religious, cultural and linguistic heritage.

The Challenges of Family Separation and Reunification

Transnational migration patterns are influenced by economic opportunities and immigration policies (Longhi, 2013). Canada has had immigration policies that encouraged migration for women doing household domestic work. This policy created a situation in which immigrants, such as those from the Caribbean, may choose to leave their children in the care of others when they travel abroad in order to improve the economic status of their family. Similar migration patterns have been documented in several national contexts (Allen, 1988; Brent & Callwood, 1993; Davison, 1962; Gopaul-McNicol, 1993; Jokhan, 2008; Lashley, 2000;

Lashley et al., 2005; Simmons & Plaza, 2007). This migration strategy is facilitated for Afro-Caribbean families because kin other than parents are often involved in the care and upbringing of children. Thus, in a given family, in addition to the child's parents, both maternal and paternal relatives may assume a degree of responsibility for the child's welfare. It is not uncommon to find that a child may live with, and be raised by, one relative while other siblings are raised by the children's parents or grandparents. Very often the relative with whom the child resides may live near the parent so that the child has daily access to his or her parents and siblings.

This separation of child and parent is usually not due to any psychological or legal inability on the part of the parents to care for the child, but may be based on complex factors, including affinity between the child and a relative, an older relative living alone for whom the child provides companionship or even the fact that the school that the child attends is closer to the relative's home than that of the parents (Gmelch, 1992). In the case of lower income families, the choice of living arrangement is most often based on economic factors, in a pattern that Rodman (1971) called "shifting," that is, the necessity to transfer the child to the care of one or more relatives as the family fortunes ebb and flow. The global mobility of the Afro-Caribbean family, therefore, is possible because of its highly plastic, open and extended structure. This structure allows migrating parents to enjoy peace of mind knowing that their children are being well cared for by extended family in familiar surroundings. However, it also means that during this time of separation, parents and children are subject to very different experiences, pressures and patterns of socialization that may lead to them to grow apart and, especially in the case of early separations, becoming strangers to each other. For parents, the child may be frozen in memory at an earlier age. For the child, attachments to the caregivers may match or exceed in intensity any primary attachments that may have formed earlier to their parents.

As a result, the process of reunification can be fraught with distress and attachment difficulties for both parents and children (Adams, 2000;

Arnold, 2006; Sewell-Coker, Hamilton-Collins, & Fein, 1985). Reunification often occurs during adolescence, a time when the child develops increased verbal and physical capacities and more sophisticated understanding of power and negotiation of autonomy/dependence needs as well as a time when relationships with peers in his/her native home are of utmost importance. These transformations may add to the challenges of migration: on the one hand, there is the strong bond that has developed with the principal caregiver and the sense of safety accorded by such a bond while, on the other hand, there is the desire to be with the natural parent and the allure of being in a country that holds the promise of immeasurable wealth and comfort.

Upon arrival in their parents' adoptive country, children may feel suddenly thrown into a world that makes little sense to them. During the separation, not only have parent and child been living separate lives but the child and family in the home country may have a very inaccurate view of the financial state of the migrant parent, especially if, during the period of separation, barrels and boxes of goods and money orders were sent home by the parent to provide for the child and others. The arrival of the child then may coincide with a profound disillusionment and sense of disappointment when the child discovers that not only does the parent not have unlimited wealth (indeed, may even be living in abject poverty) but that the child must now make similar sacrifices to insure others back home continue to receive support. Thus, reunification is often a time of strong feelings of excitement but also of grief for the loss of family in the homeland, school, peers, physical environment and the fantasy of parental wealth.

Teenagers reunited with their parents face a family with an already established routine, and parents rarely have the chance to take much time off in order to assist their children to adapt to this new situation. For their part, parents are often caught with multiple responsibilities and may have unrealistic expectations that the child will accommodate easily to the rules and regulations of a new household—a household that may not only include brothers and sisters they have never

met but often a step-parent whom the child must accept as a parent. Parents may not adequately prepare arriving children for these realties because they may not perceive these circumstances as anything other than "normal" (Arnold, 2006; Smith, Lalonde, & Johnson, 2004).

Case Vignette 13-2

The cultural consultant received a request from juvenile court for the evaluation of two brothers, Selwyn and Dacosta, 16- and 15-year-old Black males who were born in the Caribbean. Selwyn was a little over a year old and Dacosta was an infant when their parents emigrated to Canada leaving them in the care of maternal relatives but with daily access to paternal relatives who lived next door. During their stay in Canada, the parents had three younger children. When Selwyn and Dacosta reached 14 and 13 years of age respectively, their parents brought them to Canada. This reunification after almost 13 years turned out to be very difficult for all concerned.

Selwyn and Dacosta arrived in Canada in midwinter and were unaccustomed to cold weather. The day after their arrival, they were enrolled in a school whose norms they had never before encountered: the absence of school uniforms, students who argued with teachers, unfamiliar food, classes in a language (French) which they did not understand but which they had to learn in order to succeed, and, most importantly, no familiar peers. One week after they started school, both their parents returned to work. Because they would arrive home from school well before their parents, Selwyn and Dacosta were now in charge of their younger siblings until the parents returned in the evening—a situation that they deemed "unfair." They accused their parents of bringing them to the new country in order to have free baby-sitting services. They also accused their parents of favoring the younger siblings, and thus

(continued)

were often angry and argumentative with their parents.

Their parents were baffled and overwhelmed by the adolescents' behavior. They felt that the boys were ungrateful, and that they were being influenced by undesirable peers into quickly adopting the "ways and bad behaviors" of the host culture. They also thought the boys were rude and disobedient and were very concerned that their behavior would have an impact on the younger children and that, as a result, the parents would lose control over the household. Coming to the decision that talking to the boys was of no value, the parents resorted to physical discipline. Selwyn and Dacosta—who had by this time learned about the new "rights" they had in their new country—reported their parents to the school, who in turn signalled the case to social services.

Out of hurt and anger, the parents told Selwyn and Dacosta that they wished they had not brought them to their host country. The boys viewed these statements as proof that they were not wanted, leaving them with little option but to join a dysfunctional peer group or "gang" that seemed to offer unconditional acceptance. To their satisfaction, this new "family" appeared to break all the restrictive codes of their parents, and membership relieved them of the necessity of having to learn how to fit into the wider society. Eventually, both boys found themselves in the juvenile justice system because of crimes they had committed as members of this dysfunctional peer group. At their court hearing, one of the boys stated "I thought I was coming to Heaven, but I was coming to Hell!"

The estrangement and confusion that some youth feel in response to the challenges of migration and reunification make them easy targets for gangs or delinquent groups as they search for a sense of belonging. These groups provide easy identification and insulate the adolescent from an unfamiliar and sometimes harsh and rejecting world. To protect their children from this affiliation, parents may resort to threats and physical punishment, strategies that are common in many parts of the Caribbean, but that carry new meanings and consequences in most Western societies. As a result, such strategies may actually escalate rather than reduce parent–child conflict.

Like other parents in their situation, once social services became involved, the parents felt that Selwyn and Dacosta had brought humiliation and disgrace upon the family, inviting censure by the dominant society, not just of their family but, most importantly, of their whole minority group. The parents felt that the boys' conduct had tarnished the reputations of all members of the Black community. This perception was intensified by their sense that they had to be a "model minority" in order to be accepted and reduce the stereotypes and prejudice that members of the host society held concerning their group. Perceiving themselves as ostracized by both the host and heritage communities, the parents felt completely alone. It was at this point that they "extruded" the boys from the family and community, seeing them as no longer their "problem" but that of the system. They saw this rejection as necessary to "save" the three younger children from following in the footsteps of their older brothers.

As Schaafsma (2011) has observed, without an alternative means of support, such as that provided by a heritage group or community or transnational networks, migrant minorities may be more prone to suffer lasting negative effects from discrimination and prejudice. Selwyn and Dacosta's parents concern to be a "model minority" is a clear reflection of the predicament faced by minorities. Indeed, those who view themselves as powerless may be harshly judgmental towards their own group when they have no expectation of equity or authority in the wider world.

The central aims of consultation in cases like this are to stop the escalation of family conflict and reduce the adolescent's participation in gang-related criminal activities. In order to protect these vulnerable teenagers from further criminalization, in addition to other forms of interventions, cultural consultations may focus on mediation and on assisting members of the family to understand the perceptions of all of the actors. The parents need to be fully aware of the fears of the children as they attempt to confront all the new challenges they face, including inability to communicate in the new language; unfamiliar food and climate; academic institutions based on very different principles; discrimination based on radicalized identity, ethnicity or religion; potential rivalry with new siblings; new authority figures — namely, a parent they have not lived with for some time and often their new conjugal partner; and perceptions of being unloved and used as domestic help with little concern for their feelings. These children are often helped by understanding the adult's considerations about the family group that led to the decision to migrate. Often this separation involved major sacrifices made by parents and leaving older children behind to pursue better lives for the entire group was a decision made from love and hopes for the entire family, and not an act of intentional rejection or abandonment. In a safe therapeutic space, parents can also hear the children's experience of estrangement. The cultural consultant can assist the social worker to work individually and in groups with family members, to identify appropriate community-based resources (for example, youth, church and community groups) that can assist with the integration of youth into the new society. Finally, regular telephone contact can be established with the grandparents or other primary attachment figures in the home country who can positively support these youth in maintaining a sense of continuity and security in their lives. Grandparents, in turn, can join with parents to open up discussions with young people about shared concerns around integration, cultural values and behaviors and peer relations. In addition to better monitoring, the parents can be encouraged to institute rewards (e.g. an allowance) for the youths' positive contributions to the family, for example, by baby-sitting younger siblings. These behavioral interventions can also influence the hierarchical structure of the family and support effective parental authority in constructive ways.

Cultural Variations in Disciplining and Physical Punishment

Migration compels families to renegotiate child-rearing values and practices in relation to the norms and expectations of the host society. This may be difficult for some immigrant parents, not only because these norms and values are unfamiliar or at odds with their own values but also because parental values and practices are largely unconscious and affectively charged schemas that are deeply rooted in culture-specific ideologies of personhood, models of child-rearing, modes of discipline and patterns of family interaction and social relations (Chiasson-Lavoie & Roc, 2000; Hassan et al., 2008; Kim & Hong, 2007; Kleinman, 1980). Cross-cultural comparative studies have shown considerable variation in the acceptability of diverse types of disciplinary behaviors (such as hitting a child with an object) across countries and across cultural groups living in the same country (Aronson-Fontes, 2000, 2002; Buntain-Ricklefs, Kemper, Bell, & Babonis, 1994; Chao, 1994; Corral-Verdugo, Frias-Armenta, Romero, & Munoz, 1995; Elliott, Tong, & Tan, 1997; Frias-Armenta & McCloskey, 1998; Kim & Hong, 2007; McClure, Chien, Chiang, & Donahoo, 1996; McEvoy et al., 2005; Segal, 1995). An ethnic minority or immigrant parent's disciplinary behavior towards his/her child may be judged acceptable or seriously problematic by members of their heritage culture by different criteria than the norms used by professionals or majority group culture institutions (Aronson-Fontes, 2002; Ferrari, 2002; Gopaul-McNicol, 1999; Hassan & Rousseau, 2009b; Welbourne, 2002). In fact, given the heterogeneity within any ethnocultural or professional group, professional norms may not reflect the cultural beliefs of many within the majority culture (Hassan & Rousseau, 2009a; Maitra, 2008; Orhon, Ulukol, Bingoler, & Gulnar, 2006).

Although the Western literature on child maltreatment has established that recourse to physical discipline constitutes a risk factor for cycles of physical abuse (Durrant et al., 2004; Gershoff, 2002; Larrivée, Tourigny, & Bouchard, 2007), there remains a grey zone between legally "acceptable" and "abusive" physical discipline. This is an issue that is particularly important for many immigrant families. Larrivée et al. (2007) have suggested that many ethnic minority families, who consider physical discipline as an acceptable means of child-rearing, find themselves in a situation of *dysnormativity* rather than of *dysfunctionality*. In the case of dysnormativity, professionals may erroneously perceive and convey an image of the family as pathologically dysfunctional or dangerous for the child when there is in fact no family pathology but rather a clash of cultural norms and values (Hassan & Rousseau, 2009a; Mosby, Rawls, Meehan, Mays, & Pettinari, 1999).

The concept of dysnormativity is clinically important because the intensity and nature of punishment or chastisement differ significantly when dysnormative practices shade into frank abuse. These crises may be evidence of dysfunctional parenting and often related to parental mental health problems. This raises another clinical question as to whether inflicting extreme or problematic punishment is, in and of itself, evidence of a parental mental health problem. Abuse occurring in the context of parental mental health problems, therefore, is more likely to require clinical interventions with the parents and may sometimes require alternative care or resources (e.g., foster care placement or psychoeducators visiting at home) until parental mental health improves. However, the most common issues with physical discipline will respond positively to psychosocial or educational interventions that promote the family's management skills, coping with stress and use of disciplinary practices that are more acceptable in the host society. Unnecessary interventions, including placement, that assume dysfunction among dysnormative families may cause more harm than benefit for both the child and family and actually lead to new dysfunctionality in the family system. Labelling families as dysfunctional can be self-perpetuating. Thus, the history of removal of a child or "therapeutic" interventions for parents are sometimes used by professionals to justify further interventions. Although the primary objective may have been to help the child and family, erroneous interpretations of parental behaviors may, therefore, victimize the family and child.

Case Vignette 13-3

Rodrigo is a 12-year-old boy who immigrated at age 8 to Canada from Colombia with his family and two siblings. His parents had converted to a form of fundamentalist Christianity before migrating. The family had been middle class in their country of origin, and they were having difficulty adjusting to their lower economic status in Canada. The parents felt that the family should live their lives in a manner that they could not be viewed by the host society as being ungrateful or "bad" immigrants. In the parents estimation, Rodrigo did not always live up to these dictates. In particular, he was not always truthful with his siblings, parents or teachers. His mother especially was concerned that Rodrigo's lying to his teachers cast the family in a bad light and caused them to "lose face." Rodrigo received several warnings from his parents that his continued lying would result in physical punishment. On one occasion, Rodrigo provided an untruthful response to a question posed by his mother who, at the time was stirring a pot of soup with a long stainless steel spoon which she removed from the pot and used to strike him across the face and hands, leaving first degree burns. When he returned to school the next day, the teacher enquired about the nature of the injuries and, on this occasion, Rodrigo was completely truthful. As the law required, the teacher informed the authorities and the mother was charged with child abuse. The juvenile court asked for a psychological consultation during which the mother explained that the Bible was clear that sparing the rod would spoil the child. The parents also spoke of their shame concerning a child who lied, the shame this brought on the family and their fears that the host society would judge them harshly and this would increase the level of racism and discrimination which the family had already endured.

One of the major roles for the cultural consultant in cases like that of Rodrigo is to help the court contextualize the cultural difficulties faced by the family. While culture cannot be used to justify behavior that clearly harms the child, to some extent notions of harm and benefit are themselves culture-bound (Kirmayer, Rousseau, & Lashley, 2007). Understanding these issues allows the judiciary to mandate interventions that are more likely to be culturally appropriate and beneficial for the family, as well as contributing to a more open, pluralistic society. Thus, assessing the mother's behavior towards Rodrigo in context, the court suspended the placement option, and instead gave the parents a suspended sentence of 2 years and ordered them to undergo psycho-educational counselling. One of the recommendations made to the court by the consultant in Rodrigo's case, was that the therapist needed to be someone who understood the family's cultural background as well as their concerns about the host society. The consultant also recommended that a religious minister be asked to assist the mother to interpret the text of the Bible in a manner that took into account her religious beliefs and helped her to recognize areas in which her understanding may come into conflict with Canadian laws and views of the state's responsibility to children. One year later, Rodrigo's case was closed by CPS and the intervention was deemed successful.

Domestic Violence

In most Western countries, domestic violence is now legally recognized as among the risk factors that cause harm to children. In Canada, for instance, domestic violence is now legally considered as a form of child maltreatment. The arguments that justify the consideration of domestic violence as a form of child maltreatment are many, including its co-occurrence with violence towards the child and its consequences on the child and on parenting capacities (Adams, 2006; Krug, Dahlberg, Mercy, Zwi, & Lozano, 2002 ; Savard & Zaouche Gaudron, 2010). CPS are thus increasingly involved with women victims of domestic violence due to the view that

both parents, the abuser and the victim, may be unable to protect the children from the effects of the couple violence.

When domestic violence is discovered or disclosed, the actions taken by CPS—particularly when the violent spouse is noncooperative—aim to ensure that the nonabusive parent (often the mother) leaves the home, to seek refuge in a separate residence or women's shelter in order to demonstrate her willingness to protect the children from further exposure to the violence. Failure to make this commitment can jeopardize the mother's right to keep custody of her children, who may then be placed in foster care in order protect them from future episodes of violence. While the CPS professionals' mandate is to protect the children, such placement decisions may be perceived by the abused mother as punitive and disqualifying of her parental competencies. Further, the CPS position may demand that the mother accept sole responsibility for protecting her children (something she may never have envisaged) at a time when she is at her most vulnerable and struggling with fears of violence and marital collapse.

If the mother accepts the need to seek alternate accommodation, which could be the home of a relative or friend judged by CPS to be safe for the mother and the children, no professional supervision is required. However, as with many victims of domestic violence, immigrant and ethnic minority women who suffer this type of abuse tend to become isolated from extended family members or friends, making it difficult for the victims to seek support from those who may be willing to offer protection. Consequently, these women may have no other option but to seek protection in a professional shelter.

Although shelters may offer protection as well as clinical and advocacy services, some immigrant women may have difficulty accepting refuge. They may consider refuge as increasing their isolation and risking exclusion from extended family and community networks because this type of refuge may be viewed in a negative light. Women from migrant or minority groups may not express these stigma issues or other cultural concerns to staff in shelters that are not adapted to their needs. Women may choose not to disclose domestic violence for many reasons, including fear of losing custody of their children, efforts to preserve the unity of the nuclear unit as well as ties between the extended families, protecting the reputation of their husband and the challenges of socio-economic survival if the husband is the family's only mainstay for economic survival (Hassan et al., 2011). In all cases, culturally insensitive practices can contribute to the social injustices that sufferers of domestic violence experience and limit their access to much needed professional intervention. Advocacy practices that fail to consider cultural sensibilities, therefore, may contribute to a woman's return to an abusive spouse.

Cultural consultation can help uncover these additional complexities of domestic violence among immigrant women providing the contextual information needed for better understanding of the family's predicament and guiding culturally appropriate interventions.

Case Vignette 13-4

Asuntha was a 24-year-old woman from Sri Lanka who immigrated to Canada at age 18, under the sponsorship of her husband who had immigrated several years earlier. She was a distant relative of her husband who had proposed to marry her on one of his trips to Sri Lanka and then sponsored her to join him in Canada. She was living with her husband and their two daughters (ages 4 and 2) when a CPS alert was issued for psychological and physical abuse of the children. Asuntha did not work outside the home and spoke neither French nor English. With the help of an interpreter, she revealed that she and her daughters were the victims of severe physical abuse by her husband. She had previously attempted to seek help from a relative who lived in the same city, but his recommendation to her had been to "bear it and forgive." After CPS involvement, Asuntha's husband threatened to terminate her sponsorship agreement. This threat, and the complexity of the legal

procedures associated with addressing domestic violence, scared Asuntha who refused to file a criminal complaint against her husband. In order to keep custody of her daughters, she accepted the CPS requirement to leave the marital home (and abuser) and take refuge in a women's shelter. At the shelter, Asuntha expressed significant depressive symptoms and could not care for her daughters as the shelter professionals expected her to. A week later, she returned with her daughters to her abusive husband. Her daughters, who showed symptoms of PTSD, were apprehended by CPS at school, placed in foster care and given psychotherapeutic treatment. Asuntha was given the right to have supervised visits, but she was very inconsistent in attending these visits. Consequently, the court ordered a long-term placement for the daughters with the possibility of adoption by the foster family. Asuntha, who had kept the social worker's address, regularly sent cards and gifts to her daughters, but the worker judged it inappropriate to pass these items along to the girls. Two years later, Asuntha attempted again to renew supervised visits with her daughters but her application was denied. A year later, she obtained a divorce from her husband and subsequently remarried. With the help of her new spouse, she met CPS workers who congratulated her on being able to leave the abusive marriage. The new spouse was assessed by CPS workers on several occasions and considered to be a very good ally for Asuntha. She therefore made a new request to the court to allow supervised visits with her daughters and to acquaint them with their newborn half-brother. However, once again, the court denied her request.

In Asuntha's case, the cultural consultation clarified that she had joined her husband in Canada at a very young age and was under his authority both in terms of her migratory status and her access to socio-economic resources. Although this situation may not be problematic as such, it becomes difficult in cases of marital conflict and violence. In addition, Asuntha was socially isolated and had very little knowledge of the host society given that she did not speak the language. She was, therefore, particularly vulnerable to the abuse of her husband and felt unable to protect her daughters as she had no economic or social resources and nowhere to go. The CPS intervention could have been salutary in her case, had the professionals, institution and court taken into consideration the complexities of her situation and the challenges of her settlement conditions (i.e., isolation, no employment, not speaking the language, total economic dependency on her husband, no citizenship) in designing an intervention plan that could help her better meet her needs and exercise greater autonomy over her destiny, as she wished.

The relative safety of the shelter allowed Asuntha and her daughters to give expression to the traumatic experiences they had been through. Asuntha, however, felt that the major focus was on her inability, in the minds of professionals, to adequately protect her daughters, and this made her feel fearful and hopeless. She could not see her way out, and was afraid that her husband would revoke her sponsorship, and ruin her life by depriving her of her daughters. This prospect instilled so much fear in her that it overrode the risks in her mind of further jeopardy to herself and her daughters. As a result, in a desperate move, she returned to her abusive husband in order to stay close to her daughters and provide them shelter and economic well-being. CPS interpreted this as a lack of understanding and empathy for her daughters' needs, further justifying their conclusion that continued placement in a foster home would be safer for the children. The psychological experts' reports confirmed the children's trauma-related symptoms and their positive attachment to the foster family. These considerations led CPS and the court to consider that it would be in the girls' interests to cut their bonds with both biological parents. Though the court gave Asuntha the right to supervised visits with her children, her husband did not permit these visits. Three years later, when she had managed to remarry and was more secure, the court and CPS professionals refused her renewed request for supervised visits with her daughters. Their reasons for the refusal included the risk of disturbing the positive integration of the girls into their foster family, who were prepared to adopt the girls; the improvement of their psychological symptoms; the loss of the maternal language as they had become unilingual francophone (and mother did not speak French) and the fact that the daughters had no contact with their mother for 3 years.

Asuntha's case illustrates the double victimization of some ethnic minority or immigrant mothers who endure intimate partner violence. The same institutions that are meant to assist and protect women and children from violence, may themselves act in ways that are violent towards victimized mothers when they use a deficiency-focused approach, mistaking cultural boundaries as personal deficits and focusing solely on the mothers' limitations. Keeping in mind the necessity to protect children from domestic violence, cases like Asuntha's reveal the potentially devastating effects when the decisions of professionals and courts are based on oversimplification and decontextualization of the ethnic, religious, cultural and socio-economic contexts of immigrant women and children experiencing domestic violence. Asuntha's case also shows how placement decisions made without sufficient cultural awareness and attention to social context can block pathways for the transmission of linguistic, religious and ethnocultural identity. The rupture of the bonds between immigrant children placed in foster care and their families or communities of origin may affect their developing identities in many ways. In many cases, the rupture may become permanent alienation. Unfortunately, to date, very little research has investigated the consequences of such ruptures, though a growing literature on the impact of the placement of First Nations children with Euro-Canadian foster parents offer useful insights (Nuttgens & Campbell, 2010).

Asuntha's case highlights the urgency of cultural training for professionals working in legal and criminal justice systems, including health and social welfare professionals, police and judges. To be able to make decisions that are both culturally sensitive and consistent with the law, judges and other individuals or organizations involved in administering justice must be aware of the social realities of immigrants and minority groups. Cultural consultants can play a key role in training professionals and organizations to increase their cultural competence and cultural safety (Fung, Lo, Srivastava, & Andermann, 2012). The next two sections addresses some of the issues that need to be considered in developing and delivering cultural competency training in CPS and legal or criminal justice settings.

Cultural Competence Training in Social Service and Legal Settings

Training programs designed to improve practitioner and organizational cultural competence can be adapted for use with specific groups related to CPS and legal services by considering their roles and constraints. Before instituting a training program, a statement of objectives, expected outcomes and a method of evaluation should be developed. The development of training should solicit input from administrators, frontline workers and stakeholders within the community. Evaluation of the training program should examine its impact on individual workers, as well as the organization.

Although cultural competence is recognized as including the three components of knowledge, skills and values or attitudes (Dufour et al., 2012), much cultural competence training, particularly at the institutional policy level, has focused on knowledge of specific ethnocultural groups. This approach may inadvertently reinforce stereotypes of immigrant and ethnic minority families. Further, it implies that the culture of the "Other" is relatively easy to understand, that clients can state their needs clearly, or that the professional can easily identify these needs simply by paying close attention (Hassan, Fraser, Papazian, & Rousseau, 2012). However, this approach ignores the fundamentally dialectical nature of the transmission or transformation processes inherent to every culture. This approach may essentialize cultural traits, rather than enriching clinical analysis by identifying structural inequalities that mirror the imbalance of power relations between minority and majority groups (Hassan et al., 2012).

Knowledge of the family's culture must be acquired through a process of inquiry that approaches each family as unique. This inquiry can only be done when professionals begin with the recognition of their own personal biases and prejudices which may influence the helping relationship. Only by exploring one's own values, which may clash with those of the family and elicit strong emotional responses (Dufour et al., 2012), can one be open to the family's experience (Bélanger, 2002). This openness can best be achieved when workers acknowledge their ignorance of the family's culture, thus giving the family members the opportunity to tell their own story as they see it. Cultural competence training approached only through knowledge acquisition will remain a hierarchical process that reproduces the dominance of professionals and limits dialogue and exchange. Cultural competence training that focuses on issues of power, values and attitudes of professionals and institutions can foster meaningful exchange and help create cultural safety.

The establishment of a diversity training policy and standards unit within the organization can support continuous in-service training. Courses or workshops developed in collaboration with this unit would integrate cultural awareness and multicultural values throughout the training curriculum and everyday. The aim of this focus on awareness and values is to allow workers to explore their own biases in a safe, nonjudgmental and supportive environment and help change attitudes and modes of practice to insure cultural safety throughout the organization. To accomplish these aims, we suggest a three-part model based on information exchange, self-awareness (knowing one's own values and privileges) and communication skills based on empathy.

Participants need to examine their own values, beliefs and practices, and consider their own unacknowledged and unearned privileges and advantages, which those with minority status do not often enjoy. This should include discussion of the contribution of the dominant culture to the social predicaments, experiences and responses of minority groups and individuals. While it may be useful to focus training on particular populations, it is essential that consideration be given to the heterogeneity within cultural, religious and linguistic communities. Attempts to convey rules of thumb in working with specific groups too often result in stereotypes that undermine real recognition and result in individuals being misunderstood, or even insulted and alienated. In general, any specific examples must be treated as illustrations of modes of inquiry. Training should be augmented by specifics based on the most pressing needs of the organization. For example, this may include training on the implications of religious pluralism for government agencies and institutions, given the concerns of Muslim or Arab groups in many Western countries who must contend with the current international political climate. Attention to cultural issues should be coupled with discussions of human rights as reflected in international, national and local charters, statutes and provisions (Dudley, Silove, & Gale, 2012). Finally, we underline the importance of providing those at the managerial and executive levels with the training. Indeed, we would argue that such training is crucial to create systems conducive to the needs of a culturally diverse work force. Moreover, participation of senior-level managers in the training sends a message to the rest of the organization that being culturally competent is an attribute that is valued by those in authority.

In summary, training should not be viewed as a one-off event, but must consist of ongoing educational and experiential activities, reinforced and monitored over long periods of time, in order to ensure improved skills and changes in biased attitudes and actions. Moreover, organizations should demonstrate through administrative practices, including hiring, programing and promotion, that they value diversity and view it as an important component of their functioning.

Cultural Competence Training for CPS

Cultural competence and safety have been recognized as basic components of the training of social workers as well as an issue for health and social service organizations (Betancourt, Green, Carrillo, & Ananeh-Firempong, 2003; Fung et al., 2012). This training must be focused, with clearly defined objectives that each participant can reasonably expect to achieve at the end of each training session or workshop. For example, training can center on some of the typical issues addressed by CPS representatives and legal services including discipline, parental authority, child autonomy and cultural differences or variation within a specific geographical area or community.

In conducting cultural competence workshops and consultations with CPS and legal services workers, we have found that child discipline is one of the major issues commonly identified by participants. For example, some immigrant or refugee families may use disciplinary methods such as hitting a child with an object that are condoned in their cultural context of origin but that contravene child protection laws in most Western countries (Hassan et al., 2011; Pottie et al., 2011). Other cultural practices, such as scarification, coining or cupping, may be misinterpreted as signs of child abuse by clinicians (Hassan et al., 2011; Pottie et al., 2011). Some culture-specific practices, such as female circumcision, create less doubt in the minds of professional as to whether or not they constitute abuse, because these practices clearly contravene child protection and civil laws in many countries (Hassan et al., 2011; Pottie et al., 2011). Yet these practices have important cultural meanings that must be considered in determining how to intervene effectively (Grisaru, Lezer, & Belmaker, 1997; Halila, Belmaker, Abu Rabia, Froimovici, & Applebaum, 2009; Shweder, 2002). The trainer aims to help professionals learn to distinguish between parental practices that are illegal, legal but unusual or dysnormative practices and practices that may be legal or illegal but are clearly dysfunctional practices. The law defines the boundaries within which CPS interventions take place and it is within these same boundaries that culturally sensitive interventions can occur. In cases deemed to be dysnormative, professionals should inform parents of their legal rights and obligations to their child. They can then implement psychosocial interventions that help alleviate family stress, model more acceptable disciplinary practices and support the parents in acquiring new ways of establishing their authority over their children and setting appropriate limits. However, in cases of dysfunctional abusive parenting, clinical and therapeutic interventions and, sometimes, foster care placement may be necessary.

The impact of any foster placement on cultural continuity and its transmission processes, as well as identity development, must be carefully considered. For example, clinical consultations have revealed that some professionals are not aware of the fact that immigrant and refugee children placed in foster care may suffer significantly from losses and identity crises related to separation from their language of origin as well as religious, familial and cultural traditions (Hassan et al., 2011; Pottie et al., 2011). The role of religion should not be minimized as it exerts a great influence on the parent–child bond, as well as the child's evolving identity. While some attempts are made by CPS institutions to address the issues inherent in fostering children by resorting to a policy of "same-race" placements, as is the case in the United Kingdom, these practices tend to conflate geographical region with religion and skin color or other racialized "markers" of difference with culture. In such circumstances, these policies may create even more harm to the child. For example, a 15-year-old Somali boy, who was an unaccompanied minor, was placed in a Caribbean family on the assumption that he would do better in a 'Black family'. He was accustomed to having a significant amount of autonomy and reacted with anger to the more hierarchical parent–child relations in the foster home. The 'match' turned out to be a disaster. He subsequently did well in a white Québecois family, whose vision of autonomy was quite similar to Somali notions of what was appropriate for his age group.

There are instances when ethnic matching may be in the best interests of the child's well-being. There has been great concern in Canada, for example, about policies of systematic out-adoption in Aboriginal communities in the 1960s (referred as "The Sixties Scoop"; Johnston, 1983) in which CPS workers sought non-Aboriginal homes for children who they perceived as requiring placement in "good" Euro-Canadian homes (Fournier & Crey, 1997; Gough, Trocmé, Brown,

Knoke, & Blackstock, 2005). Efforts have been made in recent years to place Aboriginal children with Aboriginal families both to support their individual identity and to reduce potential damage to the larger community (Lavergne, Dufour, Trocme, & Larrivee, 2008). However, such matching must include careful consideration of relevant aspects of identity such as language, religion and ethnic groupings in ways that consider the best interest of the child and the community.

Establishing a meaningful relationship with families requires attention to the frames of reference that govern parent–child relationships, parental authority, aggression and discipline as well as determining what is a private family matter and what can be shared (Aronson-Fontes, 2002; Ben-Arieh, Khoury-Kassabri, & Haj-Yahia, 2006; Chiasson-Lavoie & Roc, 2000; Rasmussen, Akinsulure-Smith, Chu, & Keatley, 2012; Taylor, Baldwin, & Spencer, 2008). Social and mental health interventions, including CPS interventions, may gain legitimacy from the perspective of the parents if they focus on areas of convergence between the values of the family's culture and those of the institution. When the emphasis is on the cultural meaning of problematic family practices, the host country's culture tends to be regarded as superior or more "advanced" provoking defensiveness and mistrust of host society institutions (Hassan & Rousseau, 2009a). In contrast, an emphasis on shared values such as the well-being of the child, as a common goal for families and professionals, can facilitate the negotiation of differences and support the needs of the family.

When conducting assessments, language barriers present another challenge that must be taken into consideration as they can jeopardize accurate evaluation and isolate some family members from the intervention plan (Hassan et al., 2011; Pottie et al., 2011). The intricacies of language often require working with interpreters and culture brokers (see Chapters 5 and 6). With adequate communication, cultural consultation can allow the co-construction of meaning and a plan of action that incorporates knowledge from the cultural systems of the family and the professional. Working with an interpreter or culture broker raises specific process issues which the professional must take into consideration, including confidentiality, dilemma of ethnic/religious match (match may be imprecise and individuals may view members of their group with suspicion) and the impact of the interpreter as co-therapist. The professional and the brokers and/or interpreters must establish procedural rules for collaboration before engaging in their work.

Child protection laws can be confusing and difficult for parents to understand. Moreover, professionals often fail to inform parents about the local child protection laws, their legal rights and their obligations regarding children (Hassan et al., 2011; Pottie et al., 2011). In order to create a good working relationship, the child protection worker must explain his or her role in relation to the law and the rights and duties of parents. This key information will contribute to families feeling more empowered in facing the power imbalance with legal institutions such as police, CPS and courts.

Power is a central aspect of CPS work in situations where abuse or risk to the child is deemed significant. Through law enforcement and legal actions, CPS workers can compel the family to comply with recommendations. The assertion of these institutional powers can undermine parental strengths, and the tensions or contradictions between child protection and strengthening healthy family functioning must be considered in assessing placements or other interventions. Like other psychosocial and mental health practitioners, CPS workers tend to define their professional roles and identities as "good" because they help and support children and their families achieve a better future. Integrating institutional power into this idealized professional identity as a helper raises complex issues since it requires acknowledging and accepting responsibility for the potentially detrimental aspects of CPS care plans.

Immigrant and refugee parents are particularly vulnerable to the power imbalance inherent to interactions with host society institutions and professionals which undermines their voice and agency. Indeed, several qualitative studies report that parents express a deep sense of fear, apprehension and powerlessness in the face of host society legal institutions, such as child protection

agencies, child courts and the police (Corby, Millar, & Young, 1996). Obviously, mistrust of these institutions may be related to parental histories with legal authorities in their country of origin as well as the host society. As a result, legal interventions are often perceived by migrant parents as intrusive and punitive (Hassan & Rousseau, 2009b; Rao, DiClemente, & Ponton, 1992; Welbourne, 2002). Judicial interventions may be perceived as a threat to the migration project of the family, particularly among recently settled immigrants who are not familiar with host society institutions (Hassan et al., 2011; Pottie et al., 2011). The fear of punitive institutional power is multiplied for refugee parents and their families due to risk of deportation or fear of not accessing citizenship in the event of criminal proceedings such as suspected or real physical or sexual abuse (Hassan et al., 2011; Pottie et al., 2011).

Immigrant and ethnic minority families who are less familiar with host country institutions often recognize this power differential and perceive CPS and mental health professionals as "manipulating" their destinies. Consequently, they may not interact with workers in ways that convey a positive image or express gratitude for interventions. Parents may express feelings of fear, shame, victimization and powerlessness because of their vision of CPS, mental health institutions and professionals as intrusive or even violent (Hassan & Rousseau, 2008). In this context, any attempt from the family to redeem some of its power and have a say in decision making (whether through contestation, opposition or anger) may be discredited because it constitutes a threat to the image of the CPS or mental health professional's identity as competent and well-intentioned (Morneau, 1999). The professional may react by reasserting power over the family, which then leads to increased anxiety, anger and mistrust. When family and professional identities are mutually threatening, the perceptions of the "Other" becomes oversimplified, stereotyped and polarized, with each party attempting to reaffirm their identity as "good" in the face of the "bad Other" (Hassan & Rousseau, 2008). For the professional, adopting the position of keeper of the law or holder of scientific knowledge in a hierarchical expert–patient relationship, become attractive alternatives to struggling with the ambiguity and complexity of the family's situation. These dynamics further contribute to the consolidation of social control and the imbalance of power between the family, the institution and the legal system.

The trainer must enable the professionals to recognize the inherent potential violence of CPS interventions. Training must provide safe space for workers to reflect on their roles and interventions without guilt or being made to feel their actions are intentionally harmful. This safety is hard to find in most institutions given the heavy case loads, urgency of interventions and burden of administrative tasks related to clinical and legal proceedings. Nonetheless, we contend that no alliance between the worker and the family is possible if the worker does not address the "elephant in the room," which is the power differential. Thus, regardless of the institutional difficulties, every child protection worker must find an appropriate place and time to discuss the power disparity with the family. This discussion should include the direct and indirect consequences on the child, the family system, the migration situation of the family and family agendas involving the continuity of cultural and familial transmissions. Clinical encounters must promote the family's sense of empowerment and participation in the decisions that affect their own and their child's future.

Cultural Competence in the Legal System

There are other professionals, with mandates outside of health and social services, who interact with groups and individuals from ethnocultural communities and make decisions which have great impact on their functioning and view of themselves in society. The decisions and actions of police, judges or other legal professionals may also influence the mandate of health and social services professionals as they seek to assist certain families. When creating cultural competence training for these professionals, the consultant must take into consideration the particular contexts of

practice, institutional mandates, occupational roles and time constraints. The first author (ML) has been involved in developing policy and training programs for the police and juvenile justice systems. We will describe two training programs geared to such professionals to illustrate how issues of occupational role and time constraints influence program design and delivery.

Judges working within the legal systems have clearly defined schedules which are often set months ahead of the time their cases are finally heard. Reflecting these time constraints, a 1-day training session for judges and lawyers in the juvenile justice system was designed to acquaint them with many of the issues faced by youth and families who must appear in court. The goal was to expose the participants to the societal realities that affect parents and families of different ethnicities, particularly how they may perceive, interpret and address situations differently from host culture members. The purpose of training judges and others involved in the justice process was not to encourage the use of culture or ethnicity as explanations or excuses for criminal acts, but rather to integrate social and cultural considerations in sentencing and devising more effective interventions (Kirmayer et al., 2007).

Participants were presented with scenarios based on actual cases which helped them to approach these issues. For example, the historical nature of racism, discrimination and racial profiling was a focus in understanding the issues of Blacks and other racialized minorities. Case discussions were used to clarify the ways that historical factors shape collective identities and influence the response to racial or ethnic labels and attributions for youth, families and the larger society. The impact of migratory laws and policies on many communities was outlined, such as those from the Philippines and the Caribbean, in which Canadian policy favored migration of women from these communities to work as domestics in the homes of white Canadian families. As discussed earlier in this chapter, many domestics had to leave their own children in the care of others in their homeland and await reunification. The workshop discussed the problems for both parent and child inherent in the predicament of reunification after many years of separation (Arnold, 2006; Lashley, 2000; Pottinger, Stair, & Brown, 2008). These reunification experiences were discussed in the context of racism, culture change, changes in educational systems and disrupted attachments to family and friends. Although there was no formal evaluation of this 1-day workshop, it appears that judges who took part have been more likely to call for attention to cultural factors in their decisions on interventions for CPS cases complicated by these migration issues.

The second example of cultural awareness training concerns the municipal police organization in Montreal, the *Service de police de la ville de Montréal* (SPVM, the Montreal Municipal Police). As a member of the SPVM committee looking at the issue of racial profiling, the cultural consultant (ML) was able to contribute to the organization's development of teaching modules to promote cultural awareness and sensitivity towards the city's diverse communities. The organization has used these modules to provide its members with training in alternative ways of dealing with diverse citizenry rather than adopting the approach of "one size fits all." Police officers' beliefs and behaviors were challenged in a supportive manner during training which encouraged their self-awareness in approaching law enforcement interactions. Training emphasized reflection on behavior, experiences and historical perspectives that might contribute to potentially deleterious approaches to work with ethnic minorities. A parallel agenda addressed the ways that members of ethnic minority or racialized communities are perceived in public space by other citizens and host society institutions, which influences their interactions with the police. These training sessions also provided those with cultural competence skills with the support they needed to confront others within the institution in order to improve intercultural interactions—all the while validating this work as part of the basic principles of "good policing."

Exposure to the Other in non-threatening situations while enhancing understanding of how the Other may interpret the world around them, is also important for police officers. To facilitate this, in addition to the in-house training programs, the SPVM has produced a series of DVDs in which individuals from minority communities explain some of the key aspects of their religions and ethnicities. This is an ongoing program and has spawned other efforts to address diversity, such as the establishment of an advisory group that focuses exclusively on issues pertaining to mental health. Although training cannot cover every relevant variation in religion or ethnicity, training tools like these DVDs can provide an overview of the issues and, with the right facilitator, can open up dialogue and begin to foster mutual respect.

Conclusion

Cultural consultation can assist professionals and administrators in social service and legal systems in understanding issues among their clients related to social inequalities during migration and resettlement. The cultural consultant's double alliance with the family and with the child protection and legal services actors can clarify the difficulties at hand and help all involved to better understand the complexity of family and institutional situations. Agencies as well as families and communities can use cultural consultation to promote trust, facilitate negotiation and find practical solutions. These solutions may involve working through perceptions that institutions are allied with forces in the host society that have inflicted violence on the family. Negotiating meaning and finding compromises not only create the possibility of restoring some power to the family, but expands the space for dialogue between families and institutions (Hassan et al., 2012). The process of listening and recognition inherent in cultural consultation can help reduce the feelings of threat, powerlessness and mistrust that families often experience in interactions with youth protection or legal systems. By promoting the alliance with CPS workers, who sometimes feel threatened by the family and by their institution's often punitive responses to any questioning of the standardized intervention approach, the cultural consultant validates the insights and clinical intuitions of workers. This process works towards advancing a more complex understanding of the family's situation. In this space of listening and story sharing, contradictions between the family and professionals are welcomed as useful vehicles for working through possible new strategies for change and creative problem solving.

Conversely, culturally inappropriate interventions can contribute to the fragmentation of meaning and suffering of clients. Explaining social predicaments primarily in psychopathological terms places the ultimate responsibility for resolving problems on parents who have been disempowered by life circumstances and the challenges of migration (Filc, 2004; Marange, 2001). Ignoring the impact of social and structural inequalities experienced by vulnerable families, as well as minimizing the collective responsibility to remedy their plight, is an important issue for many of these families facing resettlement challenges and poor living conditions (Filc, 2004; Kirmayer, Weinfeld, et al., 2007; McClean & Shaw, 2005). By promoting recognition of these structural issues, the cultural consultant can assist in the development of a culturally safe space for families working with institutions like CPS or the courts. Cultural consultation also provides an opportunity to advance training within these agencies to insure that staff and administrators work towards fuller understanding of the needs of their clientele. In multicultural societies, training in cultural issues is essential for institutions such as child protection, police or the justice system to provide more equitable services and achieve better outcomes in their encounters with minorities.

References

Adams, C. J. (2000). Integrating children into families separated by migration: A Caribbean-American case study. *Journal of Social Distress and the Homeless, 9*(1), 143–165.

Adams, C. M. (2006). The consequences of witnessing family violence on children and implications for family counselors. *The Family Journal, 14*(4), 334–341.

Alegria, M., Atkins, M., Farmer, E., Slaton, E., & Stelk, W. (2010). One size does not fit all: Taking diversity, culture and context seriously. *Administration and Policy in Mental Health, 37*(1–2), 48–60.

Allen, E. A. (1988). West Indians. In L. Comas-Diaz & E. E. H. Griffith (Eds.), *Clinical guidelines in cross-cultural mental health* (pp. 305–333). New York, NY: Wiley.

Arnold, E. (2006). Separation and loss through immigration of African-Caribbean women to the UK. *Attachment & Human Development, 8*(2), 159–170.

Aronson-Fontes, L. (2000). Children exposed to marital violence: How school counselors can help. *Professional School Counseling, 3*(4), 231–237.

Aronson-Fontes, L. A. (2002). Child discipline and physical abuse in immigrant Latino families: Reducing violence and misunderstandings. *Journal of Counseling and Development, 80*(1), 31–40.

Barn, R. (2006). Improving services to meet the needs of minority ethnic children and families. *ECM Research and Practice Briefings: Children and Families, 13*, 1–8.

Battaglini, A., Gravel, S., Boucheron, L., Fournier, M., Brodeur, J. M., Poulin, C., et al. (2002). Quand migration et maternité se croisent: Perspectives des intervenantes et des mères immigrantes. *Service Social, 49*, 35–69.

Bélanger, M. (2002). L'intervention interculturelle. Une recherche de sens et un travail du sens. *Service Social, 49*(1), 70–93.

Ben-Arieh, A., Khoury-Kassabri, M., & Haj-Yahia, M. M. (2006). Generational, ethnic, and national differences in attitudes toward the rights of children in Israel and Palestine. *The American Journal of Orthopsychiatry, 76*(3), 381–388.

Betancourt, J. R., Green, A. R., Carrillo, J. E., & Ananeh-Firempong, O., II. (2003). Defining cultural competence: A practical framework for addressing racial/ethnic disparities in health and health care. *Public Health Reports, 118*(4), 293–302.

Brent, E. B., & Callwood, G. B. (1993). Culturally relevant care: The West Indian as a client. *Journal of Black Psychology, 19*, 290–302.

Buntain-Ricklefs, J. J., Kemper, K. J., Bell, M., & Babonis, T. (1994). Punishments: What predicts adult approval. *Child Abuse & Neglect, 18*(11), 945–955.

Chao, R. (1994). Beyond parental control and authoritarian parenting style: Understanding Chinese parenting through the cultural notion of training. *Child Development, 65*, 1111–1119.

Chen, C., Smith, P., & Mustard, C. (2010). The prevalence of over-qualification and its association with health status among occupationally active new immigrants to Canada. *Ethnicity and Health, 15*(6), 601–619.

Chiasson-Lavoie, M., & Roc, M.-L. (2000). La pratique interculturelle auprès des jeunes en difficultés. In G. Legault (Ed.), *L'intervention interculturelle*. Québec, Canada: Gaëtan Morin.

Corby, B., Millar, M., & Young, L. (1996). Parental participation in child protection work: Rethinking the rhetoric. *British Journal of Social Work, 26*(4), 475–492.

Corral-Verdugo, V., Frias-Armenta, M., Romero, M., & Munoz, A. (1995). Validity of a scale measuring the positive effects of punishing children: A study of Mexican American mothers. *Child Abuse & Neglect, 19*(2), 217–231.

Davison, R. B. (1962). *West Indian migrants*. London, England: Oxford University Press.

Dudley, M., Silove, D., & Gale, F. (2012). *Mental health and human rights: Vision, praxis, and courage.* Oxford, England: Oxford University Press.

Dufour, S., Hassan, G., & Lavergne, C. (2012). Mauvais traitements et diversité culturelle: Bilan des connaissances et implications pour la pratique. In M. Hélène Gagné, S. Drapeau, & M.-C. Saint-Jacques (Eds.), *Les enfants maltraités: de l'affliction à l'espoir. Pistes de compréhension et d'action.* Québec, Canada: Presses de l'Université Laval.

Durrant, J. E., Ensom, R., & Coalition on Physical Punishment of Children and Youth. (2004). *Joint statement on physical punishment of children and youth.* Ottawa, Ontario, Canada: Coalition on Physical Punishment of Children and Youth.

Elliott, J. M., Tong, C. K., & Tan, P. M. E. H. (1997). Attitudes of the Singapore public to actions suggesting child abuse. *Child Abuse & Neglect, 21*(5), 445–464.

Ferrari, A. M. (2002). The impact of culture upon child rearing practices and definitions of maltreatment. *Child Abuse & Neglect, 26*(8), 793–813.

Filc, D. (2004). The medical text: Between biomedicine and hegemony. *Social Science & Medicine, 59*(6), 1275–1285.

Fournier, S., & Crey, E. (1997). *Stolen from Our embrace the abduction of first nations children and the restoration of Aboriginal communities.* Vancouver, British Columbia, Canada: Douglas & McIntyre Ltd.

Frias-Armenta, M., & McCloskey, L. A. (1998). Determinants of harsh parenting in Mexico. *Journal of Abnormal Psychology, 26*(2), 129–139.

Fung, K., Lo, H. T., Srivastava, R., & Andermann, L. (2012). Organizational cultural competence consultation to a mental health institution. *Transcultural Psychiatry, 49*(2), 165–184.

Gershoff, E. T. (2002). Corporal punishment by parents and associated child behaviors and experiences: A meta-analytic and theoretical review. *Psychological Bulletin, 128*(4), 539–579.

Gmelch, G. (1992). *Double passage: The lives of caribbean migrants abroad and back home.* Ann Arbor, MI: University of Michigan Press.

Gopaul-McNicol, S. (1993). *Working with West Indian families.* New York, NY: The Guilford Press.

Gopaul-McNicol, S. A. (1999). Ethnocultural perspectives on childrearing practices in the Caribbean. *International Social Work, 42*(1), 79–86.

Gough, P., Trocmé, N., Brown, I., Knoke, D., & Blackstock, C. (2005). *Pathways to overrepresentation of Aboriginal children in care. CECW information sheet #23E.* Toronto, Ontario, Canada: University of Toronto Press.

Grisaru, N., Lezer, S., & Belmaker, R. H. (1997). Ritual female genital surgery among Ethiopian Jews. *Archives of Sexual Behavior, 26*(2), 211–215.

Halila, S., Belmaker, R. H., Abu Rabia, Y., Froimovici, M., & Applebaum, J. (2009). Disappearance of female genital mutilation from the Bedouin population of southern Israel. *The Journal of Sexual Medicine, 6*(1), 70–73.

Hassan, G., Fraser, S.-L., Papazian, G., & Rousseau, C. (2012). La psychologie clinique culturelle: une question de savoir-être. *Psychologie Québec, 29*(1), 32–34.

Hassan, G., & Rousseau, C. (2008). L'expertise Psycholégale en contexte de diversité culturelle: Luttes de pouvoir complexes autour du meilleur intérêt de l'enfant. *Revue Québécoise de Psychologie, 29*(2), 167–182.

Hassan, G., & Rousseau, C. (2009a). Quand la divergence devient exclusion: Perceptions des châtiments corporels par les parents et les adolescents immigrants. *Revue L'AUTRE, 10*(3), 292–304.

Hassan, G., & Rousseau, C. (2009b). North African and Latin American parents' and adolescents' perceptions of physical discipline and physical abuse: When dysnormativity begets exclusion. *Child Welfare, 88*(6), 5–22.

Hassan, G., Rousseau, C., Measham, T., & Lashley, M. (2008). Caribbean and filipino adolescents' and parents' perceptions of parental authority, physical punishment and cultural values and their relation to migratory characteristics. *Canadian Ethnic Studies, 40*(2), 171–186.

Hassan, G., Thombs, B. D., Rousseau, C., Kirmayer, L. J., Feightner, J., Ueffing, E., & Pottie, K. (2011). Child maltreatment: Evidence-based clinical guidelines for immigrants and refugees. *Canadian Medical Association Journal.* Retrieved from www.cmaj.ca/lookup/suppl/doi:10.1503/cmaj.090313/-/DC1

Hines, A. M., Lemon, K., Wyatt, P., & Merdinger, J. (2004). Factors related to the disproportionate involvement of children of color in the child welfare system: A review and emerging themes. *Children and Youth Services Review, 26*, 507–527.

Jokhan, M. (2008). Parental absence as a consequence of migration: Reviewing the literature. *Social and Economic Studies, 57*(2), 89–117.

Kim, E., & Hong, S. (2007). First-generation Korean-American parents' perceptions of discipline. *Journal of Professional Nursing, 23*(1), 60–68.

Kirmayer, L. J., Rousseau, C., & Lashley, M. (2007). The place of culture in forensic psychiatry. *The Journal of the American Academy of Psychiatry and the Law, 35*(1), 98–102.

Kirmayer, L. J., Weinfeld, M., Burgos, G., Galbaud du Fort, G., Lasry, J.-C., & Young, A. (2007). Use of health care services for psychological distress by immigrants in an urban multicultural milieu. *Canadian Journal of Psychiatry, 52*(4), 61–70.

Kleinman, A. M. (1980). *Patients and healers in the context of culture.* Berkeley, CA: University of California Press.

Krug, E. G., Dahlberg, L. L., Mercy, J. A., Zwi, A. B., & Lozano, R. (2002). *World report on violence and health.* Geneva, Switzerland: World Health Organization.

Larrivée, M. C., Tourigny, M., & Bouchard, C. (2007). Child physical abuse with and without other forms of maltreatment: Dysfunctionality versus dysnormality. *Child Maltreatment, 12*(4), 303–313.

Lashley, M. (2000). The unrecognized social stressors of migration and reunification in Caribbean families. *Transcultural Psychiatry, 37*(2), 201–216.

Lashley, M., Blake, C., Hussain, M., MacLean, R., Measham, T., & Rousseau, C. (2005). *Student success: The identification of strategies used by Black Caribbean youth to achieve academic success.* Retrieved from http://www.fqrsc.gouv.qc.ca/recherche/pdf/RF-MyrnaLashley.pdf

Lavergne, C., Dufour, S., Trocme, N., & Larrivee, M. C. (2008). Visible minority, Aboriginal, and Caucasian children investigated by Canadian protective services. *Child Welfare, 87*(2), 59–76.

Longhi, V. (2013). *The immigrant war: A global movement against discrimination and exploitation.* Bristol, England: The Policy Press.

Maitra, B. (2008). Post-colonial psychiatry: The promise of multiculturalism. In C. I. Cohen & S. Timimi (Eds.), *Liberatory psychiatry: Towards a new psychiatry.* Cambridge, England: Cambridge University Press.

Marange, V. (2001). *Éthique et violence: Critique de la vie pacifiée.* Paris, France: L'Harmattan.

McClean, S., & Shaw, A. (2005). From schism to continuum? The problematic relationship between expert and lay knowledge: An exploratory conceptual synthesis of two qualitative studies. *Qualitative Health Research, 15*(6), 729–749.

McClure, F. H., Chien, Y., Chiang, C., & Donahoo, S. (1996). *Cross-cultural views of maltreatment and intervention: United States versus Taiwan.* Toronto, Ontario, Canada: American Psychological Association.

McEvoy, M., Lee, C., O'Neill, A., Groisman, A., Roberts-Butelman, K., Dinghra, K., et al. (2005). Are there universal parenting concepts among culturally diverse families in an inner-city pediatric clinic? *Journal of Pediatric Health Care, 19*(3), 142–150.

Mitchell, B. A. (2005). *Canada's growing visible minority population: Generational challenges, opportunities and federal policy.* Ottawa, Ontario, Canada: Mulitculturalism Program, Department of Canadian Heritage.

Morneau, N. (1999). Réflexions sur l'intervention en maltraitance auprès des groupes culturels minoritaires. *Revue Canadienne de Service Social, 16*(2), 219–231.

Mosby, L., Rawls, A., Meehan, A., Mays, E., & Pettinari, C. J. (1999). Troubles in interracial talk about discipline: An examination of African American child rearing narratives. *Journal of Comparative Family Studies, 30*(3), 489–521.

Nuttgens, S. A., & Campbell, A. J. (2010). Multicultural considerations for counselling First Nations clients. *Canadian Journal of Counselling, 44*(2), 115–129.

Orhon, F. S., Ulukol, B., Bingoler, B., & Gulnar, S. B. (2006). Attitudes of Turkish parents, paediatric residents, and medical students toward child disciplinary practices. *Child Abuse & Neglect, 30*(10), 1081–1092.

Phalet, K., & Schonpflug, U. (2001a). Intergenerational transmission of collectivism and achievement values in two acculturation contexts: The case of Turkish families in Germany and Turkish and Moroccan families in the Netherlands. *Journal of Cross-Cultural Psychology, 32*(2), 186–201.

Phalet, K., & Schonpflug, U. (2001b). Intergenerational transmission in Turkish immigrant families: Parental collectivism, achievement values and gender differences. *Journal of Comparative Family Studies, 32*(4), 489–504.

Phinney, J. S., Ong, A., & Maden, T. (2000). Cultural values and intergenerational values discrepancies in immigrant and non-immigrant families. *Child Development, 71*(2), 528–539.

Pottie, K., Greenaway, C., Feightner, J., Welch, V., Greenaway, C., Swinkels, H., et al. (2011). Review: Evidence-based clinical guidelines for immigrants and refugees. *Canadian Medical Association Journal, 183*, E824–E925. doi:10.1503/cmaj.090313.

Pottinger, A.M., Stair, A.G., & Brown, S.W. (2008). A counselling framework for Caribbean children and families who have experienced migratory separation and reunion. *International Journal for the Advancement of Counselling, 30*(1), 15–24.

Rao, K., DiClemente, R., & Ponton, L. (1992). Child sexual abuse of children. *Journal of the American Academy of Child and Adolescent Psychiatry, 31*, 880–886.

Rasmussen, A., Akinsulure-Smith, A., Chu, T., & Keatley, K. (2012). "911" Among West African immigrants in New York city: A qualitative study of parents' disciplinary practices and their perceptions of child welfare authorities. *Social Science & Medicine, 75*, 516–525.

Rodman, H. (1971). *Lower-class families: The culture of poverty in Negro Trinidad.* New York, NY: Oxford University Press.

Saulnier, G. (2004). Immigration et parentalité. *Recherche sur la famille: Conseil de développement de la recherche sur la famille au Québec, 5*(2), 11–12.

Savard, N., & Zaouche Gaudron, C. (2010). État des lieux des recherches sur les enfants exposés à la violence conjugale. *Neuropsychiatrie de l'Enfance et de l'Adolescence, 58*(8), 513–522.

Schaafsma, J. (2011). Discrimination and subjective well-being: The moderating roles of identification with the heritage group and the host majority group. *European Journal of Social Psychology, 41*, 786–795.

Segal, V. A. (1995). Child abuse by the middle class? A study of professionals in India. *Child Abuse & Neglect, 19*(2), 217–231.

Sewell-Coker, B., Hamilton-Collins, J., & Fein, E. (1985). Social work practice with West Indian immigrants. *Social Casework: The Journal of Contemporary Social Work, 66*, 563–568.

Shweder, R. A. (2002). "What about female genital mutilation?" And why understanding culture matters in the first place. In R. A. Shweder, M. Minow, & H. Markus (Eds.), *Engaging cultural differences: The multicultural challenge in liberal democracies* (pp. 216–251). New York, NY: Russell Sage Foundation.

Simmons, A. B., & Plaza, D. E. (2007). The Caribbean community in Canada: Transnational connections and transformations. In V. Satzewich & L. Wong (Eds.), *Transnational identities and practices in Canada* (pp. 130–149). Vancouver, British Columbia, Canada: University of British Columbia.

Smith, A., Lalonde, R. N., & Johnson, S. (2004). Serial migration and its implications: A retrospective analysis of the children of Caribbean immigrants. *Cultural Diversity and Ethnic Minority Psychology, 10*(2), 107–122.

Stoltzfus, E. (2005). *Race, ethnicity and child welfare.* Washington, DC: Congressional Research Service.

Taylor, J., Baldwin, N., & Spencer, N. (2008). Predicting child abuse and neglect: Ethical, theoretical and methodological challenges. *Journal of Clinical Nursing, 17*, 1193–1200.

Vatz-Laaroussi, M., & Bessong, J.-M. (2008). Être parents en situation d'immigration: Défis, enjeux et potentiels. In C. Parent, S. Drapeau, M. Brousseau, & E. Pouliot (Eds.), *Visages multiples de la parentalité* (pp. 223–253). Québec, Canada: Université du Québec.

Welbourne, P. (2002). Culture, children's rights and child protection. *Child Abuse Review, 11*, 345–358.

Cultural Consultation in General Hospital Psychiatry

14

G. Eric Jarvis

Introduction

Cultural consultation can provide a useful adjunct to existing services in general hospital psychiatry. The cultural consultant brings a different focus than the usual approach in consultation-liaison psychiatry, inpatient psychiatry, or emergency and crises services. However, hospital emergency departments and inpatient wards may be difficult places in which to conduct cultural consultation because of time constraints, confined or awkward interviewing space, inconsistent use of language interpreters, and the severity of illness of the patients. This chapter will discuss the use of cultural consultation in general hospital psychiatry, focusing on the ways in which the context of the emergency room and inpatient wards influences the types of problems referred and the logistics of cultural consultation. I will illustrate how to use cultural consultation in these challenging settings to promote more accurate and comprehensive assessment and culturally appropriate interventions.

G.E. Jarvis, M.D., M.Sc. (✉)
Culture and Mental Health Research Unit,
Institute of Community and Family Psychiatry,
Jewish General Hospital, 4333 Cote Ste Catherine
Road, Montreal, QC, Canada H3T 1E4
e-mail: eric.jarvis@mcgill.ca

Characteristics of Hospital Settings

Hospital settings pose specific challenges for cultural consultation based on the need for timely and efficient management of patients, the dynamics of emergency departments and hospital wards, institutional policies that aim to standardize the approach to patients, and the severity of patients' conditions, which may include acute, life-threatening illness, medical comorbidity, and chronicity.

Cultural consultations with outpatients referred by community-based practitioners generally allow sufficient time to arrange for the consultations and flexibility to choose the settings for evaluation that will be most helpful to patients and their families. Outpatient consultations are organized by the Cultural Consultation Service (CCS) consultant, who controls the place, time, and format of the assessment process, modifying institutional practices that are not culturally appropriate. Ambulatory patients are usually not so severely ill that their condition impedes the communication needed to arrange and conduct the assessment.

Patients referred from inpatient psychiatry and emergency services, in contrast, may be severely ill, have limited capacity for communication, and require urgent assessment. These consultations may occur in crowded settings with other challenges that undermine the quality of the clinical encounter. The institutional context may impose priorities and constraints on the consultation that

L.J. Kirmayer et al. (eds.), *Cultural Consultation: Encountering the Other in Mental Health Care*, International and Cultural Psychology, DOI 10.1007/978-1-4614-7615-3_14, © Springer Science+Business Media New York 2014

Table 14.1 Comparison of cultural consultation in emergency department and inpatient services

Setting	Time pressure	Physical space	Interpreters	Severe illness
Emergency department	Extreme due to constant inflow and triage of new cases	Often a noisy, crowded, chaotic environment; privacy may be limited	Often not available	Degree of severity is highly variable; many acute crises, with suicidal behavior, psychosis, agitation, intoxication, and domestic violence
Inpatient services	Depends on timing of discharge	Some privacy may be possible Hospital wards have their own distinctive use of space which impacts on safety of patients and staff	May be available with proper planning	Admitted patients tend to have more severe symptoms than outpatients

may work against the process of establishing cultural safety. The involvement of multiple clinical staff or teams introduces systemic dynamics that also must be considered. Routine shift changes of staff may undermine continuity of care and make data collection and intervention more difficult.

Despite these limitations, institutional psychiatric settings also offer some advantages to the cultural consultant. Patients are continuously present and easier to meet, and the hospital can serve as a convenient place for family, community members, and psychiatric staff to come together to discuss the needs of the patient, negotiate an understanding of the illness, and plan appropriate interventions as well as post-discharge follow-up. The crisis associated with the patient's ER visit or hospitalization can mobilize the different parties involved and momentarily ease some of the resistances to change or problem solving.

Table 14.1 lists some of the specific constraints faced by cultural consultation in emergency department and inpatient hospital settings, which are discussed in more detail below.

Time Pressure

Time pressure poses challenges for cultural consultation, which requires much data gathering and negotiation and should unfold at the pace tolerated by the patient and family (Lettich, 2004; Lu, 2004). Two kinds of time constraints commonly affect cultural consultations: (1) the urgent nature of emergency or inpatient consultations and (2)

the time-consuming process of preparing the cultural consultations. Urgent emergency and inpatient consultations often arise around the need to quickly determine diagnosis and treatment plan. There is pressure for availability of beds as new patients are referred to the emergency department and psychiatric ward for urgent care. The need to discharge patients in a timely manner becomes a preoccupation that drives many clinical decisions (Rhodes, 1991). Emergency and inpatient teams need to know how to contain symptoms of psychosis or self-harm, for example, in order to manage the flow of patients appropriately. Cultural and linguistic barriers hinder this process and may precipitate an urgent referral with the expectation of rapid intervention.

The time involved in bringing together the resources needed for cultural consultation frequently limits its practical implementation in hospital settings, particularly when consultations are requested late in the patient's hospital stay and shortly before discharge. Finding a mutually convenient time for the various members of the consultation team (consultant, referring clinician, interpreter, culture broker, family members) to meet the patient can be difficult. Given the time pressure in general hospital care to discharge patients (Mizrahi, 1985), clinicians may forgo cultural consultation and settle for expedient discharge plans. When there is close cooperation and communication between the referring clinician and the consultant, however, it may be possible to modify arrangements to insure completion of the assessment.

Despite the time pressures, inpatient clinicians should be encouraged to make early referrals for cultural consultation, but the length of time required to respond may dissuade them from making use of services like the CCS. In an effort to respond quickly, more focal initial consultations can be provided, even when a culture broker or interpreter cannot be arranged, and this may sometimes help the clinical team develop intervention options that are more sensitive to cultural issues. For example, the cultural consultant can review the case and briefly write some observations and suggestions related to broad cultural themes which can be developed in more depth later. These may include the identity of the patient and languages spoken, the need for a language interpreter, possible reasons for migration from the country of origin, the patient's current status in society, general attitudes to psychiatry and medication, and the presence or absence of family in the patient's life. The Cultural Formulation Interview (CFI) in DSM-5 provides an example of a brief culturally oriented interview that can provide basic information and identify the need for more in-depth cultural evaluation and follow-up.

Challenges of the Physical Environment

A physically confined or awkward interviewing space that does not allow adequate privacy can affect the process of cultural consultation just as negatively as a lack of time. Lack of privacy prevents trust and disclosure in any patient, but this may be even more difficult for some patients referred for cultural consultation, who may be suspicious of authority because of experiences of racism, discrimination, persecution, or trauma in their countries of origin. For some refugees, being interviewed in an unfriendly, impersonal, or exposed location, such as an emergency department cubicle or inpatient nursing station, may bring back memories of interrogation or imprisonment at the hands of abusers. Ideally, these delicate interviews would be conducted in an outpatient office in relative privacy and comfort. Disclosures by patients, while difficult in the best of circumstances, may not take place at all in the hurried, public atmosphere of emergency or inpatient services. While inappropriate interviewing spaces may discourage trust

and disclosure, at other times, it may cause concern about the safety of the patient or the consultant. Even in less restrictive situations, where patients may seem to speak freely, some individuals may not feel comfortable enough to disclose or discuss key issues.

Case Vignette 14-1

Mr. A., a 37-year-old Chinese man recently arrived in Canada with his young family, was admitted to the psychiatric intensive care unit for suicide threats. The CCS interview took place in the nursing station, with staff and patients circulating at the periphery, because the patient's room was unsuitable for a team evaluation. He spoke at length about immediate concerns, such as not working and being mistreated by his landlord. However, he made no mention of other crucial issues, including a letter he had written in red ink, entitled "The Misfortune of the Happiest Immigrant Family," explaining why he planned to commit suicide. He had endured multiple humiliating losses: severe financial strain, need for government welfare, his wife's criticism for failing to provide for the family, the involvement of child protective services because his children were not being given enough food, and working as a laborer in Canada when he had been a highly paid engineer in his country of origin. Mr. A. entirely avoided discussion of these potentially shameful issues during the interview at the inpatient nursing station.

Disclosure of conflict-laden or traumatic material may be an emotionally intense experience that is difficult for many people, but for some patients the loss of face or humiliation of revealing shameful secrets before family, community, and others may be a direct contributor to feelings of despair and suicide. Consequently, creating a safe place for disclosure is not only essential for assessment but may be an important intervention in its own right. The presence of the nursing team and others in an open ward space or nursing unit may make patients feel exposed and unprotected. The informal audience creates a complex scene in which the patient may feel "on stage" and pressured to perform in ways that are at cross-purposes with the consultant's goals of exploring the meaning of illness experience. The lack of private interviewing space interacts with time pressure and demands to conform to institutional norms in ways that may not only impede trust, communication, and building a working alliance but that can aggravate the patient's underlying condition.

Availability of Language Interpreters

Although professional interpreters play an essential role in the delivery of mental health care (Lettich, 2004), interpreter services are not readily available in many hospitals (Jacobs, Sadowski, & Rathouz, 2007). Lack of professional language interpreters constitutes one of the most important impediments to cross-cultural work in hospital settings, with potentially serious consequences for patient care, including increased risk of misdiagnosis, reduced access to necessary treatment, and misunderstandings that can result in harm to the patient (Gouvernement du Québec, 2007; Sentell, Shumway, & Snowden, 2007). The following vignettes illustrate some of the basic problems that can arise due to language barriers in the emergency department.

Case Vignette 14-2

Ms. B, a 24-year-old Tamil woman from Sri Lanka, was brought to the emergency department by her husband because she had become mute. The staff psychiatrist on call interviewed her with her husband interpreting. The psychiatrist was unsuccessful in getting any history other than what the husband himself volunteered. He recorded a working diagnosis of selective mutism and recommended a sodium amytal interview. When the CCS consultant reassessed Ms. B. with the help of an interpreter, and without her husband present, she revealed a history of severe domestic abuse.

Interviewing patients through family members, while sometimes viewed as expedient in the emergency room, can lead to serious clinical errors. Use of a professional interpreter is essential to establish accurate diagnosis (see Chapter 5 for detailed guidelines). In this case, the clinical presentation should have suggested the need for an interpreter to permit assessment of potential intimate partner violence and, more broadly, because gender roles often silence women's concerns (Jack & Ali, 2010). Gender violence remains an important area of misdiagnosis and lack of appropriate intervention, especially in cases where family members are asked to interpret for one another. Neglecting to use professional interpreters can also result in impoverished clinical evaluations as the following vignette illustrates.

Case Vignette 14-3

Ms. C, a 47-year-old woman from Vietnam, came to the emergency department accompanied by her two adult children. The psychiatrist was asked to evaluate her mental status despite the fact that she only spoke Vietnamese. No mechanism existed in the hospital to provide urgent language translation, so a rudimentary examination was done using the patient's son as the interpreter. It soon became clear that the patient was distracted by what seemed to be visual hallucinations. She stared away from the interviewer at the walls and ceilings of the room, looking intently at one location and then another. When the children were asked to clarify what she was experiencing, they fell silent, preferring not to discuss their mother's behavior with the interviewer at all.

As a matter of course, the CCS uses professional interpreters, and patients are strongly encouraged to make use of the interpreter if there is any indication that their English or French is limited. Most patients are comfortable and even relieved to have this help. There are many reasons for using professional interpreters rather than family members or other volunteers: Family or others may not know how to translate language affected by severe symptoms, such as psychosis, and may be disturbed by reports of suicidal ideation, marital infidelity, or domestic abuse; family or others may be embarrassed by personal material about sexuality or other issues brought forward in the interview and may elect not to translate items that they feel should remain private; and, at times, family members are directly implicated as causes of the patient's distress, as in cases of domestic violence. Unfortunately, despite these issues, ad hoc interpreters of convenience continue to be frequently used in hospital settings. This disregard for basic parameters of clinical communication impedes access to adequate medical care and impairs the quality of services including cultural consultation, in these settings.

Cultural Consultation in Severe Mental Disorder

Emergency departments and inpatient services admit patients with relatively severe illness where they can be closely observed and monitored and receive intensive treatment and rapid follow-up. Given the limitations of hospital resources, the trend in recent years has been to admit only patients with the most severe symptoms, with the result that inpatient psychiatry wards have acquired characteristics of psychiatric intensive care units (Lu, 2004). Cultural consultation for severely ill inpatients presents unique challenges, some of which are related to the dominant models and approaches in contemporary psychiatry.

Psychiatrists increasingly view schizophrenia and other psychotic illnesses as brain disorders. This reflects a longstanding tradition in psychiatry that views biological mechanisms as central to the causes of psychopathology (*pathogenesis*) while cultural factors play a role in shaping symptomatology (*pathoplasticity*). Consistent with this perspective, Marsella (1988) proposed that the cultural variability of symptoms decreased as the importance of neuropsychiatric pathology increased. In other words, disorders with clear neurological mechanisms were presumed to be less influenced by social-environmental factors. In this view, psychotic disorders ranked just after neurological diseases in terms of the degree to which biology was

deemed important compared to the effects of culture and society. Common mental disorders like anxiety and depression were assumed to show greater shaping by culture.

One consequence of this view is that psychotic disorders, especially schizophrenia, are assumed to be universal phenomena occurring at much the same rate among all peoples, places, and times. This assumption of universality occurs even though the prevalence of most diseases varies widely with geography, ecology, demography, and other factors. Investigators in the World Health Organization (WHO) Determinants of Outcome of Severe Mental Disorders (DOSMeD) study reported that for narrowly defined schizophrenia, incidence rates were remarkably similar in all study centers, though the reported rates varied twofold from 0.7 to 1.4/10,000 (Jablensky et al., 1992).

Given the dominance of this biological view, the role of social factors in the assessment and treatment of psychosis has been pushed to the margins of psychiatric theory and practice (Jarvis, 2007). At the same time, several lines of inquiry have suggest that there are powerful effects of social context on psychosis including (1) high rates of psychosis among immigrants to the UK and Western Europe and (2) superior outcome in patients with psychosis living in some low-income countries compared to those in wealthy, better resourced nations (for a review, see Morgan, McKenzie, & Fearon, 2008).

Several important studies have reported high rates of schizophrenia and psychosis among Black migrants to Western Europe compared to native-born Whites (Cantor-Graae & Selten, 2005; Fearon et al., 2006; Kirkbride et al., 2006). These findings persist after controlling for socioeconomic status, rates of psychosis in countries of origin, obstetric complications, and other possible contributing or confounding factors (Hutchinson & Haasen, 2004; Kirkbride et al., 2008). These results point to migration-related factors including racism and discrimination in the receiving society as potential contributors to the onset of psychosis and schizophrenia (Cantor-Graae & Selten, 2005).

Studies by the WHO over the last 40 years have documented substantial variations of outcome of schizophrenia depending on setting (Harrison et al., 2001; Hopper, Harrison, & Wanderling, 2007; Jablensky et al., 1992; WHO, 1973). One consistent finding across these studies is that the outcome of psychotic illness may be better in some developing countries compared to developed nations. In more recent work, Cohen, Patel, Thara, and Gureje (2008) suggested even greater heterogeneity of outcomes through the examination of research reports on schizophrenia in 11 low- and middle-income countries. They found that there is great variation in clinical outcome among non-Western centers, and this may be of greater magnitude than the variation previously reported by the WHO between developed and developing societies. Taken together, these variations in the prevalence and course of psychotic disorders point toward a crucial role for social factors in onset and expression of psychosis as well as course and recovery (Adeponle, Whitley, & Kirmayer, 2012).

Although the research in the UK showing differences in rates of psychosis across groups has not yet been replicated in Canada, there are reasons to believe that similar phenomena may occur. There is a long heritage of colonial conquest, slavery, and persistent negative racial stereotypes in North American culture that have given rise to misattributions of psychosis to persons of African descent with other types of mental health problems (Jarvis, 2008). Patients from some racialized groups in Canada, such as those from sub-Saharan Africa and the Caribbean, encounter systematic discrimination, fewer opportunities for material advancement, and social exclusion, especially when they become distressed or ill (Satzewich, 2011). These forms of social adversity, institutionalized racism, and structural violence directly affect patterns of help-seeking and health care utilization and may contribute to the course and outcome of severe mental illness.

In patients with psychosis, it is particularly important to work with professional interpreters, rather than family members, so that problems of discrimination, social adversity, impaired cognition, and communication can be properly identified. For example, in the CCS experience, it is common for professional interpreters to report not understanding patients with thought disorder, whereas family members may downplay the problem, glossing over disorganized or incoherent statements, and filling in what they imagine the patient is trying to say. Some of the most subtle communication problems occur when it seems that the patient can speak French or English adequately.

Case Vignette 14-4

Ms. D, a 37-year-old woman of Vietnamese origin, lived with her 16-year-old son. She was admitted to the hospital after overdosing on medication and going to the subway to die where her son would not be able to find her. She lost consciousness and awoke in the hospital after having been in a coma for 2 days. The patient reported hearing the word *salope* (slut in English) repeated in her head by voices, and the inpatient team was puzzled by the meanings of these symptoms. Ms. D. spoke meager English and French and was unable to elaborate what had happened to her. The referring team asked the CCS to clarify the diagnosis, specifically, to determine if the patient had a psychotic disorder.

Through an interpreter, the patient told the following story: She had been ill for 18 months, worse for 3 months, and was unable to continue her job managing a restaurant. She was troubled by ongoing back pain, headache, and tremor or twitching of her legs. The night before the interview, she had a nightmare in which she was raped. Nightmares occurred regularly, but usually were about her living in miserable circumstances, not having enough food, etc. She was worried that her son would die of starvation. She was afraid of a female acquaintance, especially when she saw her in the street. She admitted to hearing voices on two occasions telling her to die.

After a break for a few minutes, the patient returned to the interview to discuss previously undisclosed material. Ms. D. felt deeply ashamed whenever she saw the female acquaintance because this woman had called her a prostitute. Apparently, the

(continued)

woman's husband had fallen in love with the patient and made sexual advances, and this was the source of the woman's animosity. The patient felt intensely dishonored by the innuendo and linked her physical symptoms to this shameful situation. She was tearful and tremulous and stated that she wanted to sleep and not wake up, but denied any suicide plan.

After coming to Canada, she had worked long hours in a factory sewing garments and saved enough money to buy a restaurant which she eventually sold for a substantial profit. She used much of the money to help friends in the Vietnamese community. Unfortunately, they did not repay these loans. The patient felt betrayed and guilty that she had squandered her sons' inheritance. Facing these financial losses and the innuendos about her sexual impropriety, she became suicidal and took a medication overdose.

The culture broker spoke to the patient in Vietnamese for a few minutes in order to explore her sense of shame and indignation. The patient reported sexual advances by men in the Vietnamese community, including the husband of her adversary, which were not delusional, but arose from the patient's vulnerable position as a single woman, traditional and somewhat passive. There was precedent in Vietnamese society for some men to take a second wife, or concubine, and could explain why she was approached about this in the first place. Her sense of shame and outrage was expressed in the patient's own words as *uat u'c* ("indignation") and arose from being unjustly called a prostitute by the wife of the man who had made advances to her. These problems were made worse by her having been abandoned by the father of her son 4 years earlier as well as the shame associated with the loss of her savings and her dependence on welfare. She spoke of wanting to "go to sleep" rather than face these problems.

This vignette illustrates how, with the help of language and cultural interpreters, the CCS team clarified the meaning of specific findings on the mental status examination that had suggested psychosis, to conclude that the patient was not suffering from psychotic disorder but rather from depression. The transient auditory hallucinations and the suspiciousness of members of the community could be interpreted as symptoms of psychosis, but arose instead from the stresses and strains of a single, traditional Vietnamese woman who immigrated to a new country. Alone and unsupported, she experienced overwhelming stress through a series of unfortunate events that placed her in a vulnerable position vis-à-vis the members of her own community. This was expressed through culturally distinctive idioms of distress grounded in sociosomatic theory of illness causation (Groleau & Kirmayer, 2004).

Diagnostic Issues: Distinguishing Psychosis from PTSD with Dissociative Symptoms

The CCS is often asked to clarify diagnostic issues in patients with psychotic symptoms. In a significant proportion of cases, this results in a re-diagnosis, with the psychotic symptoms reinterpreted as part of an affective disorder (major depression or bipolar disorder) or dissociative symptoms that may be part of a cultural syndrome or PTSD. The relationships among psychosis, trauma exposure, and PTSD are complicated (Mueser & Rosenberg, 2003). Epidemiologically, up to 40 % of combat veterans with diagnosed PTSD have comorbid psychotic symptoms, although misdiagnosis is common, especially in patients from cultural communities (Seedat, Stein, Oosthuizen, Emsley, & Stein, 2003). High rates of psychosis have also been observed in traumatized refugee populations (Kroll, Yusuf, & Fujiwara, 2011). Consequently, some researchers have proposed a PTSD subtype with secondary psychotic features (Hamner, 2011), although more work is needed to establish this diagnostic entity. To further complicate matters, high rates of observed dissociation in patients with PTSD (up to 30 % in women) have prompted the proposal of a dissociative subtype of PTSD (Wolf et al., 2012). Dissociation refers to experiences of altered memory, perception, and identity and is common across cultures. Dissociative experiences may be exacerbated or precipitated by trauma exposure (Seligman & Kirmayer, 2008), and the presence of dissociation predicts psychotic symptoms, such as hallucinations, in patients with a history of trauma (Kilcommons & Morrison, 2005). Many refugees have been exposed to trauma, have symptoms of PTSD, and come from ethnic and linguistic minorities where dissociative experiences may be common whether as part of religious practices or modes of expressing distress, making accurate diagnosis difficult.

To examine the impact of cultural formulation on the diagnosis of psychotic disorders, Adeponle, Thombs, Groleau, Jarvis and Kirmayer (2012) compared intake diagnoses of patients referred to the CCS to final CCS diagnoses assigned after full cultural consultation. The research team found that misdiagnosis of psychotic disorders occurred in patients of all ethnocultural backgrounds, but most especially among immigrants and refugees from South Asia. In other words, patients from India, Sri Lanka, Pakistan, and Bangladesh who were referred to the CCS with a baseline diagnosis of psychosis were significantly more likely than patients from other regions to have their diagnosis of psychosis changed to a nonpsychotic disorder, such as PTSD or adjustment disorder. There was uncertainty among referring clinicians about diagnosis in these traumatized patients, particularly as to whether or not their symptoms were psychotic or dissociative. In a qualitative companion to this study, Adeponle and colleagues (Submitted) found that clinical decision-making by the CCS team that resulted in a change in diagnosis during the clinical case conferences followed a 3-step reasoning process that included raising questions about the diagnosis of a given patient, elaborating alternate diagnoses, and either confirming or reinterpreting the diagnosis. At each step, considerations of social context and cultural variations in illness experience played a role in questioning the original diagnosis of psychotic disorder.

This process reduced but did not eliminate stereotyping or diagnostic error as illustrated in the following example.

Case Vignette 14-5

Ms. E, a 25-year-old woman from Chad, was referred from the regional refugee clinic for diagnostic assessment to rule out psychosis. She had arrived in Canada 6 months earlier and lived with her brother and his family and two of her own children (5 years old and 5 months old). The patient explained that she divorced her first husband due to conjugal violence. Her husband's family was abusive and her husband delivered severe, recurrent beatings in which she was punched and kicked until bruised and bleeding. On at least one occasion, she lost consciousness. After becoming pregnant, she feared she would be kept alive only until the child was delivered. Worried for her life, she confided in the leaders of her Church, was helped to leave the country by a circuitous route, and finally arrived in Montreal 1 month before the birth of her second child.

The patient reported the following symptoms since arrival in Canada: poor sleep, poor appetite, depressed mood, frequent tearfulness, wish to die, frequent nightmares of her husband appearing to her, auditory hallucinations of her husband and others telling her that she must die and they will take the baby, and fear of her husband to the point she rarely left the apartment. The patient also reported headache, heaviness in the head, and the sensation of heat in the head. She denied suicidal plan or intent, but said that if refused status in Canada, she would attempt suicide because she could not be sent back to Chad where her ex-husband would certainly find her.

The patient overall was downcast and lethargic, but appropriate and cooperative during most of the interview. She presented her story in a succinct, articulate manner

(continued)

without evidence of thought disorder. At one point in the interview, when the consultant was interrupted by a phone call, the patient became acutely distressed. She shouted loudly, clenched her fists, and closed her eyes. She yelled, "No! Leave her!" as if responding to internal stimuli and for the next few seconds looked around the room and out the office windows as if searching for something or someone. Ms. E. did not respond for 1–2 min, but held her head in her hands, weeping and whispering "No, no, no." At last she explained that her husband's voice had threatened again to take away her baby. She wondered if he was using sorcery to communicate with her. She sometimes also heard the voices of his family members saying similar things. She seemed convinced that her husband was nearby and was coming for her baby but was reassured and settled after 5–10 min.

The attending psychiatrist was concerned and brought her to the emergency department to rule out major depressive disorder with psychotic features. The psychiatrist suggested that in view of the young children at home, the patient needed a social work consult and possible hospital admission to initiate antipsychotic treatment. In the end, Ms. E. recovered quickly in the emergency department, and her brother took her home against medical advice. The patient refused medication despite ongoing symptoms of anxiety but allowed the CCS team to follow her on an outpatient basis, and she was seen on three later occasions. Her greatest explicit concern remained her upcoming refugee hearing.

The decision to bring Ms. E. to the emergency department was based on the psychiatrist's concern for the patient's safety as well as the safety of the young children in her brother's home. It was a difficult decision speedily made in a moment of crisis. In retrospect it was not the right decision, but one that was based on a poor understanding of the patient's symptoms, diagnosis, and the cultural context of her distress. Post hoc discussions with the culture broker and other CCS team members highlighted a number of issues. First, the patient's diagnosis was most likely PTSD with associated depressive and dissociative symptoms. Psychosis was not the principal diagnosis. The hallucinations, nightmares, and paranoid behavior represented posttraumatic dissociation with cultural overlay. The evidence for this included the form and content of the symptoms and their rapid resolution with reassurance. Second, the patient hinted that her symptoms were linked to sorcery. Her dramatic behavior was consistent with the dissociative behavior associated with spirit possession and spirit attacks (Kirmayer & Santhanam, 2001). Betrayal of social responsibilities, such as the abandonment of a husband, in Ms. E.'s eyes, resulted in spiritual retribution, possibly in the form of spirit possession or other form of attack. The manifestation of distress in this way served at least two purposes: (1) It was a vehicle to express distress about a taboo topic (abandonment of social duty in the face of conjugal violence), and (2) it served a tacit help-seeking function by drawing attention to the intensity of the patient's distress.

Hence, in this case, the patient's symptoms signified a spiritual attack for having left her husband and his family. A knowledgeable healer was not available to ward off the power of the attacking spirits sent by her husband. Usually, this would take place through the use of "counter-witchcraft," something that the CCS team clearly was not able to provide. The patient's symptoms seemed psychotic, but in cultural context were understandable and even to be expected under the circumstances. In essence, she was trying to communicate her need to the psychiatrist (healer) in the best, clearest way she knew. Instead of providing protection against vulnerability (spiritual attack), the psychiatrist pronounced her psychotic, took her to the hospital emergency department, and attempted to recommended treatment with antipsychotic medication. It was only the diligence of the patient's brother that saved her from inappropriate care.

In the end, the CCS listened to the various parties and decided upon several revised conclusions and recommendations. First, the patient's diagnosis was PTSD, not major depressive disorder with psychotic features. Referral to an ethnically matched religious or other community organization was contraindicated due to the patient's fear of meeting her husband or contacting someone he knew. The patient knew little about her rights in Canada as a woman and a mother, so it was important to explain these things to her in addition to teaching her about the immigration process in Canada. The patient's lawyer was contacted to determine the need for a letter of support for immigration purposes. The patient also was referred to local services for immigrants and to a women's group that focused on domestic violence. It was important to gain the trust of the patient's brother, if possible, in order to better understand her functioning in cultural context and to adopt an optimistic stance, explaining that the symptoms she was experiencing were to be expected in someone that has suffered so much and that she was expected to improve in time. Medications were to play an adjunctive role in symptom management depending on the clinical state of the patient.

Strategies for Inpatient Management of Patients with Severe Mental Illness

The assumption that severe mental illness represents neuropsychiatric disorders that are determined by biological dysfunction might suggest that they will respond poorly if at all to social and cultural interventions. In practice, however, there is good evidence that attention to social and cultural issues, and psychosocial interventions such as engaging family members and educating the treatment team about cultural beliefs and practices, cannot only clarify diagnoses but guide more effective treatment plans, sometimes incorporating novel interventions that lead to better outcomes and recovery (Adeponle, Whitley & Kirmayer, 2012).

Case Vignette 14-6

Ms. F, a 64-year-old woman from Haiti, was referred to the CCS by inpatient services for a lack of response to antipsychotic treatment. The inpatient team hoped the CCS would clarify the patient's diagnosis, improve the clinician–patient alliance, and propose a treatment plan. In addition to hypertension, the patient presented with the following medical problems: (1) She was on renal dialysis 3 times per week and had surgery to provide an AV shunt for the dialysis in the last year; (2) she took multiple medications, including risperidone, citalopram, olanzapine, amlodipine, atenolol, and phenytoin, among others; and (3) she had an elevated parathyroid hormone level and was scheduled for parathyroidectomy. CT scan of the head was normal except for the incidental finding of a small focal lacuna in the right basal ganglia. The patient was known to be hypertensive. The patient was concerned about the challenges of dialysis and about the side effects of her multiple medications. Her most pressing complaint, however, was none of these, but rather had to do with the bugs or insects (*bibittes*, in Québecois French, referring to a small insect and also colloquially to emotional distress or "black thoughts") crawling on and under her skin. She could not see them because they were as small as "grains of sand," but she felt them constantly and was tormented by them, repeatedly scratching and picking at her skin in an effort to remove the bugs. According to her, these bugs originated from her rectum and migrated to her vagina and other parts of her body, especially under the breasts and under the arms. She also complained that the bugs were in her hair, on her face and in her internal organs. When she lay still she could feel them burst from time to time inside her, and they emitted a foul

(continued)

odor when they broke open. The patient denied any such problem prior to returning to Montreal a month earlier from a trip to the USA. At that time her youngest daughter, whom she had sponsored to immigrate to Canada 10 years earlier, completely cut ties with her and denied access to the two young grandchildren, telling them that their grandmother had died. The patient tearfully recounted these problems and explained that she was depressed since the surgery on her arm last year, but that the feeling intensified since the return to Montreal last month. She reported poor sleep with frequent wakening during the night, decreased appetite with an 18 kg weight loss in the last 2 months, loss of pleasure doing regular activities, and social withdrawal (not attending church every week as before).

By way of background, the patient's husband initially left the Caribbean and sponsored her migration to Canada 30 years ago, although the couple later separated without divorcing. The husband had died suddenly at around the time of the CCS evaluation. When the patient immigrated to Canada, the children stayed in Haiti with the patient's aunt except for the youngest child, a daughter, who was reared instead by a cousin who mistreated her. As funds became available, reunification took place one child at a time over years until the youngest was brought to Canada only 9 years before. The patient was a practicing Baptist, but had not attended church for several months.

On examination, the patient was a thin 64-year-old woman who appeared older than the stated age. She initially presented with a bright affect despite incessant scratching and picking at her face. As the interview progressed, the patient's demeanor changed. She became tearful and sad while discussing the rupture with her daughter. Her posture became stooped, with head hung low; arms were folded in her lap;

and she was increasingly slow to respond. There was no thought disorder and no suicidal or homicidal ideation, but there were delusional preoccupations with "bibittes" and the conviction that a foul odor emanated from them whenever they burst under her skin, in her genitalia, or within her vital organs. The bibittes were associated with sensations of itching and crawling under the skin (tactile hallucinations or formication). Cognition was grossly within normal limits. Judgment was fair except that the patient was unable to stop scratching her skin in public. Insight was poor with respect to the invasion of her body by bugs. When her concern about the odor was addressed by asking, "So you sometimes feel dirty when you smell the odor?" the patient quickly answered, "I don't smell bad—it's the bugs that are dirty!"

The first recommendation of the CCS consultant was that a general medical condition had to be carefully excluded in this patient, especially physical sensations secondary to renal failure, hyperparathyroidism, or medication side effects. In the absence of medical explanations of the patient's symptoms, the working diagnosis was major depressive disorder, single episode, with psychotic features (delusional infestation, with formication). The diagnosis of primary psychotic disorder was not considered likely. Of especial importance was the loss of daughter and grandchildren precipitated by unresolved issues of reunification. In addition to increasing the antidepressant dose, the CCS team recommended to meet again with the patient and to focus on issues of mother-daughter reunification and the patient's withdrawal from religious life as precipitants and/or exacerbating factors of depression. A family meeting was proposed with the patient's son, who lived in Montreal and who was still on speaking terms with his mother.

(continued)

At the second CCS interview, 1 month later, the patient was recovering from para-thyroid surgery and experienced an exacerbation of the preoccupation with skin parasites. She sat through much of the interview picking her face and rubbing her axillae. The patient's son, who was in attendance, indicated that his mother pulled hair from her head and caused marks on her face from incessant picking. The patient initially preferred to remain alone in her hospital room, but eventually joined the meeting with her son. She was completely absorbed by somatic discomfort, but her occasional comments were appropriate and showed that she followed the conversation. Most of the session had to do with the family situation, which involved a troubled relationship with the younger daughter who was on welfare and had financially exploited her mother while attempting to block Ms F.'s access to her grandchildren. For her part, the patient missed her grand-children, who would occasionally drop by her house to visit despite their mother's prohibition. During most of the interview, especially when discussing her daughter, the patient sat with a stooped posture, head held low, tears in her eyes, and scratching and picking her face and body. On occasion, she sighed when comments were made about the family difficulties. Her affect brightened considerably, however, and she stopped the picking behavior entirely when discussing two themes: her former life in Haiti and her religious participation. The patient was passionate about her religion and derived considerable support from it. Members of the church visited her in the hospital and prayed with her.

Formication (sensations of insects crawling under the skin) is a form of paresthesia that can have many medical causes, including medication side effects, uremia, and other conditions (Blom & Sommer, 2012). The cause in this patient was uncertain, but the sensations themselves can give rise to ideas of infestation and may also occur as a form of delusional disorder (Freudenmann & Lepping, 2009). This patient's condition was clearly exacerbated by the rupture with her daughter and grandchildren, by growing debt incurred since her daughter's arrival in Canada, and by a longing to return to her home country. The recent return from a visit to the USA may have aggravated an episode of depression that began the previous autumn around the time of surgery to provide an AV shunt for renal dialysis. Underpinning the patient's sadness were problems connected to family, migration, and reunification that had only partially been acknowledged let alone redressed (see Chapter 13). Once medical causes were ruled out, these family issues directly contributed to the patient's symptoms and confirmed a final diagnosis of major depressive disorder. Treatment recommendations reflected culturally consonant themes of visiting family in Haiti, reconnecting to the Haitian community, and facilitating religious participation for the patient.

Although family systems issues may contribute to the severity or apparent intractability of severe mental illness, family members are not always available during the process of assessment or intervention. In some cases, members of the patient's local ethnocultural community may be engaged in the consultation. When differences of opinion between community members and the treatment team emerge, however, the cultural consultant needs to mediate and negotiate an acceptable compromise to assist the patient, maintain community ties, and avoid rejection by health care providers.

Case Vignette 14-7

Ms. G. was a 40-year-old woman from Trinidad, who had immigrated to Canada 10 years earlier. She was brought to the hospital by a community social worker and admitted to psychiatry for symptoms of paranoia and angry threats toward her sister. The patient complained that her sister was tampering with her cell phone and television, had been spying on her, and was

(continued)

monitoring her telephone calls by means of special technology. The patient threatened to beat up or even kill her sister and had attacked her on one occasion. Ms. G was experiencing poor sleep, with only about 3 h per night over the last 2 weeks; decreased appetite; and depressed mood. There were no suicidal thoughts, no auditory hallucinations, and no substance abuse. Her mood was dysphoric and affect was blunted. During an interview in the hospital, the patient said, "My doctor was treating me for one thing, but something else was going on." The patient expressed the hope that the CCS team would understand what she was really going through. She said, "The doctor's treatment is not working—my ears are still aching because of my sister." She explained that her sister practiced witchcraft, or Obeah. At first, the patient didn't realize that her sister was involved in the occult. Earlier in the year, when her sister went to Trinidad, the patient stayed in her apartment to tend her children. According to the patient, the house smelled like urine and caused her to sneeze. She cleaned the place thoroughly, but when her sister returned she didn't thank the patient for her hard work cleaning up the mess. Also, the sister was supposed to contact the patient's children, who still lived in Trinidad, while in the Caribbean, but she did not. As a result, long-prepared gifts were never delivered as previously agreed. The patient complained to a friend, and the relationship with her sister became strained. In this context, Ms. G. came to think that her sister was listening to her telephone conversations and blocking the telephone to prevent her from using the line. The patient knew it was witchcraft because there was music with a heavy beat coming from the telephone. She was convinced that her sister had been using witchcraft to harm her "for a long time" because of previously unexplained hot and cold sensations in her

body. The patient referred to these sensations as "spiritual attacks." She linked these attacks to other somatic complaints: "My liver is flapping, my uterus is squeezing, there is a pressure." Despite taking up to 3 mg of risperidone daily, the patient reported no improvement in her symptoms, which included hearing music in her ears, feeling heat in her body, and thinking that her sister controlled "the system in the house" and was "involved in iniquity." She said of her sister, "She's tracking me by the moving lines of the telephone."

When asked what would help her to feel better, the patient maintained that she would need to visit "a Spiritual Baptist person" where she could fast and pray and receive blessings to overcome the attacks she was enduring. She said, "To help me, someone needs to know where the attacks are coming from. I need help when I am hurting." She reported that her mother in Trinidad had a similar problem and met with "a spiritual person" to find a successful cure. The patient saw no difference in her distress with or without medication. She thought that her inpatient psychiatrist and the Euro-Canadian minister at her church did not know how to help her. When asked about the possibility of increasing the dose of risperidone, she refused and said, "Medication cannot help me—it is the iniquity thing." Iniquity, on closer questioning, referred to what the patient called "Obeah" and the spiritual attacks arising from its practice by her sister. She believed that her sister could paralyze her by supernatural means and make items vanish from her home. The patient wanted no contact with her sister and hoped that avoiding her sister would lessen the degree to which she was under her control.

At the suggestion of the CCS, the patient brought a friend from her religious community to a meeting with her inpatient treatment team, who were cautious about

(continued)

the spiritual approach to the patient's psychosis and wanted to understand what spiritual healing would entail. The patient made up her mind to seek healing from an authority in the "Spiritual Baptist faith" (as she called it). According to the friend, a healer in her own right, cure would only come by fasting and prayer. The patient believed that her symptoms represented "chastisement of the devil" and that the symptoms would only abate once she was "called back to the fold." The friend was of the opinion that the symptoms were not chastisement per se, but were something else (not fully defined in the interview) deriving from Obeah and High Science, Caribbean healing traditions. As the friend repeated several times, "constant, earnest prayer and fasting would help remove this illness." The fasting and prayer could take up to 21 days. The patient was to be secluded in a special room during this time and would be attended to by "nurses" (those who care for her, not formally trained nurses). The friend said that the patient could take prescription medication during the healing, but it might be stopped to give the spiritual healing a chance. "Bush," or plant remedies, such as aloe vera, would also be administered to the patient. Despite the planned medication holiday during healing rituals, the patient's friend agreed to help her take the medication regularly the rest of the time. The patient was determined to proceed as planned.

In this case, the culture broker explained that throughout the Caribbean islands, in addition to Christian beliefs, there was the notion that forces in the spiritual realm could affect everyday life. As Vodou was practiced in Haiti, so Obeah was practiced throughout the English-speaking Caribbean islands. "Obeah" was a traditional term for witchcraft, or folk magic based on the belief that the forces of nature can be manipulated to influence ordinary outcomes in everyday life.

For example, in Jamaica, children learned that a certain "bush" (weed, vine), when placed under a stone, would prevent the teacher from punishing students when they are late for school. Individuals such as the patient, who were poor and from rural areas, often held to these beliefs to explain misfortunes and find solutions to their troubles and afflictions. In addition, many individuals were members of charismatic churches in which prophetic preaching foretold of impending disaster if the individual member did not adhere to certain codes of behavior. As in other Christian denominations, guilt and other forms of psychological distress were expected outcomes for "a life of sin," which left one vulnerable to "iniquity" and "chastisement from the devil." These were some of the terms that the patient used to describe her situation. Traditionally, adherents to these practices tended to envisage catastrophic outcomes for individuals who for whatever reason chose to leave the group. Hence, when the spiritual healer accompanied the patient to the CCS evaluation, the healer embraced the patient as a lost sheep returning to the flock. The healer reassured the team by saying that she knew many individuals who were not amenable to spiritual healing, but the patient was likely to benefit and even recover. The team felt it was important to encourage discussion of these treatments because to do otherwise was to undermine ongoing psychiatric treatment or follow-up. By remaining involved in these decisions, the treatment team could support the patient through the process of the spiritual healing while moderating interventions that could be excessively expensive or even potentially harmful. Furthermore, continued collaboration with the patient's religious community was a way to encourage adherence to medication, remain informed of her actual medication use, and openly discuss her reasons for stopping the medication if that occurred. The clash of explanatory illness models, between the patient and the inpatient psychiatry team, caused tension and discomfort in this case, but did not give rise to gross misunderstanding, breakdown in communication, and negative stereotyping that might have taken place without the mediation provided by the CCS. In the end, the patient eventually left the hospital to have a Spiritual Baptist healing in another city. She experienced a brief improvement in symptoms but eventually returned to psychiatric care and antipsychotic medications with only partial remission. Fortunately, the patient remained on good terms with her psychiatrist and treatment team, and this allowed long-term collaboration.

In severe mental illness, much of the work of CCS involves identifying major social stressors, helping the patient and the treatment team find common ground despite divergent explanatory models, and maintaining an effective working alliance with the treatment team. However, on occasion cultural consultation can identify strategies to approach seemingly intractable problems that have exhaustive conventional psychiatric interventions.

Case Vignette 14-8

Mr. H, a 45-year-old man from a rural community in China, was referred to the CCS from the Psychiatric Intensive Care Unit, a locked ward for severely ill psychiatric patients. He was admitted 8 months earlier due to command auditory hallucinations telling him to mutilate his body. So far, he had attempted to amputate one of his hands, perforated his bowel with a knife, and delivered serious blunt trauma to his head. No treatment modality had helped, including antipsychotic medication and electroconvulsive therapy. The patient spoke of "celestial friends" or spirits that were commanding him to carry out these acts. When asked to contract not to harm himself, he said, "I am not in a position to agree with that statement." The treatment team wondered if there was a religious or cultural component to his symptoms that they were missing that might facilitate recovery.

Over the course of the consultation, the treatment team expressed concern about how the patient hoarded food in his hospital room. They noted that he wanted to give the food to his celestial friends and asked for extra money to make purchases for them. Sometimes, he left the ward without permission to stare at food in the

cafeteria. The cultural consultation team advised patience in this regard and explained that, according to Buddhist custom, it is common practice in some parts of China to offer food to the spirits of ancestors. If an ancestor is not buried properly, is not offered food or incense or clothes, or has no descendants to take care of the tomb, the spirit may become a "hungry ghost." When the spirits are hungry, they may bother human beings to prompt them to make offerings. In this light, the treatment team was advised to explore the meaning of the food offerings along the following lines: What are the food offerings for? Is the patient making offerings to his celestial friends? If yes, what will the spirits do if he stops giving them food? Is there something he can offer the celestial friends that will induce them to stop troubling him and leave him alone? The CCS team suggested that the treatment team negotiate an acceptable form of food offering with the patient. This could strengthen the treatment alliance and foster discussion about commands to self-harm before they take place.

Cases like this, with persistent self-injury, present great difficulties for inpatient psychiatric care. The challenge for the CCS was to find practical interventions that would enhance the treatment team's understanding of the patient's behavior, open up the dialogue, and ultimately reduce self-injury. In this case, the CCS identified several culturally based strategies to enhance the patient's care.

While in this particular instance the referring team was motivated to seek cultural consultation due to the lack of clinical improvement, some inpatient teams may lose hope in the face of severe symptoms that are unresponsive to standard therapies. In these cases, they may not make a referral in the belief that little more can be done and that cultural interventions can only make an impact in patients with less biologically based conditions. Even in the most severe of mental disorders, however, cultural consultation can improve clinical understanding of the patient, provide therapeutic avenues for future investigation, and strengthen the therapeutic alliance by optimizing communication between the patient and the treatment team.

A Clinical Caveat

The very existence of a cultural consultation service within a hospital makes cultural issues more salient for staff. However, cultural issues may sometimes function as "camouflage" diverting attention from personal or systemic issues that patients, families or clinicians would prefer to ignore (see Chapter 7). At the same time, focusing on culture may divert attention from underlying medical conditions.

Case Vignette 14-9

Shalini, a young Sri Lankan Hindu Tamil woman from a high caste family, presented repeatedly to the hospital emergency room for difficulty with her gait and low back pain. After many visits to the ER, she was noted to be emaciated with very poor appetite and was admitted to psychiatry with a diagnosis of probable anorexia nervosa and personality disorder. During this hospitalization, a psychiatric resident referred her for cultural consultation as a diagnostic quandary with possible posttraumatic stress disorder added to the differential diagnosis.

Shalini had survived bombings and attacks during the Sri Lankan civil war and was sponsored to come to Canada with her husband by her mother, who was working at a clothing factory in Montreal. She had an arranged married to a young man who asked for a divorce as soon as he had secured permanent resident status in Canada. He kept her large dowry and had insisted on his ownership of her mother's Sri Lankan property according to the terms of their marriage contract. Despite the loss of the family wealth, which brought profound shame to her maternal extended family, Shalini showed little concern about the divorce and remained focused on her physical pain. The treatment team saw her mother bringing her food from home and interpreted this as probable maternal enmeshment, with a working diagnosis of eating disorder. During the CCS consult, mother reported her worry that Shalini's appetite had diminished and stated that she was trying to help her daughter gain weight by bringing her Sri Lankan foods. The consultation found no signs of the food compulsions or family dynamics commonly associated with eating disorders. Since there were no symptoms of PTSD, the CCS consultant suggested a more extensive neurological workup. Subsequent neurological examination and MRI identified a spinal tumor which accounted for Shalini's gait disturbance and weight loss, followed by surgery leading to marked improvement.

As this case illustrates, the persistent dualism in biomedicine may lead to dichotomous thinking in which the presence of family systems and cultural issues interferes with the recognition of physical illness (Kirmayer, 1988; Miresco & Kirmayer, 2006). The cultural elements of the civil war, arranged marriage, divorce, loss of property, and a widowed mother had nothing to do with the medical causes of the patient's anorexia but led the treating staff to postulate an eating disorder, PTSD, conversion disorder, or malingering. Chapter 15 presents further examples from general hospital consultations of the interplay of cultural issues in medical conditions.

Lessons Learned

Patients with psychosis or other severe mental illness are challenging to assess and treat under routine conditions let alone when issues of culture and migration add layers of complexity to the clinical picture. The following rules of thumb, based on the experience of the CCS, can guide clinicians encountering culturally diverse patients in general hospital psychiatry.

Determine before the first interview whether or not an interpreter is needed. It is a good idea to inquire about language proficiency prior to the patient's first appointment so that the need for interpreters can be determined well beforehand. When working with psychotic patients, professional interpreters may have difficulty translating when the patient's language is vague or incoherent. The interpreter needs to convey this difficulty because it provides useful diagnostic information. When family members are used to interpret, they may unintentionally obscure the presence of thought disorder, and other psychotic symptoms, by filling in the gaps, leaving out nonsensical material, or organizing incoherent statements, in an effort to portray the loved one in a favorable light. Language barriers can magnify deficits and symptoms or even make them seem present when none exist. On the other hand, when the patient is given the option of speaking through a qualified interpreter in her mother tongue, language that initially seems disjointed because of limited proficiency may become clearer.

Allow sufficient time for interviews of patients who speak a different language or are from a different culture. Scheduling extra time can prevent problems caused by too rapid or compressed consultations that may prevent adequate assessment and treatment negotiation and increase the risk of clinical error. Allowing adequate time at the first meeting with a patient will pay dividends in terms of engagement and rapport, treatment adherence, and assessment of suicide and aggression risk. Typically, the consultant should allow 2 h for the first meeting with any patient requiring an interpreter.

Focus on urgent matters first. Many patients, particularly immigrants and refugees, are faced with a variety of practical dilemmas that need to be urgently addressed. Resolving these issues will go a long way to reducing the distress of patients who may otherwise seem demanding or difficult to help and for whom medication, and other standard treatment modalities, may not be working well. For example, an upcoming immigration hearing for a refugee claimant is such a momentous event that virtually every other consideration is of secondary importance. Planning ahead for the hearing, including recommending a designated representative for patients unable to relate their story unassisted and providing letters of support, may be as important as providing appropriate medication and obtaining an interpreter (see Chapter 12). Other urgent matters that cannot be neglected include finding competent legal counsel, procuring health care coverage, finding shelter and other basic necessities, and, for some patients, securing a work permit.

Adopt a respectful, nonjudgmental clinical stance. The temptation among many clinicians, when the language, culture, and religion of a patient are different from those of the treating clinician, is to assert the supremacy of the psychiatric model in the assessment and treatment of mental disorder. The complexity of the patient's experience, including their cultural idioms of distress and modes of illness experience, can be simplified by mapping them onto the signs and symptoms of specific diagnostic entities. However, straining to fit every patient with severe mental illness into the neatly demarcated categories and rubrics of psychiatry ignores much potentially vital clinical information that is associated with culturally distinctive symptoms, idioms, and explanations. Careful exploration of the patient's and family's own understanding of psychiatric symptoms and their efforts to deal with distress through culturally based coping strategies or various forms of healing practice will convey respect for the patient and their family, building trust and a working alliance, which can improve treatment adherence and clinical outcomes. In contrast, disinterest, excessive criticism, or outright dismissal of patients' alternative explanations, coping strategies, and uses of complementary or traditional treatments will risk polarization, alienation, and breakdown of the alliance, with discontinuation of treatment.

Sometimes patients or their families may reveal explanations of symptoms that strike the clinician as wrong, absurd, or even harmful. Suspending judgment long enough to understand the personal and social meaning of these explanations and their relationship to broader ethnocultural values and perspectives may be essential to maintaining a therapeutic relationship and influencing the patient's care. Traditional and alternative therapies should not be dismissed out of hand, but should be discussed and explored before endorsing or discouraging them as part of the patient's treatment. Care should be taken to show respect and genuine curiosity in relation to religious beliefs and practices of patients with mental disorders and their families so that appropriate community supports may be uncovered and mobilized. Religious communities are far more likely to be helpful resources than they are to conflict with psychiatric care, although some degree of mutual suspicion between psychiatric and traditional practitioners is common. The wise clinician will recognize that culture gives contextual meaning to symptoms, and understanding these meanings opens the way to negotiate bridges between worldviews or modes of coexistence, rather than conquering, colonizing, or converting the other to the viewpoint of biomedicine and psychiatry. In patient-centered care, the aim is shared decision-making in which appropriate treatments are offered rather than imposed and patients remain active partners in their own care and recovery.

Recognize that patients and families are usually trying the best they can, even when their efforts seem ill-informed or ineffectual. Barriers to mental health care arise when immigrants and refugees unwittingly seek help, or conduct themselves, in ways that may not be generally accepted in their new country. Examples include missing appointments or arriving late for appointments; not understanding the purpose of the consultation; forgetting to obtain medical reports, insurance forms, or other important papers; bringing small children along to the evaluation with no one to tend them; refusing to allow the interpreter into the consultation; insisting on speaking limited

English rather than speaking through the available interpreter; and refusing to divulge key information for fear that it will not be kept in confidence. All of these challenges to clinical and bureaucratic routines can be understood in relation to divergent culturally based realities and expectations, and they should not be too readily interpreted as evidence of a lack of motivation, interest, or engagement in treatment. Maintaining a respectful, sympathetic attitude toward the social predicaments of minorities, immigrants and refugees will go a long way toward gaining their trust. Most problems can be resolved, if given sufficient time and attention by sympathetic clinicians who adopt a flexible stance, within the health care system.

Appreciate that recovery will take place through understanding and respect. The assignment of psychiatric diagnoses is not only dependent on the symptoms elicited from patients during the clinical evaluation, but also on the assumptions and biases of the clinician. There is evidence for systematic biases in diagnosis due to racial stereotypes and other factors (Adeponle, Thombs, Groleau, Jarvis & Kirmayer, 2012). When working with patients from racialized groups, migrants, and other minorities with severe mental illness, caution should be the rule to avoid hasty decisions that risk misdiagnosis and inappropriate treatment. By taking the time to work with professional interpreters, and by making an effort to understand the everyday social predicaments of patients from marginalized, racialized, and other minority groups, the clinician can promote trust, respect, and positive therapeutic alliance that will allow the best possible clinical outcomes. The collaboration of family and community are essential to recovery from mental illness throughout the world, and their perspectives should be engaged to insure that patients receive appropriate support and maximize avenues to social reintegration after discharge from the hospital (Adeponle, Whitley, & Kirmayer, 2012). True recovery then will be possible as alternate explanations of illness enter the clinical dialogue and the use of the range of culturally consonant coping strategies and forms of healing,

Table 14.2 Strategies to address the constraints on cultural consultations in hospital settings

	Time pressure	Physical space	Interpreters	Severe illness
Before the consultation	Clarify when the patient is due to be discharged Be clear about when the cultural consultation can realistically be done	Clarify where the consultation will take place Request a quiet room where the evaluation can proceed in an unhurried and private manner	Explore every available resource to insure that a professional interpreter will be present, if needed	Thoroughly review the patient's chart to map the timeline of past diagnoses and treatments and reconsider the rationale for specific diagnoses and interventions
During the consultation	If needed, ask the treatment team if the patient may be kept in hospital for a few more days to allow completion of the evaluation	Make every effort to ensure the patient's comfort Make certain the cultural consultation team feels safe	Make the interpreter an integral part of the cultural consultation team	Follow the lead of the patient regarding the pace and depth of the inquiry and limit the duration of the interview accordingly
After the consultation	Comment in the report on the effect of time constraints on the consultation	Comment in the report on the effect of the physical space on the interview process	Comment in the report on how the presence (or lack) of a professional interpreter affected the cultural consultation	Comment in the report on how the severity of the patient's symptoms influenced the cultural consultation

some of which may fall outside the traditional purview of psychiatry and medicine, are given due consideration.

Conclusion

Cultural consultations in hospital settings may be especially difficult to carry out because of time constraints, confined or awkward interviewing space, lack of language interpreters, and the severity of psychiatric illness in hospitalized patients. Table 14.2 summarizes strategies to address some of the constraints of the hospital setting.

Given the time pressure inherent to emergency care, basic elements of cultural consultation, including the use of language interpreters and culture brokers, may be difficult to implement systematically. Hence, in the emergency department, the clinician may need to use generic strategies of inquiry to achieve initial crisis intervention while opening the door to more systematic evaluation at a later date.

Inpatient services, on the other hand, although lacking in privacy and preoccupied by the dis-

charge of patients, may allow a more systematic approach to the assessment of cultural factors in the diagnosis and treatment of patients. Inpatient hospitalization typically lasts for days or weeks, so that a cultural consultation team may have sufficient time to make a contribution. Hospital admission opens the opportunity for repeated meetings with the patient. Family or community members may be brought to provide additional information or contribute to discharge treatment planning. Successful consultation with inpatients requires close collaboration with the treatment team. Indeed, a systemic approach that understands the reasons for referral and impasses in treatment as arising from interactions between the patient and the treatment team may offer fresh insights and possibilities for intervention.

While the challenges of cultural consultation in hospital settings are formidable, even minor interventions can significantly influence patient diagnosis, care, and outcome. Untying the Gordian knot of cultural consultation in hospital settings is possible if the consultant adopts a patient, flexible attitude in the face of challenging diversity.

References

Adeponle, A., Groleau, D., Jarvis, G. E., & Kirmayer, L. J. (Submitted). Clinician reasoning in the use of the cultural formulation to resolve uncertainty in the diagnosis of psychosis.

Adeponle, A., Thombs, B., Groleau, D., Jarvis, G. E., & Kirmayer, L. J. (2012). Using the cultural formulation to resolve uncertainty in diagnosis of psychosis among ethnoculturally diverse patients. *Psychiatric Services, 63*(2), 147–153.

Adeponle, A. B., Whitley, R., & Kirmayer, L. J. (2012). Cultural contexts and constructions of recovery. In A. Rudnick (Ed.), *Recovery of people with mental illness: Philosophical and related perspectives* (pp. 109–132). New York, NY: Oxford University Press.

Blom, J. D., & Sommer, I. E. C. (2012). Hallucinations of bodily sensation. In J. D. Blom & I. E. C. Sommer (Eds.), *Hallucinations: Research and practice* (pp. 157–165). New York, NY: Springer.

Cantor-Graae, E., & Selten, J.-P. (2005). Schizophrenia and migration: A meta-analysis and review. *The American Journal of Psychiatry, 162*(1), 12–24.

Cohen, A., Patel, V., Thara, R., & Gureje, O. (2008). Questioning and axiom: Better prognosis for schizophrenia in the developing world? *Schizophrenia Bulletin, 34*(2), 229–244.

Fearon, P., Kirkbride, J. B., Morgan, C., Dazzan, P., Morgan, K., Lloyd, T., et al. (2006). Incidence of schizophrenia and other psychoses in ethnic minority groups: Results from the MRC AESOP study. *Psychological Medicine, 36*, 1541–1550.

Freudenmann, R. W., & Lepping, P. (2009). Delusional infestation. *Clinical Microbiology Review, 22*(4), 690–732.

Gouvernement du Québec. (2007). *Recommandations des coroners: Recherche avancée.* Quebec, Canada: Gouvernement du Quebec. Retrieved from http://www.coroner.gouv.qc.ca

Groleau, D., & Kirmayer, L. J. (2004). Sociosomatic theory in Vietnamese immigrants' narratives of distress. *Anthropology & Medicine, 11*(2), 117–133.

Hamner, M. B. (2011). Psychotic symptoms in posttraumatic stress disorder. *Journal of Lifelong Learning in Psychiatry, 9*(3), 278–285.

Harrison, G., Hopper, K., Craig, T., Laska, E., Siegel, C., Wanderling, J., et al. (2001). Recovery from psychotic illness: A 15- and 25-year international follow-up study. *The British Journal of Psychiatry, 178*, 506–517.

Hopper, K., Harrison, G., & Wanderling, J. A. (2007). An overview of course and outcome in ISoS. In K. Hopper, G. Harrison, A. Janca, & N. Sartorius (Eds.), *Recovery from schizophrenia: An international perspective*. New York, NY: Oxford University Press.

Hutchinson, G., & Haasen, C. (2004). Migration and schizophrenia: The challenges for European psychiatry and implications for the future. *Social Psychiatry and Psychiatric Epidemiology, 39*(5), 350–370.

Jablensky, A., Sartorius, N., Ernberg, G., Anker, M., Korten, A., Cooper, J. E., et al. (1992). Schizophrenia: Manifestations, incidence and course in different cultures: A World Health Organization ten-country study. *Psychological Medicine, Monograph Suppl*, 20.

Jack, D. C., & Ali, A. (Eds.). (2010). *Silencing the self across cultures: Depression and gender in the social world*. Oxford, England: Oxford University Press.

Jacobs, E. A., Sadowski, L. S., & Rathouz, P. J. (2007). The impact of an enhanced interpreter service intervention on hospital costs and patient satisfaction. *Journal of General Internal Medicine, 22*(Suppl 2), 306–311.

Jarvis, G. E. (2007). The social causes of psychosis in North American psychiatry: a review of a disappearing literature. *Canadian Journal of Psychiatry, 52*(5), 287–294.

Jarvis, G. E. (2008). Changing psychiatric perception of African Americans with psychosis. *European Journal of American Culture, 27*(3), 227–252.

Kilcommons, A. M., & Morrison, A. P. (2005). Relationships between trauma and psychosis: An exploration of cognitive and dissociative factors. *Acta Psychiatrica Scandinavica, 112*, 351–359.

Kirkbride, J. B., Barker, D., Cowden, R., Stamps, R., Yang, M., Jone, P. B., et al. (2008). Psychoses, ethnicity and socio-economic status. *The British Journal of Psychiatry, 193*, 18–24.

Kirkbride, J. B., Fearon, P., Morgan, C., Dazzan, P., Morgan, K., Tarrant, J., et al. (2006). Heterogeneity in incidence rates of schizophrenia and other psychotic syndromes: Findings from the 3-center AESOP study. *Archives of General Psychiatry, 63*, 250–258.

Kirmayer, L. J. (1988). Mind and body as metaphors: Hidden values in biomedicine. In M. Lock & D. Gordon (Eds.), *Biomedicine examined* (pp. 57–92). Dordrecht, Netherlands: Kluwer.

Kirmayer, L. J., & Santhanam, R. (2001). The anthropology of hysteria. In P. W. Halligan, C. Bass, & J. C. Marshall (Eds.), *Contemporary approaches to the study of hysteria: Clinical and theoretical perspectives* (pp. 251–270). Oxford, England: Oxford University Press.

Kroll, J., Yusuf, A. I., & Fujiwara, K. (2011). Psychoses, PTSD, and depression in Somali refugees in Minnesota. *Social Psychiatry and Psychiatric Epidemiology, 46*, 481–493.

Lettich, L. (2004). Culture and the psychiatric emergency service. In W. S. Tseng & J. Streltzer (Eds.), *Cultural competence in clinical psychiatry* (pp. 53–65). Arlington, VA: American Psychiatric Publishing.

Lu, F. G. (2004). Culture and inpatient psychiatry. In W. S. Tseng & J. Streltzer (Eds.), *Cultural competence in clinical psychiatry* (pp. 21–36). Arlington, VA: American Psychiatric Publishing.

Marsella, A.J. (1988). Cross-cultural research on severe mental disorders: issues and findings. *Acta Psychiatrica Scandinavica, Suppl, 344*, 7–22.

Miresco, M. J., & Kirmayer, L. J. (2006). The persistence of mind-brain dualism in psychiatric reasoning about clinical scenarios. *The American Journal of Psychiatry, 163*(5), 913–918.

Mizrahi, T. (1985). Getting rid of patients: Contradictions in the socialisation of internists to the doctor-patient relationship. *Sociology of Health & Illness, 7*(2), 214–235.

Morgan, C., McKenzie, K., & Fearon, P. (2008). *Society and psychosis*. New York, NY: Cambridge University Press.

Mueser, K. T., & Rosenberg, S. D. (2003). Editorial: Treating the trauma of first episode psychosis: A PTSD perspective. *Journal of Mental Health, 12*(2), 103–108.

Rhodes, L. A. (1991). *Emptying beds: The work of an emergency psychiatric unit*. Berkeley, CA: University of California Press.

Satzewich, V. (2011). *Racism in Canada*. Don Mills, Toronto, Canada: Oxford University Press.

Seedat, S., Stein, M. B., Oosthuizen, P. P., Emsley, R. A., & Stein, D. J. (2003). Linking posttraumatic stress dis-

order and psychosis: A look at epidemiology, phenomenology, and treatment. *The Journal of Nervous and Mental Disease, 191*(10), 675–681.

Seligman, R., & Kirmayer, L. J. (2008). Dissociative experience and cultural neuroscience: Narrative, metaphor and mechanism. *Culture, Medicine and Psychiatry, 32*(1), 31–64.

Sentell, T., Shumway, M., & Snowden, L. (2007). Access to mental health treatment by English language proficiency and race/ethnicity. *Journal of General Internal Medicine, 22*(Suppl 2), 289–293.

Wolf, E. J., Lunney, C. A., Miller, M. W., Resick, P. A., Friedman, M. J., & Schnurr, P. P. (2012). The dissociative subtype of PTSD: A replication and extension. *Depression and Anxiety, 29*, 679–688.

World Health Organization. (1973). *The international pilot study of schizophrenia* (Vol. 1). Geneva, Switzerland: WHO.

Cultural Consultation in Medical Settings

15

Melissa Dominicé Dao and Laurence J. Kirmayer

Clinicians working in general medical settings encounter many patients whose linguistic and cultural backgrounds are relevant to their care. Clinicians may attribute difficulties in communication, assessment, treatment negotiation or adherence to cultural factors and request a cultural consultation if this service is available. Carrying out cultural consultations in general medicine may differ in some respects from work in psychiatric settings. In this chapter, we describe some common issues and considerations in cultural consultation in general hospital and outpatient general medicine settings based on our experiences with cultural consultation services in Montreal and Geneva.

In some respects, cultural consultation is similar to other forms of consultation in medicine offered by cardiologists, endocrinologist, neurologists and many other specialists

M. Dominicé Dao, M.D., M.Sc. (✉)
Département de Médecine Communautaire, de Premier Recours et des Urgences, Consultation Transculturelle, Service de Médecine de Premier Recours, Hôpitaux Universitaires de Genève, 4, rue Gabrielle-Perret-Gentil, 1211 Genève 14, Switzerland
e-mail: melissa.dominice@hcuge.ch

L.J. Kirmayer, M.D.
Culture and Mental Health Research Unit, Institute of Community and Family Psychiatry, Jewish General Hospital, 4333 Cote Ste Catherine Road, Montreal, QC, Canada H3T 1E4
e-mail: laurence.kirmayer@mcgill.ca

(Kirmayer, Groleau, Guzder, Blake, & Jarvis, 2003). General internists and primary care physicians are accustomed to asking specialists for advice, assessment and help with the treatment of patients with complex medical problems. The consultant may simply discuss the case with the referring clinician, undertake comprehensive assessment and treatment planning, follow the patient with the referring clinician (in a form of collaborative care) or entirely take over management of the case when the problems are especially complex and/or focussed on one organ system. In hospital settings, psychiatric consultants may have liaison roles with specific units, teams or programs to provide ongoing consultation, training and support (Amos & Robinson, 2010; Stern, 2010).

Despite the familiarity of the consultation process, implementing cultural consultation in general medical settings poses unique challenges. Cultural consultation relies on the referring clinician's ability to recognise the need for cultural expertise. While physicians are trained to identify problems for which specific types of medical expertise are relevant, they usually are much less familiar with the indications for cultural consultation. Indeed, primary care physicians' conceptualizations of culture may be vague or based on common stereotypes of race and ethnicity (Rosenberg, Kirmayer, Xenocostas, Dao, & Loignon, 2007). As with referrals to any specialized service, consultation requests may sometimes mask more basic difficulties in clinical

L.J. Kirmayer et al. (eds.), *Cultural Consultation: Encountering the Other in Mental Health Care*, International and Cultural Psychology, DOI 10.1007/978-1-4614-7615-3_15,
© Springer Science+Business Media New York 2014

management or the need for resources that are scarce or difficult to find. In addition to the explicit reasons for referral, as the case unfolds, additional reasons for the consultation may emerge, including linguistic barriers, economic problems, social or administrative difficulties, patient mistrust of health professionals, institutional barriers, experiences of discrimination and untreated psychiatric conditions.

Medical diagnosis relies on identifying clusters of physical symptoms and signs and measuring biological markers or parameters with laboratory tests. Diagnosis then leads to specific treatment based on scientific evidence and expert consensus. There is a tacit assumption that the processes of diagnosis and treatment, as well as the underlying mechanisms of disease progression and treatment response, are independent of cultural factors (Taylor, 2003). While there is recognition of some variation of diseases in specific populations, this is generally understood in terms of genetic variation or environmental exposures to toxins or infectious agents. Perhaps because of this assumption of universality, cultural consultation requests in general medicine usually do not focus on diagnostic issues but tend to involve patients with very complex management issues. When explicitly cultural issues arise, these are often related to clinicians' difficulties applying the usual biomedical approach to care for the patient (Wachtler, Brorsson, & Troein, 2006). The consultation request may request help in "taking care of the cultural problem," with the assumption that once culture is dealt with, conventional biomedical knowledge will be sufficient to guide clinical care. The consultant, on the other hand, may see the need to more thoroughly rethink the nature of the patient's diagnoses and treatment. In such circumstances, the agendas of the cultural consultant and the referring physician may diverge and will need to be renegotiated. In any case, in general medicine settings, the cultural consultant acts in much the same way as a liaison consultant, keeping in mind that his main client is the referring clinician rather than the patient. The aim is to support the clinician and transfer knowledge and skills to enhance the referring clinician's capacity to provide appropriate care. Although some patients may view the consultant as a co-therapist, this is not the intended role. Rather, the cultural consultant aims to assist the referring physician in providing appropriate care by providing cultural information to contextualise the patient's problems and clinical strategies for intervention through a didactic model using the cultural formulation.

At the Montreal CCS, referring clinicians address consultation requests to an administrative coordinator, who in turn organizes the meeting between the patient, a cultural consultant and a culture broker with knowledge of the patient's cultural background and community. After one or several meetings with the patient, initial recommendations are given to the referring clinician. The referring clinician is then invited to attend the CCS multidisciplinary team meeting to further discuss the case and receive recommendations. Most clinicians are not able to attend these case conferences because of their own busy schedules, but when the case is particularly challenging, a member of the primary care team may attend. After the case conference, a written report detailing the cultural evaluation and the recommendations is prepared and sent to the referring clinician. About half of the requests for consultation come from hospital-based clinics but only about 10 % are from medical inpatient services.

At the Geneva University Hospitals (HUG), in Switzerland, a transcultural consultation service (TCS) was initiated in 2007 by the first author, a physician specialized in internal medicine and trained in cultural psychiatry, with the collaboration of a medical anthropologist, also responsible for coordinating interpreter services at the HUG (Dominicé Dao, 2009). The structure of the TCS was based on the Montreal CCS model. Some adaptations were made to fit the local setting, guided by the results of a formative research study investigating the needs of health care workers at the HUG for assistance with difficulties related to intercultural work.

Geneva has a population of about 470,000, including 40 % non-Swiss residents, the majority with long-term working permits, and a much smaller proportion of short-term international civil servants, and still smaller groups of asylum seekers and undocumented workers (Office Cantonal de la Statistique, Genève, 2012; http://www.ge.ch/statistique Bureau d'Intégration des Etrangers, 2003). Although there is a historical tradition of receiving immigrants—Geneva has had more than 30 % of foreigners for over four centuries—the federal immigration policies have often been quite restrictive. Currently, foreigners come from about 190 countries; though 75 % come from European nations, an increasing proportion are non-European immigrants.

The HUG, one of five university hospital centers in Switzerland, includes a network of eight hospitals, providing 700,000 hospital days and 900,000 outpatient consultations in 2011 (HUG, Facts and Figures of HUG, 2012). It is the only public hospital network in Geneva and receives joint financing by state subsidies and fee for service from mandatory private health insurance. Cultural diversity is strongly represented both in staff and patients, with 51 % of each group being foreigners (HUG, Réseau santé pour tous, 2012) and 39 % of patients and 18 % of staff speaking a first language other than French (Hudelson, P. Enquête de prise en charge des patients migrants, 2010 (unpublished); Données linguistiques HUG, 2012 (unpublished)). In the early 1990s, the HUG introduced interpreter services free of charge for patients (Bischoff, Tonnerre, Eytan, Bernstein, & Loutan, 1999; Loutan, Farinelli, & Pampallona, 1999). The HUG also offers facilitated access to care to specific underserved populations; consultation services for asylum seekers and for undocumented migrants were established in 1993 and 1996, respectively. There has been little institutional attention given to culture per se at the HUG, but there have been several initiatives by individuals. A pioneer consultation program in cultural psychiatry was created in 1985 by Dr. Jacques Arpin but was discontinued after his departure from the HUG. Since 2008, there has been an ethno-psychoanalysis consultation program in the Department of Child and Adolescent Health.

The Geneva TCS comprises three frontline consultants: a physician (an internal medicine specialist, trained in cultural psychiatry), a medical anthropologist and a nurse specialized in community health care. A small pool of culture brokers has been identified, in the community, among hospital interpreters and hospital personnel. Culture brokers bring their expertise to the consultation, either during the evaluation process or during the case discussion. Cases are discussed twice monthly with a multidisciplinary team of health professionals working closely with immigrant patients in Geneva. The composition of this group has varied over time and has included institutional and private psychiatrists, pediatric nurses, family doctors, a public health specialist, a sociologist and a chaplain. The referring clinician is encouraged to attend the case conference.

Because of the frequent co-occurrence of cultural and psychiatric issues, several experienced psychiatrists were included in the multidisciplinary team. The cultural consultation reports prepared by the TCS are integrated in the patient's electronic medical record at the HUG, as with other specialist consultation reports. This integration of the report in the medical record allows for the patient's personal and cultural information to be available to all hospital clinicians as needed. Exceptions to this procedure are made for confidential information about sensitive issues that the patient does not wish to reveal openly (e.g., rape, family secrets). Careful attention is given to avoid stereotyping the patient's culture and to focus attention on the patient's unique predicament. Clinicians appreciate being able to go back and read the report, especially with chronic patients who are often readmitted. Some clinicians have found the report long, and we now include a summary of key points at the end.

In Geneva, an analysis of the first 5 years of activity (2007–2011) revealed that the vast majority of consultation requests (80 %) were made by physicians, with the remaining requests coming from nurses, social workers and psychologists. The Department of Internal Medicine and the Department of Community Medicine and Primary Care requested two-thirds of the TCS consultations. Fifty-eight percent of consultations were made for hospitalized patients. In Montreal, of the patients referred to the CCS from medical wards or outpatient clinics, about 1/3 were referred by family physicians or GPs, 1/3 by nurses and 20 % from other medical practitioners. The remaining 20 % were referred by social workers or mental health professionals (psychiatrists and psychologists). Fully 77 % of referrals were labelled urgent or ASAP. The most common explicit reasons for referral were help in clarifying diagnosis (60 %), treatment planning (60 %), clinician patient communication (25 %), issues related to immigration or refugee claim (12 %) and treatment adherence (8 %). An interpreter was requested by the referring clinician in 57 % of cases and one had been used in the past in 22 % of cases.

In Geneva, the three most frequent reasons for referral were (1) difficulties understanding patients' explanatory models, expectations or comprehension of disease; (2) patient refusal of an intervention or nonadherence to treatment; and (3) the referring clinician's need for more knowledge about social and cultural factors influencing the case. Conflicts with patients or patients' families, which the referring clinician attributed to cultural issues, were also a frequent reason for referral. Diagnostic issues, whether absence of or unclear diagnosis, were less frequent reasons for referral, probably related to the fact that, unlike the Montreal CCS, the Geneva TCS is not geared toward providing psychiatric evaluations.

The cases referred to the TCS often involved wider issues that made their clinical management especially challenging, such as the presence of violence or a life-threatening illness, unresolved conflicts within the health care team itself or institutional barriers to care. These were not directly related to cultural differences between the patient and health care provider but interacted with social and cultural contextual issues. The consequences for the clinician of this complexity included feelings of distress, frustration, incompetence, helplessness and exhaustion. These emotions sometimes led clinicians to blame or discredit patients or to overemphasize cultural factors as a defence against the threat to their professional competence (Cohen-Emerique & Hohl, 2004; Leanza, 2005).

Difficulty Understanding the Patient's Explanatory Model

A very common reason for referral emerges from the referring clinician's impression that the patient's explanatory model of illness differs from the physician's biomedical paradigm, whether in terms of causes and consequences of illness, or expectations for health care and appropriate treatment. The origins and implications of these differing explanatory models have been the focus of much research in clinically applied medical anthropology (Cooper, Harding, Mullen, & O'Donnell, 2012; Dein, 2004; Helman, 1985; Kleinman, Eisenberg, & Good, 1978; Weiss & Somma, 2007; Weller, Baer, de Alba, Garcia, & Salcedo Rocha, 2012).

Case Vignette 15-1

Souleymane was a young Muslim man from Senegal who was perfectly fluent in French and finishing his Masters' degree in microbiology at a local university. He had been hospitalized with pulmonary tuberculosis without improvement despite 3 weeks of antibiotics. The infectious disease team believed his TB could be a sign of HIV co-infection, but Souleymane refused HIV testing, arguing that his long-term girlfriend tested negative and that he therefore could not possibly have the disease. He also indicated that his circumcision was a preventive factor against catching HIV and, finally, that he could tell if someone was infected by HIV. These statements shocked the health care team: they thought Souleymane would share their biomedical model of disease in light of his extensive scientific training. They were also concerned because the patient had had no visits from family or friends over the past 3 weeks of hospitalization and believed that he was quite distressed by this despite his denial.

(continued)

During the TCS evaluation, Souleymane emphasized that he belonged to a privileged social stratum in his country of origin. He raised this because it was his impression that the team stereotyped all Africans as poor and uneducated. He believed that he had caught tuberculosis through lab work with infected specimens instead of in his country of origin, as none of his relatives had been infected. He also felt that the team's hypothesis that he might have HIV was evidence of prejudice against Africans. He noted, accurately, that epidemiological data indicated that the prevalence of HIV in his country was only 1 %—a rate identical to that in Switzerland. The interview revealed that the patient's use of the biomedical model, acquired through his studies, coexisted with other explanatory models. While he recognized and employed the microbiological model of tuberculosis, he also stated that "illness was the will of God." The TCS team explored with him the possibility that he might be the target of jealousy because of his enviable socioeconomic position. In many African traditions, such envy can provoke sorcery attacks leading to illness. In fact, this was his mother's explanation for his illness; Souleymane himself, though, was not sure whether to believe it. He stated that after having lived a third of his life in Europe, he had lost familiarity with this type of traditional explanation. However, he acknowledged he was preoccupied with this possibility and was having frequent nightmares related to this fear.

He had shared the tuberculosis diagnosis with his family by telephone, but he had not informed his local friends and colleagues because he feared the stigma attached to this disease. He was very reluctant to have the HIV test because of his fear that a documented positive test would eliminate his chances of finding a job, which was essential in order to support his family.

Souleymane's story illustrates a number of issues that may provoke negative attitudes in the health care team: his rejection of conventional procedures and intervention, the divergence of his explanatory model of illness from biomedical models (despite his extensive education in biomedical principles), visible minority status, stereotypes about the high prevalence of HIV in Africans and the symbolic impact of the quarantine of a contagious patient. The combination of these factors complicated the relationship with the medical team. Indeed, Souleymane's overt mistrust of the team may have been triggered by his accurate perception of the team's negative attitudes.

Increased understanding of the patient's perspective obtained through the consultation helped the team to tolerate his refusal and diminished their stereotyping. The consultant proposed a strategy—conducting an anonymous HIV test (a standard procedure at the outpatient clinic)—which allowed the patient to control information about his HIV status. In addition, the patient's family in Senegal performed a number of traditional rituals to counteract a possible curse. The patient slowly improved and was discharged without the team learning of his HIV status. As in many cultural consultations, a crucial effect of the intervention was to avoid a polarized "either/or" situation in order to help the referring team maintain a working alliance with the patient.

Treatment Refusal and Nonadherence

Adherence to treatment is influenced by many factors including patients' own explanatory models and their understanding and acceptance of the biomedical explanation and the clinician's authority. However, adherence also reflects lifestyle, habit, routines, commitments and identities that must be renegotiated particularly with severe, chronic or life-threatening illness (Groleau, Whitley, Lesperance, & Kirmayer, 2010). Treatment refusal or nonadherence to treatment recommendations, therefore, may be related to differences in explanatory models of illness, but these differences are often intermixed with other issues such as linguistic barriers, social stressors, economic difficulties or familial roles and authority in decision-making.

Case Vignette 15-2

A request was made by the inpatient internal medicine team to evaluate Lindita, a young unmarried woman from Kosovo who was hospitalized for incapacitating dyspnea. The workup showed that she was suffering from severe arterial pulmonary hypertension with no identifiable cause. The consultation request was made because the patient refused to take the anticoagulant medication prescribed by the pulmonary specialist. The treatment team was also worried because neither Lindita nor her family would give up the idea of a future pregnancy, despite perinatal mortality rates estimated as high as 40 % in this condition. One of the pulmonary specialists feared that Lindita would disregard their medical advice and get pregnant anyway. The question to the TCS was whether cultural factors were present that influenced the patient's understanding of the diagnosis and acceptance of treatment recommendations. The medical intern in charge on the ward believed that the team's difficulties were related to the fact that Lindita's culture of origin greatly valued motherhood. The team expected the TCS to provide them with cultural information and alternative strategies to better manage the case.

Although Lindita was quite fluent in French, she had little formal education and could read neither French nor Albanian. She did not understand the nature of this disease and had a simple, mechanistic view of her body, thinking that "broken parts can be fixed." She did understand and agreed she should not get pregnant while on the medication but feared that the teratogenic effects of taking medication would be permanent, even if she eventually stopped taking the medication. Her family was extremely worried about her future marriage prospects and supported her refusal to initiate treatment. Organizing meetings between the extended family and the medical team in the presence of an interpreter,

guiding the medical team on how to deliver simplified explanations of her disease, and focusing on the illness and the threat it posed to Lindita's health, rather than on the conflict around the treatment, helped the team, the patient and her family to negotiate common treatment goals.

In the case of Lindita, the medical team was confronted with a patient who refused to take the medication prescribed and to adhere to medical recommendations to avoid pregnancy. They did not mention some of the other obviously important issues: the emotional impact of the recent diagnosis of a severe chronic, debilitating condition in a young, previously healthy woman and the difficulties the patient and her family had accepting this diagnosis and planning and providing for her future. As with many requests for cultural consultation, the referring team hoped for a cultural solution for what was, in fact, a clinical dilemma frequently encountered with patients from any background. In such cases, it may be unclear whether it is the difficult situation itself that brings clinicians to consider the cultural difference or if the cultural differences really add a layer of complexity to an already challenging situation.

In this vignette, the cultural evaluation identified several important issues that contributed to the patient's apparent non-adherence to treatment: linguistic barriers in communicating with the patient and her family, their lack of knowledge of biomedicine and bodily anatomy, strong cultural and family values surrounding marriage and fertility and group rather than individual decision-making. In many cases, the cultural formulation uncovers a divergence of explanatory models of illness between patient and health care providers (Bhui & Bhugra, 2004). Addressing divergent explanatory models is not simply a matter of education or health literacy. Explanatory models of illness are often embedded in or closely linked to wider personal and social issues that must be considered if medical information is to be conveyed in ways that are intelligible and credible to the patient and effective in changing health behavior.

Situations in which patients refuse treatment or other aspects of care are frequent reasons for cultural consultation. The referring team may have an almost magical wish that the cultural consultant will change the patient's mind. The consultant then must redefine his role as providing information that will allow a broader perspective and better understanding of the patient. Sometimes alternative strategies can be found to reach the clinician's goal of behavioral change, while in other cases an alternative goal must be negotiated.

Case Vignette 15-3

Severin, a 45-year-old man from Angola, who had left his country 10 years ago because of the civil war, had been diagnosed with HIV 4 years earlier. He had taken antiretroviral (ARV) therapy regularly until 1 year ago when he stopped taking it in the context of economic difficulties paying for his health insurance. His kidney function had declined to the point where he was in terminal renal insufficiency, for which he was admitted to hospital. The nephrologists wanted to start dialysis, but he flatly refused. He questioned the authority of the physicians, declaring that he was ready to resume taking ARVs, which he believed would undoubtedly improve his kidney function enough to avoid dialysis. The medical team requested a TCS consultation to "convince the patient to start dialysis." The consultant renegotiated the initial goal as an exploration of the patient's perspective behind the refusal.

Severin understood his medical situation quite well and acknowledged the prospect of his dying due to kidney failure in the absence of treatment. There was no language barrier. He had searched the Internet for further information and discussed the issues with his cousin who was a physician. However, he maintained an extremely optimistic view, grounded in his Christian faith which gave him hope and strength. He also pointed out that he was highly educated and held a university degree. He believed that if he took the ARV medication regularly, his kidney function would improve, arguing that he already felt better after 1 week of therapy (and indeed his blood chemistry results were improved). He gave several examples of miraculous recoveries of relatives with HIV in Africa. He also gave the example of his father, who suffered all his life from a severe chronic condition, which he believed to be inflicted by sorcery and nevertheless died of old age. Severin evaded our questions about whether sorcery could have anything to do with his own illness. He considered the doctors' attitude as paternalistic and dismissive of his faith and his university education. He sensed, quite accurately, that they did not trust that he would comply with his medication. His mother and siblings, who were continuously present during the hospitalization, supported his decision to not start dialysis. Presented with different possible outcome scenarios, he agreed that if things got worse, he would reconsider dialysis.

Several issues were at stake in this patient's rejection of dialysis: general compliance issues in chronic illness, denial or minimization of his condition, positive prototypes of illness leading to expectations of good outcome, questions of authority in decision-making and possibly alternative explanatory models (although the patient was not keen to discuss sorcery and traditional treatments with the European doctors). Again, some of these issues are inherent to any treatment of a chronic condition; others are more specifically cultural, such as the weighing of medical authority against other sources of knowledge or experience. It was also evident that the patient suffered from his loss of socioeconomic status and lack of recognition of his educational attainment in Switzerland. Recommendations made to the team reflected these multiple issues. We suggested including the hospital chaplain in the patient's care and she became a major resource for the patient and the team. We encouraged the team to consider the patient a valid partner in clinical decision-making, recognizing his active role in information seeking, by proposing relevant sources to augment his knowledge of kidney failure and bringing him to visit the dialysis unit. The team collaborated with his family doctor and negotiated regular follow-up after his discharge. Despite initial improvement, several months later, after further worsening of his blood chemistry, he accepted dialysis.

Clinicians' Requests for Cultural Information

Often clinicians request cultural information about patients, with the hope that increased knowledge of cultural context will help them understand their patient. We are particularly attentive to these requests because they may raise several problematic issues. One is that clinicians tend to consider the patient as sole recipient of "culture", neglecting their own background which is taken for granted. There is a risk of "over-culturalizing" the patient or focusing on the "exotic". Another danger of providing cultural information about a certain group is that of stereotyping and generalizing aspects of culture which may not apply to the patient.

One task of the consultation, therefore, is to clarify which specific aspects of the patient's cultural background or current context are of interest to the referring clinicians and why they believe these factors might be relevant to the patient's situation. In place of an exclusive focus on the patient's cultural background, we then attempt to frame the problem in terms of interactions between the two equally legitimate cultural contexts of the patient and the health care team. Finally, we often bring to the attention of the clinician the importance of the culture of biomedicine and how their own assumptions or routines might contribute to the current difficulty. Of course we are careful to verify with the patient the pertinence of any general statements provided by the culture broker. Most of the time, the consultation sheds light on the patient's particular personal predicament, which takes precedence over more general cultural matters.

When similar clinical difficulties arise with patients from a certain background, the request to the TCS may concern a whole group of patients or a community. This is illustrated in the following vignette.

Case Vignette 15-4

The Division of Pneumology requested a consultation after identifying a cluster of tuberculosis cases in an immigrant community and recognizing that social relationships existed between several patients. They specifically wanted to understand this community in terms of demographics, socioeconomic background, access and barriers to care. They also wanted to determine if cultural factors constituted obstacles to efficient contact tracing procedures and what culturally congruent strategies could help to overcome any obstacles. (To avoid stigmatization of this community, it will not be named.)

The TCS provided detailed information about the profile of this specific community and identified several issues that likely played a role in the difficulties related to contact tracing. First, there was intense stigma attached to the diagnosis of tuberculosis, which was considered a "dirty and sinful disease" which would bring shame and social exclusion. There were also linguistic barriers due to patients' reluctance to work with interpreters because of confidentiality issues in a small community, so that patients and health care professionals both used a third language that neither was fluent in, which undermined mutual comprehension. Differences in communication style, i.e., the fact that bad news should traditionally be given in an oblique and indirect manner, further complicated the social worker's task, as she was asked to contact all potential contacts by telephone to invite them to receive tuberculosis testing. Patients found this unacceptable and thus did not give any names of contacts.

(continued)

The TCS also commented on community features that could enhance successful contact tracing and proposed a number of strategies to bypass some obstacles: working with professional interpreters; mediation through a neutral "middle man," which was the traditionally acceptable way to deliver bad news; using alternate sources to broadcast information about TB, e.g., bulletin boards in ethnic community shops; and open TB testing of respected community figures such as esteemed clergymen during religious celebrations.

In this case knowledge of the social dynamics of the community and more specific information about the meanings and stigma attached to TB were essential to providing useful consultation to guide a public health intervention (Tardin, Dominicé Dao, Ninet, & Janssens, 2009). In several other situations, transcultural consultation requests about a specific community or repeated consultations for the same issue in similar patients revealed structural problems in the care to these patients, in addition to salient cultural issues within the patients' community (Dominicé Dao et al., 2010).

Conflicts with Patients' Families

Although family medicine explicitly acknowledges the central role of the family in primary health care, much of Western medicine is rooted in individualistic notions of the person. The patient's body is seen as the locus of disease so that diagnosis can be made without systematic attention to social context. Moreover, because the patient is seen as an autonomous individual, ethical decisions can be made without considering the implications for family and community. As a result of this individualistic approach, families are sometimes marginalized in the delivery of care. Yet families are major sources of both stress and social support. In most parts of the world, families play a key role in guiding help-seeking and making decisions about health care.

Clinicians unfamiliar with these patterns of family involvement may find it difficult to understand the patient's predicament or negotiate effective and appropriate care.

Case Vignette 15-5

A consultation request was made by the rehabilitation clinic for Senait, an elderly widow from Eritrea with advanced metastatic cancer. The family would not allow the medical team to reveal the diagnosis to their mother. The patient spoke only Tigrinya and her daughter insisted on interpreting. The family was constantly present in the room, sleeping and eating with their mother. They were very reluctant to allow the administration of morphine but insisted that the nurses continue to bathe and dress Senait and get her out of bed every morning despite her obvious and intense pain. The team was distressed with this situation and was torn between the desire to respect the family's personal and cultural values and concern about not respecting local professional, ethical and legal rules and norms for informed consent and pain relief. Some nurses stated that they felt they were "torturing" the patient by following the family's requests.

The first action of the TCS consultant was to hold a meeting with the family with the collaboration of a trained interpreter. This allowed Senait to explain that, in the absence of her husband, she wished for her eldest sons to be told the diagnosis and to make all the decisions regarding her health, but did not wish for any direct information herself. The patient, her family and the culture broker recognized this as cultural norm. The presence of the interpreter allowed her to confirm that any mobilization of her body was increasingly painful and that the low dose of morphine was not providing her adequate relief. At this point in the interview, the eldest daughter described their mother as being confused, a claim which

(continued)

was not confirmed by the interpreter. After the family meeting, the interpreter explained that morphine was associated with worsening of one's condition and rapid death in the view of the local community.

This case presented many complex medical and social issues, including language barriers, end-of-life issues, authority for decision-making, denial of the severity of mother's illness by one daughter, differences in cultural representations of morphine and culture-related family dynamics that were unfamiliar to the health care team. Indeed, end-of-life and palliative care situations are often suffused with cultural issues involving core values and beliefs (Crawley, Marshall, Lo, & Koenig, 2002; Gysels et al., 2012). The work of the cultural consultation was to support the team who continued to provide thorough and sensitive care to the mother despite major cultural barriers with potential grounds for misunderstanding and conflict. The TCS consultant also validated the clinical team's concern with pain control and their right to refuse to perform interventions that would hurt the patient without adequate analgesia. Additional specific recommendations were to have regular encounters with the patient with an interpreter and to include her children in all decision-making meetings.

Social and Economic Contexts

While certain cultural issues are salient for clinicians treating medical patients, many important contextual factors remain unrecognized until uncovered in the process of cultural consultation. These include major social determinants of health, cultural values and practices that shape coping and help-seeking, concerns about the meaning and implications of illness and expectations for care.

A common issue encountered in cultural consultations for medical patients is the presence of major stressors in the patient's life or a very precarious social or economic context that

overshadows the current medical problem for the patient but that remains largely ignored by the clinician, such as in the following example.

Case Vignette 15-6

Rebecca, a 19-year-old woman born in Europe of immigrant parents from Rwanda, suffering from poorly controlled sickle-cell disease, was referred by her haematologist because he thought her nonadherence to medication was related to her cultural belief that her illness had to do with bewitchment. More materially, her lack of compliance over the previous year was due to lack of financial means to buy the medication. The increase of sickle-cell crises prevented her from working, thus leading to further financial loss. The forced fasting that followed her lack of money for food also brought on more sickle-cell crises. Regarding her bewitchment, she explained that when she was a child, her parents had brought her to Rwanda to receive traditional treatment; this had left her free of disease for almost 5 years. She wanted to try this treatment again, but didn't know how to access it, as she was not talking (or receiving any support) from her parents after a fight linked to their disapproval of her choice of life partner. In fact, her belief in traditional treatment did not conflict with her belief in medical treatment, which she regarded as effective. She acknowledged that she sometimes just became "tired of being sick and taking medication every day since childhood" and that she would just quit for several months at a time, although she realized the negative impact of these episodes.

Rebecca's hematologist had overlooked possible socioeconomic problems and focused on the most obvious cultural difference in illness explanations. Rather than a difference in treatment perspectives, however, the cultural consultation showed that from Rebecca's perspective there were multiple concurrent treatment alternatives, if only she had the means to access them. In addition to socioeconomic barriers, issues of dealing with a chronic disabling disease were also in the forefront. The TCS evaluation led to a referral to a social worker who intervened to help Rebecca access a number of government subsidies and referral to a primary care doctor specialized in youth medicine to work on broader issues of adapting to chronic illness and the developmental passage to adulthood.

Discrimination as Source of Communication Problems or Conflict

In many settings, it is difficult for clinicians and patients to talk explicitly about experiences of racism and discrimination. Although it is not surprising, therefore, that clinicians do not identify discrimination as a motive for consultation, issues related to racial, ethnic or religious discrimination may underlie requests in situations where health care providers feel that there are communication problems or conflict with a patient.

Case Vignette 15-7

The dialysis team made a request for a TCS consultation for Negasi, an Ethiopian man in his sixties, suffering from end-stage renal failure, who had been receiving dialysis 3 times a week for 3 years. The consultation request was made to understand why he seemed constantly unsatisfied with care, whereas the team considered that they had gone out of their way to help him. The nurses believed there was a gender issue and felt he treated them "like servants". When he began dialysis, he had no legal status in Switzerland or health insurance. The social worker had helped him access a temporary residence permit on humanitarian grounds, which gave him free access to health care, social benefits and housing. He spoke Amharic and some English, but no French.

The TCS consultant met with him twice, separately from the dialysis sessions, with both an interpreter and culture broker present. He complained that the nurses and orderlies did not listen to him or respond to his requests to change dirty sheets on his bed, help him cut his food as his right arm was tied to the bed, etc. A nurse had told him: "You should be happy that you get to stay in this country and be taken care of." His was very shocked by this statement, explaining that his culture commands respect toward and welcoming of foreigners. He thought the doctors did not pay enough attention to his symptoms, especially his exhaustion after the dialysis sessions. He believed he was being discriminated against because he was not yet on the transplant list, whereas newer patients were. He wished for a transplant in order to return to Ethiopia, and he feared being sent back to his country without access to dialysis. Exploration of his background revealed that he had come to Switzerland on business and had fallen sick rapidly, preventing his return to his country and to his family. He was very sad and demoralized by this separation and his loss of social status and was ashamed of his dire living conditions. The dialysis sessions exhausted him, making it difficult to attend French classes or find a job. He was worried because he could not fulfil his role as provider for his family. Furthermore, domestic tasks were new to him and he did not know how to cook. He was well integrated in the Ethiopian Orthodox community, from whom he received occasional support.

Feedback from the TCS evaluation to the dialysis team during a weekly multidisciplinary team meeting included a discussion on the everyday discrimination encountered by African patients, especially those without legal status and suffering from a serious chronic illness. The consultant pointed out how these experiences of

(continued)

discrimination might be internalized and lead the patient to misinterpret some of the team's actions as discriminatory. The consultant also relayed the patient's distress at the doubting of his migration narrative, when team members conjectured that his was a case of "medical tourism." There were contradictory opinions about his eligibility for the transplant list, and an active debate took place within the dialysis team because it was unclear whether his temporary permit allowed him to be put on the list. His lack of mastery of French also was considered a relative contraindication for transplantation listing, because it would make post-transplant follow-up more difficult. The consultant pointed out that medical interpreters were readily available, and that refusal to consider his eligibility would constitute a health care inequity. Ultimately, the head of the Division supported his enlisting for transplantation.

Several issues coexist in this complex situation. Paramount was the language barrier, especially with the nurses and orderlies who did not always speak English and had trouble communicating with the patient but also with the doctors as the patient's English did not allow full discussion of complex medical problems. There were obvious discriminatory reactions from some members of the team, probably exacerbated by language and cultural misunderstandings and by the context of recently enacted tougher immigration laws and political campaign messages by a nationalist party portraying asylum seekers as abusers of the system or even criminals. Differences in expectations about the roles of patient and health care workers also played a role. The "grey zone" of transplant list criteria put the doctors in the uncomfortable position of having to make health care rationing decisions that might have political overtones or implications. Finally, it became evident that an undiagnosed and untreated depressive disorder contributed to the patient's fatigue, as well as to the general clinical picture. The TCS consultant recommended that the dialysis team have regular interviews with interpreters present, arrange a formal evaluation for depression by the team psychiatrist, include a family doctor in his care to address both medical and social issues and ensure the patient participated actively in all major decisions regarding his health.

Diagnostic Issues

A number of cultural consultations in general medical settings involved patients that were initially referred for clarification of cultural issues but were found to have unrecognized or untreated mental illness, in particular depression or posttraumatic stress disorder. Related to the difficulties in diagnostic assessment and treatment were issues of cultural differences in the expression of affect, patient's representation of mental illness and their fear of stigmatization, availability and differential expectations of mental health care or clinician reluctance to discuss patient's traumatic history (Kirmayer, 2001). Because of the psychiatric setting of the Montreal CCS, issues of clarification of psychiatric diagnosis are more common there but also occur occasionally in the Geneva TCS. When this is the case, collaboration with consultation-liaison psychiatry is essential, as in the following case.

Case Vignette 15-8

Mahmoud and his 85-year-old mother Parvin were referred for a cultural consultation by their family doctor because of increased conflict between the two and Mahmoud's exhaustion in caring for his mother. The consultation question was whether personality disorder or dementia might explain the mother's difficult behavior. The TCS conducted two interviews with both the cultural consultant and the consultation-liaison psychiatrist present, as well as a Farsi interpreter and culture broker: the first interview with Mahmoud, the second one with Parvin alone and then with her son.

(continued)

Mahmoud came to Europe from Iran as a teenager to study and made his life there as a university professor. He was married to a Swiss woman and the father of four adult and independent children. After being widowed, Mahmoud's mother came from Iran to live with him. Conflict rapidly developed between his mother and his wife. The two women did not share a common language or culture, and communication between them relied on Mahmoud's translation. The situation had worsened since Parvin became physically entirely dependent upon her son and daughter-in-law for all aspects of her care including bathroom routines. He described his mother as always having what he considered to be a "very strong Persian character" which manifested in her accusing people of wrongdoing without any evidence and offering irrational opinions which, as a scientist, irritated him profoundly. He minimized her recent uninhibited behavior and paranoia as part of the same character traits. He appeared to deny the severity of his mother's illness and her imminent end of life. He was exhausted by the constant care he provided to his mother but also was overwhelmed by guilt and shame at the prospect of placing her in an institution, which was personally and culturally unacceptable. His marriage was jeopardized by this situation, which added further stress. His psychiatric evaluation revealed major depressive symptoms that warranted treatment.

Assessment of the mother revealed probable dementia with confusion, abnormal and uninhibited behavior, and loss of recent memory. She seemed nevertheless both aware and at peace with the idea that this was the end of her life.

Clarification of the mother's diagnosis helped the family doctor proceed with adequate follow-up care for Parvin and position himself clearly vis-à-vis her son and daughter-in-law. The consultation also helped the family doctor realise the severity of Mahmoud's depression, raising concern about possible worsening of this condition upon the mother's death. A long process of negotiation was initiated to help Mahmoud accept practical help for his mother and psychiatric help for himself and to focus on providing his mother with the best possible end of life. To accomplish this, the family doctor had to take into account the cultural obligation that children had to look after elders. This knowledge helped the physician offer relevant support to Mahmoud.

In this situation, it was mostly language barriers and complex family dynamics that prevented the family doctor from making adequate assessments of the condition of both mother and son. Beyond language and family dynamics, cultures vary in modes of emotional experience and expression. In some cases seen by the TCS, the clinical assessment and treatment have been compromised because physicians have had difficulty identifying cultural variations in expression of emotions. In particular, clinicians may take at face value the

---

Case Vignette 15-9

Rosa, a 54-year-old woman, originally from the Philippines, was referred to the TCS by her family doctor who was concerned about her poor adherence to treatment prescribed for severe asthma. She was separated from her husband and had a 10 year-old daughter. Rosa had met her husband in Manila and they came back to live in his home country of Switzerland. Rosa left her husband, after years of verbal and physical abuse from him, when their daughter was 3 years old. She had worked as a domestic helper in a family but had to quit 2 years ago because of her health problems. Her diffuse joint pains and severe asthma were too incapacitating to allow her to return to work, and a disability claim was pending.

Her family doctor requested a TCS consultation, because he believed that cultural factors, namely, differences in perspectives of illness, could explain her noncompliance

(continued)

with asthma medication and failure to consult her family doctor during flare-ups of her asthma. In recent months, she had visited the emergency several times in respiratory distress after progressive worsening over the previous week and, on one occasion, she had to be monitored in the intensive care unit. Her family doctor felt very frustrated, because he had asked her to call him as soon as she felt worse and had even given her his personal cell phone number, which she never used. In the consultation request, he asked for information about the patient's explanatory model of asthma and possible cultural barriers to her medical management.

The TCS consultant met with Rosa twice, the first time conversing in English and a little French, the second time with a Tagalog interpreter. She appeared very light-hearted and gay, smiling, talking and laughing a lot, but inquiries into her personal situation revealed a tremendous amount of distress related to the continuous conflict with her ex-husband regarding their daughter's custody and his reluctance to pay her alimony, as well as her own economic difficulties because of lack of income. She expressed intense guilt because her mother in the Philippines was severely ill and her own financial situation did not allow her either to visit or send money for her mother's health care. Regarding her medical problems, she said that she was used to the chronic pain but that she was very discouraged by the impact of asthma on her daily activities. In fact, at the end of the second interview, she revealed that she had recurrent suicidal ideation. A month earlier she had poured herself a glass of bleach, but the sudden arrival of her daughter in the kitchen had prevented her from drinking it. Further questioning revealed she met diagnostic criteria for major depression.

superficial good humor expected in some cultures. This is illustrated by the case of Rosa.

Rather than a difference in cultural explanatory models, the main issue in Rosa's case involved differences in cultural modes or styles of presentation of distress, which accounted for the nonrecognition of the severity of her mood disorder by her family doctor. For Rosa, this lack of overt expression of distress resulted from her preoccupation with saving face and the fatalistic optimism she adopted, as well as the fact that expression of negative emotions is discouraged and mental illness shamed and stigmatized in Filipino society (Sanchez & Gaw, 2007). Congruent with her cultural background, Rosa's allusions to her distress were made indirectly, through cues that her physician did not pick up on. The TCS consultant interpreted the noncompliance to her medication and her lack of action on the worsening of her asthma as signs of her depression, an interpretation that Rosa confirmed. The TCS consultant along with her family doctor negotiated a referral to a culturally competent mental health care professional, in conjunction with a referral to the primary care clinic's social worker for evaluation of possible financial subsidies and to a volunteer legal consultant to help implement the divorce judgement.

Medically Unexplained Symptoms

A frequent reason for requesting cultural consultation has to do with the problem of medically unexplained symptoms (MUS) in immigrant patients. MUS are defined by the presence of somatic symptoms in the absence of a medical diagnosis after adequate investigations (Kirmayer, Groleau, Looper, & Dao, 2004). They are often associated with emotional distress. These symptoms pose dilemmas in Western biomedical health care systems that tend to separate mental and physical illnesses (Miresco & Kirmayer, 2006). There is a rich literature on understanding the physiological, attentional, affective and cognitive-interpretive mechanisms that may contribute to MUS (Kirmayer & Looper, 2007). Techniques from cognitive behavior therapy have been found useful in treatment (Looper & Kirmayer, 2002). These can be adapted for cross-cultural use by incorporating culture-specific explanatory models and coping strategies.

Treating a patient suffering from MUS originating from an unfamiliar culture or background constitutes a double difficulty for the clinician. Referral of these patients to the cultural consultant may be triggered by a number of factors, including hope for the existence of a cultural syndrome that would explain the unfamiliar symptoms, the clinician's feelings of frustration and inability to help the patient and the patient's refusal of psychiatric referral. Kim's predicament is a striking example of a transcultural case of MUS.

Case Vignette 15-10

Kim was a married women in her late forties, of Vietnamese background, whose youngest son had been diagnosed with paranoid schizophrenia. She had immigrated from Vietnam to Switzerland over 20 years ago. Her husband worked as an orderly; she had not worked since the birth of her children. She suffered from acute and diffuse joint and bone pain, fatigue and depression. She had been treated for years by a family doctor and recently by a psychiatrist, without any improvement. Her depression became worse after her disability claim was rejected. The medical expert reviewing her case for the claim stated that "factors other than medical, predominantly social and cultural, were impeding her ability to work."

She was referred for cultural consultation by her psychiatrist who wanted better understanding of Kim's cultural and family context. The referring psychiatrist was convinced that taking care of her son was exhausting Kim and that he should be placed in an institution for Kim to have "more time for herself." The psychiatrist was frustrated by Kim continuously bringing the discussion back to her somatic symptoms.

A careful history obtained through an interpreter revealed that Kim had been orphaned during the Vietnam War, which led her and her siblings to live with her father's younger brother. She reported being treated as a slave by this man and his wife, who beat her regularly. Her only ally was her paternal grandmother, who tried to protect and nurture her as best she could. Kim escaped Vietnam in the early 1980s in a daunting journey on a small boat and was granted asylum in Switzerland where she met her husband, also a Vietnamese refugee. When she was pregnant with her youngest son, her grandmother died in Vietnam, leaving her inconsolable. She believed that her intense feelings of bereavement had harmed her son and thus explained his diagnosis of schizophrenia. She also believed that this was a punishment for not taking care of her grandmother in old age. She felt very stigmatized by her son's psychiatric illness and hid it from the community. He required her constant care because of suicidal ideation and inappropriate behavior. She felt supported by her husband and the medical team and found some solace in her Catholic faith. But she was reluctant to speak about her suffering, saying that *"cởi áo cho ngườ i xem lưng"* ("One does not bare one's back for other's to see"), a proverb equivalent to the idea that you should keep your problems private and "not wash your linen in public." Nevertheless, she did quite spontaneously bare her body to show the consultant the striking stigmata of her child-time abuse.

Kim's symptoms seem to act as an idiom of distress and closely resembled the Vietnamese malady *uất ức*, which has been described as a sociosomatic idiom or explanation for bodily illness caused by extreme social indignation or injustice that cannot be openly disclosed (Groleau & Kirmayer, 2004). She was abused by the very people who owed her and her siblings respect as children of the eldest son. They had also deprived them of their inheritance: their uncle sold the family land and did not share the benefits with her and her siblings. The rejection of her disability claim was the final injustice. When the term was mentioned to her, Kim denied having heard of *uất ức*, but she did not reject our explanation. For her physician, Kim's symptoms could thus be better understood in cultural perspective and hopefully more easily managed. The TCS team recommended a number of culturally congruent resources that the physician could include in the care of this patient: Buddhist meditation that was offered at the outpatient psychiatry clinic and referral to a Catholic hospital chaplain familiar with psychiatric illness. We clarified Vietnamese family dynamics and roles and explained to her doctors that placing her son in an institution would be in complete contradiction with Kim's moral and familial obligations and might even bring on additional distress. The patient appreciated the cultural evaluation, and the knowledge that her psychiatrist would have a better understanding of her plight helped reinforce this therapeutic relationship.

Misattribution of Clinical Problems to Culture

Requests for cultural consultations are often triggered by an intuition that "something cultural" is at stake, although it may be difficult for the referring clinician to identify the exact role of culture. There may also be situations where culture actually plays little or no role in the complexity of the clinical situation, but because the patient appears in some way "different" from the majority, a cultural consultation referral is initiated. This recognition of difference means that cultural issues are important for the medical team

Case Vignette 15-11

Brigitte was hospitalized for a pulmonary infection complicated by a pleural effusion. A 50-year-old mother of four children, she had emigrated from Cameroon over 25 years earlier. Her lengthy medical history included hypertension, hepatitis C secondary to blood transfusions and an episode of erythema multiforme (Stevens-Johnson syndrome), a life-threatening allergic hypersensitivity reaction to an antibiotic prescribed for an infection 4 years earlier. Since that allergic reaction, she had become suspicious of any medication and had not been compliant with the drugs prescribed for hypertension. The referring medical team was concerned she would not continue the antibiotics once she left the hospital and also that she was experiencing complications from her poorly controlled blood pressure. They requested a TCS consultation to explore cultural factors that might be influencing the patient's understanding of the disease and her perceived lack of adherence to treatment.

When we met with her, she had many questions regarding her illness. She could not understand why the physicians wanted to discharge her because she still had pain in her chest and her legs were swollen. Exploration of her background revealed that she had been able to attend only very little schooling and that she had little notion of anatomy or body organs. According to her, the body was a single receptacle bordered by her skin, and she did not acknowledge any internal boundaries (such as organs). Thus the fact that her legs were swollen (in reality from a touch of heart failure) was a sign that the doctors had not finished their job, since "all the water had not been taken out." She openly expressed mistrust of any medication but directly related this to severe reaction she had experienced from the antibiotics prescribed for another infection.

or health care system, whether or not they are at the root of the patient's health problems.

In this situation, more than a cultural barrier, there was an educational barrier and an understandable response to the life-threatening side effects of medication that led to persistent mistrust and communication problems. The team did not suspect that the patient was illiterate and believed that the terms they employed like "lung", "lung envelope", "heart" and "infection with pus" were simple enough that the patient would understand them and could visualize what they meant. In situations like this, exploring the patient's body image through drawing and unpacking the meaning of specific metaphors can be helpful (Saint Arnault & Shimabukuro, 2012).

The medical team also minimized the impact of the severe iatrogenic episode of the Stevens-Johnson syndrome and did not want to acknowledge the responsibility that the patient attributed to health care professionals for what she considered to be a serious medical error. The TCS consultant underlined how coherent and appropriate the mistrust was, from the patient's point of view. The TCS made recommendations to openly discuss the mistrust and its consequences, look for allies in the outpatient team already caring for the patient and offer creative ways to adequately explain the key aspects of her illness and the necessity of continuing the antibiotics once she left the hospital.

Conclusion

Cultural consultation in general hospital medicine can provide a useful adjunct to routine care, supporting clinical teams in responding to the diversity of patient populations. The focus on practical solutions for pressing issues in care provides an opportunity to convey strategies of inquiry, communication and negotiation that can be used by the clinical teams in their daily work.

The clinical vignettes presented in this chapter illustrate how each TCS consultation leads to the unpacking of several different issues, which may or may not be related to the patient's culture. These issues frequently coexist and interact in ways that increase complexity to the point where the clinician in charge is impelled to request external advice. Of course, many of the same complexity factors can be found with non-immigrant patients, where culture and ethnicity may be less salient. Often, complexity may be related to aspects of the culture of biomedicine or to local institutional cultures. In these multilayered situations, the cultural component is only one source of complication. But clinicians often entertain the hope that "solving the cultural problem" will allow them to proceed with "medicine as usual." To some extent, this hope reflects an attitude brought to many innovative or specialized services, but it may also reflect a more pervasive view of culture as creating obstacles to standard practice. This view of culture as erecting barriers to standard care is problematic because it tends to hide structural problems in the health care system or prejudices of the institutions and practitioners associated with the "dominant" or "mainstream" cultural groups. The focus on obstacles also may downplay or ignore the positive dimensions of culture as the constituting the roots of individual and collective identity and esteem as well as providing resources for adaptation, resilience and creative diversity.

Our experience practicing cultural consultations in medical settings reveals a number of common problems encountered by individual physicians and institutions caring for patients of diverse origins. One issue is the tendency to overestimate patients' fluency in host country languages and, consequently, to underutilize trained interpreters, even when they are made available by the institution (Hudelson & Vilpert, 2009). In these situations, communication is obviously hindered by lack of shared vocabulary. Another difficulty is insufficient knowledge of clinicians of their patients' non-medical history and of personal, social and cultural factors influencing present care. Often, when clinicians believed there was a cultural barrier, we uncovered a social or personal problem reflecting structural issues (lack of health insurance, financial difficulties, social isolation, etc.) that constituted a barrier to care and/or contributed to the medical illness. This difficulty in recognizing social and cultural issues was partly related to clinicians" lack of training and the lack of a model for the systematic evaluation of cultural factors in the clinical encounter (Rosenberg, Kirmayer, et al., 2007). Furthermore, clinicians tended to focus primarily on their patients as bearers of culture and ignored their own personal cultural background, the role of the culture of medicine, and that of the institutions that shaped their own belief systems, values and practices (Taylor, 2003).

Clarifying the cultural component of these difficulties, whether related to the patient or the health care professional; providing clinicians with additional cultural and social data about the patient; and referring them to local resources were the main interventions in these cultural consultations. The Cultural Formulation (Mezzich, Caracci, Fabrega, & Kirmayer, 2009), which is the guide used to interview patients in both consultation services, offers a practical and didactic model that the clinicians can learn to apply in future clinical encounters. Hospital teams often ask for several consecutive cultural consultations, until the model is sufficiently integrated into their practice and they feel competent to explore these topics on their own. Our experience with cultural consultation in medical settings points to the obvious need for additional and mandatory medical training in cultural competence and in particular in learning to access and assess the social and cultural contexts of patients and their families.

References

Amos, J. J., & Robinson, R. G. (2010). *Psychosomatic medicine: An introduction to consultation-liaison psychiatry.* Cambridge, England: Cambridge University Press.

Bhui, K., & Bhugra, D. (2004). Communication with patients from other cultures: The place of explanatory models. *Advances in Psychiatric Treatment, 10*, 474–478.

Bischoff, A., Tonnerre, C., Eytan, A., Bernstein, M., & Loutan, L. (1999). Adressing language barriers to health care: A survey of medical services in Switzerland. *Social & Preventive Medicine, 44*(6), 248–256.

Bureau d'Intégration des Etrangers. (2003). *Comment l'immigration évolue et modifie Genève.* Genève, Switzerland: Cahiers du BIE n°2.

Cohen-Emerique, M., & Hohl, J. (2004). Les réactions défensives à la menace identitaire chez les professionnels en situations interculturelles. *Cahiers Internationaux de Psychologie Sociale, 61*, 21–34.

Cooper, M., Harding, S., Mullen, K., & O'Donnell, C. (2012). 'A Chronic disease is a disease which keeps coming back … it is like the flu': Chronic disease risk perception and explanatory models among French- and Swahili-speaking African migrants. *Ethnicity and Health.* doi:10.1080/13557858.2012.740003.

Crawley, L. M., Marshall, P. A., Lo, B., & Koenig, B. A. (2002). Strategies for culturally effective end-of-life care. *Annals of Internal Medicine, 136*(9), 673–679.

Dein, S. (2004). Explanatory models of and attitudes towards cancer in different cultures. *The Lancet Oncology, 5*(2), 119–124.

Dominicé Dao, M. (2009). Consultation transculturelle en milieu hospitalier. In B. Goguikian Ratcliff & O. Strasser (Eds.), *Clinique de l'exil: Chronique d'une pratique engagée* (pp. 59–71). Geneva, Switzerland: Georg.

Dominicé Dao, M. I., Ferreira, J. F., Vallier, N., Roulin, D., Hirschel, B., & Calmy, A. (2010). Health perceptions of African HIV-infected patients and of their physicians. *Patient Education and Counseling, 80*(2), 185–190.

Groleau, D., & Kirmayer, L. J. (2004). Sociosomatic theory in Vietnamese immigrants' narratives of distress. *Anthropology & Medicine, 11*(2), 117–133.

Groleau, D., Whitley, R., Lesperance, F., & Kirmayer, L. J. (2010). Spiritual reconfigurations of self after a myocardial infarction: Influence of culture and place. *Health & Place, 16*(5), 853–860.

Gysels, M., Evans, N., Meñaca, A., Andrew, E., Toscani, F., Finetti, S., et al. (2012). Culture and end of life care: A scoping exercise in seven European countries. *PLoS One, 7*(4), e34188.

Helman, C. G. (1985). Communication in primary care: The role of patient and practitioner explanatory models. *Social Science & Medicine, 20*(9), 923–931.

Hudelson, P., & Vilpert, S. (2009). Overcoming language barriers with foreign-language speaking patients: A survey to investigate intra-hospital variation in attitudes and practices. *BMC Health Services Research, 9*, 187.

Kirmayer, L. J. (2001). Failures of imagination: The refugee's narrative in psychiatry. *Anthropology & Medicine, 10*(2), 167–185.

Kirmayer, L. J., Groleau, D., Guzder, J., Blake, C., & Jarvis, E. (2003). Cultural consultation: A model of mental health service for multicultural societies. *Canadian Journal of Psychiatry, 48*(2), 145–153.

Kirmayer, L. J., Groleau, D., Looper, K. J., & Dao, M. D. (2004). Explaining medically unexplained symptoms. *Canadian Journal of Psychiatry, 49*(10), 663–672.

Kirmayer, L. J., & Looper, K. J. (2007). Somatoform disorders. In M. Hersen, S. Turner, & D. Beidel (Eds.), *Adult psychopathology.* New York, NY: John Wiley & Sons.

Kleinman, A., Eisenberg, L., & Good, B. (1978). Culture, illness, and care: Clinical lessons from anthropologic and cross-cultural research. *Annals of Internal Medicine, 88*(2), 251–258.

Leanza, Y. (2005). Le rapport à l'autre culturel en milieu médical: l'exemple de consultations pédiatriques de prévention pour des familles migrantes. *Bulletin de l'ARIC, 41*, 8–27.

Looper, K. J., & Kirmayer, L. J. (2002). Behavioral medicine approaches to somatoform disorders. *Journal of Consulting and Clinical Psychology, 70*(3), 810–827.

Loutan, L., Farinelli, T., & Pampallona, S. (1999). Medical interpreters have feelings too. *Médecine Sociale et Préventive, 44*(6), 280–282.

Mezzich, J. E., Caracci, G., Fabrega, H., Jr., & Kirmayer, L. J. (2009). Cultural formulation guidelines. *Transcultural Psychiatry, 46*(3), 383–405.

Miresco, M. J., & Kirmayer, L. J. (2006). The persistence of mind-brain dualism in psychiatric reasoning about clinical scenarios. *The American Journal of Psychiatry, 163*(5), 913–918.

Rosenberg, E., Kirmayer, L. J., Xenocostas, S., Dao, M. D., & Loignon, C. (2007). GPs' strategies in intercultural clinical encounters. *Family Practice, 24*(2), 145–151.

Saint Arnault, D., & Shimabukuro, S. (2012). The clinical ethnographic interview: A user-friendly guide to the cultural formulation of distress and help seeking. *Transcultural Psychiatry, 49*(2), 302–322.

Sanchez, F., & Gaw, A. (2007). Mental health care of Filipino Americans. *Psychiatric Services, 58*(6), 810–815.

Stern, T. A. (2010). *Massachusetts general hospital handbook of general hospital psychiatry* (6th ed.). Philadelphia, PA: Saunders/Elsevier.

Tardin, A., Dominicé Dao, M., Ninet, B., & Janssens, J. P. (2009). Tuberculosis cluster in an immigrant community: Case identification issues and a transcultural perspective. *Tropical Medicine & International Health, 14*(9), 995–1002.

Taylor, J. S. (2003). Confronting "culture" in medicine's culture of no culture. *Academic Medicine, 78*, 555–559.

Wachtler, C., Brorsson, A., & Troein, M. (2006). Meeting and treating cultural difference in primary care: A qualitative interview study. *Family Practice, 23*(1), 111–115.

Weiss, M. G., & Somma, D. (2007). Explanatory models in psychiatry. In D. Bhugra & K. Bhui (Eds.), *Textbook of cultural psychiatry* (pp. 127–140). Cambridge, England: Cambridge University Press.

Weller, S. C., Baer, R. D., de Alba, G., Garcia, J., & Salcedo Rocha, A. L. (2012). Explanatory models of diabetes in the U.S. and Mexico: The patient-provider gap and cultural competence. *Social Science & Medicine, 75*(6), 1088–1096.

Conclusion: The Future of Cultural Consultation

Laurence J. Kirmayer, Jaswant Guzder, and Cécile Rousseau

In this chapter we reflect on the lessons learned from over a decade of work by the cultural consultation service. We consider the challenges of implementation and evaluation, the evidence for impact on health outcomes the implications for mental health policy, the design of health care systems, the training of professionals and everyday clinical practice.

The findings from the CCS project are important because they indicate significant unmet needs for mental health services for Indigenous peoples, immigrants, refugees and asylum seekers. At the same time, the CCS project suggests that outpatient consultation provides an effective means of responding to some of these needs. A service like the CCS can support mainstream health care, provide ongoing training within clinical institutions and create a context that allows professionals from diverse backgrounds to make systematic use of their linguistic and cultural expertise.

As seen in many of the case vignettes presented in this volume, the cultural consultation service has documented serious errors in diagnosis and inadequate treatment of mental health problems that reflect a lack of clinical attention to culture and social context. Systematic attention to these issues can lead to more comprehensive assessment, more effective treatment and better clinical outcomes.

Outpatient consultation is a familiar process for health professionals. Family physicians are accustomed to referring patients for specialist evaluation, and collaborative care models provide a natural way to incorporate attention to culture in mental health services. The dilemma, of course, is that a referring clinician must recognize the need for consultation, convey this to the patient in an acceptable way, find the appropriate resources and be able to apply any recommendations effectively. All of this presumes a substantial degree of cultural awareness or competence on the part of the referring clinician. This requires training in cultural aspects of mental health. The virtue of the consultation approach is that it works with the existing health system framework and improves continuity of care by reducing segmentation and there can be a spillover effect from consultations so that other patients in the clinician's practice benefit from new knowledge and skills.

L.J. Kirmayer, M.D. (✉)
Culture & Mental Health Research Unit, Institute of Community & Family Psychiatry, Jewish General Hospital, 4333 Cote Ste Catherine Road, Montreal, QC, Canada H3T 1E4
e-mail: laurence.kirmayer@mcgill.ca

J. Guzder, M.D.
Center for Child Development and Mental Health, Institute of Community and Family Psychiatry, 4335 Cote St. Catherine Road, Montreal, QC, Canada H3T 1E4
e-mail: jaswant@videotron.ca

C. Rousseau, M.D., M.Sc.
Directrice scientifique, Centre de recherche et de formation, CSSS de la Montagne, 7085 Hutchison, Local 204.2, Montréal, QC, Canada H3N 1Y9
e-mail: cecile.rousseau@mcgill.ca

L.J. Kirmayer et al. (eds.), *Cultural Consultation: Encountering the Other in Mental Health Care*, International and Cultural Psychology, DOI 10.1007/978-1-4614-7615-3_16, © Springer Science+Business Media New York 2014

Globalization is increasing the rate and intensity of culture contact and exchange. Rather than resulting in a standardization or homogeneity of experience, however, these exchanges are leading to the emergence of new forms of hybrid identity. At the same time, the networks that bind people together through the Internet and social media are providing opportunities for new forms of identity and community. Along with this come changes in the meanings of culture itself. Recent years have seen significant changes in the demography of Canadian cities, which have made issues of culture more salient. While Canada has always been a nation of immigrants, the older waves of mainly European immigrants have shifted to be predominately people from the Asian and southern countries. Many of these cultures have substantially different values at the levels of individual psychology, family structures and community— all of which affect the nature of mental health problems and solutions.

At the same time, the post 9/11 environment of anxiety has contributed to new waves of xenophobia and restrictive immigration legislation in many countries. Commitments to the protection of refugees have weakened, undermining both the right of asylum and the conditions for productive resettlement. Recently, the Canadian Federal government increased the use of detention for refugee claimants and, simultaneously, drastically cut their health care coverage. There are ongoing legal challenges to this retrograde policy. However, in the meantime, failed refugee claimants and other migrants with precarious status, who arrived in Canada as temporary workers or with a visa, are likely to form an increasingly important group of undocumented persons in need of health care. These vulnerable individuals and families constitute an important challenge for the health system.

While globalization has broken down barriers between nations and cultures and encouraged cultural exchange, intermixing and hybridization, it has not resulted in a global monoculture (Burke, 2009). Indeed, one reaction to this exchange has been the reassertion of local ethnic identities and boundaries to exclude the cultural "Other." In many jurisdictions, there have been increasing calls for less accommodation and more assimilation

of immigrant and refugee communities. Even within Canada, there are notable regional differences in policies and attitudes toward migration and cultural diversity. For example, Quebec has a provincial government that is currently proposing a "charter of secularism" to insure that religious values and symbols are kept out of the public sphere. This is consistent with laicism and republicanism in France but very much counter to the spirit of multiculturalism. On the other hand, Québec is the only provincial government that has officially stated that it will cover the cost of health care for refugees, because the federal policy is unacceptable in terms of Québec values. This illustrates the local paradoxes in facing otherness and the complex ties between welcoming policies and collective history.

There is increasing recognition of the importance of culture in psychiatry. The US National Institute of Mental Health sponsored a culture and diagnosis work group that made many recommendations for DSM-IV only some of which were incorporated, most notably the outline for cultural formulation (Mezzich et al., 1999). DSM-5 has expanded on this with a cultural formulation interview and supplementary modules that provide a way to collect clinically relevant information about illness experience, culture and context. To make effective use of this information, however, clinicians need better understanding of the biological, psychological and social processes through which culture influences normal development, psychopathology and adaptation. The ongoing revisions of ICD-10 have also emphasized the importance of culture and its interaction with clinical utility. It will be interesting to see how the growing body of work on cultural idioms of distress and local nosological systems influences this international document.

Paths to a Culturally Safe and Competent Mental Health Care System

Cultural consultation provides a way to improve the overall competence of practitioners and institutions. The case centered approach fits with the explicit mandate, everyday tasks and practical concerns of health care institutions. At the same time, discussion of issues of social and cultural context in specific cases highlights systemic issues and implications of standard practice in health care institutions. In a sense, it reveals the culture of the institution, pushing back against medicines "culture of no culture" (Taylor, 2003).

Recognition of culture points to the need for adaptation of service models and interventions and a variety of approaches have been developed (Bhui, Warfa, Edonya, McKenzie, & Bhugra, 2007). Unfortunately, there have been no comparative evaluation studies of the merits and limitations of any of these models, so that it remains difficult for planners to choose from among the different approaches and models for the development and maintenance of specialized services (Bhui et al., 2007; Renzaho, Romios, Crock, & Sonderlund, 2013). This is a general problem with applying evidence-based approaches in the area of cultural diversity (Whitley, Rousseau, Carpenter Song, & Kirmayer 2011). In the absence of evidence for a specific model, the CCS has followed the main trends in contemporary psychiatry and psychology in terms of effective psychosocial and psychotherapeutic interventions but has also built on the experiential and cultural knowledge of its clinicians and cultural brokers to expand the repertoire of available interventions and adapt them for particular patients. There is a need for more work developing innovative interventions that may rely on different mechanisms of healing and adaptation rooted in social processes of culture and community and for rigorously evaluating these practices.

Access to Services

The CCS experience documented important gaps in the delivery of mental health care to refugees, immigrants and First Nations peoples. Many of the patients referred to the CCS had needs for services that went beyond what was available to them in the health care. These cases required more time and more resources (e.g., interpreters, culture brokers, meetings with extended family,

linkage with community organizations) than comparable cases from Canadian-born patients to accomplish basic clinical tasks of diagnostic assessment and treatment planning. Given this greater demand and the technical and logistical complexity of conducting an adequate assessment, in many cases a basic assessment with an interpreter had never been attempted even though patients had been in the treatment system for many years. The use of the cultural formulation and strategies for working with cultural difference are still not widely known by clinicians and have not been given sufficient attention in professional training or continuing education.

The CCS facilitated access to services in several ways. Through its collaboration with the regional refugee clinic and other community organizations, the CCS provided service for underserved groups who usually do not receive mental health care. For patients already in the health care system, the CCS provided links to clinicians, interpreters, culture brokers and community organizations with knowledge and expertise in working with specific ethnocultural groups. By providing access to specialized consultation that increased the knowledge and clinical skills of clinicians, the service improved the quality of care of patients. Finally, by creating a place for professionals from different disciplines to learn to use cultural perspectives in their work, the CCS contributed to building capacity to respond to diversity within the mainstream health care system.

The development of a specialized resource like the CCS also brings with it certain problems. Increasing clinicians' awareness of and sensitivity to cultural issues leads to an increase in demands, which can quickly exceed the capacity of the team. It may also lead clinicians to think that cultural issues are outside their areas of competence and should all be referred. Regulating intake by adjusting the catchment area or criteria for referral reduces accessibility for those who may be in greatest need. The CCS also raises expectations in terms of the need for various forms of specialized treatment that may not exist, e.g., psychotherapy or family therapy in different languages and expertise in working with survivors of torture. This can exert useful pressure on the health care system, motivating the development of new services, but it can also create frustration in settings where resources are limited. Interestingly, however, many of the basic CCS recommendations fall within the range of nonspecialized interventions recommended by the WHO in the Mental Health Gap Action Program (mhGAP) modules, designed to be feasible in low-income countries (World Health Organization, 2010). This reflects the role of cultural consultation in addressing basic needs that are sometimes displaced by technical interventions in high-resource settings with specialized health care. In many cases, CCS consultations emphasize providing psychological first aid built on cultural coping strategies, family and community-based psychosocial care and restoring the ruptured social networks that are essential for recovery and well-being.

The CCS increasingly recognized the need to offer time-limited treatment interventions and long-term follow-up to meet the needs of referring clinicians and patients to have access to basic care. On the other hand, the Transcultural Clinic at the MCH, which offered comprehensive treatment and longer-term therapy from the start, found that it quickly became backlogged and was unable to respond to its unique populations (including refugee children). As a result of this and of the difficulty of sustaining a specialized transcultural clinic in a hospital setting, the MCH considered a move toward more consultative services based on supporting care providers in other parts of the hospital and other institutions or community settings. Thus, both services, although starting out with different models, converged on a mix of consultation-liaison (mainly diagnostic assessment and treatment planning) and direct treatment provision (including various forms of individual and family therapy and aspects of case management, coordinating care from many providers). The ideal situation would seem to be a service that primarily serves consultation and training functions but has the capacity to follow complex cases with a network of diverse providers.

Person-Centered Medicine and Communication

There has been much recent interest in person-centered care as a counterbalance to the tendency in biomedicine to focus on treating the disease rather than the person (Mezzich et al., 2010). The work of the CCS fits squarely with this person-centered approach but expands it by focusing not only on individual illness experience but on the family, community and social-systemic contexts of suffering and healing. The CCS assessment process attends to the voice of patients and clinicians to identify their most pressing needs and concerns. The consultant views patient and clinician as embedded in social systems and institutions—including health care, social services, education, immigration and community organizations—that frame their concerns and present them with a limited set of options. By providing a place to consider diverse perspectives on illness and healing and think outside the limits of conventional frameworks, the CCS has promoted the use of innovative interventions for mental health problems.

The CCS approach reflects core values, global strategies and specific clinical tactics. At the level of values, the CCS adopts an ethical stance that grants the primacy and validity of patients' own stories, which include both illness narratives and autobiographical accounts that situate their personal predicaments and aspirations in their life trajectories. Eliciting and understanding this story requires adequate communication which, in turn, entails the use of interpreters and culture brokers to insure that patient and clinician can grasp each other's meaning and intentions. Interpreters are integrated into the CCS team as partners in the assessment and treatment process. While recognizing that interpreters cannot provide an unbiased view or perfect window onto patients' experience, they are nevertheless absolutely essential to go beyond the imprecision and error found when there are significant linguistic barriers to communication. Full communication is the basis for the CCS assessment and any subsequent intervention.

The CCS approach is based on an epistemological view that recognizes the fluidity and multiplicity of narratives and perspectives so that, contrary to the juridical view of the refugee review board and other institutions, no one story suffices or can be privileged as the "final" truth. This multiplicity is found not only in the illness narratives of patients and their families but also among members of the health care team. It is reflected in the composition of the CCS team and the discussions that take place at the CCS case conferences. The aim in this colloquy is not to reach a simple consensus but to elicit and hold a range of hypotheses or options that provide potential trajectories for interventions that can promote healing and recovery.

Given the problems that the CCS regularly identifies in routine care and the health care system as a whole, its work necessarily involves a stance of advocacy. This is expressed both through actions on behalf of individual patients or ethnocultural communities and through an ongoing research program that aims to document the vital importance of cultural consideration for improving quality of care.

problem, as mutual understanding, common goals and new forms of collaboration can emerge. Even when the relevant professionals and concerned parties are unable to meet face to face, the CCS team may act as a go-between through successive conversations with different stakeholders and can identify intersectoral issues where collaboration can resolve shared problems and bring mutual benefits.

The CCS thus challenges the tendency for segmentation of care and, by focusing on a set of issues that lie beyond the expertise of any single professional or institution, encourages open dialogue, collaboration and partnership. This is important not only in remote rural communities, where such segmentation seems especially absurd, but also in highly resourced urban milieus where institutions may compete for resources or struggle to protect their turf and areas of responsibility.

The experience of the CCS also shows how building links with the community can identify resources to untangle complicated cases and provide opportunities for treatment and social reintegration that go beyond the limitations of conventional mental health care.

Service Integration and Continuity of Care

The work of the CCS cuts across sectors of the health and social service systems and so can contribute to improving continuity of care. The service works with many different types of health care and social service providers, accepting referrals from both frontline and specialty settings. In the process of making sense of a given case, the CCS may convene workers from several different institutions representing sectors of health, social services, education and legal systems. The CCS case formulation often identifies multilevel or multi-system problems that call for the expertise of several professions and the need for collaboration across institutions and with community organizations. Getting some of these people together around the same table to discuss a difficult case often has ramifications beyond the immediate clinical

Health Outcomes and Cost-Effectiveness

Due to the extremely heterogeneous nature of the cases seen by the CCS, the relatively brief intervention and the lack of direct patient contact in many cases, it has proved difficult to demonstrate the impact of the CCS on specific health outcomes and evaluate its cost-effectiveness. For many or most patients seen by the CCS, it appears there were significant changes in service use, diagnosis and treatment in individual cases that had dramatic impact both on their long-term well-being and functioning and on the ultimate costs of their care to the health and social service systems. Although there are cases in which the CCS assessment and recommendations clearly had an immediate, dramatic effect, for most cases other situational factors also played an important role in the outcome. A report from Jacques Ramsay, coroner in Quebec, based in part on consultation with the CCS, described six cases of mortality directly related to obstacles in accessing health care for migrant refugee or undocumented patients (Gouvernement du Québec, 2007). While language barriers and the lack of appropriate use of interpreters were major reasons for these tragic outcomes, other issues including institutional racism, prejudice and discrimination, cultural misunderstandings and the politics of migratory status were all significant contributors to these deaths, which illustrate the risks of cultural blindness and ethnocentrism in clinical practice.

Some of the cases seen by the CCS had received no mental health evaluation or treatment, despite lengthy periods of contact with health care, and were clearly costing the system much more because of this neglect than they would have if effective treatment had been provided at the outset. Problems that may be amenable to a relatively brief intense intervention, like having an interpreter available to make a proper diagnosis at the start, may become more complicated and refractory to treatment over time as errors occur, trust in care providers and institutions erodes and the functioning of the individual and family deteriorates.

The CCS has also seen many patients who have been in treatment for lengthy periods of time but never received a culturally oriented assessment with an interpreter. Reassessment often led to substantial changes in diagnosis and treatment plan. In many cases, patients who had not been receiving any effective treatment for their conditions were accurately diagnosed and enrolled in appropriate treatment. In some cases, this involved children who had been incorrectly diagnosed due to a lack of use of interpreters and cultural expertise and who had been treated for years with inappropriate medications and other interventions. The personal and social cost of this systematic mismanagement is enormous. Of course, this is not only an economic or health care issue but also an ethical and human rights concern.

The existence of the CCS raised awareness about a host of issues related to culture throughout the health care system. Among the unanticipated effects of the service was a great increase in interest in training in cultural psychiatry among students in medicine, psychiatry, social work and nursing. The opportunity to participate in the CCS has attracted trainees from psychiatry, psychology, social work and other disciplines to McGill postgraduate programs. The availability of this type of clinical experience may have a major impact on the skills and orientation of future generations of mental health practitioners.

Obstacles to Implementation and Sustainability

Our experience with the CCS identified important obstacles to the implementation of cultural consultation services and culturally sensitive care more generally. Some of these obstacles stem from limited resources and time pressure in the health care system, but there are subtler obstacles that reflect ambivalence in the broader society that is reflected in the local values and practices of health care institutions and professionals. Hospitals, clinics and other social service institutions that initially welcomed the effort to provide culturally responsive care found it difficult to understand and integrate the social perspectives and interventions provided by the CCS, which fell outside the framework of routine practice. This problem was especially evident when the CCS uncovered institutional biases or structural problems that required substantial change in standard practices or bureaucratic routines. It also occurred when professionals accustomed to working with limited models and treatment algorithms were required to think more contextually and integrate multilevel and multisectoral interventions into their practice.

The CCS followed a consultation model with the aim of supplementing existing mental health care and upgrading the skills of practitioners throughout the health care system. However, because of problems in access to psychiatry and other mental health services throughout the system, there was pressure to replace the consultation-liaison model with an outpatient treatment team approach that could provide basic care to take some of the load off existing services. There was also pressure to respond to crises or emergencies (e.g., imminent deportation) or provide quick consultations to expedite disposition of cases.

Finding the requisite resources (consultants with expertise in cultural psychiatry, culture brokers, interpreters, community supports) for patients from particular cultural backgrounds was sometimes difficult, especially when the local immigrant community in question was small, which was the case for many newcomers.

One barrier to addressing cultural diversity in mental health care is the prevalent ethnocentrism of health care providers and planners. For example, some clinicians asserted that they did not need to consider culture explicitly because they treated every patient equitably and on their own terms. Unfortunately, this liberal "colour blindness" often was expressed in clinic routines and procedures that did not accommodate important variations in patients' needs and expectations.

This lack of accommodation of the patient's reality was also evident in attitudes toward language. Despite the clear indications in the literature and potential medico-legal implications of inadequate communication, many hospitals and clinics underutilize existing interpreter resources because practitioners are satisfied with a minimal level of communication with their patients or find it too difficult logistically to obtain the requisite help. This is sometimes justified by claiming that newcomers need to adapt by learning to speak the host country language. In the context of Quebec, this claim is reinforced by a general concern with the need to protect and promote French as the official language.

There was also a tendency to reframe social structural and economic problems in cultural terms and so divert attention from larger issues that demand political action. For example, issues related to Aboriginal health have been framed in terms of culture when there are obvious social structural problems related to poverty, marginalization and disempowerment that are major determinants of health disparities in this population (King, Smith, & Gracey, 2009; Reading & Wien, 2009). At the same time, explicit attention to culture may be very appropriate as much of the oppression endured by Aboriginal peoples

involved deliberate devaluing and suppression of their traditions (Kirmayer, Brass, & Valaskakis, 2008). Similarly, many families from racialized minorities referred from youth protection face structural problems related to patterns of migration and discrimination within Canadian society (Chapter 13). Yet valorizing and supporting bicultural identities and the traditions of their parents and grandparents can be an important component of helping migrants strengthen a sense of individual identity and collective belonging.

By insisting that cultural issues are important and demonstrating that culturally competent care requires specific knowledge and skills, the CCS also challenged the complacency of existing institutions. The focus on cultural competence and safety as relevant to patient care implied that professionals needed to acquire new knowledge and skills and new ways of doing their work and this sometimes evoked apprehension and resistance to change. Insuring that consultations were framed in accessible language and emphasized the transfer of skills and strategies reduced this apprehension. In many cases, it was possible to present cultural information within the framework of family theory and therapy, which reinforced clinician's sense of competence and made interventions easier to understand and integrate into existing treatment plans.

Reflecting the current dominance of reductionist biological models and pharmacological treatments in psychiatry, some psychiatrists did not recognize social, cultural, economic or other structural issues as important dimensions of psychiatric care. Others did not see the consultation as useful even for difficult cases, usually because they viewed it as too time-consuming or intrusive. Concerns voiced by clinicians who had not used the service included the impression that such consultations would increase their workload, were too lengthy, would take too long to arrange and therefore would not respond to the need for timely resolution of clinical problems. Many of these clinicians would prefer to hand over difficult cases altogether rather than go through the consultation process and perhaps receive recommendations that required that they work in unfamiliar ways.

Sustainability has been a challenging issue for the CCS. In particular, funding has remained difficult to secure. In large part, this reflects the continuing perception by many policy makers, administrators and clinicians that culture is peripheral to the goals and methods of mental health services. As a result, a service like the CCS is not a budgetary priority.

In the Quebec version of the Canadian system of universal health insurance (Medicare), funding for psychiatrists is covered by the state on a fee-for-service basis, but support for other mental health professionals (i.e., psychologists, nurse practitioners, social workers) must come from hospital or clinic budgets or else be paid by the client directly. As a result, it is difficult to sustain an interdisciplinary team without commitment from a hospital administration or comprehensive community clinic. As well, because cultural consultation often requires coordinating the efforts of multiple consultants, interpreters, culture brokers, patients and their families, there is a need for skilled clinical administrative staff who can provide telephone intake and triage and organize the work of the service. Finally, building collaborative relationships with ethnocultural community organizations takes time and effort that may not meet immediate clinical needs but lays the groundwork for effective interventions at a later time.

Transferability: Implementing Cultural Consultation in Other Settings

Although the CCS was developed in a particular context, we believe that it can be easily adapted to different settings and health care systems. In fact, similar services have been developed in other cities with modifications based on the needs of the local communities and practitioners. The basic requirements to transfer of the model include:

1. An explicit commitment (ideally long term) on the part of regional health and social service authorities and institutions to improving the quality of mental health services by addressing cultural diversity.

2. Information about the kinds of diversity in the local population and the specific service needs of particular groups. It is important to recognize that lack of use of services does not indicate lack of need. Minority groups often underutilize mental health services because they fear stigma or discrimination. Insuring cultural safety of institutions and addressing negative attitudes toward mental health services in the community will eventually increase use of services by marginalized groups. Hence, the initial effect may be an increase in cost. When this is averaged over time, however, better access will lead to more efficient use of services and better health outcomes.

3. A willingness to work closely with representatives of ethnocultural communities and community organizations to identify unmet needs and potential resources for the delivery of culturally appropriate mental health care. This requires understanding the internal diversity of cultural communities and provides the opportunity to build up a network of resources that can be deployed in the assessment and management of specific cases. This process can also contribute to reducing psychiatric stigma and educate the community to be more effective consumers of available services. This work must scrupulously respect issues of confidentiality, which are particularly delicate in small ethnocultural communities.

4. The process of implementation involves identifying staff with the requisite skills and obtaining infrastructure support (consulting rooms for individual and family meetings, administrative and secretarial support, telecommunications, videoconferencing, Internet access). It is important to locate the service in a place within the health care system that makes it acceptable to both patients and clinicians, preferably a nonpsychiatric setting that is easily accessible to the cultural communities and clinicians who are being served.

5. The core staff for the service will generally include an individual or small group of clinicians with expertise in cultural psychiatry or cultural-clinical psychology. This includes familiarity with the elements of cultural

assessment and formulation and the techniques of consultation-liaison work. Usually, clinicians obtain this expertise by training in specialized programs and by ongoing efforts to reflect on their own ethnocultural background and learn from clinical experiences with diverse populations.

6. The ready availability of a pool of professional medical interpreters is essential for work with newcomers or others with limited proficiency in the languages of mainstream institutions. Ideally, these interpreters should have specific training in mental health issues to allow more accurate assessment of mental status, deal with complex cases of trauma and manage their own emotional reactions and countertransference.

7. Similarly, the service requires a group of culture brokers (some of whom may be bilingual, bicultural clinicians or interpreters) who can serve as go-betweens in clinical communication and provide information on relevant cultural context and background. Funding, supervision and support must be arranged for each of these types of collaborators.

8. The vitality of the service will be greatly enhanced by assembling a multidisciplinary team of culturally diverse professionals open to rethinking standard practices. In addition to adding to the available expertise and ability to respond to specific populations, this team can also provide the solidarity and support needed to challenge and transform existing institutional policies and practices.

9. Given the innovative clinical model and interventions of the CCS, there is a need for a flexible institutional framework that can adapt to the pragmatic aspects of cultural consultation including changes in the number and type of patients referred to the service, the need to engage extended families and community organizations in decision-making processes and the need to collaborate with other institutions.

Policy Implications

The CCS documented significant unmet need for services among ethnocultural minorities, including immigrants, refugees and Indigenous peoples.

The analysis of cases seen in the cultural consultation services and transcultural clinics indicates that language, cultural background and racism all diminish access to mental health care or undermine the relevance and reception of conventional care. Many of the cases seen in our clinics had inadequate treatment for mental health problems, in some cases despite having been "in the system" for years. In a significant number of cases, the absence of interpreters or culture brokers and the cultural complexity of the cases prevented adequate assessment in conventional mental health care settings.

Given the great diversity of immigration to Canada, ethnospecific clinics are not practical for most groups, in most regions. For small communities, specialized clinics may also be undesirable because they cannot provide the requisite privacy and anonymity for patients, since everyone in the community knows everyone else.

While there are grassroots community initiatives that address the mental health needs of immigrants and refugees, there remains a significant lack of coordination of resources as well as a lack of a coherent structure to manage the needs of an increasingly diverse population. As well, there are too few clinical consultants available to support primary care and frontline workers in the community.

Our results suggest that there is a need to balance three sources of help for culturally diverse populations: (1) to increase awareness and skills at the level of primary care, (2) to support community services and improve liaison with professional mental health care and (3) to provide specialized teams with cultural knowledge and language skills essential to work with patients who require a high level of expertise to diagnose and treat their problems.

The model we advocate involves the development of specific cultural consultation services which can provide assessment and treatment planning as well as networking with community resources for clinicians in primary care, psychiatry, social services and other mental health disciplines. This service can also contribute directly to the training of interpreters and culture brokers as well as developing links with helping resources within the cultural communities. Given the need for similar resources (clinicians from specific backgrounds, interpreters, culture brokers) for both consultation and treatment, the most useful services will allow a combination of consultation with the availability of intervention and follow-up for complex cases or those requiring specialized resources.

Health care and social service institutions must enable clinicians who have specific cultural knowledge and skills to devote time to cultural consultation and to train other clinicians in this domain. They should also make it easier for practitioners to access and use interpreters and culture brokers. This requires supporting the additional time and personnel needed to work interculturally and across languages as well as recognizing (and recruiting) clinicians with diverse backgrounds and linguistic skills. This includes budgeting funds and establishing systems to remunerate culture brokers for their time and expertise.

There is a need to support community services and improve their liaison with professional mental health care as well as to develop culture brokers who can work closely with clinicians to mediate clinical encounters and identify appropriate resources to assist with the social care of patients.

Implications for Training

An important goal of the CCS is to increase the cultural competence of the mental health care system as a whole by addressing the training needs of frontline workers in primary care and mental health. Much of the training effort of the CCS has gone on through case conferences and consultations responding to the immediate clinical concerns of referring individuals and organizations. To address broader training needs, we reviewed training models and developed teaching materials and in-service training workshops for health and social service professionals.

The review of training approaches used three strategies: (1) a systematic review of available literature on cultural competence training using PsychLit, PubMed and Google Scholar search engines; (2) a brief survey questionnaire and subsequent conversations with international leaders in the field addressing pedagogical philosophy, methods, models, trends and gaps in cross-cultural training in mental health; and (3) on-site visits to local, national and international programs. The initial version of this review appeared as an appendix in the CCS evaluation report (see www.mcgill.ca/ccs).

A growing body of literature supports the need for cultural competence training in mental health. Although there is general agreement that the notions of race, ethnicity and culture have been conflated and inappropriately applied in clinical settings, there are various training models emphasizing different issues, including antiracism, cultural awareness, cultural competence, cultural safety and culture-specific or generic approaches (Kirmayer, 2012a). Training manuals have been developed for use in university programs, continuing education and clinical settings. Most follow a modular format with readings and exercises to address a spectrum of issues related to cultural awareness and skill development. However, there is limited evidence to support the effectiveness of most training programs in terms of either cognitive and attitudinal changes or ultimate impact on clinical skills and practice.

Much of the work on cultural competence comes from the United States, Australia and the UK where concepts and categories of ethnocultural and racialized identity differ substantially from those in Canada and other places (Kirmayer, 2012a). In recent years, the Mental Health Commission of Canada and Aboriginal groups have adopted the notion of cultural safety as a rubric under which to develop training and intervention models (Mental Health Commission of Canada, 2009, 2012; Smye, Josewski, & Kendall, 2010). This recognizes the continuing legacy of colonialism and state policies that have disempowered and oppressed Indigenous peoples. Immigrants, refugees and racialized ethnic minorities also experience systematic disadvantage that must be addressed in creating institutions and modes of practice that are culturally safe and respond to the needs of patients, families and communities. Cultural safety will require attention to specific social structural and historical issues in each setting. Table 16.1 lists some of the strengths and limits of different

Table 16.1 Levels of cultural competence

	Institution	Practitioner	Technique
Strategy	Organizational cultural competence	Clinical cultural competence	Cultural adaptation of interventions
Examples	Institutional policies of equity, antiracism, cultural diversity awareness Insuring that administration and staff are representative of ethnocultural composition of communities served Engaging communities in policy making, planning, and regulation of services	Ethnic matching of clinician and patient Training of professionals in specific and generic cultural knowledge, skills and attitudes Referral to other professionals and helpers in the community Use of culture-brokers or mediators	Adjusting style of interaction and communication to patient Matching intervention to patient Cultural adaptation of interventions Adoption of new interventions Referral to other sources of help or healing
Benefits	Can organize systems and services in ways that are responsive to needs of specific groups Can address issues of power and discrimination, empowering community and resulting in greater equity, safety and trust in institution Can improve access and acceptability through community relationship to the institution and through design of specific programs	Can facilitate initial trust Linguistic match facilitates communication Shared cultural background knowledge facilitates mutual understanding Can provide role of modelling of successful or resilient individuals from similar background	Can tailor intervention to take into account specific psychological or social issues and processes May improve acceptability of intervention Can mobilize personal and community cultural resources for resilience and recovery Can identify culture-specific goals and outcomes that require alternative therapeutic approaches
Limitations	If focus is primarily on representativeness of governance and staff, actual delivery of services may be conventional Institutional policies may not result in actual changes in behaviors of staff Ethnospecific services may constitute a form of social segregation and fail to transform the general health care system	Match may be crude or approximate (owing to differences in ethnicity, subculture, social class, education, dialect, etc.) Clinician may not know how to apply their own tacit cultural knowledge to clinical care Clinicians may be feel typecast, professionally limited or marginalized Patients may feel singled out, racially categorized, stereotyped Patients may feel exposed to scrutiny by their own community and may wish for the psychological distance or privacy associated with meeting a cultural "outsider"	Adaptation may be superficial or purely cosmetic May lose elements essential for efficacy Culturally-grounded methods may not address issues related to cultural hybridity or culture change Culture-specific or traditional methods may be socially conservative and do not allow patients opportunity to escape from culturally mediated or rationalized forms of oppression Interventions may not be familiar or appealing to patients who eschew tradition and value other ("modern," scientific) approaches

approaches to cultural competence and safety in training and the organization of health systems (Kirmayer, 2012b).

To address the need for locally appropriate training approaches, the CCS established a multidisciplinary group to assess the education needs of different professionals and develop specific training activities in (1) primary care, (2) interpreter and culture-broker programs and (3) graduate training programs. The primary care work group comprised physicians, social workers and frontline workers who identified cultural training needs in their respective disciplines. The group met regularly to coordinate these activities.

Group members have been active in intercultural training. They organized workshops to increase the competence of clinicians in the domain of culture and mental health, particularly for refugee services, and to know how to make appropriate use of specialized services. An interpreter training subgroup included administrators from the Regional Board of Health and Social Services, who were responsible for the training and deployment of interpreters throughout the health care system. This group made recommendations for improving the training of interpreters in the domain of mental health. It also interfaced with the primary care group to help train practitioners to make appropriate use of interpreters, since there was evidence of underutilization of interpreters.

A subgroup addressed postgraduate training for psychiatrists and mental health professionals as well as with philosophy and methods of training and education at a more global level. This group organized an Advanced Study Institute on Models of Training in Culture and Mental Health in May 2001 as part of the annual McGill Summer Program in Social and Cultural Psychiatry (www.mcgill.ca/tcpsych). Papers from a subsequent workshop on "Rethinking Cultural Competence from International Perspectives," held in April 2010, have appeared in *Transcultural Psychiatry* (Kirmayer, 2012b). This work culminated in the framing of guidelines for training in cultural psychiatry produced by the Section on Transcultural Psychiatry of the

Canadian Psychiatric Association (CPA-TPS) and endorsed by the CPA Standing Committee on Education (Kirmayer, Fung, et al., 2012). These guidelines are available online and are being supplemented with training materials including readings, video lectures and links to other training resources (see: www.transcultural-psychiatry.ca). Table 16.2 summarizes some of the major themes and content areas in these guidelines, which are deliberately broad and inclusive and which can be adapted for other professions.

In collaboration with the McGill Division of Social and Transcultural Psychiatry and specific teaching hospitals, the CCS has supported monthly seminars for mental health professionals in the community. A series based at the Montreal Children's Hospital entitled "Culture and Clinic Rounds" used case-based presentations to focus on clinical assessment issues including trauma and organized violence, family separation and reunification, psychotherapy with South Asian women and boundary issues in transcultural psychiatry. A second series of monthly meetings based at the Jewish General Hospital (where the CCS is located) on "Culture & Community Mental Health" focused on research and clinical issues in community psychiatry. Topics included minority origin professionals in health and social services; women, racism and the mental health system; rape as a crime of war; linkages between community organizations and mental health professionals; dilemmas of ethnic match; and the asylum-seeking process.

An integral goal of the CCS has been to promote dialogue with existing community resources in culture and mental health. To that end, CCS consultants have met with staff involved with training in community organizations to identify training needs and plan relevant workshops and other activities. Partners in these activities have included the regional network providing treatment and supervision for those working with survivors of torture (Réseau d'Intervention auprès des personnes victimes de violence organisée, RIVO); the regional coordinating group for immigrant refugee organizations (Table de Concertation des organismes de Montréal au service des réfugiés et

Table 16.2 Core knowledge, skills and attitudes for training in cultural consultation

Knowledge

Prevalence of mental health among specific ethnocultural groups and populations

Cultural variations in idioms of distress, symptom presentation, illness explanatory models and cultural syndromes

Ethnic differences in response to medications, including pharmacokinetics (metabolism) and pharmacodynamics (drug response, susceptibility to side effects)

Interactions of culture with gender, age and social status

Sociocultural stressors, including migration, poverty and discrimination

Skills

Conduct and organize a culturally oriented assessment

Ability to negotiate sociocultural factors, such as healer–patient role expectations and power dynamics, that influence clinical engagement and alliance

Conduct a culturally valid mental status examination

Produce a cultural formulation

Consider cultural issues and present an integrative biopsychosocial–spiritual understanding

Develop a culturally appropriate treatment plan

Cultural adapt psychotherapy, pharmacotherapy and other interventions

Appropriate management of ethnic differences when using pharmacotherapy and somatic therapy

Direct patients to relevant community resources

Modify style of communication to facilitate rapport with patients and their families

Appropriate use of linguistic and cultural interpreters

Work with interpreters and culture brokers

Consult and collaborate effectively with other physicians, health care professionals, agencies, religious leaders, community leaders and cultural consultants as appropriate

Attitudes

Reflect on and recognize one's own biases and assumptions

Demonstrate integrity, honesty, compassion and respect for diversity

Understand ethical issues that concern diverse populations

Recognize power differences and dynamics in professional collaborative relationships

Demonstrate respect for diversity in working with teams

Aware of power dynamics and take appropriate steps to address inequity owing to sociocultural forces within teams

Participate in and promote quality assurance that takes into account cultural and equity issues

Ensure equitable allocation of health care resources and access to care

Identify and understand the impact of racism, access barriers and other social factors leading to mental health sequelae and health disparities in disadvantaged groups

Knowledge of major regional, national and international advocacy groups in mental health care

Ability to engage in effective mental health promotion strategies, including community educational talks and workshops

Advocate effectively for the biopsychosocial, cultural and spiritual needs of patients and their families within the health care system and community

Based on Kirmayer, Fung, et al. (2012)

immigrantes, TCRI); a training center for organizational cultural competence (Institut Interculturel de Montréal, IIM); the local branch of the Canadian Mental Health Association, a lay advocacy group; a regional coalition of about 80 cultural community organizations (Alliance des Communautés Culturelles pour L'égalité dans la Santé et des Services Sociaux, ACCESSS); and a social service organization for immigrants (Centre sociale d'aide aux immigrants). We identified areas of potential collaboration with these organizations, including training mental health professionals in intercultural awareness and skills, information and resource sharing and the development of a mechanism for providing ongoing clinical consultations for mental health professionals working in an intercultural context. Often groups working on intercultural mental health care were unaware of the contributions of other groups locally, nationally and internationally.

Cross-cultural training is a necessary component of clinical training for all mental health professionals. However, in most educational and practice settings, it remains largely undeveloped. In particular, most mental health professionals receive no training on how to work with interpreters and culture brokers and no systematic education in cross-cultural assessment or intervention.

Clearly, there is a need to strengthen training of mental health practitioners in concepts of culture and strategies of intercultural care. This should include recognition of the value of clinician's own linguistic and cultural background knowledge as added skills. Professional training should provide explicit models for integrating tacit cultural knowledge and current best practices in mental health care. Trainees should be given opportunities to reflect on and make use of their own cultural backgrounds and to employ their linguistic skills in working with patients.

There is a particular need to train mental health practitioners to work with interpreters. This must become a standard part of all graduate training programs in psychology, psychiatry, nursing, social work and other health and social service professions. In-service training and continuing education programs should be provided for practitioners to refine their skills in intercultural communication and collaboration with medical interpreters.

Interpreting in the context of mental health care is especially demanding because of the technical need to transmit not only the gist of what someone is saying but its precise form and quality (set against a backdrop of cultural norms) in order for the clinician to assess the patient's mental status. Mental health interpreting also involves emotionally intense and challenging situations that may affect all participants. Interpreters therefore need additional training in mental health as well as supervision and support to work with potentially distressing or traumatizing situations.

There is also a need to develop training for clinicians, interpreters and other knowledgeable community members who can play an important role as culture brokers. This requires addressing specific ethical issues that challenge the narrow role currently assigned to interpreters (Chapter 6).

Finally, quality assurance and accreditation standards for training programs must specify the components of cultural safety and competence in detail (e.g. knowledge, skills and attitudes) and insure they are addressed in training program curricula, evaluation and recertification. Only formal monitoring can insure that these issues are fully integrated into training and certification of professionals so that knowledge, skills and attitudes essential for cultural safety and competence become part of the core expertise of every mental health professional.

From Consultation and Clinical Services to Advocacy

As we have shown throughout this book, the political dimensions of culture are very often at the forefront in the consultation process. Intergroup power relations and the stresses and injury that stem from social exclusion—whether through the structural violence of poverty, micro-aggressions of discrimination in daily interactions, institutionalized racism or as a result of restrictive policies of immigration and asylum—are sources of social suffering that may be expressed as mental health problems or complicate the course of recovery. From the perspectives of public health, clinicians have a responsibility to advocate for changes in social policy that will promote mental well-being, prevent illness and facilitate recovery. In the same way that clinicians advocate for anti-bullying measures and for restricted access to firearms, clinicians working with ethnocultural minorities, immigrants or refugee must advocate to improve the quality of services, recognition and protection and to decrease the social adversity that vulnerable groups confront.

While advocacy for individual cases to support a refugee claim or facilitate access to services is highly valuable, clinicians should also advocate as a group to improve the way in which their societies welcome immigrants and refugees and support their resettlement. In a context of increasing xenophobia, this can be a challenging endeavour, and the creation of international networks of advocacy can help local advocates persist, despite institutional pressures, to keep human rights issues on government agendas. These rights include not only the protection of the right of asylum but also the right to health, education and the protection of the child's best interest. Recognizing that we are fundamentally cultural beings and require hospitable communities and participation in traditions to flourish, there are also international rights to culture itself (Kirmayer, 2012b). Mental health services that work with culture as a resource for individual and collective resilience can contribute to the protection of this right.

Building Communities of Practice

In 2007, a meeting of about 200 clinicians and leaders of government and community organizations from across Canada produced a set of recommendations for addressing health disparities and cultural diversity in health care (National Transcultural Health Conference, 2007). The recommendations emphasized the concept of cultural safety, achieved through explicit attention to cultural issues in health care, including the development of the skills of cultural competence, the use of trained interpreters and culture brokers, involving both linguistic translation and cultural mediation; ready availability of culturally appropriate information on illness and treatment in multiple languages through oral, written and visual materials accessible through Internet websites, social media or standalone audiovisual kiosks; building on cultural knowledge through partnerships with communities; and the development of local, regional and national networking. Many of the ideas from this conference have been incorporated into subsequent work by the CCS, particularly through the development of Internet web-based resources for training and clinical services.

To insure that the work of cultural consultation has maximum impact, frontline workers need easy access to resources and support to provide culturally appropriate care. One efficient way to achieve this is through the use of web-based resources and other information communication technologies which offer several advantages for promoting intercultural care. First, they allow for networking, creating links between community groups, clinicians and government organizations. Secondly, they allow for much wider accessibility, making these materials and tools available in rural or remote locations. Specific resources can be determined through needs assessment and during ongoing consultation with stakeholders but would likely include (1) training and self-assessment materials for continuing education in cultural competence (Lim, Hsiung, & Hales, 2006); (2) multilingual mental health information resources for patients, families and professionals; (3) specific material on key issues including ethnocultural variations in diagnostic and neuropsychological assessment and response to psychiatric medication; (4) guidelines for the design and implementation of cultural consultation, community-based collaborative care and ethnospecific mental health services; and, eventually, (5) consultation for specific clinical and organizational issues related to cultural diversity in mental health care.

Intercultural work can be both exceptionally demanding and rewarding. Many practitioners concerned with cultural issues find themselves a lone voice in their local health care system. There is a need to develop a community of practice through networking to bring together and support individuals who can spearhead the development of services like the CCS and who are actively engaged in intercultural work. This network can exchange information and support a national clearing house for models of intervention, clinical resources and training materials. This network can also sponsor interdisciplinary training activities and collaborative research across centers.

With support from the Mental Health Commission of Canada, we have developed a web-based Multicultural Mental Health Resource Centre (www.mmhrc.ca). The MMHRC is essentially an Internet portal to provide easy access to material useful for intercultural mental health

Table 16.3 Contents of a Web-based resource for multicultural mental health

For health care providers

- Guidelines for working with interpreters and culture brokers and for specific patient populations or clinical problems (e.g. immigrants, refugees, survivors of torture)
- How to locate resources needed for intercultural care (e.g. interpreters, culture brokers, community organizations)
- Self-study and assessment materials for cultural competence
- Updates from current clinical and research literature on culture and mental health

For patients and their families

- Mental health information factsheets in multiple languages
- Self-help materials

For community organizations

- Information on mental health services
- Stigma reduction materials for diverse groups

For policymakers, planners and administrators

- Information on policies, law and human rights declarations related to diversity in mental health care at different levels of jurisdiction (i.e. local health care systems, regional, national)
- Criteria and measures for organizational cultural safety and cultural competence
- Demographic information on ethnocultural communities
- Models and approaches to the design of services for culturally diverse populations

Source: www.mmhrc.ca

care (Table 16.3). The website brings together links to resources and other sites useful to primary care and mental health practitioners, patients and their families, community organizations and policy makers. For clinicians, the site provides information on cultural assessment and formulation, migration-related health issues, methods for the use of interpreters and culture brokers and ways of helping patients to access community resources. For patients and their families or caregivers, there is multilingual information on common mental disorders and materials for self-care and information on health resources as well as links to local and national community organizations. For health administrators and planners, the site serves as a clearing house for information on models of care and best practices in addressing cultural diversity in psychiatry and mental health care. This includes bringing

together materials developed in other countries to give a comparative perspective on available strategies and facilitate local, national and international networks for knowledge exchange in this area. An associated e-mail listserv provides a vehicle to announce programs and make requests to the network for information. Video podcasts, a blog and other social media are used to share ideas within the network and can attract a wider audience to enlarge the community of practice.

Conclusion: Valuing Cultural Diversity

Every culture has its own styles of reasoning and raison d'etre rooted in certain core values and ways of life. Culture is of value for each individual as it is essential to the realization of one's full personhood with a range of competencies that build on collective history and accomplishments. Culture is of value to the group or community as a means of weaving people together with common purpose and coordinated roles in a larger system capable of creating institutions that far outreach the capacity of any individual. Beyond culture as a primary good for each individual or collectivity, we can recognize the diversity of cultures itself as a good, on analogy to the ecological role of biological diversity in insuring the viability of ecosystems in situations of stress and change. This global diversity can be valuable even to a relatively homogeneous or monocultural society. Every language and cultural tradition offers us imaginative possibilities that may help us adapt to new circumstances or address some of the limitations, injustices and inequities in our own way of life.

Recognizing the creative value of the encounter between different traditions works against the stale and stultifying arguments for exclusion or assimilation that arise from limited imagination and engagement with others. When the other is viewed only in terms of problematic difference, we miss the creativity of exploring a new worldview that can challenge and invigorate our own, whether through dialogue or hybridization. Rather than viewing others from a distant, disengaged and uninformed view of their experience, which inevitably leads to stereotyping and prejudice (and sometimes is used to justify our own fearful reactions and aggression), we can engage them directly in dialogue and in the process enlarge our imagination of what it is to be human.

If we value diversity for any or all of these reasons, we must work to create forms of community that can sustain it. Along the way, we must do our best to protect the global diversity that is our collective cultural capital. Our willingness to work for this diversity, at home and internationally, reflects the level of our interest in and respect for others—and for the other in ourselves, born of our own hybrid histories, identities and experiences. The politics of alterity shapes our social world but it also has echoes in the recesses of each individual's psyche as we write and rewrite our personal stories of identity. Health services are crucial arenas where diverse people come together in times of crisis with an openness born of the urgency of their predicament and the commitment to a compassionate response. The appropriateness and effectiveness of this response depends on recognizing the person in their individuality, which, in turn, draws from their participation in multiple cultural communities. Multicultural mental health care allows us the opportunity to explore cultural identities and engage communities to in an effort to understand and help others in ways that are grounded in recognition of both our common humanity and our essential differences.

References

Bhui, K., Warfa, N., Edonya, P., McKenzie, K., & Bhugra, D. (2007). Cultural competence in mental health care: A review of model evaluations. *BMC Health Services Research, 7*, 15.

Burke, P. (2009). *Cultural hybridity*. Cambridge: Polity.

Gouvernement du Québec. (2007). *Recommandations des coroners: Recherche avancée*. Quebec, Canada: Gouvernement du Quebec. Retrieved from http://www.coroner.gouv.qc.ca

King, M., Smith, A., & Gracey, M. (2009). Indigenous health part 2: The underlying causes of the health gap. *The Lancet, 374*(9683), 76–85.

Kirmayer, L. J. (2012a). Rethinking cultural competence. *Transcultural Psychiatry, 49*(2), 149–164.

Kirmayer, L. J. (2012b). Culture and context in human rights. In M. Dudley, D. Silove, & F. Gale (Eds.), *Mental health and human rights* (pp. 95–112). Oxford, England: Oxford University Press.

Kirmayer, L. J., Brass, G. M., & Valaskakis, G. G. (2008). Conclusion: Healing/invention/tradition. In L. J. Kirmayer & G. Valaskakis (Eds.), *Healing traditions: The mental health of aboriginal peoples in Canada* (pp. 440–472). Vancouver, British Columbia, Canada: University of British Columbia Press.

Kirmayer, L. J., Fung, K., Rousseau, C., Lo, H. T., Menzies, P., Guzder, J., et al. (2012). Guidelines for training in cultural psychiatry. *Canadian Journal of Psychiatry, 57*(3), Insert 1–16.

Lim, R. F., Hsiung, B. C., & Hales, D. J. (2006). Lifelong learning: Skills and online resources. *Academic Psychiatry, 30*(6), 540–547.

Mental Health Commission of Canada. (2009). *Toward recovery and well-being: A framework for mental health strategy for Canada*. Ottawa, Ontario, Canada: Mental Health Commission of Canada.

Mental Health Commission of Canada. (2012). *Changing directions, changing lives: The mental health strategy for Canada*. Ottawa, Ontario, Canada: Mental Health Commission of Canada.

Mezzich, J. E., Kirmayer, L. J., Kleinman, A., Fabrega, H., Jr., Parron, D. L., Good, B. J., et al. (1999). The place of culture in DSM-IV. *The Journal of Nervous and Mental Disease, 187*(8), 457–464.

Mezzich, J. E., Salloum, I. M., Cloninger, C. R., Salvador-Carulla, L., Kirmayer, L. J., Banzato, C. E. M., et al. (2010). Person-centered integrative diagnosis: Conceptual basis and structural model. *Canadian Journal of Psychiatry, 55*(11), 701–708.

National Transcultural Health Conference. (2007). *Recommendations from the national transcultural health conference*. Montreal, Quebec, Canada: Montreal Children's Hospital.

Reading, C. L., & Wien, F. (2009). *Health inequalities and social determinants of Aboriginal peoples' health*. Victoria, British Columbia, Canada: National Collaborating Centre for Aboriginal Health.

Renzaho, A. M., Romios, P., Crock, C., & Sonderlund, A. L. (2013). The effectiveness of cultural competence programs in ethnic minority patient-centered health care—A systematic review of the literature. *International Journal for Quality in Health Care*. doi:10.1093/intqhc/mzt006.

Smye, V., Josewski, V., & Kendall, E. (2010). *Cultural safety: An overview*. Ottawa, Ontario, Canada: First Nations, Inuit and Métis Advisory Committee, Mental Health Commission of Canada.

Taylor, J. S. (2003). Confronting "culture" in medicine's culture of no culture. *Academic Medicine, 78*, 555–559.

Whitley, R., Rousseau, C., Carpenter Song, E., & Kirmayer, L. J. (2011). Evidence-based medicine: Opportunities and challenges in a diverse society. *Canadian Journal of Psychiatry, 56*.

World Health Organization. (2010). *MhGAP intervention guide for mental, neurological and substance use disorders in non-specialized health settings: Version 1.0*. Geneva, Switzerland: World Health Organization.

Index

A
Aboriginal, 5, 7, 35, 115, 119, 223, 229, 283, 339, 342
Acculturation, 37, 38, 69, 72, 75, 97, 141, 154, 156, 158, 164, 166, 167, 175, 176, 185, 207, 208
Adherence, 4, 10, 34, 38, 39, 41, 43, 59, 77, 82, 90, 103, 118, 300, 307, 313, 316, 317, 325, 328
Adjustment disorder, 36, 37, 72, 186, 298
Adolescent, 12, 56, 75, 82, 98, 125, 145, 151, 152, 156, 157, 167, 172–174, 211, 212, 235, 237, 252, 270, 274, 315
African, 6, 8, 35, 36, 66, 91, 92, 123, 125, 126, 128, 129, 132, 142, 146, 185–193, 195, 197, 296, 317, 323
Afro-American, 119
Afro-Canadian, 183, 191–193
Afro-Caribbean, 6, 191, 273
Allophone, 22, 23
Anglophone, 193
Antidepressant, 12, 142, 148–150, 174, 256, 301
Antipsychotic, 131, 153, 299, 300, 305
Anxiety, 15, 17, 36, 37, 78, 79, 169, 186, 196, 213, 214, 237, 248–252, 255, 261, 263, 284, 295, 299, 334
Arab, 270, 282
Asian
    East, 35, 132
    South, 22, 27, 35, 36, 97, 133, 140, 142, 143, 154, 156, 157, 163–180, 298, 344
    Southeast, 35, 132
Assimilation, 8, 118, 141, 146, 165, 176, 228, 229, 334, 348
Asylum, 7, 9, 12, 16, 34, 35, 38, 42, 75, 77, 92, 93, 124, 148, 245, 247, 248, 251, 252, 315, 324, 327, 333, 334, 344, 346, 347
Attachment, 15, 97, 107, 127, 140, 142, 146, 155, 157, 165, 177, 178, 210, 215, 237, 251, 252, 273, 276, 280, 286
Attention deficit, hyperactivity disorder (ADHD), 76, 80
Australia, 5, 7, 29, 71, 90, 119, 153, 164, 226, 228, 250, 342
Avicenne clinic, 82, 85

B
Bicultural, 12, 29, 52, 58, 83, 117, 120, 132, 133, 152, 156, 158, 175, 208, 339, 341
Bipolar disorder, 262, 297

Black, 6, 22, 118, 154, 164, 170, 184, 186, 188, 189, 191–197, 200, 269, 274, 275, 283, 285, 295, 300
Black and minority ethnic (BME), 6, 118
Boundary violations, 177, 344
Buddhist, 17, 305, 328

C
Camouflage, cultural, 152–155, 173, 306
Canadian Coalition for Immigrant and Refugee Health (CCIRH), 207
Caste, 54, 57, 143, 146, 165, 166, 177, 179, 306
CBT. *See* Cognitive behavioral therapy (CBT)
CCIRH. *See* Canadian Coalition for Immigrant and Refugee Health (CCIRH)
Centre Georges Devereux, 122–123
Centre Minkowska, 106
Centro Franz Fanon, 122–124
Child
    development, 75, 81
    maltreatment, 207, 276, 278
    protection, 77, 82, 123, 127, 156, 269–287
Chinese, 7, 22, 35, 36, 151, 152, 207, 293
Class, 78, 92, 102–104, 126, 134, 164, 166, 167, 183, 189, 191, 194, 199, 274, 277, 323, 343
CLSC, 25–27, 33, 75, 76, 79, 186
Cognitive behavioral therapy (CBT), 47, 105–106, 255
Collaborative care, 73, 76, 80, 86, 91, 150, 203–218, 225, 230, 235, 238, 239, 313, 333, 347
Collectivism, 146
Colonialism, 117, 164, 208, 225, 342
Community
    remote, 119, 223–241, 337, 347
    rural, 119, 223–227, 230–232, 235, 240, 275, 337
Compliance. *See* Adherence
Conduct disorder, 154
Confidentiality, 36, 38, 51, 53, 89, 91, 93, 95–99, 107, 164, 169, 176, 192, 224, 227, 228, 232–234, 239, 270, 284, 320, 340
Countertransference, 24, 107, 108, 141, 163, 164, 195, 238, 341
Courts, 12, 246, 271, 274, 275, 277–280, 284, 285, 287
Creole, 22, 24, 65, 66, 104
Creolization, 116, 186, 191

L.J. Kirmayer et al. (eds.), *Cultural Consultation: Encountering the Other in Mental Health Care,*
International and Cultural Psychology, DOI 10.1007/978-1-4614-7615-3,
© Springer Science+Business Media New York 2014

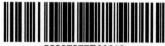
Made in the USA
Middletown, DE
17 November 2017